ISOLATED
AND CULTURED
HEPATOCYTES

RESEARCH IN

ISOLATED AND CULTURED HEPATOCYTES

**André Guillouzo and
Christiane Guguen-Guillouzo**

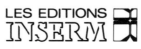

LES EDITIONS INSERM

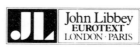

John Libbey
EUROTEXT
LONDON · PARIS

British Library Cataloguing in Publication Data
Isolated and cultured hepatocytes. — (Research in —; v. 1)
   1. Liver cells   2. Cell culture
   I. Guillouzo, André   II. Guguen-Guillouzo, Christiane
   III. Series
   612'.35   QP185

   ISBN (John Libbey & Co. Ltd) 0 86196 078 5
   ISBN (INSERM) 2 85598 289 8

Research in —/Recherches en — is a series of books published
in simultaneous English and French editions.

   Isolated and cultured hepatocytes (Research in —)
   is published in French as:

   Hépatocytes isolés et en culture (Recherches en —)

   ISBN (John Libbey & Co. Ltd) 0 86196 079 3
   ISBN (INSERM) 2 85598 290 1

First published by

John Libbey & Company Ltd
80/84 Bondway, London SW8 1SF, England. (01) 582 5266
John Libbey Eurotext Ltd
6 rue Blanche, 92120 Montrouge, France. (1) 47 35 85 52
ISBN 0 86196 078 5

Institut National de la Santé et de la Recherche Médicale
101 rue de Tolbiac, 75654 Paris Cedex 13, France. (1) 45 84 14 41
ISBN 2 85598 289 8

Typeset by Deltatype
Printed in Great Britain by Whitstable Litho Ltd, Whitstable, Kent
Bound by The Standard Bookbinding Co. Ltd, London NW10

Preface

The liver is characterized by its cellular heterogeneity and by the multiplicity of its biological function. Most of these functions are expressed in the hepatocyte, although this cell type represents only two-thirds of the total liver cell population. Because of this, simple *in-vitro* systems were soon developed to study liver function. Among them, isolated perfused liver, tissue slices and subcellular fractions have been widely used for some time. However, the short life-span of these systems (a few hours) was one of their most severe shortcomings.

During the last ten years, suspensions of hepatocytes isolated by enzymatic perfusion of the liver have been used increasingly. Although this model has not allowed studies exceeding a few hours, it has fostered significant progress in the understanding of hepatocyte function and regulation.

Cultured hepatocytes are the only *in-vitro* model suitable for long-term studies, provided that the cells retain their differentiated state. Much research has been done to establish the right culture conditions, focusing on the importance of soluble factors (hormones, growth factors, trace elements etc), extracellular matrix components and cell-to-cell interactions and it is now possible to maintain functional hepatocytes in primary culture for days or even months.

Today, freshly isolated or cultured hepatocytes constitute suitable model systems to investigate the biology and pathology of the liver, including the human liver. These systems should also be useful in molecular biology and specific genetic studies. Their applications include pharmacology, toxicology, cancer, and parasitology.

The main objectives of this book are to summarize recent progress in the isolation and culture of differentiated hepatocytes, to provide a wide state-of-the-art view of recent findings obtained with isolated and cultured hepatocytes, and to stimulate new research and novel applications.

Publication of this book has been made possible by the collaboration of many specialists from France and elsewhere, and by the initiative of INSERM, together with John Libbey Eurotext who have launched this new series of books — *Research in . . . .* We thank Dr Ph. Lazar, director of INSERM, the Publications Committee and its president Professor S. Bonfils, and we are grateful to Mrs S. Mouchet (head of the Publications Department), Mrs C. Geynet and finally Professor C. Matuchansky, Scientific advisor for INSERM publications.

We are indebted to Georges Baffet, Jean-Marc Bégué, Bruno Clément, Jean-Marc Fraslin, Philippe Gripon, Michel Kraemer, Gérard Lescoat and Damrong Ratanasavanh for their help in the translation of

English manuscripts, as well as to Professor J. Kruh and Drs G. Gellaen and Y. Laperche who kindly reviewed some chapters.

We thank our secretaries Mrs M. André and A. Vannier for their invaluable assistance in the preparation of this book.

We also wish to express our sincere appreciation to Professor M. Bourel who initiated and provided continuous advice on our personal work, to Professors P. Brissot and J. P. Campion, and to all our colleagues and collaborators who contributed to the development of the hepatocyte culture studies performed in our laboratory.

André Guillouzo
Christiane Guguen-Guillouzo

Contents

Research in *Isolated and cultured hepatocytes* A. Guillouzo & C. Guguen-Guillouzo eds. pp. 1–12.
© 1986 John Libbey Eurotext Ltd./INSERM.

1

Methods for preparation of adult and fetal hepatocytes

Christiane GUGUEN-GUILLOUZO and André GUILLOUZO

Unité de Recherches Hépatologiques, INSERM U49, hôpital Pontchaillou, 35033 Rennes Cedex, FRANCE

SUMMARY

During the last few years, the two-step *in situ* collagenase perfusion method for isolation of viable adult hepatocytes has been applied to various species, including man, and high cell yields with a very good viability were obtained. Hepatocyte suspensions can be further fractionated according to their density (periportal *vs* centrilobular cells) or their volume (ploidy). Fetal livers are also easily dissociated by collagenase treatment. The major limitation of hepatocyte suspensions is a short life-span (a few hours) and the difficulty in isolating fetal mammalian and human hepatocytes with a high percentage of single cells. For longer term survival, parenchymal cells must be maintained in culture attached to a substratum.

Introduction

The problems raised by both the cellular heterogeneity of the liver and the determination of the role of endogenous and exogenous factors on the different hepatic functions have early led investigators to devise *in vitro* techniques for the study of liver functions in purified cell populations. The techniques used to obtain isolated hepatocytes were originally based on mechanical means, then on the use of chelating agents such as citrate, ethylenediaminetetracetic acid (EDTA) or tetraphenylboron to remove the Ca^{++} and K^+ which strengthen the intercellular bonds and finally on a treatment using enzyme solutions: trypsin, papain, lysozyme, neuraminidase or pepsin. Under these conditions, the cell yield did not exceed five per cent of the total cell population and the functional properties of the majority of the cells were lost (38).

A considerable step forward in isolation of intact adult rat hepatocytes was made by the introduction of collagenase and hyaluronidase as dissociating agents (22). Berry & Friend (5) established the basic protocol involving a two-step perfusion of the liver *in situ*, first with calcium-free buffer, followed by a calcium-supplemented buffer containing collagenase. Many authors still use this original protocol which includes Hanks buffer and recirculation of the perfusates. However, a number of investigators have simplified the original technique. The major modifications include omission of oxygenation of the perfusate and the use of HEPES buffer (27, 39). The influence of these various modifications on the cell yield and metabolic activities of freshly isolated rat hepatocytes have been extensively reviewed by Seglen (40). The two-step *in situ* collagenase perfusion is now a widely used method for obtaining viable dispersed hepatocytes from various species. Moreover, since isolated adult hepatocyte suspensions are an heterogenous cell population regarding the degree of ploidy and functional activities, several methods have been devised for the separation of different hepatocyte classes.

Basic protocols for the disaggregation of fetal livers also involve the use of proteolytic enzymes. Both collagenase and trypsin, albeit unsuitable for the adult organ, are usually used.

This article is devoted to a review of the current procedures for obtaining hepatocyte suspensions from adult and fetal livers of various species as well as those for the separation of hepatocyte subpopulations.

Isolation of adult hepatocytes

Rat

The two-step *in situ* collagenase perfusion technique has been primarily developed for disaggregation of the adult rat liver. The method presently used in our laboratory is based on that of Seglen (40). Rats weighing 180–200 g are used and are anaesthetized by intraperitoneal injection of Nembutal (1.5 ml/kg). Heparin (1000 IU) is injected into the femoral vein and the abdomen is opened. The liver is first washed via the portal vein with a calcium-free HEPES buffer, pH 7.65 at 37°C and at a flow rate of 30 ml/min for 10–15 min. The composition of HEPES buffer is as follows: 160.8 mM NaCl; 3.15 mM KCl; 0.7 mM Na_2HPO_4, 12 H_2O, 0.33 mM HEPES. The second step is performed with the same buffer containing 0.025% collagenase and 0.075% $CaCl_2$ at a flow rate of 20 ml/min for 15 min.

At the end of the perfusion the collapsed organ is removed and washed with HEPES buffer. The cells are dispersed in L_{15} Leibovitz enriched medium with 0.2% bovine serum albumin after disruption of the surrounding Glisson's capsule and gentle dissociation of the organ with a spatula.

The original cell suspension is filtered through gauze and allowed to sediment for 20 min. The cells are then washed three times by slow centrifugation (50 g) in order to remove cell debris, damaged cells and non-parenchymal cells. Cell yields range between 400 and 600×10^6 hepatocytes with a viability often greater than 95% as determined by the well-preserved refringent shape or the trypan blue exclusion test. Very few non-parenchymal cells are still present in the final cell preparation.

Other rodents

The basic two-step perfusion procedure has been also used for obtaining viable hepatocytes from various other rodents, including mouse (25, 32, 36), rabbit (10), guinea pig (1, 12) and hamster (32).

Man

For a long time, adaptation of the two-step *in situ* collagenase perfusion to the human liver remained unsuccessful. This can be explained by difficulties due to the size of the organ and the additional problem of obtaining adequate samples. Recently, independently, three groups have developed techniques to enable the isolation of viable human adult hepatocytes by perfusing either a portion of the whole liver (15) or biopsies (9, 35, 43). Whole organs were obtained from kidney donors. Liver pieces were resected from patients undergoing partial hepatectomy or from kidney donors. In our experiments, the age of the donors varied from 18 months to 60 years, although the majority were aged between 18 and 30 years. Most of the kidney donors died following road traffic accidents and had received little medication before organ removal.

Dissociation of a portion of the whole liver. Immediately following kidney removal, the anterior branch of the left portal vein is dissected free and a polyethylene cannula is rapidly inserted. The perfusion is confined to a limited area of the left lobe which usually represents 5 to 10% of the whole organ (Fig. 1). The liver is first washed with

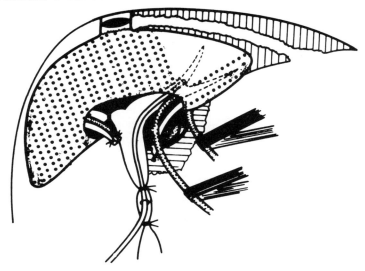

Fig. 1. Schematic drawing of an adult human liver during the perfusion process. The blanched area indicates the perfused portion of the liver (drawn by Professor J. P. Campion).

HEPES buffer at 75 ml/min at 37°C for 20 min then with a HEPES buffered solution containing 0.05% collagenase and 5 mM $CaCl_2$ at 50 ml/min for 20 min (9, 14, 15). Perfusion is improved by clamping hepatic arteries, and solutions are neither oxygenated nor recirculated. At the end of the perfusion, the well perfused part of the liver is transferred to L_{15} Leibovitz medium containing 0.2% bovine albumin. Cells are dispersed by gentle shaking and cell aggregates can be further dissociated by incubation for 30 min in HEPES-buffered collagenase solution at 37°C with stirring.

Dissociation of liver biopsies. Liver pieces are taken from an edge of the organ in order to force the perfusates to recirculate. Just after resection, a silicon paediatric catheter (0.5 to 1.0 mm in diameter) is inserted into the largest vascular orifice. The flow rate of the perfusion depends on the weight of liver pieces. Those weighing 6–10 g are perfused with 150 ml of HEPES buffer at 16–18 ml/min, then with 100 ml of the enzymatic solution at 8–10 ml/min (9). For larger pieces, weighing 10 g or more, flow rates are increased up to 60 ml/min. It is important to minimize the time between liver resection and perfusion in order to obtain high cell yields. However, liver pieces can still be successfully perfused 30–45 min after resection. To increase well-perfused areas, Strom *et al.* (43) perfused liver pieces through several orifices (3 to 5 per piece weighing 6 to 12 g). This perfusion procedure with wedge biopsies of the liver can also be used for isolating liver parenchymal cells from various animal species (35, 43).

Cell suspensions obtained by both procedures are filtered through gauze and allowed to sediment for 20 min in order to eliminate cell debris, blood and sinusoidal cells. The cells are then washed three times by centrifugation at 50 g (Fig. 2A).

A cell yield of between 1 and 12×10^8 hepatocytes with a viability of 70 to 90% is obtained by perfusing the left hepatic lobe of the whole organ or large liver pieces

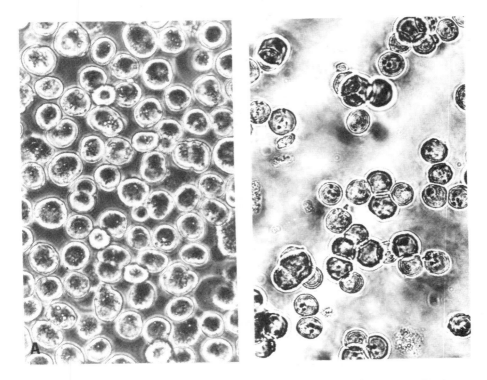

Fig. 2. Phase-contrast micrographs of freshly isolated human (A) and trout (B) hepatocytes (Magnification × 340).

while perfusion of small liver pieces (6 to 15 g) yields 20 to 80×10^6 hepatocytes with a viability of 75 to 95%.

Other mammals

Hepatocytes from other mammals can be isolated according to the procedures described for human and rat liver from either biopsies or portions of whole livers (18) or whole livers (33) depending upon the size of the organs.

Birds

The perfusion is essentially as used for rats. To disaggregate Japanese quail liver, a retrograde perfusion through the hepatic vein is made since the portal vein is inaccessible (23). For the chicken liver, perfusion is done via a mesenteric vein (26).

Amphibians

Hepatocytes from adult bullfrogs weighing 200–350 g can be isolated by using the two-step perfusion introduced by Berry & Friend (5) with slight modifications (42). Animals are injected with 500 IU heparin and 50 mg pentobarbital/250 g body weight before perfusion. The liver is perfused via the post-cava with buffer at a flow rate of 7.5–8.0 ml/min and then with collagenase solution at a flow rate of 4.5–5.0 ml/min without recirculation. Both solutions are maintained at 40°C and continuously gassed with 95% O_2–5% CO_2. Digestion is usually complete after 200 ml of the collagenase solution have been perfused.

Fish

Isolated hepatocytes have been obtained from trout (13, 31, 45), eel (21), carp (6) and catfish (7, 24). The following protocol is used for dispersion of trout hepatocytes in our laboratory (31). The fish receives 2000 IU heparin by intracardiac injection and the portal intestinal vein is ligatured. The liver is first washed with 400 ml of calcium-free HEPES buffer pH 7.65 at 10–15°C at a flow rate of 10–12 ml/min then with 250 ml of buffer containing 0.026% collagenase and 6.67 mM $CaCl_2$ at the same flow rate and at room temperature. The solutions are not oxygenated and are allowed to run to waste through a cut made in the heart. At the end of the perfusion, the gall-bladder is removed and the liver washed with HEPES buffer. The following operations are similar to those described for the rat liver.

Separation of hepatocyte subpopulations

Separation of centrilobular and periportal hepatocytes

Centrilobular and periportal rat hepatocytes can be separated by submitting whole hepatocyte suspensions to density gradient centrifugation. Castagna & Chauveau (8) first reported the separation of hepatocytes into subfractions on Ficoll density gradients. In an extensive study using 15 to 40% Ficoll density gradients, Drochmans et al. (11) separated two types of hepatocytes: one (lighter cells) had a mean density of 1.10 and a mean diameter of 20.5 μm; the other (heavier cells) had a mean density of 1.14 and a mean diameter of 19.0 μm. By stereological and electron microscopic analysis, lighter hepatocytes which represented a small proportion of the total cell population, were considered to correspond to centrilobular cells and heavier hepatocytes to cells located in other regions of the lobule. More than 80% of the cells were normal in appearance. A better efficiency in the separation of the two hepatocyte subpopulations was obtained by treating the rats with phenobarbital before cell isolation (47). The barbiturate promoted proliferation of smooth endoplasmic reticulum in centrilobular parenchymal cells.

Problems with osmolarity and viscosity which occur with Ficoll gradients are reduced by using metrizamide gradients (3). The group used linear (1.07–1.12 g/cm^3 at 20°C) and iso-osmotic (290–305 mosmol/kg water) gradients. The light and heavy solutions were prepared by mixing cell suspension, buffer and 30% metrizamide solution in appropriate proportions giving an equal concentration of about 2×10^6 cells/ml. After centrifugation at 130 g for 5 min, fractions were collected and combined into five populations (P$_1$ to P$_5$). P$_1$ corresponding to the cells of lowest density was judged to contain an excess of centrilobular hepatocytes and P$_4$ an abundance of periportal hepatocytes. P$_2$ and P$_3$ mainly comprised midlobular cells. By using slightly different conditions, Gumucio et al. (20) and Stacey & Klaassen (41) separated two enriched cell fractions. The metrizamide gradient was prepared by layering equal volumes of 35, 25, 20 and 15% metrizamide solutions in buffer and gradients were centrifuged at 3300 g for 30 min. Viability remained high (around 95%) after cell fractionation (41).

Separation of hepatocyte subpopulations according to the degree of ploidy

There is a close correlation between hepatocyte volume and the degree of ploidy and although ploidy increases from periportal to the centrilobular region of the lobule, diploid cells are present in different parts of the lobule. Two main techniques have been used to separate hepatocyte populations into different ploidy classes: velocity sedimentation at unit gravity and elutriation (counterflow) centrifugation. These methods have been devised for the separation of rat hepatocyte subpopulations.

Velocity sedimentation at unit gravity. Rat hepatocytes suspended in calcium-free Hanks medium are layered onto a linear 1–4% Ficoll density gradient. Ficoll of 70 000 molecular weight is preferred to Ficoll with an average molecular weight of 400 000 since sedimentation proceeds faster. Since the viscosity is lower, fractionation is completed in 60–70 min. After centrifugation, hepatocyte subpopulations are resuspended in Hanks medium containing bovine serum albumin. The purity of diploid and tetraploid cell populations is respectively 80% and 99%. Cell viability is about 80% (44).

Elutriation. The elutriation procedure involves counterflow centrifugation of hepatocytes suspended in a nutrient medium (4, 29, 30). Rat hepatocytes (50 to

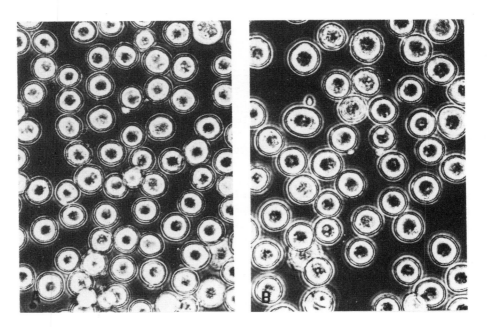

Fig. 3. Phase-contrast micrographs of elutriated rat hepatocytes: A, diploid cells; B, tetraploid cells (A, B: Magnification × 400) (taken from reference 29).

70×10^6) are introduced at a flow rate of 10 ml/min into the elutriation separating chamber of a JE-6 rotor running at 840 rpm in a J21B Beckman centrifuge. The cells are separated at room temperature into five subpopulations by increasing the flow rate successively from 15 to 20, 25, 30 and 40 ml/min. Two elutriations can be performed within 3 h after collagenase dissociation of the liver. The first fraction with a mean cell diameter of 19 μm is considered to represent diploid hepatocytes, and the third fraction with a mean diameter of 22 μm tetraploid hepatocytes. Other fractions are more heterogeneous. From two elutriations $15–20 \times 10^6$ diploid cells and $40–70 \times 10^6$ tetraploid cells are recovered. The 2n and 4n fractions have a purity of about 85 and 95% and their viability is about 85 and 98% respectively (30) (Fig. 3).

Isolation of fetal hepatocytes

Rodent and human hepatocytes

Although trypsin was the first enzyme used successfully to isolate hepatocytes from fetal rat liver (34), collagenase is now most often employed for dissociating rodent and human fetal liver (17, 19, 28). This enzyme has been combined with trypsin or hyaluronidase but is now used alone. The following technique is routinely used in our laboratory for dissociating rat and human fetal liver (17, 19). Liver fragments are washed three times with HEPES, pH 7.6 and incubated in the dissociating medium for 10 min at 37°C with gentle stirring. The first supernatant containing mainly blood cells is discarded. Two further stirrings, each lasting 10 min, are carried out and, when necessary, the remaining packed cells separated by straining through a glass syringe or pipette. Fetal rat livers are not minced prior to enzymatic digestion. The dissociating medium is that used for adult rat liver perfusion. For the isolation of liver cells from fetuses of 15 and 19 days gestation, livers from 15 and 6 litters respectively are dissociated in 50 ml of enzymatic solution. The supernatants are collected and centrifuged at low speed (50 g) for 1 min. The cells are washed three times with the Eagle's minimum essential medium, deficient in arginine as described by Leffert & Paul (28) and supplemented with 10% fetal calf serum. The percentage of single cells is usually low, less than 50%; small cell aggregates are commonly observed.

Embryonic chick hepatocytes

Livers are minced and placed in a sterile mixture of 0.05% collagenase and 0.05% hyaluronidase. The material is shredded with a Pasteur pipette until no lumps are visible. After 10–15 min at room temperature a cell suspension consisting mainly of single cells is obtained. Prior perfusion of embryos through the heart allows depletion of red blood cells. One to 1.5 ml of enzymatic solution is required to disaggregate the liver of a 17-day-old embryo (37).

Conclusions

Today, the basic two-step *in situ* collagenase perfusion method is routinely used for isolation of viable hepatocytes from various species. The most critical parameters for obtaining high yields of viable cells are the temperature, the pH and the flow rate of the solutions which must be carefully controlled. There is no need for these solutions to be oxygenated or recirculated.

Collagenase preparations, which are crude extracts of *Clostridium histolyticum* have been claimed to have different dispersion efficiencies. Several categories of crude collagenase with different content of proteolytic enzymes are available. The best categories for liver dispersion are now well known and there is only little variation in efficiency of different batches. When low cell yields are obtained, those are improved by changing the calcium concentration.

The highest cell yields are obtained by perfusion of either whole livers or a portion of whole livers. However, the two-step perfusion technique may be successfully applied to liver biopsies from various species (35, 43). Viable hepatocytes can also be isolated by enzymatic digestion of liver slices but cell yields are lower than with the perfusion method. Bellemann *et al.* (2) improved the yields by using buffers supplemented with glucose and aerated with a mixture of oxygen and carbon dioxide.

A number of criteria have been proposed as an indicator of the viability of freshly isolated hepatocytes. No one criterion may be regarded as ideal. The most commonly used criterion of cellular integrity is the trypan blue exclusion test but it is often misinterpreted (40). Hepatocytes with a well-defined refractive shape can be considered as well preserved cells (Fig. 2).

Isolated hepatocytes exhibit the typical fine structure of *in vivo* cells but specialized membrane domains, eg intercellular junctions and bile canaliculi, are no longer visible (9, 46). Loss of various intracellular compounds such as amino acids and limited functional alterations have been reported during cell isolation. However, most of these alterations are reversible and isolated hepatocytes express specific functions at levels which depend upon the *in vitro* environment, eg medium composition.

To survive for longer than a few hours, hepatocytes must attach to a substratum. In conventional culture conditions, they survive for a few days or weeks but rapidly lose their most differentiated functions. Prolongation of hepatocyte survival and of expression of specific functions is obtained by various modifications of the medium and/or the support. However, up to now, long-term prolongation of cell survival with maintenance of active specific liver functions has been successful only by co-culturing hepatocytes with another liver cell type, indicating that an environment close to that existing *in vivo* must be recreated *in vitro* (16). All these aspects are developed in the following chapters.

ACKNOWLEDGEMENTS

The authors wish to thank Mrs A. Vannier for typing the manuscript. The personal research described in the chapter was supported by INSERM.

REFERENCES

1 Arinze I. J., Rowley D. L.: Gluconeogenesis by isolated guinea pig liver parenchymal cells. *Biochem. J.* 1975, **152**: 393–399.

2 Bellemann P., Gebhardt R., Mecke D.: An improved method for the isolation of hepatocytes from liver slices. *Anal. Biochem.* 1977, **81**: 408–415.

3 Bengtsson G., Kiessling K. H., Smith-Kielland A., Morland J.: Partial separation and biochemical characteristics of periportal and perivenous hepatocytes from rat liver. *Eur. J. Biochem.* 1981, **118**: 591–597.

4 Bernaert D., Wanson J. C., Mosselmans R., De Parmentier F., Drochmans P.: Separation of adult rat hepatocytes into distinct subpopulations by centrifugation elutriation. Morphological, morpho-metrical and biochemical characterization of cell fractions. *Biol. Cell* 1979, **34**: 159–174.

5 Berry M. N., Friend D. S.: High-yield preparation of isolated rat liver parenchymal cells. A biochemical and fine structural study. *J. Cell Biol.* 1969, **43**: 506–520.

6 Bouche G., Gas N., Paris H.: Isolation of carp hepatocytes by centrifugation on a discontinuous Ficoll gradient. A biochemical and ultrastructural study. *Biol. Cell* 1979, **36**: 17–24.

7 Campbell J. W., Aster P. L., Casey C. A., Vorhaben J. E.: Preparation and use of fish hepatocytes. *In: Isolation, Characterization and Use of Hepatocytes*, R. A. Harris, N. W. Cornell (Eds): Elsevier, New York, 1983, pp 31–40.

8 Castagna M., Chauveau J.: Separation of metabolically distinct cell fractions from isolated rat hepatocytes. *Exp. Cell Res.* 1969, **57**: 211–222.

9 Clement B., Guguen-Guillouzo C., Campion J. P., Glaise D., Bourel M., Guillouzo A.: Long-term co-cultures of adult human hepatocytes with rat liver epithelial cells: modulation of active albumin secretion and accumulation of extracellular material. *Hepatology* 1984, **4**: 373–380.

10 Corona G. L., Santagostino G., Facino R. M., Pirillo D.: Cell membrane modifications in rabbit isolated hepatocytes following a chronic amitryptiline treatment. *Biochem. Pharmacol.* 1973, **22**: 849–856.

11 Drochmans P., Wanson J. C., Mosselmans R.: Isolation and subfractionation of Ficoll gradient of adult rat hepatocytes. Size, morphology and biochemical characteristics of cell fractions. *J. Cell Biol.* 1975, **66**: 1–22.

12 Elliot K. R. F., Pogson C. L.: Preparation and characterization of isolated parenchymal cells from guinea pig liver. *Mol. Cell. Biochem.* 1977, **16**: 23–29.

13 French C. J., Mommensen T. P., Hochacka P. W.: Amino acid utilisation in isolated hepatocytes from rainbow trout. *Eur. J. Biochem.* 1971, **113**: 311–317.

14 Guguen-Guillouzo C., Baffet G., Clement B., Begue J. M., Glaise D., Guillouzo A.: Human adult hepatocytes: isolation and maintenance at high levels of specific functions in a co-culture system. *In: Isolation, Characterization and Use of Hepatocytes*, R. A. Harris, N. W. Cornell (Eds): Elsevier, New York, 1983, pp 105–110.

15 Guguen-Guillouzo C., Campion J. P., Brissot P., Glaise D., Launois B., Bourel M., Guillouzo A.: High yield preparation of isolated human adult hepatocytes by enzymatic perfusion of the liver. *Cell Biol. Int. Rep.* 1982, **6**: 625–628.

16 Guguen-Guillouzo C., Clement B., Baffet G., Beaumont C., Morel-Chany E., Glaise D., Guillouzo A.: Maintenance and reversibility of active albumin secretion by adult rat hepatocytes co-cultured with another liver epithelial cell type. *Exp. Cell Res.* 1983, **143**, 47–54.

17 Guguen-Guillouzo C., Marie J., Cottreau D., Pasdeloup N., Kahn A.: Isozyme shift in cultured fetal human hepatocytes: a study of pyruvate kinase and phosphofructokinase. *Biochem. Biophys. Res. Commun.* 1980, **93**: 528–533.

18 Guguen-Guillouzo C., Seignoux D., Courtois Y., Brissot P., Marceau N., Glaise D., Guillouzo A.: Amplified phenotypic changes in adult rat and baboon hepatocytes cultured on a complex biomatrix. *Biol. Cell* 1982, **44**: 101–110.

19 Guguen-Guillouzo C., Tichonicky L., Szajnert M. F., Kruh J.: Changes in some chromatin and cytoplasmic enzymes of perinatal rat hepatocytes during culture. *In Vitro* 1980, **16**: 1–10.

20 Gumucio J. J., DeMason L. J., Miller D. L., Krezoski S. O., Keener M.: Induction of cytochrome P–450 in a selective subpopulation of hepatocytes. *Am. J. Physiol.* 1978, **234**: C102–C109.

21 Hayashi S., Ooshiro Z.: Preparation of isolated cells of eel liver. *Bull. Jap. Soc. Fish.* 1978, **44**: 499–503.

22 Howard R. B., Christensen A. K., Gibbs F. A., Pesch L. A.: The enzymatic preparation of isolated intact parenchymal cells from rat liver. *J. Cell Biol.* 1967, **35**: 675–684.

23 Katz J., Wals P. A., Golden S.: Carbohydrate and lipid metabolism in hepatocytes of Japanese quail. *In: Isolation, Characterization and Use of Hepatocytes*, R. A. Harris, N. W. Cornell (Eds): Elsevier, New York, 1983, pp 505–516.

24 Klaunig J. E.: Establishment of fish hepatocyte cultures for use in *in vitro* carcinogenicity studies. *Natl. Cancer Inst. Mon.* 1984, **65**: 163–173.

25 Klaunig J. E., Goldblatt P. J., Hinton D. E. Lipsky M. M., Chacko J., Trump B. F.: Mouse liver cell culture. I. Hepatocyte isolation. *In Vitro* 1981, **17**: 913–925.

26 Kuhlenschmidt M. S., Schmell E., Slife C. W., Kuhlenschmidt T. B., Sieber F., Lee Y. C., Roseman S.: Studies on the intercellular adhesion of rat and chicken hepatocytes. Conditions affecting cell-cell specificity. *J. Biol. Chem.* 1982, **257**: 3157–3164.

27 Le Cam A., Guillouzo A., Freychet P.: Ultrastructural and biochemical studies of isolated adult rat hepatocytes prepared under hypoxic conditions. Cryopreservation of hepatocytes. *Exp. Cell Res.* 1976, **98**: 383–395.

28 Leffert H. L., Paul D.: Studies on primary cultures of differentiated fetal liver cells. *J. Cell Biol.* 1972, **52**: 559–568.

29 Le Rumeur E., Beaumont C., Guillouzo C., Rissel M., Bourel M., Guillouzo A.: All normal rat hepatocytes produce albumin at a rate related to their degree of ploidy. *Biochem. Biophys. Res. Commun.* 1981, **101**: 1038–1046.

30 Le Rumeur E., Guguen-Guillouzo C., Beaumont C., Saunier A., Guillouzo A.: Albumin secretion and protein synthesis by cultured diploid and tetraploid rat hepatocytes separated by elutriation. *Exp. Cell Res.* 1983, **147**: 247–254.

31 Maitre J. L., Valotaire Y., Guguen-Guillouzo C.: Estradiol-17 β stimulation of vitellogenin synthesis in primary culture of male rainbow hepatocytes. *In Vitro* 1986, (In press).

32 Maslansky C. J., Williams G. M.: Primary cultures and the levels of cytochrome P–450 in hepatocytes from mouse, rat, hamster and rabbit. *In Vitro* 1982, **18**: 683–693.

33 Pangburn S. H., Newton R. S., Chang C. H., Weinstein D. B., Steinberg D.: Receptor-mediated catabolism of homologous low density lipoproteins in cultured pig hepatocytes. *J. Biol. Chem.* 1981, **256**: 3340–3347.

34 Plas C.: Recherches sur la différenciation fonctionnelle chez le foetus de rat. Séparation et culture des hépatocytes à partir d'une suspension cellulaire. *C. R. Acad. Sci. (Paris)* 1969, **268**: 143–146.

35 Reese J. A., Byard J. L.: Isolation and culture of adult hepatocytes from liver biopsies. *In Vitro* 1982, **17**: 935–941.

36 Renton K. W., Deloria L. B., Mannering G. J.: Effects of polyriboinosinic acid-polyribocytidylic acid and a mouse interferon preparation on cytochrome P–450-dependent monooxygenase systems in cultures of primary mouse hepatocytes. *Mol. Pharmacol.* 1978, **14**: 672–681.

37 Sassa S., Kappas A.: Induction of δ-aminolevulinate synthase and porphyrins in cultured liver cells maintained in chemically defined medium. *J. Biol. Chem.* 1977, **252**: 2428–2436.

38 Schreiber G., Schreiber M.: The preparation of single cell suspensions from liver and their use for the study of protein synthesis. *Subcell. Biochem.* 1973, **2**: 321–383.

39 Seglen P. O.: Preparation of rat liver cells. III. Enzymatic requirements for tissue dispersion. *Exp. Cell Res.* 1973, **82**: 391–398.

40 Seglen P. O.: Preparation of isolated rat liver cells. *Meth. Cell Biol.* 1975, **13**: 29–83.

41 Stacey N. H., Klaassen C. D.: Uptake of galactose, ouabain and taurocholate into centrolobular and periportal enriched hepatocyte subpopulations. *J. Pharmacol. Exp. Ther.* 1981, **216**: 634–639.

42 Stanchfield J. E., Yager J. D. Jr.: An estrogen responsive primary amphibian liver cell culture system. *Exp. Cell Res.* 1976, **116**: 239–252.

43 Strom S. C., Jirtle R. L., Jones R. S., Novicki D. L., Rosenberg M. R., Novotny A., Irons G., McLain J. R., Michalopoulos G.: Isolation, culture and transplantation of human hepatocytes. *J. Natl. Cancer Instit.* 1982, **68**: 771–778.

44 Tulp A., Welagen J. J. M. N., Emmelot P.: Separation of intact rat hepatocytes and rat liver nuclei into ploidy classes by velocity sedimentation at unit gravity. *Biochem. Biophys. Acta* 1976, **451**: 567–582.

45 Walton M. J., Cowey C. B.: Gluconeogenesis by isolated hepatocytes from rainbow trout salmo Gairdneri. *Comp. Biochem. Physiol.* 1979, **62B**, 75–79.

46 Wanson J. C., Bernaert D., May E.: Morphology and functional properties of isolated and cultured hepatocytes. *In*: *Progress in Liver Diseases*, H. Popper, F. Schaffner (Eds): Grune & Stratton, New York, 1979, Vol. 6, pp 1–22.

47 Wanson J. C., Drochmans P., May C., Penasse W., Popowski A.: Isolation of centrolobular and perilobular hepatocytes after phenobarbital treatment. *J. Cell Biol.* 1975, **66**: 23–41.

Research in *Isolated and cultured hepatocytes* A. Guillouzo & C. Guguen-Guillouzo eds. pp. 13–38.
© 1986 John Libbey Eurotext Ltd./INSERM.

2

Hepatocyte proliferation in culture

Joan A. McGOWAN

Shriners Burns Institute, 51 Blossom Street, Boston MA 02114, USA

SUMMARY

DNA synthesis, as well as cell proliferation, can be stimulated in adult rat liver parenchymal cells maintained in monolayer culture. This unique differentiated cell can be used *in vitro* to dissect and scrutinize the many factors that may be involved in the regulation of liver growth. Techniques are available to facilitate the study of hepatocyte growth in the absence of non-parenchymal liver cells and their products. Under optimal conditions, more than 80 per cent of hepatic parenchymal cells undergo at least one round of replicative DNA synthesis. The most active hepatotrophic factors now under investigation include epidermal growth factor (EGF), insulin, glucagon, and arginine vasopressin. Hepatocyte proliferation is also stimulated by serum factors, with rat serum far exceeding other types of sera in activity. The dissection of rat serum into its component activities has uncovered several new hepatocyte growth factors, including a rat platelet-derived factor, or factors, that act(s) synergistically with the other components of plasma. Many other substances and conditions modulate the response of hepatocytes to growth stimuli *in vitro*, including components of the basal medium (especially pyruvate, lactate, and proline), cell density, the extracellular matrix material used as substratum and, possibly, cell-derived autocrine factors. Thus, investigations with a homogeneous and responsive hepatic parenchymal cell population continue to identify hepatoproliferative factors and will facilitate studies of the general mechanism of growth factor action on these primary cells.

Introduction

Much of the research on the proliferation of hepatocytes *in vitro* has been inspired and motivated by the studies of liver regeneration *in vivo*. The factors that initiate and regulate the replication of adult mammalian liver cells following partial resection of this organ have been a topic of intense scrutiny for several decades (12, 13, 58, 62, 113).

The development of techniques for the isolation and maintenance of liver parenchymal cells in culture has made possible study of the direct effects of growth factors and hormones on hepatocytes. In this way, some of the complexity of whole animal physiology may be circumvented. As several other chapters have indicated, however, *in vitro* biology has its own unique complexity. Since it has been a goal to study a single, defined cell population — the parenchymal cell — and to do so under controlled environmental conditions, this review will focus on studies that have been conducted under stringently controlled conditions of cell isolation and maintenance and carried out with adult rat hepatocytes, isolated by collagenase perfusion *in situ*. These techniques permit the isolation of highly viable preparations of parenchymal cells with very low contamination by other cell types. Maintained in short-term culture (less than one week), in a defined medium, the hepatic parenchymal cells undergo DNA synthesis and mitosis in the presence of growth factors. Substantial information is now accumulating about the hormone, nutrient and growth factor interactions that regulate hepatocyte growth *in vitro*.

Methods of approach

A clear picture of the specific environmental factors that influence hepatocyte proliferation *in vitro* has sometimes been clouded by the disparate methods used to approach the problem. There has not been, nor should there be, a single approach to establishing and maintaining hepatocyte growth *in vitro*. It is extremely important, however, that investigators understand and continue to re-evaluate their techniques as well as those of colleagues. This section focuses on the different approaches used to assess proliferation and on some of the problems that most frequently interfere with clear interpretations of experimental data. Two general areas are discussed: 1) the problem of selecting for the differentiated hepatic parenchymal cell in culture, and 2) the specific techniques used to assess proliferation *in vitro*.

Cell type selection

For two reasons, it has been important for investigators to develop techniques for performing experiments on nearly homogeneous preparations of hepatocytes: 1) to establish that the hepatic parenchymal cells are indeed proliferation-competent *in vitro*, and 2) to preclude the physical or paracrine influence of other cell types.

The heterogeneity of cell types in the liver poses a problem for studies of hepatocyte proliferation *in vitro*. Early studies demonstrated that non-parenchymal cells could divide rapidly in explant culture, whereas differentiated hepatocytes failed to proliferate (33, 102). Consequently, there can be a dramatic change in the cellular composition of such cultures within one week after plating.

Table 1. The cellular distribution of non-parenchymal and parenchymal liver cells.

	Parenchymal cells (% of total)	Non-parenchymal cells (% of total)
Cytoplasmic volume	92.5	7.5
Cell number	65.0	35.0
Nuclear volume	86.8	13.2

Adapted from Blouin *et al.* (9) and Van Berkel (119).

The figures in Table 1 show the relative contribution of parenchymal and non-parenchymal cells to the total liver. As Table 1 indicates, the cytoplasmic volume of the parenchymal cells exceeds 90%, whereas these cells constitute only 65% of the total number of cells. The binuclearity and polyploidy of parenchymal cells is reflected in the enhanced nuclear volume when compared with cell number.

A great deal of interest and controversy has arisen over the origin of the cell types observed in mixed liver cell cultures maintained for more than one week in serum-containing medium. These arguments are pertinent to the subject of parenchymal cell proliferation. Grisham (32, 118) has presented evidence that many of the epithelial cell lines derived from the liver, as well as the major growth fraction of long-term hepatic cultures, arise from the epithelium of the bile ductules, an extremely small component (less than 1%) of the initial cell isolate. As they develop into lines, these cells characteristically express one or several of the differentiated characteristics of mature liver cells. Moreover, they are clonogenic, whereas parenchymal cells are not (32). The bile duct epithelial cells arise from the diverticulum of the foregut, as do the hepatocytes (123). This shared embryologic origin, as well as their isozyme patterns (32), further suggests that the bile duct epithelial cells may be facultative stem cells, which can mature and express some of the functional characteristics of hepatocytes. Recent evidence also indicates that a relationship may exist between the cells that grow out from normal liver in long-term culture and the 'oval' cells induced by certain liver carcinogens (39, 107, 118).

Thus, the real threat of 'overgrowth' in liver cell cultures comes not from the easily distinguished sinusoidal liver cells or fibroblasts, but rather from cells present at very low concentration in initial plating samples, which have the capacity to acquire parenchymal cell-like characteristics.

Selective isolation. Several simple procedures and practices can be used to promote the isolation of nearly homogeneous hepatic parenchymal cells and inhibit the growth of other cells types. The most important of the procedures contributing to the selective isolation of parenchymal hepatocytes is the *in situ* collagenase perfusion as described by Seglen (105). Perfusion techniques are generally more gentle than tissue dissolution techniques that expose extirpated tissue to the crude enzymes in solution. This latter method is the only one available for fetal tissue (46, 59, 60) and has been widely applied to neonatal liver (1, 2). In non-perfused preparations the parenchymal cells are damaged due to the contaminating proteolytic enzymes in the crude collagenase as well as mechanical injury. This tends to enhance the contribution of the non-parenchymal cells, which are notably more resistant to proteases (8, 45). Marceau and his collaborators have recently developed techniques for perfusing neonatal rat liver and have begun a careful and much needed comparison of neonatal and adult rat liver using comparable procedures (66).

After *in situ* perfusion, the parenchymal cells may be further selected on the basis of size and density, using either gravity sedimentation, low speed centrifugation or, to best advantage, centrifugal elutriation (39, 61). Hepatic parenchymal cells attach to tissue culture plastic or to collagen-coated plates within 30 minutes; therefore, short attachment times offer another means for separation, especially from endothelial cells, which require much longer attachment times (8). These commonly used procedures generally yield an initial plating sample of greater than 98–99% parenchymal cells (7).

Selective media. One of the most powerful ways to select for a particular cell type in tissue culture is the use of specific culture media. By manipulating components in the media, based on the functional capabilities of the desired cell, one can preclude the survival of other cell types. For example, the use of an arginine-free medium for the culture of hepatocytes was first proposed by Sato *et al.* (102) and later popularized by Leffert, Paul & coworkers (46, 48, 59, 60). The basis for the selectivity of arginine-free medium is the liver's unique capacity to synthesize arginine from ornithine via the urea cycle. Liver cells, and, to a lesser extent, the epithelial cells of the intestinal mucosa contain the mitochondrial enzyme, ornithine carbamoyl transferase (OCT), which converts ornithine to citrulline (92). Thus, replacing arginine with ornithine in the basal tissue culture medium inhibits the survival of cells that do not contain the enzyme, OCT, since these cells will be starved for arginine.

In a similar manner, glucose may be deleted from the hepatocyte culture medium since parenchymal cells contain the enzyme glucose-6-phosphatase and can produce glucose from gluconeogenic precursors. Thus, hepatocyte cultures may be maintained in the absence of glucose with no deleterious effect upon ATP concentration (McGowan, unpublished observations). The absolute selectivity of these deletions must, however, be viewed with caution.

Cross-feeding is a possibility in cultures that are initially largely parenchymal in composition. Thus, cells producing either arginine (from ornithine) or glucose may export, as do hepatocytes *in vivo*, enough of these substrates to maintain limited colonies of other cell types.

The unique cellular distribution of these enzymes, ornithine carbamoyl transferase and glucose-6-phosphatase, has also been questioned. Wagle *et al.* (120) demonstrated arginine synthesis from radioactive ornithine in isolated rat Kupffer cells. Moreover, if longer term cultures of hepatocytes become contaminated, not with sinusoidal liver cells but with putative stem cells, such as the bile duct epithelia, these cells may express these 'uniquely' parenchymal enzyme activities, due either to their embryological relationship with hepatocytes, or alternatively, they may acquire such activity during maturation in culture. For example, epithelial cell lines derived from rat liver begin to express up to 50% of the glucose-6-phosphatase activity found in normal liver (32).

In addition to the manipulation of glucose and arginine, Marceau *et al.* (65) demonstrated that dexamethasone drastically inhibits the growth of fibroblasts in hepatocyte cultures. Moreover, the absence of serum impedes the survival of cell types other than the parenchymal cell (23).

Length of time in culture. The best assurance that one is dealing with hepatic parenchymal cell proliferation is to minimize the length of time that the cell cultures are maintained. Short-term cultures may also circumvent, to some extent, the issue of phenotypic stability, although some investigators have described a very rapid decline in the transcriptional activity of genes for differentiated hepatic functions (19).

Numerous investigators have described the loss of differentiated functional activities suffered by hepatocytes with increasing time in culture (7, 34, 91, 111, 112) and maintenance of differentiated function in monolayer cultures of hepatocytes remains one of the most interesting and active aspects of hepatocyte research (see other contributions to this volume).

The recent, successful extension of phenotypic expression using co-culture of hepatocytes with liver epithelial cells (4, 34, 35) suggests that it may be important to scrutinize hepatocyte proliferation under such *controlled* mixed culture conditions.

Growth assessment

Before approaching the problem of proliferation, it is useful to keep in mind the *in vivo* model of liver cell replication. Following the classic partial hepatectomy, in which two-thirds of the rat liver are removed, the remnant cells (one-third of the original tissue) undergo tissue-wide replication. In young adult animals, greater than 90% of the parenchymal cells replicate at least once and other non-parenchymal cells also replicate at a somewhat later time than the parenchymal cells (12, 31). The original mass of the tissue is restored within one week. Clearly, if 90% of parenchymal cells replicate once, a subset of cells must undergo a second round of replication. In the most simple case, if 100% of the hepatocytes replicate during the first cycle, 50% of the cells replicating twice would restore the total initial number of cells. *In vivo*, each cell replicates only a very limited number of times to complete a cycle of regenerative restoration. Thus, the focus of most investigators studying hepatocytes *in vitro* has been on the proliferation-initiating factors, utilizing techniques to measure the initiation of DNA synthesis, the extent of cellular participation and whether the cells *in vitro* complete the cell cycle including mitosis and cytokinesis.

The techniques for assessing the liver growth of hepatocytes are similar to those developed for studying other cell types in culture or indeed for studies of liver growth *in vivo*. They are: 1) the incorporation of a radioactive precursor, usually tritiated thymidine, into cellular DNA; 2) the measurement of the increase in DNA per culture; 3) mitotic indices; and, 4) the increase in cell number or number of nuclei. Several of these techniques actually measure different parts of the cell cycle.

Incorporation of tritiated thymidine into DNA. This technique has been widely adopted to measure the DNA synthesis phase of the cell cycle. Cells in culture, or tissues in whole animals, are exposed to ^{3}H-thymidine for a period of time. At the end of the labelling period, the incorporation of the precursor into the product, DNA, may be measured chemically or by autoradiography.

Because of its specificity for DNA, thymidine is an optimal precursor. When assessing DNA synthesis by chemical isolation and analysis of the radioactivity per unit of tissue, several factors should be considered. First, since exogenous thymidine must be phosphorylated to thymidine triphosphosphate (TTP) and enter a cellular pool of TTP, largely derived from *de novo* synthesis, the specific activity (radioactivity/mole) of thymidine must be carefully selected. Generally, about 3 μM thymidine in the medium is sufficient to stabilize the endogenous TTP pool and permit the reliable assessment of DNA synthesis. High concentrations of thymidine, greater than 10 μM, will inhibit overall DNA synthesis due to the feedback inhibition of ribonucleotide reductase. The inhibition of this enzyme drastically reduces the availability of deoxycytidine triphosphate, the other pyrimidine precursor for DNA synthesis (20).

A second source of possible artifact in the interpretation of data from ^{3}H-thymidine incorporation is the spurious appearance of ^{3}H-counts in non-DNA fractions of cell isolates. This problem is especially exacerbated by long labelling times. Studies by Schneider & Greco (103) and Morley & Kingdon (79) have indicated that both non-specific binding of ^{3}H-species to protein as well as actual incorporation of the breakdown products of ^{3}H-thymidine into lipids, protein and RNA also can occur during labelling periods as short as sixty minutes. McGowan *et al.* (72), using a long (24-hour) incorporation period for ^{3}H-thymidine in hepatocyte cultures also obtained evidence that spurious incorporation must be monitored. To avoid these problems, samples for DNA analysis should undergo washes with trichloroacetic acid and alcohol, as well as alkaline hydrolysis, to avoid the appearance in the final isolated DNA of radioactivity from nucleosides, lipids or RNA (80).

A third problem with the use of tritiated thymidine incorporation into chemically isolated DNA is that this method does not distinguish replicative from repair DNA synthesis. Replicative DNA synthesis may be blocked by either hydroxyurea, which inhibits ribonucleotide reductase, or aphidicolin, which blocks DNA polymerase α.

The values for the incorporation of ³H-thymidine in the presence of either inhibitor, subtracted from incorporation in their absence, yields the true replicative incorporation rates. Use of these inhibitors as controls in each experimental group also precludes errors due to incorporation of tritium into non-DNA. Alternatively, the isolated DNA may be separated on $CsCl_2$ gradients (111).

The fourth and last consideration in the chemical analysis of ³H-thymidine incorporation is that this technique does not distinguish the cell type that is undergoing DNA synthesis. Thus, in mixed cultures, which are often used in fetal and neonatal as well as adult liver cell preparations, maintained for longer than one week, the chemical determination of ³H-thymidine incorporation is never sufficient to prove parenchymal cell replication.

Because of these considerations, autoradiographic analysis to confirm DNA synthesis in true parenchymal cells is of paramount importance. In addition to showing the incorporation of labelled precursor into nuclear DNA in morphologically distinct hepatocytes, autoradiographic techniques also can be used to determine the extent of cell participation in replication and to distinguish replicative from repair synthesis. This approach can determine directly the percentage of the hepatocytes undergoing DNA replication during a distinct period. As indicated by Fig. 1, the nuclei of cells undergoing replicative DNA synthesis are uniformly dark with individual grains often obscured and no grains over non-replicating nuclei. Repair synthesis, on the other hand, would have the appearance of a few grains per nucleus. An additional advantage of autoradiography has been indicated by Michalopoulos (75), who combined autoradiography with histochemical staining for glucose-6-phosphatase to further certify the parenchymal nature of the cells undergoing DNA replication.

A further consideration in growth assessment by means of ³H-thymidine incorporation is the timing of the response. Many factors such as age, stress and nutrition affect the timing as well as the extent of the *in vivo* response of the liver to

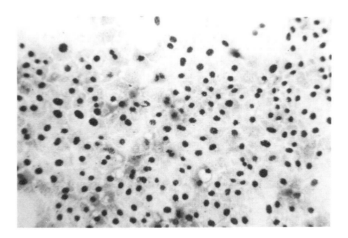

Fig. 1. Autoradiograph of hepatocytes cultured for 72 hours in the presence of serum-free medium containing epidermal growth factor (100 ng/ml) insulin (20 mU/ml), pyruvate (20 mM) and ³H-thymidine (1 μCi/ml, 3 μM). Magnification ×125.

growth stimulation (13). Since this may be the case as well *in vitro*, it is possible to mis-assess a growth regulatory agent by looking at too short a labelling period.

With all of its obvious advantages, autoradiographic analysis of DNA replication is more tedious and labour intensive than chemical analysis, which can be automated.

Increase in DNA per culture. If DNA replication has occurred, DNA per culture dish should increase. However, as pointed out by Baserga (6), 'Division of cells does not necessarily mean multiplication.' In this passage, he is referring to the situation *in vivo*, where cell replication is often balanced by cell loss yielding no net increase in cells. The same can be said of hepatocyte cultures, where cellular attrition often occurs at the same time as DNA synthesis. The advantage of isotopic methods is that they do not require accumulation to assess replication. Thus, increases in DNA per culture are very good evidence that DNA synthesis has occurred. A lack of increase may, however, be due to continuing cellular attrition, which is often noted, especially on untreated plastic surfaces. Prolonged attachment of hepatocytes has been reported on surfaces coated with liver derived extracellular matrix (23, 93, 95).

Increases in mitoses. After DNA synthesis, the cells would normally progress to mitosis and cell division, completing one turn of the cell cycle. However, a variety of studies of hepatocytes in culture indicated little mitotic activity, despite high rates of DNA replication (28, 36, 37, 42, 72, 94, 117). This finding had suggested to some investigators that perhaps other factors or cell conditions are necessary for the cell to complete mitosis. More recently, several laboratories have reported mitoses in hepatocytes in culture, and the explanation for the promotion of mitoses has varied among the different laboratories. Hasegawa *et al.* (38) have suggested that a low Ca^{++} concentration (<0.2mM) is required for mitotic division, whereas we have seen high rates of mitosis with normal Ca^{++} (0.8–1.0 mM) but high concentrations of intermediary metabolites (70, 72). Michalopoulos *et al.* (75) have

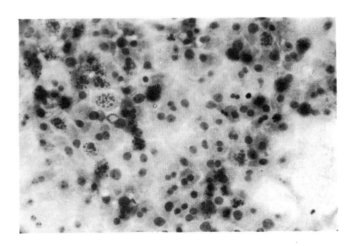

Fig. 2. Cells maintained as in Fig. 1, without ^{3}H-thymidine, but including 1 μM colcemid during the last 18 hours in culture. Giemsa stained. Magnification ×125.

quantitated mitoses in cultures in the presence of 50% of rat serum and observe that under these conditions, most of the cells undergoing replicative DNA synthesis also go through mitosis. Another factor may be the cell density. The appearance of mitotic figures is especially prominent at low seeding densities (75, 85).

Mitoses can be readily observed, as shown in Fig. 2, if colcemid is added to stimulated cells during the last 12 to 18 hours in culture. The cells that have entered mitosis during that period are seen either with very densely stained chromatin, or, if the cell entered mitosis early in the exposure to colcemid, with numerous micronuclei. Figure 2 supports the contention of several investigators that substantial mitotic activity occurs in hepatocyte cultures stimulated by growth factors.

Increases in nuclei or total cell counts. Measurement of increases in cell count or number of nuclei over a period of time would obviously circumvent many of the problems associated with isotopic incorporation studies or the counting of mitoses. Once again, certification of the replicating cell is a necessity, and cellular attrition complicates such analyses. Moreover, it is difficult to perform accurate cell counts on hepatocytes that have remained in culture for several days. After exposure to EDTA-trypsin, hepatocytes come off in sheets and fail to form single cell suspensions. It has been reported that 0.1% collagenase in buffer will remove cells from all surfaces except biomatrix (23). Isolated liver cell nuclei may be quantitatively prepared by exposure of hepatocyte cultures to 0.1 M citric acid containing 1% Triton X-100 (85). These may then be counted in an electronic particle counter, by hemocytometer or subjected to flow cytometry.

Some unique aspects to liver cell replication *in vivo* should be recognized as they become an object of study *in vitro*. While rat liver cells are mononuclear and diploid at birth, further growth of the liver during development involves the formation of up to 30% binucleate cells and about 70% of nuclei that contain double the normal diploid number of chromosomes (12). The initial cell isolate of adult rat liver may reflect this composition or may even be enhanced for the larger binucleate and/or tetraploid cells due to the particular isolation method.

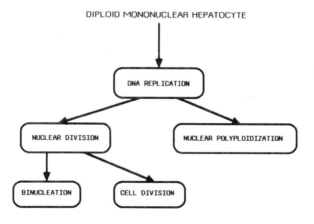

Fig. 3. Possible pathways of hepatocyte replication.

As outlined in Fig. 3, following the replication of DNA, there are several paths that the individual diploid mononuclear cell may follow, leading to nuclear polyploidization, nuclear division without cytokinesis, or complete cell division. It is not known to what extent each of these steps may be independently controlled by environmental factors.

Bissell & Guzelian (7), studying isolated quiescent cells from both normal and regenerating liver, noted no changes in ploidy with time in culture up to 48 hours. Whereas, when hepatocytes are maintained in a stimulatory mixture of insulin and EGF, the percentage of 2N (diploid) nuclei decrease, while 4N (tetraploid) nuclei remain about the same and the 8N (octaploid) nuclei, increase with time in culture (117). Studies by Enat *et al.* (23) also suggest that increases in DNA observed in hepatocyte culture may not correspond to increases in cell number. The parameters of DNA content, number of nuclei and cell number thus need to be carefully scrutinized to determine the characteristic pattern of cell replication *in vitro* and to see if the pattern itself is subject to environmental manipulation.

In any event, several studies suggest that the size of the cell as well as the total protein content are related to the ploidy (24, 81). Le Rumeur *et al.* (61) have measured albumin secretion by hepatocytes of different ploidy classes separated by centrifugal elutriation and have found that the amount of albumin secreted is proportional to the amount of DNA in the nucleus. This suggests that for the liver cell the primary event in responding to a growth stimulus may be the replication of DNA, which is correlated with and may direct both the increase in functional cell mass and the increase in enzymatic activity in consonance with the nuclear content of DNA.

The role of serum and serum factors

Heterologous sera

Most cell lines in culture require serum for growth, and early investigations with cultured hepatocytes included fetal calf serum. While some of these studies have suggested that hepatocytes proliferate readily in monolayer culture in the presence of calf serum (46, 48, 59, 60, 90), most investigators found little evidence of hepatic parenchymal cell growth with fetal calf serum alone (94, 117). Hepatocytes do require serum for attachment, spreading and to maintain viability over several days in culture (40). Fibronectin, at 5 to 10 μg/ml, substitutes for the attachment and spreading functions of serum but less so for the maintenance of viability. However, bovine pituitary trypsin inhibitor can serve to prolong viability (4). Hasegawa & Koga (37) also report a requirement for serum to maintain attachment over several days in culture but observe that pyruvate at 5 to 30 mM is equally effective.

In addition to attachment, spreading factors and non-specific anti-protease activity, serum is considered to be a source of specific hormones and growth factors. The successful approach of Sato and his colleagues to the serum-free maintenance of a variety of cell types is based on the development of cell type-specific hormonal/growth factor cocktails (5).

Enat *et al.* (23) have suggested that calf serum has several deleterious effects on hepatocytes in monolayer culture. This group observes that when liver cell cultures, which initially contain a few per cent of non-parenchymal cells, are maintained in serum-containing medium, there is selection for the non-parenchymal cells, which proliferate in the presence of serum. In addition, bovine serum appears to suppress the expression of specific differentiated hepatocyte functions (19, 23), suggesting that much of the growth reported to occur in serum-containing medium, especially in long-term cultures, may be due to the contribution of the non-parenchymal cells. Although this problem has sometimes been insufficiently addressed by investigators claiming hepatocyte growth, there are several studies using fetal calf serum in which the replicating cells are clearly identified as hepatic parenchymal cells by auto-radiographic analyses (28, 85, 94). However, although some replicative DNA synthesis can occur in the presence of calf serum, Strain *et al* (115) observed that bovine sera (fetal, newborn and calf), as well as other heterologous sera (horse, mouse, human), were less effective in stimulating DNA synthesis in hepatocytes than either a serum-free medium supplemented with insulin and EGF or medium containing rat serum.

Rat serum

Studies *in vivo* have indicated that following partial liver resection, the hepatotrophic stimulus can be transferred from the animal with the liver deficit to another animal with an intact liver by the establishment of rapid cross-circulation between the two animals (63, 78). These studies suggest the presence of a humoral factor in the blood of the partially hepatectomized animal.

A number of *in vitro* studies, beginning with those of Paul *et al.* (90) have thus sought to use hepatocytes in culture as a model system to identify the elusive humoral stimulator of hepatic regeneration. Paul and his collaborators observed that serum from partially hepatectomized rats was more active in stimulating fetal liver growth in culture than was serum from animals with intact livers. Supporting this finding, Michalopoulos has reported enhanced stimulation of DNA synthesis in adult hepatocytes using serum of animals partially hepatectomized 24 to 48 hours earlier, when compared to control serum (75). The parenchymal nature of the cells responding in short-term culture was fastidiously identified by Michalopoulos *et al.* (75) by combined autoradiography and histochemical staining for glucose 6-phosphatase. The stimulatory substance, which also is present in the serum of normal rats, appears to be more active in regenerating serum. The activity can be separated into high (>120 000) and low (<3000) molecular weight species that act synergistically in serum (76).

Using sera derived from control animals, as well as from animals subjected to partial hepatectomy at various times before serum collection, Strain *et al.* (115) observed no consistent difference between normal and regenerating rat serum. Nakamura *et al.* (82) confirm the variability among lots of sera and the lack of specific hepatotrophic activity in the whole serum of partially hepatectomized animals. However, this group observes that following serum purification by gel filtration, an active fraction of the hepatectomized serum contains almost twice the stimulatory activity of the normal serum. Moreover, the activity of these fractions is low when initially prepared but increases during storage. The increase in activity does not occur when the whole serum is stored or if the fractions are stored in the presence of protease inhibitors, suggesting that the hepatotrophic factor(s) may circulate in an inactive form.

Debate is certain to continue on the presence or absence of regeneration-specific growth factors in the blood of partially hepatectomized animals. Further insights must await purification and identification of the putative growth factors themselves.

Platelet factors

The search for purified growth factors from rat serum may be thwarted by unknown but important synergistic interactions. It may be difficult to show the activity of any one particular fraction unless other required components are also present. Nevertheless, in addition to the advances in the dissection of serum, rat platelets have been identified as a source of the hepatotrophic activity of rat serum. Strain *et al.* (115) observed that the removal of platelets prior to clotting reduced the DNA synthesis stimulating activity of rat plasma by 50%. As further investigated by Russell *et al.* (99, 100), a lysate of rat platelets restores the full activity of serum when combined with platelet-poor serum. The stimulatory activity of rat platelets immediately suggests comparison with the well-known human platelet-derived growth factor (PDGF). Differences in several biological and physical characteristics, as summarized in Table 2, indicate that the hepatocyte-stimulating activity in rat serum is not due to rat PDGF.

Table 2. Comparison of rat platelet factor (RPF) with platelet-derived growth factor (PDGF).

Similarities	*Differences*	
	RPF	*PDGF*
Platelet derived		
Cationic		
Trypsin sensitive	Heat labile (>65°C)	Heat stable (100°C)
Inactivated by disulfide bond reduction	65 000 MW (tentative)	30 000 MW
Acts synergistically with plasma factors	No somatomedin requirement	Requires somatomedin
	Stimulates hepatocytes	No hepatotrophic activity

Based on data from Russell *et al.* (111, 112) and Stiles *et al.* (114).

Paul & Piasecki (89) have recently confirmed the observation of the hepatotrophic activity of rat platelets and show that this activity is secreted in response to thrombin.

Clearly, any activity in rat serum derived from normal or partially hepatectomized animals may be difficult to unmask due to the concurrent presence of both stimulator and inhibitor factors. The success of several groups of investigators with various factors isolated from whole serum and platelets indicates that further purification of rat serum factors may lead to some new and possibly physiologically relevant growth factors.

Hormones and growth factors in serum-free media

The development of a serum-free medium for hepatocytes has been a longstanding aim. It can be argued that with a completely defined medium it will be possible to assess the growth-promoting properties of a variety of putative growth regulatory substances. Indeed, this is the approach to be discussed in this section. A cautionary note, however, seems appropriate in order to avoid some potential sources of misinterpretation of data. First, not all substances that stimulate growth *in vitro* will have a physiological role in growth regulation. Such substances may still be useful, on the other hand, in the overall investigation of growth mechanisms. Second, the growth activity of other regulatory factors may not be observed in the hepatocyte culture system due to deficiencies or defects in the components of the basal medium. Liver cells *in vivo* are exposed to the very rich environment of portal vein plasma. Growth regulatory substances may act, or depend, upon a variety of synergistic interactions which are, at this stage of hepatocyte culture techniques, largely unknown. Nevertheless, a great deal has been learned in the last several years about the actions and interactions of growth factors and hormones in the stimulation of hepatocyte DNA synthesis. Interpreting the experimental evidence cautiously, it may be possible to move from what *can* stimulate hepatocyte growth *in vitro* to what *does* so *in vivo*.

Epidermal growth factor (EGF)

Epidermal growth factor, a 6045 dalton (53 amino acid) polypeptide, has been the subject of several recent reviews (21, 26, 101). Isolated from the submaxillary glands of the male mouse, this growth factor has wide ranging mitogenic activity on cells in culture. Richman *et al.* (94) were the first investigators to show that EGF, especially in combination with insulin and glucagon, could stimulate DNA synthesis in isolated hepatocytes maintained in monolayer culture. Bucher *et al.* (15) then showed that EGF promotes growth in the liver of whole animals. This raises the question of the role this factor may play in normal liver growth and regeneration.

   Circulating levels of EGF in the rat are about 1 ng/ml (58), and the factor shows stimulatory activity in hepatocyte cultures at levels ranging from 1 to 100 ng/ml, especially in combination with other growth promoting hormones. Although there has been no evidence to date that the plasma concentration of EGF changes following partial hepatectomy, Earp & O'Keefe have reported that EGF receptors 'down regulate', that is, they are diminished on hepatocyte membranes following partial hepatectomy (22), suggesting binding and subsequent internalization of EGF. EGF is rapidly taken up by the liver cells *in vivo* (101). A bolus of radioactively labelled EGF is completely taken up by one pass through the liver. The uptake of EGF is highest in the area surrounding the portal tract. St Hilaire & Jones (101) have shown that internalized EGF is processed by the hepatocyte *in vivo* by two main pathways: one involving lysosomal degradation of the ligand and the other secretion of intact EGF into the biliary circulation. This has suggested that the liver may play a role in the steady state concentration of EGF via enterohepatic circulation and differential channeling to either the lysosomal or direct biliary secretion.

   The definitive mechanism of action of EGF in stimulating cell growth is unknown, although a variety of activities on cell physiology have been described (21). The binding of EGF stimulates phosphorylation of its own receptor (a 170 000 dalton glycoprotein) by a receptor associated tyrosine-specific protein kinase (21, 96). Other

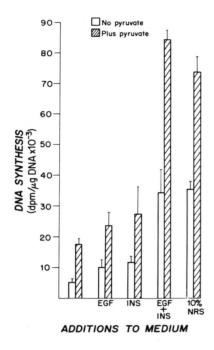

Fig. 4.
Hormones in serum-free medium. The effect of insulin (INS) 20 mU/ml, EGF 10 ng/ml and normal rat serum (NRS) 10% on DNA synthesis in the presence and absence of 20 mM pyruvate. ^{3}H-thymidine was present during the last 24 hours in culture and cells were harvested at 72 hours. From McGowan *et al.* (82), with permission.

cellular proteins may also be phosphorylated by the action of EGF but these have not yet been identified.

As shown in Fig. 4, EGF requires other growth promoting hormones and nutrients for maximal activity in stimulating DNA synthesis in hepatocytes in culture, and these will be discussed in the subsequent sections.

Insulin

In vivo studies have indicated that insulin plays a role in promoting liver growth, but that it is not necessary *per se* (12–17, 113). Animals deprived of insulin still respond to partial hepatectomy with liver growth that is less vigorous than that in normal animals (17).

The portal and systemic venous concentrations of insulin decline after partial hepatectomy, while glucagon is elevated (14). Nevertheless, infusion of combinations of insulin and glucagon to partially hepatectomized rats, whose liver growth is dramatically slowed due to total evisceration, restores near normal growth rate (17). The role of the pancreatic hormones, insulin and glucagon, may thus be considered not as primary growth factors but as major parts of the background hormonal activity in which normal liver cell growth occurs. Their action *in vitro* as indicated by Fig. 4, further suggests such a supportive role.

In hepatocyte cultures, insulin alone generally increases the rate of DNA synthesis by about two-fold and acts synergistically with EGF (see Fig. 4) and a variety of other growth stimulatory substances, which are discussed below (28, 41, 42, 50, 70–72, 94).

The concentration of insulin generally used to promote growth in hepatocyte cultures (1×10^{-8}M to 1×10^{-6}M) (28, 42, 72, 94) is hyperphysiologic, which has led to the suggestion that the growth promoting activity of insulin may be due to the cross reactivity of high concentrations of insulin with cellular receptors for other insulin-like growth factors, particularly insulin-like growth factor 1 (IGF-1), which is identical to somatomedin C (Sm-C). The type I somatomedin receptor is structurally similar to the insulin receptor. The neutral rat somatomedin, MSA (homologous to human IGF-II), has little affinity for insulin or IGF-1/Sm-C (68). Koch *et al.* (49) have compared the effects of insulin and the insulin-like growth factors on liver growth *in vitro* and have observed growth stimulation by physiological concentrations of insulin and IGF-1 but not by MSA. The low hepatic concentration of IGF-1/Sm-C receptors (68), and the fact that hepatocytes produce IGF-1/Sm-C in culture (51), suggest that insulin promotes the growth of hepatocytes through interaction with its own receptor.

Glucagon and β-adrenergic agonists

Glucagon is generally regarded as a catabolic hormone because of its effects on liver carbohydrate and lipid metabolism. Studies *in vivo* have indicated that insulin and glucagon in combination promote liver growth under some circumstances where neither hormone alone is stimulatory (13). They combine to accelerate hepatic growth in partially hepatectomized, eviscerated rats (17), which lack portally derived stimulatory factors. In addition, Lieberman and colleagues have used glucagon in combination with triiodothyronine, amino acids, and heparin to induce growth in intact (non-hepatectomized) rat liver (108, 109).

In view of these activities observed *in vivo* it is not surprising that several groups (23, 28, 36, 72, 94) report that insulin and glucagon combine synergistically to enhance hepatocyte DNA synthesis in the presence of EGF. These effects are observed in medium containing fetal calf serum (28, 94) as well as in serum-free medium (23, 36, 72). Moreover, the effects of glucagon can be replaced by exogenous cyclic AMP (28) or dibutyryl cAMP (72).

There is not universal agreement that glucagon is growth stimulatory (117). We have observed that the effectiveness of glucagon in stimulating DNA synthesis in hepatocytes may depend upon a variety of environmental factors, including the condition of the rat before perfusion. Hepatocytes isolated from animals maintained on a strict feeding schedule (4-h feeding period) are stimulated to undergo DNA synthesis by 1.4×10^{-7}M glucagon, whereas hepatocytes from animals fed *ad libitum* either fail to respond or show inhibition of DNA synthesis by glucagon (16).

Brønstad *et al.* (10) have recently reported that both glucagon and dibutyryl cyclic AMP can inhibit as well as stimulate DNA synthesis in hepatocytes. This group has pointed out that the stimulatory effects of glucagon are sensitive to both the concentration of the hormone as well as the cell density under the conditions of their experiments.

A number of agents mimic the activity of glucagon by raising intracellular cyclic AMP. Glucagon and the β-adrenergic agonists, isoproterenol, epinephrine and, to a lesser extent, norepinephrine may be grouped due to their action in elevating intracellular cyclic AMP. Friedman *et al.* (28) reported that, in addition to glucagon and cyclic AMP, epinephrine and isoproterenol effectively stimulate the labelling of hepatocyte nuclei. The effects of all these agents were enhanced in the presence of 3-methyl-isobutyl xanthine (MIX) which inhibits cAMP phosphodiesterase, a further indication that these agents act through raising the cyclic AMP levels in the cell.

In a similar study, using a serum-free medium, McGowan *et al.* (72) showed the growth promoting efficacy of dibutyryl cyclic AMP, isoproterenol, as well as cholera toxin, which irreversibly activates adenylate cyclase. In addition, the phosphodiesterase inhibitor, MIX, added alone, also stimulated DNA synthesis. It is interesting to note, in view of these positive effects of β-adrenergic agents on hepatocyte DNA synthesis, that adult rat hepatocytes *in vivo* have very few β-adrenergic receptors, whereas these receptors are high in fetal and neonatal animals. Indeed, Nakamura *et al.* (86) have shown that freshly isolated hepatocytes have very low β-adrenergic receptors, which rise with time in culture. Freshly isolated cells do not respond to isoproterenol with an elevation of cyclic AMP. The responsiveness to isoproterenol develops and is maximal by two days after plating in normal hepatocytes. Hepatocytes isolated from regenerating livers exhibit increased sensitivity to β-adrenergic stimulation (11).

Alpha-adrenergic agonists and vasopressin

Substances acting on α-adrenergic receptors as well as vasopressin promote enhanced DNA synthesis in the presence of other growth regulatory substances (28, 98). The action of the α-adrenergic agonists and vasopressin has been linked to calcium as a secondary messenger. Recently, however, it has been shown that changes in membrane polyphosphoinositide metabolism precede those in calcium concentration. Apparently, occupancy of these specific receptors can generate two putative intracellular secondary messengers: 1) diacylglycerol, which has been used directly on cells and stimulates the protein kinase C; and, 2) inositol triphosphate, which directs the release of Ca^{++} from intracellular storage sites (67).

Alpha-adrenergic receptor activation has been linked to hepatocyte growth by the observation of Michalopoulos *et al.* (76) that norepinephrine promotes DNA synthetic activity when added to normal rat serum. Furthermore, norepinephrine can stimulate DNA synthesis in combination with epidermal growth factor and insulin in serum-free medium. This stimulation by norepinephrine is blocked by the α_1-adrenergic antagonist prazosin, indicating action through the α_1-adrenergic receptor (Michalopoulos, personal communication). Phenylephrine, another α_1 agonist, also actively stimulates DNA synthesis (28). Nakamura *et al.* (88) have shown that although adult liver cells *in vivo* contain high concentrations of α-adrenergic receptors, 80% of which are the α_1 type, the number of these receptors declines with time in culture and is reduced by one-third during the first two days in culture. Thus the α_1 receptors undergo changes reciprocal to those of the β receptors as the cells adapt to monolayer culture conditions.

Adult rat liver hepatocytes *in vivo* can be expected to show low responsiveness to the classical β-adrenergic agonist, isoproterenol, and much greater responsiveness to the α agonist norepinephrine; whereas, in culture, hepatocytes become more responsive to β stimulation and less to α adrenergic stimulation.

Russell & Bucher (98) have reported that arginine vasopressin (AVP) augments the activity of other growth factors, especially when the other growth factors are at suboptimal concentrations. Thus, vasopressin stimulates DNA synthesis in hepatocytes with low concentrations of EGF or rat serum but is ineffective at high growth factor concentration. Hepatocytes contain AVP receptors of the V_1 type, which are calcium-linked and regulate pressor-like activities in other cell types.

The observation that AVP stimulates hepatocyte DNA synthesis in culture led Russell & Bucher (97) to examine the process of liver regeneration in the vasopressin-deficient Brattleboro rat. They observed a depressed proliferative response to partial hepatectomy in the AVP-deficient animals compared with control animals of the Long Evans strain, from which the Brattleboro was derived. Replacement therapy with arginine vasopressin, delivered via indwelling osmotic pumps for three days prior to partial hepatectomy successfully restored the regenerative response in some but not all animals tested. This line of research indicates the potential of this culture system for revealing hitherto unknown regulators of liver growth.

Other factors

The glucocorticoids, hydrocortisone and dexamethasone, promote both initial and prolonged cell attachment (55), possibly through the stimulation of hepatocyte-derived cell attachment proteins (4). However, there has been no evidence that these steroid hormones directly stimulate DNA synthesis. Some investigators remove the glucocorticoids after an initial plating period (36, 42), whereas others maintain the cells in the presence of glucocorticoids during the whole growth stimulatory period (72). Glucocorticoids increase the binding of radiolabelled EGF to hepatocytes, and this effect is counteracted by insulin (64).

Hepatocyte growth stimulation by prostaglandins has been suggested by the work of Armato and his collaborators (1, 2). Their work with neonatal rat liver cells has indicated that prostaglandins of the F series $PGF_{1\alpha}$ and $PGF_{2\alpha}$ stimulate both DNA synthesis and mitosis (2).

Thyroid hormone (T_3) has been used by Short & Lieberman (109) and their collaborators as part of a mixture containing glucagon, amino acids and heparin which stimulates DNA synthesis in the intact livers of rats *in vivo*. No direct role for any of the thyroid hormones in hepatocyte growth stimulation has been indicated in *in vitro* studies using T_3 (27, 117).

Other growth modulating factors

In addition to hormonal and growth factor effects on hepatocyte proliferation, there are a variety of other factors that influence the cells' responsiveness to growth stimulation. It is difficult to distinguish which of these factors may be a part of the primary signal to replicate and which may be circumstantially or even artifactually related to the specific culture conditions.

The role of intermediary metabolites in promoting hepatocyte replication

A role for pyruvate in *in vitro* hepatocyte metabolism was first suggested by Seglen *et* al. (106). The addition of high concentrations of pyruvate to freshly isolated hepatocytes improves the strongly negative nitrogen balance that is observed in serum-free unsupplemented medium. Early studies of Hasegawa & Koga further suggested that supplementation of media with pyruvate prevents the cellular deterioration observed in the absence of serum (37), and enhances DNA synthesis stimulated by insulin and glucagon (50). McKeehan & McKeehan (74) have shown that pyruvate and several other 2-oxocarboxylic acids can replace serum proteins and facilitate the serum-free growth and maintenance of fibroblasts. Lactate and other reduced forms of the oxocarboxylic acids are inactive on the fibroblasts, whereas lactate is as active as pyruvate in stimulating hepatocyte replication (69). As indicated in Fig. 4, addition of 20 mM pyruvate enhances the growth stimulating activity of basal medium, insulin, EGF, or combinations of insulin and EGF, as well as that of normal rat serum (69–71).

While the mechanism by which high concentrations of pyruvate and lactate promote hepatocyte growth remains largely unknown, this phenomenon raises the question of the extent to which 'functional overload' may prime liver cells for growth. *In vivo* following partial hepatectomy, the liver remnant is subjected to increased metabolic work with a drastically reduced number of functional units. The liver generally acts as an exquisite metabolostat, responding to the metabolic needs of the whole organism. Growth promotion by metabolic feedback is suggested by the stimulation of liver growth in non-hepatectomized animals by a sequence of protein deprivation and refeeding with a high protein diet (14, 108). While such an experimental protocol will obviously involve hormones and possibly growth factors, the metabolic and nutritional stimuli are an important driving force in regenerative liver growth.

Composition of basal media

The components of any basal medium may be categorized broadly as: salts and electrolytes, amino acids, vitamins and minerals (including trace minerals), buffering agents, glucose or some other carbohydrate energy source and, in some media, a lipid source. There has been very little investigation of how these various components interact either to promote prolonged survival of hepatocytes or to support growth. There have, nevertheless, been several media specifically designed for liver cells, including Williams' E and G (122), Koga's L (50), Seglen's SM-1 (104). Most recently, Enat et al. (23) have proposed a serum-free medium for hepatocyte proliferation based on RPMI 1640. In addition, Waymouth's MAB 87/3 (121) has been used as the basis of the serum-free medium used by McGowan & Bucher (70–72) to achieve high rates of DNA replication.

Nakamura et al. (84) have compared a variety of basal media* for their efficacy in promoting DNA replication in the presence of insulin and EGF. Under the conditions of their experiments, little DNA replication is stimulated by EGF and insulin using L-15, Dulbecco's Modified Eagle's Medium, or Minimal Essential Medium. However, with Williams' E, McCoy's 5A, or Ham's F12 comparably high levels of stimulation are observed. As suggested earlier by Hasegawa et al. (38), proline is a requirement for active hepatocyte DNA synthesis. The addition of

---

* For specifications of all basal media, see Grand Island Biological Co catalogue, 1984.

proline to the deficient media noted above caused DNA synthesis to be enhanced. Speculating that the lack of proline may inhibit collagen synthesis since proline is such a large component of the collagen molecule, these investigators showed, further, that specific inhibition of collagen synthesis by *cis*-hydroxyproline caused a dose-dependent inhibition of hepatocyte DNA replication (84).

These observations suggest that another function of media components may be to promote hepatocyte synthesis of its own extracellular matrix components, thereby facilitating growth induction. The role of extracellular matrix in hepatocyte growth and differentiation has been described by Reid and her collaborators (23, 93, 95; see also Reid *et al.*, Chapter 11 of this volume).

The differences among the basal media currently in use may explain some of the conflicting results that appear in the literature. There may also be components of the basal medium which are inhibitory. We have observed that glutamine (>2 mM) and also alanine (>2 mM) inhibit DNA synthesis (69). Although there has been no evidence reported for the efficacy of lipid components in media for hepatocytes, several of the commonly used media do contain supplements of linoleic acid, namely, Williams' E (0.03 μg/ml), Enat *et al.* (23) (5 μg/ml), Ham's F12 (0.084 μg/ml) and Koga's L (1 μg/ml).

A major focus in the development of Seglen's medium SM-1 (104) was to establish amino acid requirements that could optimally stimulate protein synthesis and inhibit protein degradation. In the course of these studies they described a rationale for the inclusion of pyruvate and high concentrations of amino acids based on protein turnover. They also found that high osmolality of the medium promotes survival during culture. We have also observed that increasing the osmolality of the basal medium by adding 50 to 100 mM additional sodium chloride actually enhances growth factor stimulation of DNA synthesis in both serum-containing (100) and serum-free medium (McGowan, unpublished observations).

The possible relevance of sodium (Na^+) ion fluxes to hepatocyte growth *in vitro* has been emphasized by the work of Leffert & Koch (47, 56, 57), who first demonstrated the inhibitory effect of amiloride, a potent inhibitor of sodium fluxes on growth factor stimulated DNA synthesis in cultured liver cells. In a recent review, Glaser *et al.* (29) have discussed the relevance of Na^+/H^+ exchange in the mitogenic response of cells to growth factors. The activation of Na^+/H^+ antiport activity by growth factors or high extracellular Na^+ also increases intracellular potassium, since the increased intracellular sodium will be exchanged for potassium by the activity of Na^+/K^+ ATPase. Burns & Rozengurt (18) have shown a very high correlation of mitogenic activity with intracellular K^+ concentration. In addition, since the sodium ions are exchanged for hydrogen ions, cytoplasmic alkalinization may affect a variety of enzyme systems sensitive to small changes in pH. Both gluconeogenesis and ureogenesis are strongly dependent on the intracellular pH (44). Therefore, the metabolic activation noted upon exposure to growth factors may be related to intracellular pH.

Cell density

Several investigators have suggested that plating density may determine hepato-cellular responsiveness to growth factor stimulation (10, 28, 72, 75, 85). Nakamura *et al.* (83, 85) observed that the response of hepatocytes to the stimulatory activity of insulin and EGF decreases as the cell density is increased with no stimulation above 5×10^4 cells per cm^2. The importance of low plating densities is also suggested by Michalopoulos *et al.* (75) in studies using rat serum. This raises the issue of a specific inhibitor of hepatocyte growth, produced by the hepatocyte itself. Nakamura *et al.* (87) have reported hepatocyte growth inhibiting activity derived from membrane fractions of mature hepatocytes.

One mechanism for the control of liver growth suggests that the liver, as well as other highly differentiated tissues, may produce growth inhibitory substances called 'chalones' which suppress cellular growth. Partial resection of the liver or loss of functional units by any means would then decrease the production of the 'chalone' and thereby permissively support growth until enough units producing the inhibitory substance had been restored, thereby shutting-off growth (43, 52, 110).

Although this hypothesis and the evidence cited above would suggest that hepatocytes generate an inhibitory substance in culture, which controls growth, other investigators (28) have reported that both higher cell densities and high cell concentration per ml of medium promote DNA synthesis. In the experiments of Friedman *et al.* (28), hepatocyte conditioned medium promotes DNA replication in the presence of insulin, glucagon and EGF and, indeed, renewal of medium each day depresses the replicative response. This would imply that hepatocytes either produce an autostimulatory factor or, alternatively, actively detoxify some inhibitory substance in the medium. LeBrecque (53, 54) has reported a substance, hepatic stimulator substance (HSS), that can be extracted from the liver of either partially hepatectomized or weanling rats by sequential heat treatment (65°C) and alcohol precipitation. HSS is heat stable (100°C) and stimulates the incorporation of tritiated thymidine into liver DNA of non-hepatectomized adult rats. Further studies by Francavilla *et al.* (27), using LaBrecque's isolation procedure, have indicated that production of HSS can also be stimulated by injection with T$_3$. This group has tested the effectiveness of HSS on Novikoff hepatoma cells as well as hepatocytes. The maximal stimulation is a 128% increase in DNA synthesis, and higher concentrations of HSS are inhibitory.

The relevance of these tissue-derived factors to the regulation of liver growth rests on the evidence that: 1) the active stimulatory substance is found only in growing (weanling or regenerating) or hormonally stimulated (T$_3$), but not in adult non-growing, liver; and, 2) its activity appears to be specific for liver tissue *in vivo* or liver derived cells (hepatoma) *in vitro* (53).

Other cell-derived stimulatory or autocrine factors produced by hepatocytes, which influence growth, may be the products of oncogene activation. Oncogenes are cellular genes that, upon activation, cause the malignant transformation of some cell types. During the *in vivo* response of the liver to partial hepatectomy, there is a five-fold increase in the expression of the cellular oncogene *ras* (30). The expression of both *myc* and *ras* is increased prior to DNA synthesis, suggesting a possible relationship between the activity of these genes and the onset of the hepatic growth response (25). This mechanism may further serve as an intracellular amplification system, acting in response to extracellular signals and fine-tuned to the specific cytoplasmic environment.

Conclusions

Clearly, great progress has been made in the last decade to facilitate the isolation, maintenance and even proliferation of hepatocytes. A realistic picture is emerging of the true difficulties of long-term maintenance and growth of the hepatocyte in culture. The challenge of the next several years is to improve the environmental conditions of the isolated hepatocyte in culture. As emphasized by the other contributors to this book, the concept of environment must now be expanded beyond the nutrients, hormones, growth factors and other components of the tissue culture media to the physical and possibly chemical influences of other cell types as well as the components of the extracellular matrix.

The current success with the stimulation of high rates of DNA replication in hepatocytes should lead to further progress radiating in two different directions. First, since it is now possible to stimulate at least the onset of growth in hepatocyte cultures, scrutiny of the pre-replicative period should intensify. A major question that arises from review of the hepatocyte growth regulatory substances relates to the mechanism of growth stimulation. Beyond growth factor/receptor interaction, what are the major intracellular events or processes that lead to the onset of DNA synthesis? Is there a unique, cell-specific, critical path or do several different sequences lead to replication? Secondly, while currently hepatocytes may be observed to undergo from one to several cycles of replication *in vitro*, growth to confluence and sub-culturing has not been possible with cultures of purely parenchymal cells. It is undoubtedly a hope, if not a dream, of dedicated hepatoculturists that the already mentioned and forthcoming improvements in the environmental conditions of the isolated cells will lead both to long-term maintenance of differentiation as well as to prolonged and continuing growth.

ACKNOWLEDGEMENTS

The author is grateful for the critical reviews of Dr Nancy Bucher and Dr William Russell and for the research support of the Shriners Hospital for Crippled Children (Grant #15851).

REFERENCES

1 Andreis P. G., Whitfield J. F., Armato U.: Stimulation of DNA synthesis and mitosis of hepatocytes in primary cultures of neonatal rat liver by arachidonic acid and prostaglandins. *Exp. Cell. Res.* 1981, **134**: 265–272.

2 Armato U., Andreis P. G.: Prostaglandins of the F series are extremely powerful growth factors for primary neonatal rat hepatocytes. *Life Sci.* 1983, **33**: 1745–1755.

3 Asami O., Nakamura T., Mura T., Ichihara A.: Identification of trypsin inhibitor in bovine pituitary extracts as a survival factor for adult rat hepatocytes in primary culture. *J. Biochem.* 1984, **95**: 299–309.

4 Baffet G., Clement B., Glaise D., Guillouzo A., Guguen-Guillouzo C.: Hydrocortisone modulates the production of extracellular material and albumin in long-term cultures of adult rat hepatocytes with other liver epithelial cells. *Biochem. Biophys. Res. Comm.* 1982, **109**: 507–512.

5 Barnes, D., Sato, G.: Serum-free cell culture: a unifying approach. *Cell* 1980, **22**: 649–655.

6 Baserga R.: *Multiplication and Division in Mammalian Cells*: Marcel Dekker Inc, New York, 1976, p 189.

7 Bissell D. M., Guzelian P. S.: Phenotypic stability of adult rat hepatocytes in primary monolayer culture. *Ann. N.Y. Acad. Sci.* 1980, **349**: 85–98.

8 Blomhoff R., Smedsrød B., Eskild W., Granum, P., Berg T.: Preparation of isolated liver endothelial cells and Kupffer cells in high yield by means of an enterotoxin. *Exp. Cell Res.* 1984, **150**: 194–204.

9 Blouin A., Bolender R. P., Weibel E. R.: Distribution of organelles and membranes between hepatocytes and nonhepatocytes in the rat liver parenchyma. *J. Cell. Biol.* 1977, **72**: 441–455.

10 Brønstad G. O., Sand T. E., Christoffersen T.: Bidirectional concentration-dependent effects of glucagon and dibutrrylcyclic AMP on DNA synthesis in cultured adult rat hepatocytes. *Biochim. Biophys. Acta* 1983, **763**: 58–83.

11 Brønstad G., Christoffersen T.: Increased effect of adrenaline on cyclic AMP formation and positive beta-adrenergic modulation of DNA-synthesis in regenerating hepatocytes. *FEBS Lett.* 1980, **120**: 89–93.

12 Bucher N. L. R., Malt R. A.: *Regeneration of the Liver and Kidney*: Little, Brown & Co, New York, 1971, pp 1–278.

13 Bucher N. L. R., McGowan J. A.: Regeneration: regulatory mechanisms. *In: Liver and Biliary Disease: A Pathophysiological Approach*, R. Wright, K. Alberti, S. Karran, H. Millward-Sadler (Eds): W. B. Saunders, London, 1979, pp 210–227.

14 Bucher N. L. R., McGowan J. A., Patel V.: *In: ICN/UCLA Symposia on Molecular and Cellular Biology*, Vol. 12, E. R. Dirksen, D. M. Prescott, C. F. Fox (Eds): Academic Press, New York, 1978, pp 661–670.

15 Bucher N. L. R., Patel V., Cohen S.: Hormonal factors concerned with liver regeneration. *In: Hepatotrophic Factors*, Ciba Foundation Symposium No. 55 (New Series): Elsevier/Excerpta Medica/North-Holland, New York, 1978, pp 95–107.

16 Bucher N. L. R., Russell W. E., McGowan J. A.: Aspects of hormonal influence on liver growth. *In: Glucagon in Gastroenterology and Hepatology*, J. Picazo (Ed.): MTP Press Limited, Boston, 1982, pp 141–153.

17 Bucher N. L. R., Swaffield M. N.: Regulation of hepatic regeneration in rats by synergistic action of insulin and glucagon. *Proc. Natl. Acad. Sci.* 1975, **72**: 1157–1160.

18 Burns C. P., Rozengurt E.: Extracellular Na^+ and initiation of DNA synthesis: role of intracellular pH and K^+. *J. Cell. Biol.* 1984, **98**: 1082–1089.

19 Clayton D. F., Darnell J. E.: Changes in liver-specific compared to common gene transcription during primary culture of mouse hepatocytes. *Molec. Cell. Biol.* 1983, **3**: 1552–1561.

20 Cleaver J. E.: *Thymidine Metabolism and Cell Kinetics*: North Holland Publishing Co, Amsterdam, 1967, pp 1–259.

21 Das M.: Epidermal growth factor: mechanisms of action. *Int. Rev. Cytol.* 1982, **72**: 233–256.

22 Earp H. S., O'Keefe E. J. O.: Epidermal growth factor receptor number decreases during rat liver regeneration. *J. Clin. Invest.* 1981, **67**: 1580–83.

23 Enat R., Jefferson, D. M., Ruiz-Opazo N., Gatmaitan Z., Leinwand L. A., Reid L. M.: Hepatocyte proliferation *in vitro*: its dependence on the use of serum-free hormonally defined medium and substrata of extracellular matrix. *Proc. Natl. Acad. Sci.* 1984, **81**: 1411–1415.

24 Epstein C.: Cell size, nuclear content, and the development of polyploidy in the mammalian liver. *Proc. Natl. Acad. Sci.* 1967, **57**: 327–334.

25 Fausto N., Shank P.: Oncogene expression in liver regeneration and hepatocarcinogenesis. *Hepatology* 1983, **3**: 1016–1023.

26 Fox C. F., Linsley P. S., Wrann M.: Receptor remodeling and regulation in the action of epidermal growth factor. *Fed. Proc.* 1982, **41**: 2988–2995.

27 Francavilla A., Ove P., Nanthiel D., Coetzee M., Wu S-K., Diko A., Starzl T.: Induction of hepatocyte stimulating activity by T_3 and appearance of the activity despite inhibition of DNA synthesis by adriamycin. *Horm. Metabol. Res.* 1984, **16**: 237–242.

28 Friedman D., Claus T., Pilkis S., Pine G.: Hormonal regulation of DNA synthesis in primary cultures of adult rat hepatocytes — Action of glucagon. *Exp. Cell Res.* 1981, **135**: 283–290.

29 Glaser L., Whiteley B., Rothenberg P., Cassel D.: Mitogenic polypeptides control ion flux in responsive cells. *Bio. Essays* 1984, **1**: 16–20.

30 Goyette M., Petropoulos C. M., Shank P. R., Fausto, N.: Expression of a cellular oncogene during liver regeneration. *Science* 1983, **219**: 510–512.

31 Grisham J. W.: Morphologic study of deoxyribonucleic acid synthesis and cell proliferation in regenerating rat liver: Autoradiography with thymidine -H^3. *Cancer Res.* 1962, **22**: 842–849.

32 Grisham J. W.: Cell types in long-term propagable cultures of rat liver. *Ann. N.Y. Acad. Sci.* 1980, **349**: 128–137.

33 Grisham J. W., Thal S. B., Nagel A.: Cellular derivation of continuously cultured epithelial cells from normal rat liver. *In: Gene Expression and Carcinogenesis in Cultured Liver*, L. E. Gershensen, E. B. Thompson (Eds): Academic Press, New York, 1975, pp 1–23.

34 Guguen-Guillouzo C., Guillouzo, A.: Modulation of functional activities in cultured rat hepatocytes. *Mol. Cell Biochem.* 1983, **53–54**: 35–56.

35 Guguen-Guillouzo, C., Clement B., Baffet, G., Beaumont, C., Morel-Chany E., Glaise D., Guillouzo A.: Maintenance and reversibility of active albumin secretion by adult rat hepatocytes co-cultured with another liver epithelial cell type. *Exp. Cell Res.* 1983, **143**: 47–54.

36 Hasegawa K., Namai K., Koga, M.: Induction of DNA synthesis in adult rat hepatocytes cultured in a serum-free medium. *Biochem. Biophys. Res. Commun.* 1980, **95**: 243–249.

37 Hasegawa K., Koga M.: A high concentration of pyruvate is essential for survival and DNA synthesis in primary cultures of adult rat hepatocytes in a serum-free medium. *Biomed. Res.* 1981, **2**: 217–221.

38 Hasegawa K., Watanabe K., Koga M.: Induction of mitosis in primary cultures of adult rat hepatocytes under serum-free conditions. *Biochem. Biophys. Res. Commun.* 1982, **104**: 259–265.

39 Hayner N. T., Brown L., Yaswen P., Brooks M., Fausto N.: Isozyme profiles of oval cells, parenchymal cells, and biliary cells isolated by centrifugal elutriation from normal and preneoplastic livers. *Cancer Res.* 1984, **44**: 332–338.

40 Horiuti Y., Nakamura T., Ichihara A.: Role of serum in maintenance of functional hepatocytes in primary culture. *J. Biochem (Tokyo)* 1982, **92**: 1985–1994.

41 Ichihara A., Nakamura T., Tanaka K.: Use of hepatocytes in primary culture for biochemical studies on liver functions. *Mol. Cell Biochem.* 1982, **43**: 245–260.

42 Ichihara A., Nakamura T., Tanaka K., Tomita Y., Aoyama K., Kato S., Shinno H.: Biochemical functions of adult rat hepatocytes in primary culture. *Ann. N.Y. Acad. Sci.* 1980, **349**: 77–84.

43 Iype P. T., McMahon J. B.: Hepatic proliferation inhibitor. *Mol. Cell. Biochem.* 1984, **59**: 57–80.

44 Kashiwagura T., Deutch C., Taylor J., Erecinski M. , Wilson D.: Dependence of gluconeogenesis, urea synthesis and energy metabolism of hepatocytes on intracellular pH. *J. Biol. Chem.* 1984, **259**: 237–243.

45 Knook D. L., Wisse E. (Eds): *Sinusoidal Liver Cells*: Elsevier Biomedical Press, Amsterdam, 1982, pp 1–358.

46 Koch K., Leffert H. L. : Growth control of differentiated fetal rat hepatocytes in primary monolayer culture. VI. Studies with conditioned medium and its functional interactions with serum factors. *J. Cell Biol.* 1974, **62**: 780–791.

47 Koch K. S., Leffert H. L.: Increased sodium ion influx is necessary to initiate rat hepatocyte proliferation. *Cell* 1979, **18**: 153–163.

48 Koch K. S., Leffert H. L.: Growth control of differentiated adult rat hepatocytes in primary culture. *Ann. N.Y. Acad. Sci.* 1980, **349**: 111–127.

49 Koch K. S., Shapiro P., Skelly H., Leffert H. L.: Rat hepatocyte proliferation is stimulated by insulin-like peptides in defined medium. *Biochem. Biophys. Res. Comm.* 1982, **109**: 1054–1060.

50 Koga M., Namai K., Hasekawa K.: Induction of DNA synthesis in primary culture of rat hepatocytes. *Dokkyo J. of Med. Sci.* 1979, **6**: 69–75.

51 Kogawa M., Takano K., Asakawa K., Hizuka N., Tsushima T., Shizume K.: Insulin stimulation of somatomedin A production in monolayer cultures of rat hepatocytes. *Acta. Endocrinol. (Copenh).* 1983, **103**: 385–390.

52 Kuo C., Yoo T.: *In vitro* inhibition of tritiated thymidine uptake in Morris hepatoma cells by normal rat liver extract: A possible liver chalone. *J. Natl. Cancer Inst.* 1977, **59**: 1691–1695.

53 LaBrecque D. R.: *In vitro* stimulation of cell growth by hepatic stimulator substance. *Am. J. Physiol.*, 1983, **242**: G289–295.

54 LaBrecque D. R., Bachur N. R.: Hepatic stimulator substance: physiochemical characteristics and specificity. *Am. J. Physiol.* 1983, **242**: G281–288.

55 Laishes B. A., Williams G. M.: Conditions affecting primary cell cultures of functional adult rat hepatocytes. II. Dexamethasone enhanced longevity and maintenance of morphology. *In Vitro* 1976, **12**: 821–832.

56   Leffert H. L., Koch K. S.: Regulation of growth of hepatocytes by sodium ions. *Prog. Liver. Dis.* 1979, **6**: 123–134.

57   Leffert H. L., Koch K. S.: Ionic events at the membrane initiate rat liver regeneration. *Ann. N.Y. Acad. Sci.* 1980, **339**: 201–215.

58   Leffert H. L., Koch K. S., Moran T., Rubalcava B.: Hormonal control of rat liver regeneration. *Gastroent.* 1979, **76**: 1470–1482.

59   Leffert H. L., Paul D.: Studies on primary cultures of differentiated fetal liver cells. *J. Cell. Biol.* 1972, **52**: 559–568.

60   Leffert H. L., Paul D.: Serum dependent growth of primary cultured differentiated fetal rat hepatocytes in arginine-deficient medium. *J. Cell Physiol.* 1973, **81**: 113–124.

61   LeRumeur E., Beaumont C., Guillouzo C., Rissel M., Bourel M., Guillouzo A.: All normal rat hepatocytes produce albumin at a rate related to their degree of ploidy. *Biochem. Biophys. Res. Comm.* 1981, **101**: 1038–1046.

62   Lesch R., Reutter W. (Eds): *Liver Regeneration after Experimental Injury*: Stratton Intercontinental Medical Book Corporation, New York, 1975, pp 1–364.

63   Lieberman I.: Studies on the control of mammalian deoxyribonucleic acid synthesis. *In: Biochemistry of Cell Division*, R. Baserga (Ed.): C. C. Thomas, Springfield, Illinois, 1969, pp 119–137.

64   Lin Q., Balisdell J., O'Keefe, E. J., Earp H. S.: Insulin inhibits the glucocorticoid-mediated increase in hepatocyte EGF binding. *J. Cell Physiol.* 1984, **119**: 267–272.

65   Marceau N., Goyette R., Valet J. P., Deschenes J.: Dexamethasone drastically inhibits the growth of fibroblasts. *Exp. Cell Res.* 1980, **125**: 497–502.

66   Marceau N., Noel M., Deschenes J.: Growth and functional activities of neonatal and adult rat hepatocytes cultured on fibronectin coated substratum in serum-free medium. *In Vitro* 1982, **18**: 1–11.

67   Marx J. L.: A new view of receptor action. *Science* 1984, **224**: 271–274.

68   Massague J., Czech M. P.: The subunit structures of two distinct receptors for insulin-like growth factors I and II and their relationship to the insulin receptor. *J. Biol. Chem.* 1982, **257**: 5038–5045.

69   McGowan J. A., Bucher N. L.: Pyruvate promotion of DNA synthesis in serum-free primary cultures of adult rat hepatocytes. *In Vitro* 1983, **19**: 159–166.

70   McGowan J. A., Bucher N. L. R.: Hepatotrophic activity of pyruvate. *In: Isolation, Characterization and Use of Hepatocytes*, R. A. Harris, N. W. Cornell (Eds): Elsevier, New York, 1983, 165–170.

71   McGowan J. A., Russell W. E., Bucher N. L.: Hepatocyte DNA replication: effect of nutrients and intermediary metabolites. *Fed. Proc.* 1984, **43**: 131–133.

72   McGowan J. A., Strain A. J., Bucher N. L.: DNA synthesis in primary cultures of adult rat hepatocytes in a defined medium: effects of epidermal growth factor, insulin, glucagon, and cyclic-AMP. *J. Cell. Physiol.* 1981, **108**: 353–363.

73   McMahon J., Iype T.: Specific inhibition of proliferation of nonalignment rat hepatic cells by a factor from rat liver. *Cancer Res.* 1980, **40**: 1249–1254.

74   McKeehan W., McKeehan K.: Oxocarboxylic acids, pyridine nucleotide-linked oxidoreductases and serum factors in regulation of cell proliferation. *J. Cell. Physiol.* 1979, **101**: 9–16.

75   Michalopoulos G., Cianciulli H. D., Novotny A. R., Kligerman A. D., Strom S. C., Jirtle R. L.: Liver regeneration studies with rat hepatocytes in primary culture. *Cancer Res.* 1982, **42**: 4673–4682.

76   Michalopoulos G., Houck K. A., Dolan M. L., Luetteke C.: Control of hepatocyte replication by two serum factors. *Cancer Res.* 1984, **44**: 4414–4419.

77   Michalopoulos G., Pitot H. C.: Primary culture of parenchymal liver cells on collagen membranes. *Exp. Cell. Res.* 1975, **94**: 70–78.

78   Moolton F. L., Bucher N. L. R.: Regeneration of rat liver transfer of humoral agent by gross circulation. *Science* 1967, **158**: 272–274.

79   Morley C. G. D., Kingdon H. S.: Use of ^{3}H-thymidine for measurement of DNA synthesis in rat liver — a warning. *Anal. Biochem.* 1972, **45**: 298–305.

80   Munro H. N., Fleck A.: The determination of nucleic acids. *In: Methods of Biochemical Analysis*, Vol. 14, D. Glick (Ed.): Interscience/John Wiley, New York, 1966, pp 113–176.

81   Nadal C., Zajdela F.: Polyploidie somatique dans le Foie de rat. *Exp. Cell Res.* 1966, **42**: 99–116.

82 Nakamura T., Nawa K., Ichihara A.: Partial purification and characterization of hepatocyte growth factor from serum of hepatectomized rats. *Biochem. Biophys. Res. Comm.* 1984, **122**: 1450–1459.

83 Nakamura T., Tomita Y., Noda C., Ichihara A.: Density-dependent controls of growth and various cellular activities of mature rat hepatocytes in primary cultures. *In: Isolation, Characterization and Use of Hepatocytes*, R. A. Harris, N. W. Cornell,(Eds): Elsevier, New York, pp 193–198.

84 Nakamura T., Teramoto H., Tomita Y., Ichihara A.: L-Proline is an essential amino acid for hepatocyte growth in culture. *Biochem. Biophys. Res. Commun.* 1984, **122**: 884–891.

85 Nakamura T., Tomita Y., Ichihara A.: Density-dependent growth control of adult rat hepatocytes in primary culture. *J. Biochem. (Tokyo).* 1983, **94**: 1029–1035.

86 Nakamura T., Tomomura A., Noda C., Shimoji M., Ichihara A.: Acquisition of a beta-adrenergic response by adult rat hepatocytes during primary culture. *J. Biol. Chem.* 1983, **258**: 9283–9289.

87 Nakamura T., Yoshimoto K., Nakayama Y., Tomita Y., Ichihara A.: Reciprocal modulation of growth and differentiated functions of mature rat hepatocytes in primary culture by cell–cell contact and cell membranes. *Proc. Natl. Acad. Sci.* 1983, **80**: 7229–7233.

88 Nakamura T., Tomomura A., Kato S., Noda, C., Ichihara A.: Reciprocal expressions of α- and β-adrenergic receptors, but constant expression of glucagon receptor by rat hepatocytes during development and primary culture. *J. Biochem.* 1984, **96**: 127–136.

89 Paul D., Piasecki A.: Rat platelets contain growth factor(s) distinct from PDGF which stimulate DNA synthesis in primary adult rat hepatocyte cultures. *Exp. Cell. Res.* 1984, **154**: 95–100.

90 Paul D., Leffert H., Sato G., Holley R. W.: Stimulation of DNA and protein synthesis in fetal rat liver cells by serum from partially hepatectomized rats. *Proc. Natl. Acad. Sci.* 1972, **69**: 374–377.

91 Pitot H. C., Sirica A. E.: Methodology and utility of primary cultures of hepatocytes from experimental animals. *Methods in Cell Biol.* 1980, **21**: 441–456.

92 Raijman L.: Citrulline synthesis in rat tissues and liver content of carbomoyl phosphate and ornithine. *Biochem. J.* 1974, **138**: 225–232.

93 Reid L., Gaitmaitan Z., Arias I., Ponce P., Rojkind M.: Long-term cultures of normal rat hepatocytes on liver biomatrix. *Ann. N.Y. Acad. Sci.* 1980, **349**: 70–76.

94 Richman R. A., Claus T. H., Pilkis S. J., Friedman D. L.: Hormonal stimulation of DNA synthesis in primary cultures of adult rat hepatocytes. *Proc. Natl. Acad. Sci.* 1976, **73**: 3589–3593.

95 Rojkind M., Gatmaitan Z., MacKensen S., Grambrone M. A., Ponce P., Reid L. M.: Connective tissue biomatrix: its isolation and utilization for long-term cultures of normal rat hepatocytes. *J. Cell Biol.* 1980, **87**: 255–263.

96 Rubin R. A., O'Keefe E. J., Earp H. S.: Alteration of epidermal growth factor-dependent phosphorylation during rat liver regeneration. *Proc. Natl. Acad. Sci.* 1982, **79**: 776–780.

97 Russell W. E., Bucher N. L. R.: Vasopressin modulates liver regeneration in the Brattleboro Rat. *Am. J. Physiol.* 1983, **245**: G321–324.

98 Russell W. E., Bucher N. L. R.: Vasopressin as a regulator of liver growth. *In: Isolation, Characterization and Use of Hepatocytes*, R. A. Harris, N. W. Cornell (Eds): Elsevier, New York, 1983, pp 171–176.

99 Russell W. E., McGowan J. A., Bucher N. L. R.: Biological properties of a hepatocyte growth factor from rat platelets. *J. Cell Physiol.* 1984, **119**: 193–197.

100 Russell W. E., McGowan J. A., Bucher N. L. R.: Partial characterization of a hepatocyte growth factor from rat platelets. *J. Cell Physiol.* 1984, **119**: 183–192.

101 St. Hilaire R. J., Jones A. L.: Epidermal growth factor: Its biological and metabolic effects with emphasis on the hepatocyte. *Hepatology* 1982, **2**: 601–613.

102 Sato G., Zaroff L., Mills S. E.: Tissue culture populations and their relation to the tissue of origin. *Proc. Natl. Acad. Sci.* 1960, **46**: 963–972.

103 Schneider W. C., Greco A. E.: Incorporation of pyrimidine deoxyribonucleotides into liver lipids and other components. *Biochim. Biophys. Acta.* 1971, **228**: 610–626.

104 Schwarze P. E., Solheim A. E., Seglen P. O.: Amino acid and energy requirements for rat hepatocytes in primary culture. *In Vitro* 1982, **18**: 43–54.

105 Seglen P. O.: Preparation of isolated rat liver cells. *In: Methods in Cell Biology*, Vol. 13, D. M. Prescott (Ed.): Academic Press, New York, 1976, pp 29–83.

106 Seglen P. O., Solheim A. E., Grinde B., Gordon P. B., Schwarze P. E., Gjessing R., Poli A.:

Amino acid control of protein synthesis and degradation in isolated rat hepatocytes. *Ann. N.Y. Acad Sci.* 1980, **349**: 1–17.

107 Sell S., Osborn K., Leffert H-L.: Autoradiography of 'oval cells' appearing rapidly in the livers of rats fed N-2-fluorenylacetamide in a choline devoid diet. *Carcinogenesis* 1981, **2**: 7–14.

108 Short J., Armstrong N. B., Kolitsky M. A., Mitchell R. A., Zemel R. A., Lieberman I.: *In: Control of Proliferation in Animal Cells*, B. Clarkson, R. Baserga (Eds): Cold Spring Harbor Laboratory, New York, 1974, pp 37–48.

109 Short J., Brown R. F., Husakova J. R., Gilbertson J. R., Zemel R., Lieberman I.: Induction of DNA synthesis in the liver of the intact animal. *J. Biol. Chem.* 1972, **147**: 1757–1766.

110 Simard A., Corneille Y., Deschamps Y., Nerly G.: Inhibition of cell proliferation in livers of hepatectomized rats by a rabbit hepatic chalone. *Proc. Natl. Acad. Sci.* 1974, **71**: 1763–1766.

111 Sirica A. E., Richards W., Tsukada Y., Sattler C. A., Pitot H. C.: Fetal phenotypic expression by adult rat hepatocytes on collagen gel/nylon meshes. *Proc. Natl. Acad. Sci.* 1979, **76**: 283–287.

112 Spence J-T., Haars L., Edwards A., Bosch A., Pitot H-C.: Regulation of gene expression in primary cultures of adult rat hepatocytes on collagen gels. *Ann. N.Y. Acad. Sci.* 1980, **349**: 99–110.

113 Starzl T. E., Terblanche J.: Hepatotrophic substances. *Prog. Liver Disease* 1979, **6**: 135–151.

114 Stiles C. D., Capone G. T., Sher C. D., Antoniades H. N., Nan Wyk J. J., Pledger W. J.: Dual control of cell growth by somatomedins and platelet-derived growth factor. *Proc. Natl. Acad. Sci.* 1979, **76**: 1279–1283.

115 Strain A. J., McGowan J. A., Bucher N. L.: Stimulation of DNA synthesis in primary cultures of adult rat hepatocytes by rat platelet-associated substance(s). *In Vitro* 1982, **18**: 108–116.

116 Strom S. C., Michalopoulos G.: Collagen as a substrate for cell growth and differentiation. *Methods Enzymol.* 1982, **82**: 544–555.

117 Tomita Y., Nakamura T., Ichihara A.: Control of DNA synthesis and ornithine decarboxylase activity by hormones and amino acids in primary cultures of adult rat hepatocytes. *Exp. Cell. Res.* 1981, **135**: 363–37x.

118 Tsao M-S., Smith J., Nelson K., Grisham J.: A diploid epithelial cell line from normal adult rat liver with phenotypic properties of 'oval' cells. *Exp. Cell Res.* 1984, **254**: 38–52.

119 Van Berkel T. J. C.: Functions of hepatic non-parenchymal cells. *In: Metabolic Compartmentation*, H. Sies (Ed.): Academic Press, New York, 1982, pp 437–482.

120 Wagle S. R., Hofmann F., Decker K.: Studies on urea synthesis, insulin degradation, and phagocytosis by isolated Kupffer cells. *Biochem. Biophys. Res. Comm.* 1976, **72**: 448–455.

121 Waymouth C.: Preparation of medium MAB 87/3 for primary cultures of epithelial cells. *TCA Manual* 1976, **3**: 521–525.

122 Williams G. M., Bermudez E., Scaramuzzino D.: Rat hepatocyte primary cell cultures. III. Improved dissociation and attachment techniques and enhancement of survival by culture medium. *In Vitro* **13**: 809–817.

123 Wilson J. W., Groat C. S., Leduc E. H.: Histogenesis of the liver. *Ann. N.Y. Acad. Sci.* 1963, **111**: 8–22.

Research in *Isolated and cultured hepatocytes* A. Guillouzo & C. Guguen-Guillouzo eds. pp. 39–61.
© 1986 John Libbey Eurotext Ltd./INSERM.

3

The cytoskeleton of cultured hepatocytes

Normand MARCEAU, Hélène BARIBAULT, Lucie GERMAIN
and Micheline NOEL

*Laval University Cancer Research Center and Department of Medicine,
Laval University, Quebec, CANADA*

SUMMARY

The present review summarizes recent findings on the composition and organization of the various cytoskeletal systems of cultured hepatocytes and hepatocyte-related cells, especially those of rats. Like other normal adherent mammalian cells, hepatocytes seeded on various substrata and cultured in the presence of hormonal factors that promote cell growth or differentiation undergo morphological changes. Such hormonally-induced modifications in cell shape are associated with changes in the organization of microfilaments, cytokeratin filaments and microtubules. In addition, other studies on cultured suckling rat hepatocytes have shown that dexamethasone can modulate the synthesis of cytokeratins and that such changes could be correlated to a large extent with the capacity of the hepatocytes to perform differentiated functions. Data presented here indicate that cytokeratins can, in fact, be used as markers of hepatocyte differentiation. Finally, the recent findings on the cytoskeletal modifications associated with the neoplastic transformation of hepatocyte-related cells are reviewed, particularly in relation to the differential effects of calcium deprivation on the cytoskeleton arrangement of cultured normal versus tumorigenic hepatic epithelial cells. In spite of such an advance in our knowledge of the biochemistry and immunology of the various cytoskeletal systems, as is the case for other mammalian cells, the understanding of their role in normal hepatocyte functioning is still at its infancy.

Introduction

Like other normal adherent mammalian cells, hepatocytes, in the presence of hormonal factors that promote cell growth or differentiation, undergo morphological changes upon seeding and subsequent culture on various substrata. Recent studies of fibroblasts and epithelial cells cultured as monolayers indicate that changes in cell shape constitute a very dynamic phenomenon related to the ability of the cells to deform, to form intercellular contacts, to attach to culture substrata and to migrate. The evidence accumulated so far points to the fact that all of these processes are most likely to be controlled by the cytoskeleton (24, 29, 85).

The cytoskeleton is a complex cytoplasmic structure composed of four fibrillar systems: microfilaments, intermediate filaments, microtubules and the still controversial microtrabecular lattice. In turn, each system is composed of several constituent proteins, and in recent years a major advance has been made in their biochemical and immunochemical characterization. However, much remains to be learned about the role of these fibrillar systems in normal cell function (24, 29, 79).

The purpose of this review is to summarize recent data on the composition and ultrastructural organization of cytoskeletal elements of cultured hepatocytes, especially those of the rat. The findings will be discussed in the context of what is known about these elements in other mammalian cells with regard to the cell shape and the modulation of cytoskeletal expression in apparent correlation with induced changes in functional activity. The variations in their intrinsic composition during the course of hepatocyte differentiation and neoplastic transformation is also considered.

The cytoskeleton and cell shape of substratum-dependent cultured cells

The characteristic shape and functional organization of eukaryotic cells is based largely on the extent of cell adhesion and on the defined arrangement of the cytoskeleton (1, 2, 54). Numerous studies have been concerned with the adhesive behaviour of various cultured cell types to each other and to the substratum (35). The data show that spreading results from progressive cell contacts and attachment to a substratum and is influenced by the presence of extracellular matrix components such as collagen, laminin and fibronectin (9). The influence of biomatrix on hepatocyte growth and functional activity will be covered in details by others (Chapters 11 and 12).

The importance of the contribution of cytoskeletal components to cell shape is perhaps best demonstrated by the fact that the typical cellular morphology of cells attached to culture substrata can still be recognized after extraction of the non-ionic detergent soluble cellular components and membranes (20).

The cytoskeleton is regarded as a network composed of three major classes of fibre proteins: microfilaments, microtubules and intermediate filaments. A fourth component, the still controversial microtrabecular lattice, may be integrally associated with the other three (69).

In non-muscle cells, microfilaments include the major protein actin and a variety of associated proteins. Microfilaments are often seen to interact with the surface membrane (7, 8), and recent data have indicated that the interaction involves distinct actin-binding proteins which differ depending on the regional specialization of the membrane. For example, fibroblasts attach to culture substratum via adhesion plaques (7) which contain vinculin (7, 29). Another actin-binding protein, the non-erythrocyte spectrin, is a subplasmallemnal, lattice-forming protein and is immunologically cross-reactive with erythrocyte α-spectrin (8, 32). Its role in relation to cell shape is ill defined.

Besides its localization at the surface membrane level, actin has also been identified in chromatin and other nuclear elements extracted from various cell types (4, 11, 33, 51). With respect to the functional significance for the presence of actin in nuclei, recent evidence from work on HeLa cells and amphibian oocytes indicates that it could represent a transcription initiation factor for RNA polymerase II (18, 74). However, the exact relationship between cytoplasmic and nuclear actin remains unclear.

Cytoplasmic microtubules are composed of α and β tubulins and various associated proteins (MAPs), the best known being the MAP2 and Tau proteins which are necessary for the polymerization of tubulins (for a review see references 83 and 85). MAP2 is apparently involved in the interaction between microtubules and actin-containing filaments (37, 38) and there is strong evidence that these interactions are important for cell shape.

Although the molecular composition of microfilaments and microtubules does not differ in different cell types, at least five major cell type-specific classes of intermediate filaments have been described (for a review see references 47 and 48). Vimentin is a specific marker of mesenchymal cells *in vivo* and in culture, while cytokeratins constitute a family of highly insoluble proteins characteristic of epithelial cells and cells of epithelial origin (for a review see reference 65).

In the context of the present review, cytokeratins represent cytoskeletal elements of major interest. There are 20 different cytokeratin polypeptides in human and rat tissues (65, 75). Gel electrophoretic analyses of cytoskeletal polypeptides (obtained by lysis of cultured cells and extraction with non-ionic detergent in high salt buffers) have shown that cytokeratins are major cell proteins in many cell types. It should be stressed that cytokeratins are present in different combinations in distinct epithelial cell types (65, 75, 82).

Although the role of cytokeratins is not well defined, it has been suggested that their specific composition is important for the performance of differentiated functions in epithelial cells (68). Cytokeratin filaments interact with several structural elements and with desmosomes at the surface membrane (24, 26) which supports the view that intermediate filaments may represent a mechanical integrator of the cytoplasm and a modulator of cell shape (48).

Hepatocytes as functionally organized units in culture

In the liver, hepatocytes are organized in a three-dimensional lobular architecture. One of their morphological features is the regional specialization of their surface membrane corresponding to portions that are exposed to sinusoids on one side and to bile canaliculi on the other. Microvilli are prominent in the canaliculi lumen and the membrane interfaces between adjacent hepatocytes are attached by desmosomes (26, 67).

The ability of cultured hepatocytes to perform cell-type specific functions requires conditions that generate, within a short period, intercellular contacts and cellular

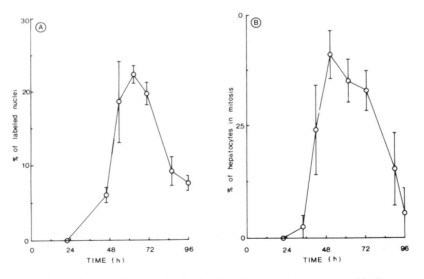

Fig. 1. **Kinetics of entry into S-phase and mitosis of suckling rat hepatocytes.** Medium was changed 2 h after plating to medium supplemented with EGF (10 ng/ml) and glucagon (600 nM). The hormonal factors were added at the same concentrations at 24, 48 and 72 h after the initial stimulation. [^{3}H]–TdR (1 μCi/ml) (A) or colchicine (0.12 mM) (B) were added at various times for 8 h after which cells were fixed and processed for autoradiography or Hoechst staining. The per cent of labelled nuclei (A) and mitotic hepatocytes (B) at various times after stimulation are shown. Points of the curve (the mid point of the 8 h labelling period) are the means±SEM of triplicate dishes of 2 (A) and 4 (B) separate experiments.

arrangements equivalent to those *in vivo*. This implies that *in vitro* maintenance of cellular functions is somehow linked to preservation of cellular shape and ultrastructure (49, 56).

To study this relationship, systems of primary cultures of rat hepatocytes have been developed in attempts to approximate *in vivo* cellular organization. In recent years, the major concern has been the search for the extracellular factors responsible for the adaptation, growth and maintenance of rat hepatocytes in culture. Initial

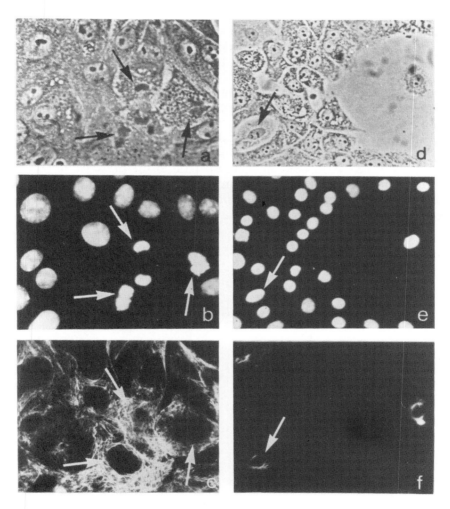

Fig. 2. Hepatocytes were cultured in the presence of EGF plus glucacon, fixed with ethanol 100% at −20°C for 10 min and processed for immunofluorescence and Hoescht staining. A view of the same field shows that mitotic cells in hepatocytes assemblies (A–B) are positive to anti-cytokeratin A (C) and anti-vimentin negative (D–E–F). Phase contrast shows that mitotic hepatocytes never round up (A). Note the presence of vimentin positive cells (D–E–F).

studies had shown that serum was required for the attachment of hepatocytes to plastic substratum but had no long-term beneficial effect on hepatocyte survival (50). Hence, the first approach has been to add various factors to either supplement or replace serum. For example, fibronectin can replace the serum requirement for hepatocyte attachment to plastic (12, 56). The other factors that have been tested were insulin, glucagon and EGF, hormonal factors which are probably involved in rat liver regeneration (6). The result has been that, although various combinations of EGF, insulin and glucagon (with or without serum) stimulate adult rat hepatocytes to enter the S-phase, in most cases very few mitoses have been observed (62–64, 70). Recent work in our laboratory has shown that under culture conditions identical to those of adult rat hepatocytes, suckling rat hepatocytes massively enter S-phase (Fig. 1) and undergo mitosis (Figs 1 & 2). The main parameter that distinguishes suckling from adult rat hepatocytes is their ploidy level, an increase in ploidy being associated with normal liver differentiation (5, 16).

Cessation of AFP production occurs during the normal differentiation of suckling rat hepatocytes (3). *In vivo* studies have shown that at this time of development the injection of glucocorticoids inhibits the production of AFP, but not of albumin. In this respect, these steroids are considered to be differentiation-promoting factors.

We have examined the effects of dexamethasone on cultured suckling rat hepatocytes seeded on fibronectin-coated plastic in the presence of insulin and/or EGF. Albumin production was maintained at a high and constant level over a 5-day period in the presence of insulin, EGF and dexamethasone (Fig. 3). When EGF was omitted, the production remained constant, but at a lower level, over a 3-day period.

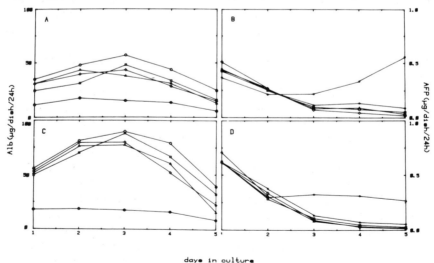

days in culture

Fig. 3. Effect of combination of EGF, insulin and dexamethasone on albumin (A, C) and alpha-fetoprotein (B, D) production. Suckling rat hepatocytes were seeded at a cell density of $1 \times 10^5/cm^2$ (A, B) or $2 \times 10^5/cm^2$ (C, D) and cultured in the presence of insulin (0.1 μg/ml) in all cases and EGF (10 ng/ml) (●), dexamethasone (1 μM) (□), dexamethasone (10 μM) (△), EGF (10 ng/ml) and dexamethasone (1 μM) (○) or EGF (10 ng/ml) and dexamethasone (10 μM) (◇). The medium was changed every day. The rate of production of albumin and alphafetoprotein is expressed as μg/dish/24 h of culture. Values are the average of triplicate dishes in 3 (A, C) or 2 (B, D) separate experiments.

In the absence of dexamethasone, albumin production was low whereas AFP production remained high (Fig. 3).

Long-term maintenance of functional activities requires more elaborate hepatocyte culture systems. These include the use of liver specific extracellular matrix elements as coating material of plastic substratum (71), the establishment of spheroidal aggregate cultures following seeding of hepatocytes on non-adherent substratum (44, 45), and the co-culture of hepatocytes with epithelial cells also isolated from the liver and which can be propagated in conventional monolayer culture (13, 41). Under these conditions, the expression of differentiated functions, such as albumin production, can be maintained for at least a few months (see Chapters 11 and 12 for further discussion).

Nevertheless, the point to stress here is that rat hepatocytes cultured on fibronectin-coated plastic in the absence of serum offers a reliable means to evaluate the modulation of hepatocyte shape and cytoskeleton organization by growth and differentiation-promoting factors.

Hormonally-induced changes in cell shape and cytoskeletal organization in cultured rat hepatocytes

One major observation in rat hepatocytes *in situ* is the occurrence of a compact microfilament network concentrated around bile canaliculi. This network was found to contain actin (25). Clusters of microfilaments have also been observed along the sinusoidal face of the hepatocytes. To our knowledge, no data are available on the occurrence or on relative amounts of the various actin-binding proteins, such as vinculin and spectrin, in rat hepatocytes.

We have examined the modulating effect of dexamethasone and insulin on the shape and cytoskeletal organization of rat hepatocytes cultured on fibronectin precoated surfaces. In the absence of either hormone or in the presence of insulin, hepatocytes spread extensively. Microfilaments were organized as cables in the cytoplasm and, as there were few clusters beneath the surface membrane, at the interface with the medium (Fig. 4). The degree of organization increased with time. Cytokeratin filaments showed a relatively low degree of organization and microtubules were arranged as a fine mesh extending throughout the cytoplasm (57). In the presence of dexamethasone or dexamethasone and insulin, hepatocytes formed a more compact monolayer. Microfilaments accumulated in a ring-like fashion around intercellular spaces at the cell interface with the substratum and as numerous clusters at the medium interface (Fig. 5). Anti-prekeratin reacted with fine fibrils in the cytoplasm, with a stronger staining at the edge of the intercellular spaces. A low concentration of microtubules was observed in the perinuclear region. Electron micrographs confirmed the presence of compact microfilament networks around the intercellular spaces along with some intermediate filaments and microfilament clusters beneath the surface membrane (Fig. 6). Desmosomes and some large mitochondria were observed close to these structures (Fig. 6).

Interestingly, the ring-like organization of actin-microfilaments around the intercellular spaces resembles the well developed network of microfilaments observed *in situ* around the bile canaliculi (26). The accumulation of actin as clusters

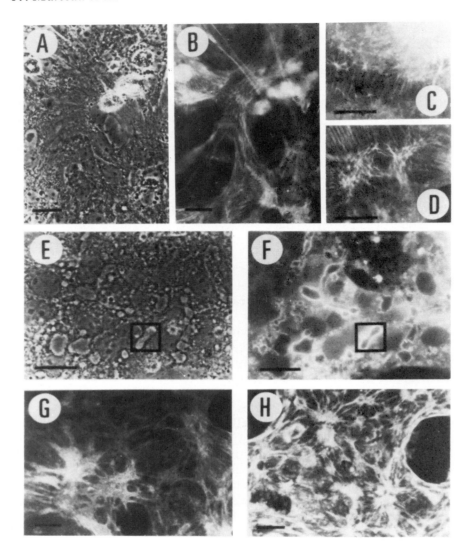

Fig. 4. Indirect immunofluorescence microscopy of adult rat hepatocytes in culture stained with anti-actin. Hepatocytes were cultured in absence (A–D) or presence (E–H) of 1 μM dexamethasone. A and E are phase contrast micrographs while B–D & F–H are the staining patterns. Note the cluster formation (B), the bridging filaments at cell-cell interface (C, arrow) and the geodome-like formation (D). In presence of dexamethasone, intercellular spaces are formed and the anti-actin intensely delineated the contour (E and F, insets). Some microfilaments accumulated beneath the surface membrane at the interface with the culture medium at 72 h (G) and even more at 168 h (H). Bars = 25 μm.

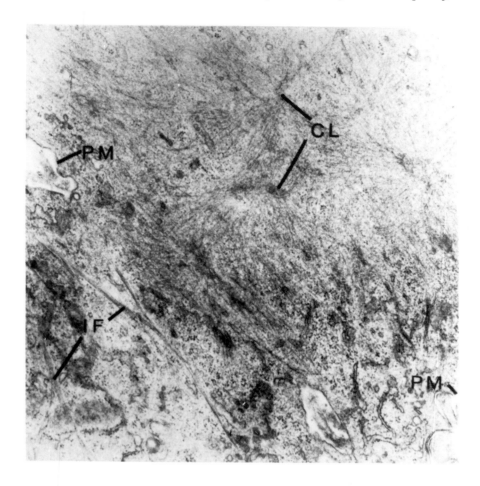

Fig. 5. Electron micrograph showing a portion of an hepatocyte after 72 h in culture. Beneath the cell surface, microfilaments seem to radiate from local complexes (CL). Bundles of intermediate-sized filaments can also be observed (IF). PM denotes the plasma membrane. Magnification: ×37 500.

beneath the surface membrane at the interface with the culture medium could well be imitative of the dense accumulation of actin-microfilaments along the sinusoid portions of the surface membrane *in situ* (23, 34).

Similar experiments have been performed on cultured rat hepatocytes following the addition of various combinations of EGF, insulin and dexamethasone (Fig. 7). These studies suggest that the glucocorticoid is the main modulator of hepatocyte shape and cytoskeletal organization.

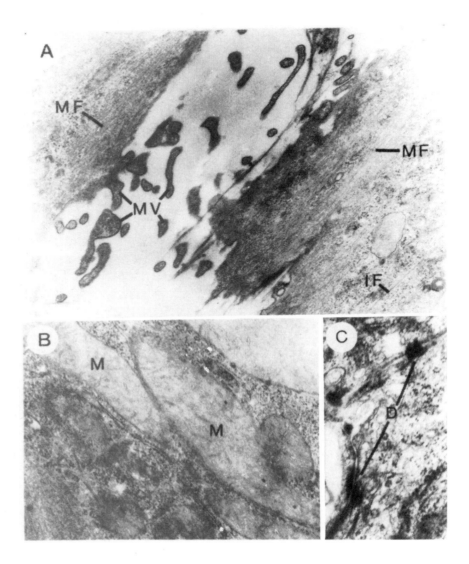

Fig. 6. Electron micrograph showing portions of dexamethasone-treated hepatocytes after 96 h in culture. (A) Microfilaments (MF) are present in large amount at the periphery of two cells. Intermediate-sized filaments are also found (IF). Magnification × 28 500. Note the presence of microvilli (MV) in the intercellular space. (B) Very large mitochondria (M) are frequently observed in the cytoplasm of these cells. Magnification: ×26 000 (C) At the junction of hepatocytes, numerous desmosomes D are generally present. Magnification: ×28 500.

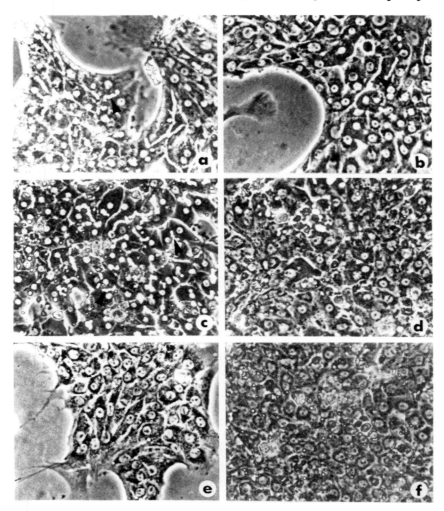

Fig. 7. Effects of combination of EGF, insulin and dexamethasone on rat hepatocyte culture morphology. Suckling rat hepatocytes were plated at a cell density of $1 \times 10^5/cm^2$ (*a, b, e*) or $2 \times 10^5/cm^2$ (*c, d, f*) and cultured for 3 days in the presence of insulin (0.1 µg/ml) (*a–f*) and dexamethasone (1 µM) (*a, c*) dexamethasone (10 µM) (*b*), EGF (10 ng/ml) and dexamethasone (1 µM) (*d*), EGF (10 µg/ml) (*e, f*). Note the presence of canaliculi-like structures (arrowheads). Phase contrast micrographs at 200×.

Hormonal modulation of cytokeratin synthesis in cultured differentiating rat hepatocytes

As discussed in the previous sections, glucocorticoids and insulin, in the absence of serum, modulate the ability of cultured rat hepatocytes to perform differentiated functions (56). This modulation of cellular functions is somehow linked to a preservation of cellular shape and a proper arrangement of microfilaments and cytokeratin filaments. Rat hepatocytes contain 6–7 cytokeratin components of 40 000 to 55 000 MW (21), assembled as tonofilaments interacting with various organelles and with desmosomes at cell-cell junctions (26, 90). Despite the biochemical and immunological characterization of rat hepatocyte cytokeratins (21), direct evidence for a role in modulating the action of hormones on cell function is still lacking.

We have recently performed studies to examine the synthesis and organization of cytokeratins in differentiating suckling rat hepatocytes cultured under conditions that promote cell growth or differentiation in response to hormonal stimulation. Dexamethasone added to suckling rat hepatocytes cultured in serum-free medium supplemented with insulin and EGF caused a selective dose-dependent increase in cytokeratin synthesis (Fig. 8). The response was dependent on the initial hepatocyte density. For example, at 5×10^4 hepatocytes/cm^2 a concentration of 1 or 10 μM dexamethasone, in the presence of insulin, enhanced the synthesis of a 55 000 MW cytokeratin and to a lesser degree a 49 000 MW cytokeratin, whereas at 10^5 hepatocytes/cm^2 10 μM dexamethasone preferentially stimulated a 51 000 MW cytokeratin. Preferential synthesis of the 51 000 MW component also occurred when either 1 or 10 μM dexamethasone was added to cultures seeded at 2×10^5 hepatocytes/cm^2. The inclusion of EGF along with dexamethasone and insulin in cultures at 2×10^5 cells/cm^2 yielded a differential effect of dexamethasone concentration equivalent to that observed at the lower cell density in the absence of EGF. Under conditions where increased cytokeratin synthesis was observed, the hepatocytes maintained a high production of albumin and lost their capacity to produce AFP (Fig. 3), a change in gene expression associated with the normal differentiation of suckling rat hepatocytes. In contrast, no enhancement of cytokeratin synthesis was observed in hepatocytes following the addition of EGF and insulin, a condition that promoted hepatocyte growth and the maintenance of AFP production (Table 1 & Fig. 3). The dexamethasone-induced enhancement of cytokeratin synthesis was still present at day 3 post-seeding. At this time, morphological observations by phase contrast and immunofluorescent microscopy using monoclonal antibodies against the 55 000 and 49 000 MW components revealed that under growth-promoting

Table 1. **Effect of hormone combination, dexamethasone concentration and cell density on DNA synthesis in cultured rat hepatocytes.** Suckling rat hepatocytes were seeded on fibronectin-precoated plastics in serum-free William's E medium. Hormonal factors were added to the medium at 24 h and [^{3}H]-TdR (1 μCi/ml) was added between 24 and 48 h post-seeding and cells were fixed and processed for autoradiography. Values represent the mean (SEM) of triplicate dishes in 3 separate experiments.

Hormonal factors	% of labelled nuclei	
	1×10^5 cells/cm^2	2×10^5 cells/cm^2
None	5.3 (5.2)	0.3 (0.3)
EGF, insulin	61.3 (3.4)	7.3 (8.8)
EGF, insulin, dexamethasone (1 μM)	49.9 (6.2)	7.8 (6.9)
EGF, insulin, dexamethasone (10 μM)	56.3 (10.3)	1.0 (1.4)
Insulin, dexamethasone (1 μM)	8.3 (2.2)	1.3 (1.8)

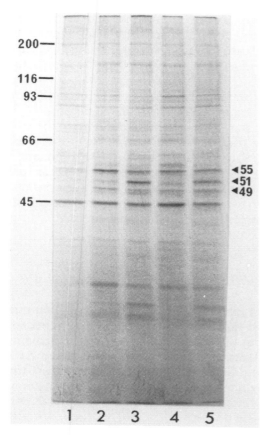

200 —
116 —
93 —
66 —
45 —

◀55
◀51
◀49

1 2 3 4 5

Fig. 8.
Effect of the concentration of insulin and dexamethasone on protein synthesis of cultured rat hepatocytes. Autoradiogram of 10% SDS-polyacrylamide slab gel of total proteins extracted from suckling rat hepatocytes seeded at a cell density of $10^5/cm^2$ and incubated for 2 h in the presence of $[^{35}S]$-methionine, after 24 h in the absence of supplements (lane 1); in the presence of insulin (0.1 μg/ml) and dexamethasone (1 μM) (lane 2); insulin (1 μg/ml) and dexamethasone (10 μM) (lane 3); insulin (1 μg/ml) and dexamethasone (1 μM) (lane 4) or insulin (0.1 μg/ml) and dexamethasone (10 μM) (lane 5); 1.5×10^5 cpm were applied to each well.

conditions the hepatocytes were spread and the cytokeratin filaments were stretched, whereas under differentiation-promoting conditions the cultures constitute a compact monolayer of cells exhibiting highly ordered filaments. Therefore, on the whole, these data suggest a close relationship between synthesis and organization of cytokeratins and promotion of differentiation of suckling rat hepatocytes by glucocorticoids.

One striking feature of cytokeratin filaments in cultured rat hepatocytes is that following successive extractions of cultured hepatocytes with Triton X-100, KCl, RNAse and DNAse, immunofluorescence microscopy with using antibodies CK55 and CK49 reveals patterns of cytokeratin filaments very similar to those observed in intact hepatocytes (60). This means that, as in the case of intermediate filaments in other similarly treated cells (20), hepatocyte cytokeratin filaments comprise a scaffold structure that extends throughout the entire hepatocyte monolayer and maintains the spatial localization of nuclei and intercellular junction complexes, even after the hepatocytes have lost their phospholipids, nucleic acids and a large portion of their proteins.

Cytokeratins are encoded by a multigene family (27, 44) and it remains to be determined whether a change in the rate of transcription, of post-transcriptional processing or in the stability of the mRNA is responsible for the observed modulation in cytokeratin synthesis levels in hepatocytes treated with dexamethasone. It is generally accepted that glucocorticoids act by altering the rate of transcription of specific genes (66), as is the case for AFP expression in the liver (3), although they may stimulate accumulation of specific mRNAs by inducing an RNA processing factor that would allow production of stable transcripts (84). Whatever the mechanism(s) regulating cytokeratin expression in cultured rat hepatocytes, the fact remains that a growth-promoting factor such as insulin is necessary for dexamethasone to exert its modulating action.

The significance of the requirement of a peptide hormone which acts at the cell surface in the modulating effect of glucocorticoid on specific gene expression is still unclear. Furthermore, it is interesting that events occurring at the cell surface are not restricted to insulin action since we found that EGF can intervene in this hormone interaction and that glucagon can to a certain extent replace the requirement for insulin (Baribault & Marceau, in preparation). How this information received at the cell surface is processed in the cell remains to be elucidated.

Cytokeratins as markers of hepatocyte differentiation *in situ* and in culture

The hepatocyte appears as a distinct cell type at around day 12 of gestation and immediately after birth the cell already expresses many of its differentiated characteristics (36, 80). There are a number of functional and metabolic elements that can be used as markers of its differentiation status. For example, AFP production and gamma-glutamyltransferase (GGT) expression are high during the fetal period and both decrease to extremely low levels during the first 1–2 weeks of life. In contrast, tyrosine aminotransferase (TAT) is induced only after birth and albumin production increases with increasing post-natal age (80).

The precursor of hepatocytes is ill defined. There is, however, some evidence that they may originate from bile ducts (15, 30, 90). Such an origin, which is a currently accepted possibility, is based on data obtained from studies of rats treated with hepatocarcinogens. An early response to virtually any hepatocarcinogen consists of

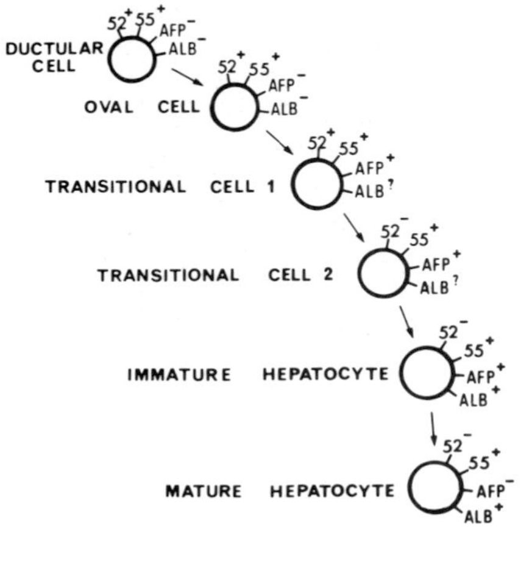

Fig. 9.
Putative differentiation link between bile duct cells, oval cells, transitional cells and hepatocytes on the basis of cytokeratins, AFP and albumin expression. It shows that oval cells have a cytokeratin composition identical to that of bile ductular cells. Two types of transitional cells are distinguished on the basis of a differential expression of AFP and CK52 cytokeratins. The same differentiation markers, when used in combination with albumin (ALB), would distinguish transitional cells from immature and mature hepatocytes.

proliferation of the epithelial cells lining the bile ducts and (sometimes) the intralobular ducts (15). These rapidly dividing cells have been designated 'oval' cells, they express GGT, a property of the epithelial cells of the bile duct, and are different from transitional cells which have been characterized as cells producing at least two hepatocytic proteins — albumin and AFP (72, 73). Still, the analysis using AFP for example as a cell marker provides little information on liver cell lineage since bile ductular cells are non-AFP producers.

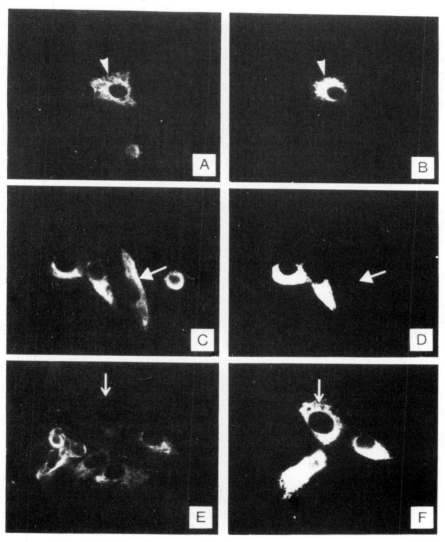

Fig. 10. Double immunofluorescence labelling of CK52 (A, C, E) and AFP (B, D, F) on cells of the fraction IV, following velocity sedimentation of cells isolated from the liver of rats fed 3'-Me-DAB for 4 weeks. Three patterns were observed: cells labelled with the 2 antibodies (▶), or only one: anti-CK52 antibody (➤), anti-AFP antibody (→). Magnification ×500.

Using single and double indirect immunofluorescence microscopy, we recently analysed the CK52/CK55 cytokeratin and AFP/albumin expression in the various cell types emerging at the early stage of rat hepatocarcinogenesis, and in normal newborn and adult rat hepatocytes (30). The analysis, conducted *in situ* and *in vitro* on isolated liver cell preparations, shows that CK55 is present not only in hepatocytes but also in bile ductular cells and oval cells (30), thus suggesting a common lineage between these liver epithelial cell types. Moreover, CK52 was detected only in bile ductular cells and oval cells. Thus the differential expression of these hepatic cytokeratins provides evidence for a direct relationship between oval cells and bile ductular epithelial cells (30).

The combined results of analyses using anti-CK52-, CK55- and AFP-antibodies suggest a link between oval cells, transitional cells and immature hepatocytes (Fig. 9). The presence of CK55 in oval cells expressing CK52 and in AFP- and albumin-producing hepatocytes isolated from newborn rats is an indication of a relationship between oval cells and immature hepatocytes. Besides the cell population containing CK52 only (oval cells), the double antibody technique revealed cells expressing both CK52 and AFP and cells strongly expressing AFP, with very little or no CK52 (Fig. 10). On the basis of morphological data reported by others (62), the epithelial cells expressing both CK52 and AFP would represent a class of transitional cells related to oval cells while those expressing only AFP are suggestive of a second class of transitional cells at a stage close to that of immature hepatocytes (Fig. 9).

However, the normal liver is a complex tissue, composed not only of hepatocytes but also of several additional cell types (36). The presence of these non-parenchymal cells becomes particularly evident when attempts are made to establish liver cells in culture (39, 40). Primary cultures of rat liver cells may contain mostly hepatocytes during the first week post-seeding (40, 87), but during long-term culture they are usually replaced by small cells, some of which are epithelial in character (40, 87) while others resemble endothelial cells (40). The epitheloid cells can often be subcultured and established as cell lines (10, 14, 31, 39, 53, 79, 87). Although it is not possible at present to unequivocally identify all types of cells that emerge in long-term cultures, it would seem that the hepatic epithelial cells originate from cells in the non-parenchymal cell population rather than from altered hepatocytes in the culture. These cultured hepatic epithelial cells contain cytoplasmic organelles, ultrastructurally resembling those of terminal biliary duct or intermediate cells *in vivo* (40). They may express, partially and variably, some of the differentiated functions of hepatocytes, such as AFP and/or albumin, suggesting the existence of clones derived from cells *in vivo* that express various degrees of hepatocyte differentiation (40).

A recent analysis of the expression of cytokeratins in such hepatic epithelial cell lines has shown that they contain CK52 and CK55, two cytokeratins present in bile ductular cells (Fig. 11). Further studies on such cells after treatments with differentiation-promoting factors, should help in our further understanding of hepatocyte development and differentiation.

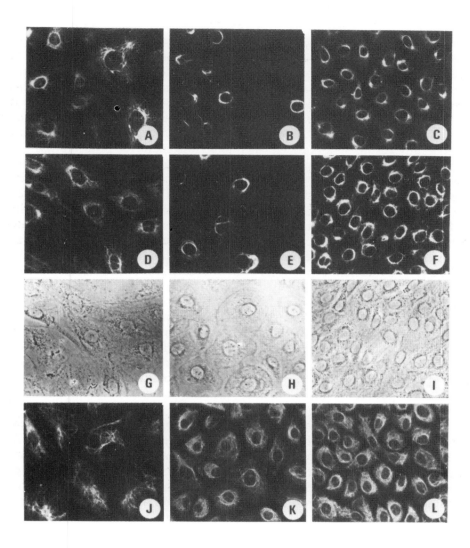

Fig. 11. Immunofluorescence staining of CK55 (A, B, C), CK52 (D, E, F), vimentin (J, K, L) on 3 cell lines: rat liver epithelial cells (A, D, G, J) mesothelial-like cells (B, E, H, K), T51B (C, F, I, L). G, H, I are phase contrast micrographs corresponding to *D, E, F*, respectively. Magnification ×400.

Cytoskeletal events associated with the neoplastic transformation
of hepatocyte-related cells

A large number of studies have been done on the response of cultured epithelial cells derived from liver (mainly from rats) (2, 40, 55, 77, 87) to chemical carcinogens. In most cases the persistent morphological alterations resulting from the chemical transformation were changes in cell shape and size, focal multilayered growth, major disturbance in cytoskeletal organization and a reduction in the number of cells displaying a primary cilium. As with many other cell types, neoplastic transformation generally results in a reduced calcium requirement for proliferation (17, 76). Because of the involvement of calcium in the organization and distribution of cytoskeletal elements (see reference 59 for a recent review), we studied the cytoskeletal changes induced by calcium deprivation in normal and tumorigenic rat liver cells in culture (76). Interestingly, in spite of the differential inhibition of growth of normal as opposed to tumorigenic cells caused by calcium deprivation, our studies demonstrated that calcium deprivation induces dramatic but different changes in the morphology of normal epithelial cells and hepatoma cells (77).

Loss of cell contact and retraction of the cytoplasm following calcium deprivation are observed in both cell types but it occurs immediately in normal cells and gradually (over a 24 h period) in hepatoma cells. Transmission electron micrographs of epidermal and carcinoma cells in a low calcium environment reveal a disruption of desmosomes and their subsequent internalization as hemidesmosomes. Scanning electron micrographs of normal and hepatoma cells after 24 h in low calcium show that the cell surface of normal cells is induced to contract following calcium deprivation and remains smooth with only few microvilli, whereas the induced cell-rounding in hepatoma cultures is accompanied by marked formation of blebs and microvilli.

These induced changes in cell shape and morphology are accompanied by marked changes in the organization of cytoskeleton components. The changes are different in the normal and tumorigenic liver epithelial cell types (78). First of all, it should be stressed that the cytoskeleton of normal cells growing in standard (1.8 mM calcium) medium is highly organized, with parallel actin microfilament bundles and extending networks of microtubules and intermediate filaments, whereas these components in hepatoma cells are generally irregular and disorganized even in standard medium (78).

After 24 h in low calcium, the microtubule and vimentin networks of normal cells are contracted, diffuse and disorganized. Cytokeratin filaments are retracted from the cell periphery to a more perinuclear position (78), a reorganization associated with the loss of desmosomes which has also been observed in other cells. On the other hand, in low calcium, microtubules and cytokeratin filaments of hepatoma cells are unaffected.

The most striking changes are observed in the distribution of actin-containing microfilaments. Following a 24 h exposure to low calcium, the microfilaments bundles of normal cells become concentrated at attachment sites at the periphery, parallel to the cell axis (78), whereas the disorganized microfilament bundles of the hepatoma cells (largely disrupted even in standard calcium medium) appear as intense regions of actin in a non-filamentous form at blebs and/or contact regions.

Since only the growth of normal cells but not the hepatoma cells, is inhibited in low calcium, one is tempted to conclude that the differential responses of the cytoskeleton of normal and neoplastic liver cells to calcium deprivation may be linked to proliferative events.

All of these findings on the differential response of normal versus cancerous cells have been discussed recently (59) in the light of the known interaction between this Ca^{2+} and serum growth factors in the initiation of DNA synthesis and mitosis, the direct involvement of calcium and its partner cAMP, in the control of the integrity of the cytoskeleton, the activation of distinct protein kinases by all of these factors, the role played by various cytoskeletal proteins as substrates for phosphorylation (59). Finally, a means by which neoplastic cells can bypass normal protein kinase regulatory pathways has been proposed based on recent data showing that the product of some oncogenes are protein kinases (59).

Conclusions

In the light of what is known about the expression, structure and functions of the cytoskeleton in mammalian cells, our knowledge of the hepatocyte cytoskeleton is still incomplete. That cultured hepatocytes contain actin-microfilaments, microtubules and cytokeratin filaments is well established. Very little, however, is known about the presence of various actin-binding proteins, such as spectrin and vinculin, the tubulin-associated proteins such as MAP2 and the actual expression of vimentin. As is the case for other mammalian cells, our understanding of the intrinsic roles played by the various cytoskeletal systems in normal hepatocyte functioning is still in its infancy.

ACKNOWLEDGEMENTS

We thank Dr William I. Waithe for critical reading of the manuscript, and Elisabeth Lemay and Chantal Bedard for their secretarial assistance. Hélène Baribault was the recipient of a studentship from the Cancer Research Society and Lucie Germain received one from the Medical Research Council of Canada. This work was supported in part by the National Cancer Institute of Canada.

REFERENCES

1 Aplin J. D., Bardsley W. G., Niven V. M.: Kinetic analysis of cell spreading. *J. Cell Sci.* 1983, **61**: 375–388.
2 Bannikov G. A., Guelstein V. I., Montessan R., Tint I. S., Tomatis L., Troyanovsky S. M., Vasiliev J. M.: Cell shape and organization of cytoskeleton and surface fibronectin in nontumorigenic and tumorigenic rat liver cultures. *J. Cell Sci.* 1982, **54**: 47–67.
3 Bélanger L., Baril P., Guertin M., Gingras M. C., Gourdeau H., Anderson A., Hamel D., Boucher J. M.: Oncodevelopmental and hormonal regulation of α_1-fetoprotein gene expression. *In*: *Advances in Enzyme Regulation*, G. Weber (Ed.): Pergamon Press, New York, 1983, Vol. 21, pp 73–99.
4. Boschek C. B., Jockusch B. M., Friis R. R., Back R., Grundmann E., Bauer H.: Early changes in the distribution and organization of microfilaments proteins during cell transformation. *Cell* 1981, **24**: 175–184.

5   Brodsky W. Y., Uryvalva I. V.: Cell polyploidy: its relation to tissue growth and function. *Int. Rev. Cytol.* 1977, *50*: 275–332.

6   Bucher N. L. R., Patel U., Cohen S.: Hormonal factors concerned with liver regeneration. *In: Hepatotrophic Factors*, Ciba Foundation Symposium No. 55, 1977: Elsevier/Excerpta Medica/ North-Holland, New York, pp 95–107.

7   Burridge K., Feramisco J. R.: Microinjection and localization of a 130K protein in living fibroblasts: a relationship to actin and fibronectin. *Cell* 1980, *19*: 587–595.

8   Burridge K., Kelly T., Mangeat P.: Nonerythrocyte spectrins: actin-membrane attachment proteins occurring in many cell types. *J. Cell Biol.* 1982, *95*: 478–486.

9   Carlsson R., Engvall E., Freeman A., Ruoslahti E.: Laminin and fibronectin in cell adhesion: enhanced adhesion of cells from regenerating liver to laminin. *Proc. Natl. Acad. Sci.* 1981 **78**: 2403–2406.

10 Chessebeuf M., Olsson A., Bournot P., Desgres J., Guiguet M., Maume G., Maume B. F., Perissel B., Padieu P.: Long-term cell culture of rat liver epithelial cells retaining some hepatic functions. *Biochimie* 1974, *56*: 1365–1379.

11 Clark T. G., Rosenbaum J. L.: An actin filament matrix in hand-isolated nuclei of *X. laevis* oocytes. *Cell* 1979, *18*: 1101–1108.

12 Deschênes J., Valet J. P., Marceau N.: Hepatocytes from newborn and weanling rats in monolayer cultures: isolation by perfusion, fibronectin-mediated adhesion, spreading and functional activity. *In Vitro* 1980, *16*: 722–730.

13 Clement B., Guguen-Guillouzo C., Campion J. P., Glaise D., Bourel M., Guillouzo A.: Long-term co-cultures of adult human hepatocytes with rat liver epithelial cells: modulation of albumin secretion and accumulation of extracellular material. *Hepatology* 1984, *4*: 373–380.

14 Coon H.: Clonal culture of differentiated cells from mammals: rat liver cell culture. *Carnegie Institute Washington Year Book* 1969 *67*: 419–421.

15 Dempo K., Chisaka N., Yoshida Y., Kaneko A., Onoe T.: Immunofluorescent study on α-fetoprotein-producing cells in the early stage of 3′-methyl-4-dimethylaminoazobenzene carcinogenesis. *Cancer Res.* 1975, *35*: 1282–1287.

16 Deschenes J., Valet J. P., Marceau N.: The relationship between cell volume, ploidy and functional activity in differentiating hepatocytes. *Cell Biophys.* 1981, *3*: 321–334.

17 Durham A. C. H., Walton J. M.: Calcium ions and the control of proliferation in normal and cancer cells. Biosci. Rep. 1982, *2*: 15–30.

18 Egly J. M., Myamoto N. G., Moncollin V., Chambon P.: Is actin a transcription initiation factor for RNA polymerase B. *Embo J.* 1984, *3*: 2363–2371.

19 Farber E.: Similarities in the sequence of early histological changes induced in the liver of the rat by ethionine, 2-acetylaminofluorene, and 3′-methyl-4-dimethylaminobenzene. *Cancer Res.* 1956, **16**: 142–149.

20 Fey E. G., Wan K. M., Penman S.: Epithelial cytoskeletal framework and nuclear matrix-intermediate filament scaffold: Three-dimensional organization and protein composition. *J. Cell Biol.* 1984, *98*: 1973–1984.

21 Franke W. W., Denk H., Kalt R., Schmid E.: Biochemical and immunological identification of cytokeratin proteins present in hepatocytes of mammalian liver tissue. *Exp. Cell Res.* 1981, *131*: 299–318.

22 Franke W. W., Schiller D. L., Moll R., Winter S., Schmid E., Engelbrecht, I.: Diversity of cytokeratins. Differentiation specific expression of cytokeratin polypeptides in epithelial cells and tissues. *J. Molec. Biol.* 1981, **153**: 933–959.

23 Franke W. W., Schmid E., Kartenbeck J., Mayer D., Hacker H. J., Bannash P., Osborn M., Weber K., Denk H., Wanson J. C., Drochmans P.: Characterization of the intermediate-sized filaments in liver cells by immunofluorescence and electron microscopy. *Biol. Cell* 1979, *34*: 99–110.

24 Franke W. W., Schmid E., Moll R.: The intermediate filament cytoskeleton in tissues and in cultured cells: differentiation specificity of expression of cell architectural elements. *In: Human Carcinogenesis*, C. Curtis, H. Herman, N. Autrup (Eds): Academic Press, New York, 1983, pp 35–84.

25 French S. W., Davies P. L.: Ultrastructural localization of actin-like filaments in rat hepatocytes. *Gastroenterology* 1975, *68*: 765–774.

26 French S. W., Kondo I., Irie T., Ihrig T. J., Benson N., Mann R.: Morphological study of intermediate filaments in rat hepatocytes. *Hepatology* 1982, **2**: 29–38.
27 Fucks E., Coppock S. M., Green H., Cleveland, D. W.: Two distinct classes of keratin genes and their evolutionary significance. *Cell* 1981, **27**: 75–84.
28 Geiger B.: A 130K protein from chicken gizzard: its localization at the termini of microfilaments bundles in cultured chicken cells. *Cell* 1979, **18**: 193–205.
29 Geiger B.: Membrane-cytoskeleton interaction. *Biochim. Biophys. Acta* 1983, **737**: 305–341.
30 Germain L., Goyette R., Marceau N.: Differential cytokeratin and α-fetoprotein expression in morphologically distinct epithelial cells emerging at the early stages of rat hepatocarcinogenesis. *Cancer Res.* 1985, **45**: 673–681.
31 Gerschenson L. E., Casanello D.: Metabolism of rat liver cells cultured in suspension insulin and glucagon effects on glycogen level. *Biochem. Biophys. Res. Commun.* 1968, **33**: 584–589.
32 Glenney J. R. Jr., Glenney P., Weber K.: Erythroid spectrin, brain fodrin, and intestinal brush border protein (TW-260/240) are related molecules containing a common calmodulin-binding subunit bound to a variant cell type-specific subunit. *Proc. Natl. Acad. Sci.* 1982, **79**: 4002–4005.
33 Goldtein L., Rubin R., Ko C.: The presence of actin in nuclei: a critical appraisal. *Cell* 1977, **12**: 601–608.
34 Goodenough D. A., Revel J. P.: A fine structural analysis of intercellular junctions in the mouse liver. *J. Cell Biol.* 1970, **45**: 272–290.
35 Gospodarowicz D., Greenburg G., Birdwell C. R.: Determination of cellular shape by the extracellular matrix and its correlation with the control of cellular growth. *Cancer Res.* 1978, **38**: 4155–4171.
36 Greengard O., Federman M., Knox W. E.: Cytomorphometry of developing rat liver and it application to enzymic differentiation. *J. Cell Biol.* 1972, **52**: 261–282.
37 Griffith L. M., Pollard T. D.: Evidence for actin filament-microtubule interaction mediated by microtubules-associated proteins. *J. Cell Biol.* 1978, **78**: 958–965.
38 Griffith L. M., Pollard T. D.: The interaction of actin filaments with microtubules and microtubule-associated proteins. *J. Biol. Chem.* 1982, **257**: 9143–9151.
39 Grisham J. W., Thal S. B., Nael A.: Cellular derivation of continuously cultured epithelial cells from normal rat liver. *In: Gene Expression and Carcinogenesis in Cultured Liver*, L. E. Gerschenson, E. B. Thompson (Eds): Academic Press, New York, 1975, pp 1–23.
40 Grisham J. W.: Cell type in rat liver cultures: their identification and isolation. *Molec. Cell. Biochem.* 1983, **53/54**: 23–33.
41 Guguen-Guillouzo C., Clement B., Baffet G., Beaumont C., Morel-Chany E., Glaise D., Guillouzo A.: Maintenance and reversibility of active albumin secretion by adult rat hepatocytes co-cultured with another liver epithelial cell type. *Exp. Cell Res.* 1983, **143**: 47–54.
42 Guguen-Guillouzo C., Seignoux D., Courtois Y., Brissot P., Marceau N., Glaise N., Guillouzo A.: Amplified phenotype changes in adult rat and baboon hepatocytes cultured on a complex biomatrix. *Biol. Cell* 1982, **46**: 11–20.
43 Iype P. T.: Cultures from adult rat liver cells. I. Establishment of monolayer cell cultures from normal liver. *J. Cell Physiol.* 1971, **78**: 281–288.
44 Kim K. H., Rheinwald J. G., Fuchs E. V.: Tissue specificity of epithelial keratins: differential expression of mRNAs from two multigene families. *Molec. Cell. Biol.* 1983, **3**: 495–502.
45 Landry J., Freyer J. P.: Regulatory mechanisms in spheroidal aggregates of normal and cancerous cells. *In: Recent Results in Cancer Research*, Vol. 95: Springer-Verlag, Berlin & Heidelberg, 1984, pp. 50–60.
46 Landry J., Bernier D., Ouellet C., Goyette R., Marceau N.: Spheroidal aggregate culture of rat liver cells: histotypic reorganization, biomatrix deposition and maintenance of functional activities. (Submitted to *J. Cell Biol.*)
47 Lazarides E.: Intermediate filaments as mechancial integrators of cellular space. *Nature* 1980, **283**: 249–256.
48 Lazarides E.: Intermediate filaments: chemically heterogeneous developmentally regulated class of proteins. *Ann. Rev. Biochem.* 1982, **51**: 219–250.
49 Lee F., Mulligan R., Berg Y., Ringold G. M.: Glucocorticoids regulate expression of dihydrofolate reductase cDNA in mouse mammary tumor virus chorionic plasmids. *Nature*, 1981, **294**: 232–288.
50 Leffert H. L., Man T., Bronstein R., Koch K. S.: Procarcinogen activation and hormonal control

of cell proliferation in differentiated primary adult rat liver cell cultures. *Nature* 1977, **267**: 58–61.

51 LeStourgeon W. M.: The occurrence of contractile proteins in nuclei and their possible functions. *In: The Cell Nucleus*, Vol. 6, H. Busch (Ed.): Academic Press, New York, 1978, pp 305–326.

52 Leroux-Nicollet I., Noel M., Baribault H., Goyette R., Marceau N.: Selective increase in cytokeratin synthesis in cultured rat hepatocytes in response to hormonal stimulation. *Biochem. Biophys. Res. Commun.* 1983, **114**: 556–563.

53 Marceau N., Robert A., Mailhot D.: The major surface protein of epithelial cells from newborn and adult rat livers in primary cultures. *Biochem. Biophys. Res. Commun.* 1977, **75**: 1092–1097.

54 Marceau N., Goyette R., Deschenes J., Valet J. P.: Morphological differences between epithelial and fibroblast cells in rat liver cultures and the roles of cell surface fibronectin and cytoskeletal element organization in cell shape. *Ann. N.Y. Acad. Sci.* 1980, **349**: 138–152.

55 Marceau N., Goyette R., Guidoin R., Antakly A.: Hormonally induced formation of extracellular biomatrix in cultured normal neoplastic liver cells. Effect of dexamethasone. *In: Scanning Electron Microscopy*: SEM Inc, 1982, AMF O'Hare, Chicago, Ill.

56 Marceau N., Noel M., Deschenes J.: Growth and functional activities of neonatal and adult rat hepatocytes cultured on fibronectin coated substratum in serum-free medium. *In Vitro* 1982, **18**: 1–11.

57 Marceau N., Goyette R., Pelletier G., Antakly T.: Hormonally-induced changes in the cytoskeleton organization of adult and newborn rat hepatocyte cultured on fibronectin precoated substratum. Effect of dexamethasone and insulin. *Cell. Mol. Biol.* 1983 **29**: 421:435.

58 Marceau N., Goyette R., Noel M.: Monoclonal antibodies specific to rat cytokeratins A and D. *J. Cell Biol.* 1983, **97**: 230.

59 Marceau N., Swierenga S. H. H.: Cytoskeletal events during Ca^{++} or EGF-induced initiation of DNA synthesis in cultured rat liver cells: role of protein phosphorylation and clues for neoplastic transformation. *In: Cell and Muscle Motility*, Vol. VI, R. M. Dowben, J. W. Shay (Eds): Plenum Press, New York, 1984, pp 97–140.

60 Marceau N., Baribault H., Leroux-Nicollet I.: Dexamethasone can modulate the synthesis and organization of cytokeratin in cultured differentiating rat hepatocytes. *Can. J. Biochem. Cell Biol.* 1985, **63**: 448–457.

61 Marceau N., Germain L., Goyette R., Noel M.: Cell origin of distinct cultured epithelial cells, as typed by cytokinase and surface component selective expression (submitted).

62 McGowan J. A., Strain A. J., Bucher N. L. R.: DNA synthesis in primary cultures of adult rat hepatocytes in a defined medium. Effects of epidermal growth factor, insulin, glucagon and cyclic-AMP. *J. Cell. Physiol.* 1981, **108**: 353–363.

63 McGowan J. A., Bucher N. L. R.: Pyruvate promotion of DNA synthesis in serum-free primary cultures of adult rat hepatocytes. *In Vitro* 1983, **19**: 159–166.

64 Michalopoulos G., Cianciulli H. D., Novotny A. R., Kligerman A. D., Strom S. C., Jirtle, R. L.: Liver regeneration studies with rat hepatocytes in primary culture. *Cancer Res.* 1982, **42**: 4673–4682.

64 Moll R., Franke W. W., Schiller D. L., Geiger G., Krepler R.: The catalog of human cytokeratins: patterns of expression in normal epithelia, tumors and cultured cells. *Cell* 1982, **31**: 11–24.

66 Murvill E. R., Le Pennec J. P., Chambon P.: Chicken oviduct progesterone receptor: location of specific regions of high affinity binding in cloned DNA fragments of hormone-responding genes. *Cell* 1982, **28**: 621–632.

67 Oda M., Price V. M., Fisher M. M., Philips M. J.: Ultrastructure of bile canaliculi, with special reference to the surface coat and the pericanaliculi web. *Lab. Invest.* 1974, **31**: 314–323.

68 Osborn M., Weber K.: Intermediate filaments: cell-tye specific markers in differentiation and pathology. *Cell* 1982, **31**: 303–306.

69 Porter K. (Chairman): The cytoplasmic matrix and the integration of cellular function. *J. Cell Biol.* 1984, **99**: 1s–246s.

70 Richman R. A., Claus T. H., Pilkis S. J., Friedman D. L.: Hormonal stimulation of DNA synthesis in primary cultures of adult rat hepatocytes. *Proc. Natl. Acad. Sci.* 1976, **73**: 3589–3589.

71 Rojkind M., Gatmaitan Z., MacKensen S., Biambrone M. A., Ponce P., Reid L. M.: Connective tissue biomatrix: its isolation and utilization for long-term cultures of normal rat hepatocytes. *J. Cell Biol.* 1980, **87**: 255–263.

72 Sell S.: Distribution of α-fetoprotein and albumin-containing cells in the livers of Fischer rats fed

four cycles of N-2-fluorenylacematime. *Cancer. Res.* 1978, **38**: 3107–3113.

73 Sells M. A., Kaytal S. L., Shinozuka H., Estes L. W., Sell S., Lombardi B.: Isolation of oval cells and transitional cells from the livers of rats fed the carcinogen DL-ethionine. *J. Natl. Cancer Inst.* 1981, **66**: 355–362.

74 Scheer U., Hinssen H., Franke W. W., Jockusch F. M.: Microinjection of actin-binding proteins and actin antibodies demonstrates involvement of nuclear actin in transcription of lampbrush chromosomes. *Cell* 1984, **39**: 111–122.

75 Sun T. T., Eichner R., Schermer A., Cooper D., Nelson W. G., Weiss R. A.: Classification, expression and possible mechanisms of evolution of mammalian epithelial keratins: a unifying model. *In: Cancer Cells, 1. The Transformed Phenotype*, A. J. Levin, G. F. V. Woude, W. C. Topp, J. D. Watson, (Eds): Cold Spring Harbor Laboratory, 1984.

76 Swierenga S. H. H., Whitfield J. F., Morris H. P.: The reduced extracellular calcium requirement for proliferation by neoplastic hepatocytes. *In Vitro*, 1978, **14**: 527–535.

77 Swierenga S. H. H., Whitfield J. F., Boynton A. L., MacManus J. P., Rixon R. H., Sikorska M., Tsang B. K., Walker P. R.: Regulation of proliferation of normal and neoplastic rat liver cells by calcium and cyclic AMP. *Ann. N.Y. Acad. Sci.* 1980, **349**: 294–307.

78 Swierenga S. H. H., Goyette R., Marceau N.: Differential effects of calcium deprivation on the cytoskeleton of non-tumorigenic and tumorigenic rat liver cells in culture. *Exp. Cell Res.* 1984, **153**: 39–49.

79 Takaoka T., Yasumoto S., Katsuta H.: A simple method for the cultivation of rat liver cells. *J. Exp. Med.* 1975, **45**: 317–326.

80 Tsanev R.: Cell cycle and liver function. *In: Cell Cycle and Cell Differentiation*, J. Reinert, H. Holtzer (Eds): Springer-Verlag, New York, 1975, **7**: 197–248.

81 Trump B. F., Berezesky I. K., Phelps P. C., Saladino A. J.: Ion regulation and the cytoskeleton in preneoplastic and neoplastic cells in human carcinogenesis, C. Curtis, C. Harris, N. Autrup (Eds.): Academic Press, New York, 1983, pp 3–33.

82 Tseng S. C. G., Jarvinen M. J., Nelson W. G., Huang J. W., Mitchell J. W., Sun T. T.: Correlation of specific keratins with different types of epithelial differentiation: monoclonal antibody studies. *Cell* 1982, **30**: 361–372.

83 Tucker R. W.: Role of microtubules and centrioles in growth regulation of mammalian cells. *In: Cell and Muscle Motility*, R. M. Dowben, J. W. Shay (Eds): Plenum Press, New York, 1981, pp 259–295.

84 Vannic J. L., Taylor J. W., Ringold G. M.: Glucocorticoid-mediated induction of α_1-acid glycoprotein: evidences for hormone-regulated RNA processing. *Proc. Natl. Acad. Sci.* 1984, **81**: 4241–4245.

85 Weatherbee J. A.: Membranes and cell movement: interactions of membranes with the proteins of the cytoskeleton. *Int. Rev. Cytol.* (Suppl. 12) 1981, 113–176.

86 Williams G. M., Gunn J. M.: Long-term cell culture of adult rat liver epithelial cells. *Expl. Cell Res.* 1974, **89**: 139–142.

87 Williams G. M.: Primary and long-term culture of adult rat liver epithelial cells. *In: Methods in Cell Biology*, D. M. Prescott (Ed.): Academic Press, New York, 1978, **14**: 357–364.

88 Wu Y. J., Parker L. M., Binder N. E., Beckett M. A., Simard J. H., Griffiths C. T., Rheinwald J. G.: The mesothelial keratins: a new family of cytoskeletal proteins identified in cultured mesothelial cells and nonkeratinizing epithelia. *Cell* 1982, **31**: 693–703.

89 Yasmen P., Hayner N. T., Fausto N.: Isolation of oval cells by centrifugal elutriation and comparison with other cell types purified from normal and preneoplastic livers. *Cancer Res.* 1984, **44**: 324–331.

90 Yokota S., Fahimi H. D.: Filament bundles of prekeratin type in hepatocytes revealed by detergent extraction after glutaraldehyde fixation. *Biol. Cell.* 1979, **34**: 119–126.

Research in *Isolated and cultured hepatocytes* A. Guillouzo & C. Guguen-Guillouzo eds. pp. 63–86.
© 1986 John Libbey Eurotext Ltd./INSERM.

4

Gluconeogenesis and its regulation in isolated and cultured hepatocytes

Louis HUE and Jean GIRARD

Hormone and Metabolic Research Unit, University of Louvain Medical School, and International Institute of Cellular and Molecular Pathology, Avenue Hippocrate 75, B-1200 Brussels, BELGIUM (LH) and Centre de Recherches sur la Nutrition, 9 rue Jules Hetzel, 92190 Meudon-Bellevue, FRANCE (JG)

SUMMARY

Gluconeogenesis is the *de novo* synthesis of glucose from non-glucidic precursors. It occurs in liver and kidney and it is absolutely required for the maintenance of blood glucose during starvation. The development of techniques on isolated organs, such as liver perfusion and especially isolated hepatocytes in suspension or culture, represents a major breakthrough and allowed significant progresses to be accomplished. The main physiological glucose precursors are lactate/pyruvate, glycerol and alanine. Gluconeogenesis is controlled at several levels which include (i) control by the supply of precursors; (ii) inhibition by the end-product, glucose; (iii) short-term stimulation and inhibition by several hormones and (iv) long-term adaptive regulation by hormones and nutritional factors. Control is achieved by regulating substrate and metabolite transport and by modifying the activity of enzymes involved in the fructose 6-phosphate/fructose1,6-bisphosphate and the pyruvate/phosphoenolpyruvate cycles. The activity of these key enzymes are modulated by stimulators or inhibitors (e.g. fructose2,6-bisphosphate), by covalent modification of enzymes (e.g. phosphorylation by cyclic AMP dependent protein kinase) and by changes in the rate of synthesis of enzymes (e.g. pyruvate kinase and phosphoenolpyruvate carboxykinase).

Introduction

The liver plays a central rôle in the maintenance of blood glucose homoeostasis. This function is achieved by its unique ability to release or remove glucose from the bloodstream depending on the concentration of the hexose and on the hormonal status of the organism (63, 147). When food is in excess, as in the post-absorptive state, the liver is concerned with the salvage of glucose, some being stored as glycogen, the rest being transformed into fatty acids. When blood glucose concentration is low, the liver produces glucose for the benefit of extrahepatic tissues that have an absolute requirement for the sugar. Glucose is indeed the main fuel of the brain and the renal medulla, and is the only energy source for the erythrocytes and retina (96). This glucose comes from glycogen. However, the liver glycogen stores are limited and exhausted after a few hours of fasting. The glucose supply relies then on its synthesis from non-glucidic precursors such as lactate, pyruvate, glycerol and some amino acids. The metabolic process by which glucose is synthesized from these precursors is called gluconeogenesis. Whereas glycolysis occurs in all living cells, gluconeogenesis operates only in liver and renal cortex.

The role of gluconeogenesis is not restricted to the provision of glucose for extrahepatic tissues, it also contributes to the utilization of amino acids which, in the post-absorptive state, are coming from the intestine or which are released by exercising muscle. The liver is also the main organ for the disposal of lactate which is continuously produced by glycolysing erythrocytes or which accumulates during intense exercise.

Gluconeogenesis is controlled by the supply of gluconeogenic substrates, by its end-product, glucose, and by hormones. In the whole animal all these effects are interrelated so that hormones may affect both the supply of gluconeogenic substrates from extrahepatic tissues and the gluconeogenic capacity of the liver itself. In this chapter we will consider mainly the intrahepatic regulation of gluconeogenesis. More detailed information on enzyme regulation and hormonal control is given in several recent reviews (65, 68, 95, 119).

Glycolysis and gluconeogenesis have several enzymes in common (Fig. 1). These enzymes catalyse reversible reactions and have little influence on the overall flux.

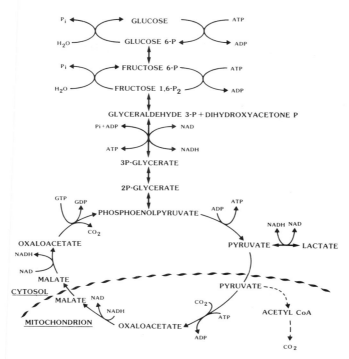

Figure 1. The pathways of glycolysis and gluconeogenesis in the liver.

The unidirectionality of gluconeogenesis is ensured by a few reactions displaced far from equilibrium, the so-called key steps. These reactions are opposed by other 'irreversible' reactions, which are the key steps of glycolysis and which determine the net glycolytic flux. If these opposite, non-equilibrium, reactions operate simultaneously and at the same rate, there is no net flux of metabolites but a 'futile' recycling, the net balance of which appears to be the wasteful expenditure of energy. Three such cycles exist in the glycolytic/gluconeogenic pathway: the glucose/glucose 6-phosphate cycle, the fructose 6-phosphate/fructose 1,6-bisphosphate cycle and the pyruvate/phosphoenolpyruvate cycle (68, 69, 83). A net gluconeogenic (unidirectional) flux occurs when the rates of the key gluconeogenic steps prevail over the corresponding glycolytic reactions.

The fructose 6-phosphate/fructose 1,6-bisphosphate and the pyruvate/phosphoenolpyruvate cycles control the first committed steps of glycolysis and gluconeogenesis respectively, and, as expected, it appears that the regulation of the gluconeogenic flux is exerted mainly at the level of these cycles. Theoretically, if these cycles are operative, a stimulation of gluconeogenesis can be achieved either by a stimulation of the activity of the gluconeogenic enzymes or by an inhibition of the glycolytic enzymes or by a combination of both. These mechanisms are indeed observed in the liver. The activity of the key enzymes in the cycles can be controlled by various means including stimulators or inhibitors, covalent modification of enzymes and synthesis or degradation of enzymes. In addition, since the gluconeo-

genic pathway is located in different subcellular compartments (cytosol, mitochondria and endoplasmic reticulum), control may be exerted at these various
permeability barriers.

Experimental approaches

Different experimental models are currently used for the study of the regulation of
liver gluconeogenesis. These are, in order of decreasing relevance to the *in vivo*
situation, studies in the intact animal, perfusion of isolated livers, incubation of
isolated hepatocytes, cultures of liver cells and incubation of liver homogenates.
Among these methods, isolated hepatocytes are the most commonly used (10, 31, 59,
152). They offer several advantages: they are easy to obtain, the method of
preparation is reproducible, their maximal gluconeogenic capacity is close to the
physiological rates, and various experimental conditions can be tested in one single
experiment. On the other hand, they have lost several characteristics of the *in vivo*
situation: the fine *in vivo* equilibrium between the various neural and hormonal
influences is lost, as is the *in situ* polarity and the metabolic zonation of the liver
(perivenous glycolytic zone and periportal gluconeogenic zone) (82). In addition,
several metabolic intermediates and amino acids (eg lysine which is required for a
rapid onset of gluconeogenesis from lactate (23)) are washed out during the
preparation.

Gluconeogenesis is measured by the rate of formation of glucose from gluconeogenic precursors. This is readily measured in the livers of starved animals which do
not contain glycogen. In livers of fed animals, however, the intense glycogenolysis
precludes any measurement of gluconeogenesis by the net formation of glucose. In
this case, the incorporation of radioactive precursors into glucose is often taken as a
measurement of the gluconeogenic flux. This incorporation does not represent net
gluconeogenesis because of the operation of futile cycles and the isotopic dilution of
the precursor by unlabelled pools of metabolites (65, 68, 83). The interpretation of
the results is, therefore, difficult and sometimes even impossible. In the intact
animal, the measurement of gluconeogenesis by the incorporation of radioactive
precursors into blood glucose is further complicated by the turnover rate of the
precursor and of the glucose formed, and by the importance of the injection and
sampling sites (66, 85, 114).

Control steps in gluconeogenesis can be identified by measuring the changes in the
pattern of metabolite concentration induced by a stimulation of gluconeogenesis. A
more quantitative approach can be used to evaluate the amount of control exerted by
each enzyme of a pathway on the overall flux through this pathway. This approach,
which is based on the 'control strength' theory developed by Kacser & Burns (91)
and by Heinrich & Rapoport (60) has recently been applied in the quantitative
analysis of control of gluconeogenesis (53, 54).

Gluconeogenic substrates

Types of substrates

In perfused rat livers or in isolated rat hepatocytes, the highest rates of gluconeogenesis are observed with fructose or dihydroxyacetone which enter the pathway at the level of the triose-phosphates (see Table 1). Lactate and pyruvate are less effective than fructose or dihydroxyacetone. This suggests that gluconeogenesis from lactate and pyruvate is limited by a reaction between pyruvate and triose-phosphates. Alanine and the other amino acids are poor precursors with rates smaller than that from lactate.

Table 1. Rates of net formation of glucose from gluconeogenic precursors in perfused livers and isolated liver cells from starved rats. The concentration of substrate was 5–10 mM.

Substrate	Glucose formed ($\mu mol/min$ per g of liver)
Fructose	2.56
Dihydroxyacetone	1.45
Lactate	0.71
Pyruvate	0.83
Serine	0.62
Glycerol	0.56
Alanine	0.50
Glutamine	0.43
Galactose	0.36
Propionate	0.18

Based on references: 32, 70, 100, 130, 145.

The rate of gluconeogenesis depends, among other factors, on the concentration of gluconeogenic precursors and half maximal rates occur at concentrations of lactate, pyruvate, alanine or glycerol which are greater than the physiological range. Therefore, an increased supply of gluconeogenic precursors from extrahepatic tissues results in a stimulation of their transformation into glucose in the liver. With sorbitol or glycerol as gluconeogenic substrates, the NADH which is formed should be reoxidized in the mitochondria. Since the rate of conversion of sorbitol into glucose is the same as for fructose, reoxidation of NADH is therefore not rate-limiting. However, when hepatocytes are incubated in the absence of Ca^{2+}, gluconeogenesis from fructose and glycerol is greatly diminished (92, 181). In isolated hepatocytes from guinea pigs and sheep, maximal rates of gluconeogenesis are obtained with fructose and propionate whereas lactate and pyruvate are less good substrates (32, 145). Propionate, which is the main gluconeogenic substrate for the ruminant *in vivo*, enters the pathway at the level of oxaloacetate thus bypassing the pyruvate carboxylase step. This step is, therefore, rate-limiting when lactate or pyruvate are the substrates.

Hormonal control of amino acid transport

Transport across the plasma membrane is the first step in amino acid metabolism. There are eight distinct systems in normal hepatocytes for transport of the amino acids (18, 88, 138). Most of these systems are not regulated by nutritional or hormonal factors and will not be discussed here.

In contrast, the system A, which transports very efficiently gluconeogenic amino acids, is finely regulated by nutritional and hormonal factors. System A-mediated transport represents the rate limiting step in the catabolism of alanine (39, 102, 142) and its activity is increased in diabetes, starvation and after a high-protein diet (4, 39, 40, 133). It is, however, decreased after adrenalectomy (89).

Glucagon, catecholamines and glucocorticoids increase amino acid uptake both in perfused livers and in isolated or cultured hepatocytes (88, 138). System A is responsible for the glucagon-mediated increase in transport of amino acids in isolated or cultured hepatocytes (101, 116). Glucagon increases the maximal velocity (V_{max}) of the high affinity system (41, 87). The effects of glucagon are rapid and persist for several hours (116). The initial effect is independent of *de novo* protein synthesis (30) whereas after 30 min the synthesis of new transport proteins is necessary for further enhancement of amino acid transport by glucagon (101, 116). The nucleus and microtubules are involved in the stimulation of amino acid transport by glucagon (25, 120).

Catecholamines stimulate amino acid uptake in isolated or cultured rat hepatocytes via alpha-adrenergic receptors (15, 117). This results from an increase in the V_{max} of the A system of amino acid transport and requires *de novo* protein synthesis (117). Glucocorticoids also stimulate amino acid transport in freshly isolated hepatocytes (15). In contrast, glucocorticoids alone produce no stimulation of amino acid transport in cultured hepatocytes, they are, however, permissive for the stimulation of amino acid transport by glucagón and catecholamines (116, 86).

Regulation of futile cycles

Changes in tissue levels of metabolites observed when the liver switches from glycolysis to gluconeogenesis indicate that two sequences in the pathway are possible sites of control: the pyruvate/phosphoenolpyruvate cycle and the fructose 6-phosphate/fructose 1,6-bisphosphate cycle (36, 135, 174). The importance of the first cycle in the regulation of gluconeogenesis has also been confirmed in a recent study of the quantitative analysis of control (53, 55). In this latter study, it was found that, in hepatocytes from starved rats, the fructose 6-phosphate/fructose 1,6-bisphosphate cycle exerted much less control on the overall flux than pyruvate carboxylase which displayed the highest flux control coefficient (53). This is probably explained by the fact that liver cells from starved rats were incubated without glucose. Under these conditions, the concentration of fructose-2,6-bisphosphate, lactate release and the cycling between glucose and triose-phosphates are negligible (74, 166). This is not the case in well-fed rats.

Pyruvate/phosphoenolpyruvate cycle

The recycling of pyruvate is influenced by hormones and by the nature of the gluconeogenic substrate. As a rule, the cycling is more intense in well-fed animals and with pyruvate as a substrate. The effect of glucagon is to decrease recycling and is directly related to its stimulation of gluconeogenesis. At least two mechanisms are responsible for the effect of glucagon on this cycle. The first one is the inactivation of pyruvate kinase and the second is the stimulation of the mitochondrial metabolism of pyruvate. A comprehensive review of all the regulatory mechanisms as well as the description of the kinetic properties of the enzymes is beyond the scope of this chapter and for detailed information the reader should refer to other reviews (see references 28, 33, 65, 68, 119). Type L pyruvate kinase is an interconvertible enzyme which is inactivated through phosphorylation by cyclic AMP-dependent protein kinase and reactivated by a phosphatase (33, 68, 119). Treatment of isolated liver preparations with glucagon causes dose-dependent changes in the kinetic properties and phosphorylation state that are similar to those found with the purified enzyme. In addition, the fact that the inactivation of pyruvate kinase by glucagon, cyclic AMP and adrenaline in hepatocytes is parallel with the stimulation of gluconeogenesis strongly suggests that phosphorylation of this enzyme plays a role in the hormonal control of gluconeogenesis (42). By contrast, α-adrenergic agonists and vasopressin cause little, if any, change in the activity of pyruvate kinase (13, 16, 21, 48, 71, 148, 154), although they stimulate the phosphorylation of the enzyme (48, 49, 108, 148). Attempts so far to phosphorylate and inactivate pyruvate kinase in the presence of Ca^{2+} but in the absence of cyclic AMP (165) have been unsuccessful. It is also noteworthy that the phosphorylation state of pyruvate kinase was not affected in cells incubated with phorbol esters (49) which are known to activate protein kinase C (110).

The inactivation of pyruvate kinase by cyclic AMP-dependent kinase offers an explanation, in biochemical terms, for the accumulation and re-routing of phosphoenolpyruvate towards glucose as well as for the decreased pyruvate and lactate production. However, it does not explain how pyruvate transport and metabolism are accelerated in the presence of a decreased concentration of pyruvate. This is probably achieved by the effect of glucagon on mitochondria which indirectly results in a stimulation of pyruvate transport and metabolism (28, 56, 57, 139). Haynes and coworkers have shown that mitochondria from liver cells treated with glucagon, adrenaline, cyclic AMP or cortisol, display an increased rate of pyruvate metabolism, including a faster rate of pyruvate carboxylation (1, 47). Later on, evidence has been presented that several hormonal effects found in the isolated mitochondria depended on the conditions of isolation and incubation of the mitochondria and could, therefore, be artifactual (139, 140). However, some of the changes induced by glucagon, such as an increase in respiration, ATP concentration and glutamate utilization, were also found in intact liver or hepatocytes and thus were not subject to the same criticism (139, 140). A more recent study indicates that glucagon might influence mitochondria by changing phosphate metabolism in liver cells (141). Whatever the exact molecular mechanism involved, the fact remains that the metabolism of pyruvate is stimulated by several hormones and that their effect contributes to the overall stimulation of gluconeogenesis.

Fructose 6-phosphate/fructose 1,6-bisphosphate cycle

Recent reviews on that subject have been published recently (see references 22, 64, 65, 164).

Phosphofructokinase and fructose 1,6-bisphosphatase, the two enzymes of the cycles, are substrates of the cyclic AMP-dependent protein kinase. However, phosphorylation of these proteins causes little change in their kinetic properties and does not affect their activity (65). The regulation of this cycle results mainly from the allosteric control by fructose 2,6-bisphosphate. Fructose 2,6-bisphosphate was discovered in 1980 as a low-molecular-weight stimulator of liver phosphofructokinase (166, 167). It is formed in the liver after a glucose load and disappears after glucagon treatment. Fructose, 2,6-bisphosphate stimulates all mammalian phosphofructokinase tested so far and it is a potent inhibitor of fructose 1,6-bisphosphatase, and its effect on both enzymes is synergistic with that of AMP. Therefore, any increase in fructose 2,6-bisphosphate will favour glycolysis whereas a decrease will result in a stimulation of gluconeogenesis at the level of the fructose 6-phosphate/fructose 1,6-bisphosphate cycle. Its concentration in the liver of fed rats is 10–20 μM and reaches very low values (<0.1 μM) during fasting.

In liver, fructose 2,6-bisphosphate is synthesized from fructose 6-phosphate and ATP by a 6-phosphofructo 2-kinase or phosphofructokinase-2. It is hydrolysed into fructose 6-phosphate and Pi by a fructose 2,6-bisphosphatase. The two enzyme activities are borne on the same protein. Cyclic AMP dependent protein kinase phosphorylates these two enzymes and, by so doing, activates the phosphatase and inactivates the kinase. This will result in the disappearance of fructose 2,6-bisphosphate and, therefore, explains the action of glucagon on this cycle.

Besides cyclic AMP, fructose 6-phosphate is an important regulator of the cycle and it explains the effect of glucose to increase fructose 2,6-bisphosphate in hepatocytes. Fructose 6-phosphate is the precursor of fructose 2,6-bisphosphate and it is a very strong inhibitor of the fructose 2,6-bisphosphatase. Therefore, an increase in fructose 6-phosphate concentration, as it occurs after glucose in hepatocytes, will result in an increase in fructose 2,6-bisphosphate except when cyclic AMP is present. Under the latter conditions, the effect of cyclic AMP prevails over that of glucose and the concentration of fructose 2,6-bisphosphate is decreased.

Glycogenolytic agents like α-adrenergic agents and vasopressin, which do not act via cyclic AMP, increase the concentration of fructose 2,6-bisphosphate, and stimulate glycolysis as a result of a stimulation of glycogen breakdown and fructose 6-phosphate accumulation.

In isolated hepatocytes from fed rats, high concentrations (20 mM) of gluconeogenic precursors such as fructose, lactate, pyruvate and alanine decrease the concentration of fructose 2,6-bisphosphate (65). The mechanism(s) responsible for this fall is not well understood. However, as a result of the decrease in fructose 2,6-bisphosphate, gluconeogenesis is favoured and the glycolytic flux is inhibited at the level of phosphofructokinase. A similar effect is obtained with glycerol even at low concentration. This effect is due to the accumulation of *sn*-glycerol 3-phosphate which is an inhibitor of phosphofructokinase-2 and an activator of fructose 2,6-bisphosphatase. In hepatocytes from starved rats, low concentrations ($\leqslant 2$ mM) of fructose, lactate, pyruvate, alanine and dihydroxyacetone slightly increase the concentration of fructose 2,6-bisphosphate (74).

Hormonal control

Short-term control by cyclic AMP, glucagon and catecholamines

The stimulation of liver gluconeogenesis by glucagon was first reported by Schimassek & Mitzkat (135) in 1963. It has since been confirmed by numerous groups and a stimulation is obtained in isolated hepatocytes with concentrations of glucagon which are within the physiological range (38, 78, 130, 175). Glucagon stimulates gluconeogenesis not only from lactate and pyruvate but also from substrates like glutamate, glutamine and propionate, which enter the pathway at the level of oxaloacetate (thus bypassing the step catalysed by pyruvate carboxylase), or like fructose, glyceraldehyde and dihydroxyacetone which are converted to triose-phosphates (65, 70, 145). There is, however, no stimulation of gluconeogenesis from high concentrations (above 5 mM) of fructose or, at least in the fasted state, from glycerol. This could be explained by the decrease in fructose 2,6-bisphosphate which is observed in the absence of glucagon: since these precursors already decrease fructose 2,6-bisphosphate to very low values, glucagon cannot further decrease the concentration of the stimulator. It therefore appears that the presence of fructose 2,6-bisphosphate is important for the expression of the glucagon effect on gluconeogenesis from substrates entering the pathway at the level of triose-phosphates (70).

There is general agreement that the stimulation of gluconeogenesis by glucagon is mediated through changes in the concentration of its secondary messenger, cyclic AMP, which in turn promotes the activation of protein kinase (38). As stated above, protein kinase will phosphorylate and inactivate pyruvate kinase and phospho-fructokinase-2, and activate fructose 2,6-bisphosphatase (5). The glycolytic flux will therefore be blocked by this dual lock. However, when glycogen is present, this lock imposed by glucagon is not sufficient to block completely the flux from glycogen through phosphofructokinase and some cycling persists between fructose 6-phosphate and fructose 1,6-bisphosphate (166).

Whereas an inactivation of pyruvate kinase is always observed after glucagon and is probably essential for the hormonal expression when lactate is the substrate, a fall in the concentration of fructose 2,6-bisphosphate is not always obtained. This is the case for livers from fasted animals in which the concentration of fructose 2,6-bisphosphate is already very low and cannot be further decreased. Under these conditions, the flux through phosphofructokinase is already minimal and the stimulation of gluconeogenesis results from the inactivation of pyruvate kinase which prevents the cycling of phosphoenolpyruvate and so orientates the flux towards glucose (70).

Adrenaline also increases the concentration of cyclic AMP in the liver, although much less than glucagon; phenylephrine, an α-adrenergic agonist, has a similar effect only when hepatocytes are incubated in the absence of calcium (13, 16, 71). The stimulation of gluconeogenesis by adrenaline is less than 50% of that by glucagon and it is predominantly mediated via the α-adrenergic receptors.

Short-term control by α-adrenergic agents, vasopressin and angiotensin

The main effect of these agents is to stimulate glycogen breakdown by a mechanism which is independent of cyclic AMP (35, 178). The current view is that this effect could result from a stimulation of phospholipid breakdown leading to the formation of inositol 1,4,5-trisphosphate which, in turn, could favour the liberation of Ca^{++} from intracellular stores (9, 81). An increased cytosolic concentration of Ca^{++} stimulates, via calmodulin, the activity of phosphorylase kinase which then activates phosphorylase.

In hepatocytes from fed rats, the stimulation of glycogen breakdown by these agents increases the concentration of hexose 6-phosphates and fructose 2,6-bisphosphate (72, 73). Such an increase in fructose 2,6-bisphosphate is expected since these agents do not increase cyclic AMP, which would otherwise prevent the formation of fructose 2,6-bisphosphate. In addition, since the effect of these agents on pyruvate kinase is minimal, they will cause an increase in lactate output (72, 77, 171). This offers an explanation in molecular terms for the unexpected stimulatory effect of α-adrenergic agonists on glycolysis. However, under the same conditions, these agents slightly stimulate the incorporation of radioactive gluconeogenic precursors into glucose thus demonstrating the occurrence of a relatively large cycling of metabolites (61, 62, 157, 170). This slight stimulation of the gluconeogenic flux might result from the small inactivation of pyruvate kinase or, more likely, from a stimulation of the first gluconeogenic steps (68, 113). Because phenylephrine and vasopressin also activate pyruvate dehydrogenase and stimulate recycling at the level of pyruvate/phosphoenolpyruvate, the stimulation of lactate output is less than expected from the increase in fructose 2,6-bisphosphate.

In hepatocytes from fasted rats, glycolysis is not stimulated except in the presence of high, non-physiological (10 mM or above) concentrations of glucose (72). In the absence of glucose, these agents cause a 30–50% increase in gluconeogenic rates measured both by isotopic method and by the net formation of glucose (65).

It has been claimed that adrenaline caused a Ca^{++}-dependent inactivation of phosphofructokinase-2 and activation of fructose 2,6-bisphosphate (123, 124). This has not been confirmed (5) and the discrepancy is difficult to interpret; however, it should be noted that the response of rat hepatocytes to adrenaline is known to depend on the age and the sex of the animals (12, 150).

Hormonal control of gene expression

During the last five years considerable progress has been made concerning the regulation of the synthesis of two enzymes involved in the regulation of hepatic glycolysis (pyruvate kinase) and gluconeogenesis (phosphoenolpyruvate carboxy-kinase). This adaptative, long-term regulation is often opposed to the so-called 'short-term' regulation (see above). However, these two types of regulation should be regarded as integral parts of the hormonal control of gluconeogenesis.

Pyruvate kinase. The activity of type L pyruvate kinase (L–PK) fluctuates markedly according to nutritional and hormonal status. It is decreased in fasted and diabetic rats and in rats fed high protein or high fat diets. Refeeding fasted rats with a high carbohydrate diet, or insulin administration to diabetic rats fed a high carbohydrate diet, restored the L–PK activity to normal values (105, 119). These alterations are due to changes in the rate of enzyme synthesis (L–PK half life, 50–75 hours), and are paralleled by changes in the level of translatable mRNA of this enzyme (20, 111, 169). In cultured hepatocytes, glucagon decreases whereas insulin increases total L–PK activity (34, 46). The effect of insulin is antagonized by glucagon (34) and synergistic with that of dexamethasone (106). Using cloned cDNA probes, the mRNAs of L–PK are barely detectable by hybridization in the liver of fasted or diabetic rats, while refeeding fasted rats with a high carbohydrate diet, or insulin administration to diabetics, gives a marked increase of liver L–PK mRNAs (112, 169). Insulin, glucocorticoids and thyroid hormones are required for the normal induction of liver L–PK mRNA synthesis in response to carbohydrate feeding (107).

As liver L–PK mRNAs are found to be low in several situations associated with high plasma glucagon (starvation, diabetes and feeding a high protein diet), this suggested that glucagon may play a role in regulating L–PK mRNA synthesis. Indeed, the induction of L–PK mRNAs by carbohydrate feeding is abolished by administration of glucagon or cyclic AMP (107). Moreover, it has been shown that glucagon blocks the transcription of the gene coding for L–PK (168). Thus, glucagon inhibits both the expression of the L–PK gene and the activity of the enzyme by phosphorylation (see above).

Phosphoenolpyruvate carboxykinase. The activity of cytosolic phosphoenolpyruvate carboxykinase (PEPCK) undergoes rapid changes depending on the nutritional and hormonal status of the rat (145, 155). It is increased by starvation, diabetes and feeding a high protein diet, and is decreased by feeding a high carbohydrate diet. Glucagon, catecholamine or cAMP administration to fed rats cause a rapid increase in liver PEPCK, while insulin administration to diabetic animals causes an equally rapid decrease of liver PEPCK.

In cultured hepatocytes from adult rats, PEPCK activity declines rapidly during the first 24 hours in hormone-free medium; thereafter, glucagon, catecholamines and cyclic AMP increase PEPCK activity when thyroid and glucocorticoid hormones are present (115, 121, 151). Insulin antagonizes the effects of glucagon (121).

The rapid alterations *in vivo* of liver PEPCK activity are accompanied by parallel changes in the rate of enzyme synthesis (155) and in the level of translatable mRNA (2, 6, 75, 90, 109).

In isolated rat hepatocytes maintained in suspension for up to 8 hours, glucagon or cyclic AMP increase the rate of enzyme synthesis, and the level of translatable mRNA coding for PEPCK (132). In this system, dexamethasone or triiodothyronine (T3) alone have no substantial effect, but they markedly amplify the effects of glucagon. Thus, glucocorticoids and thyroid hormones exert a permissive effect on the expression of the PEPCK gene by glucagon (76).

By hybridization techniques with PEPCK cDNA probes, the PEPCK mRNA has been found to be increased by starvation, diabetes and after injection of glucagon or cAMP to fed rats (182). Refeeding glucose to starved rats or administration of insulin to fed diabetic rats caused a marked decrease in PEPCK mRNAs (7, 8, 19).

In cultured H4-II-E hepatoma cells, cyclic AMP also increase PEPCK mRNA, as measured by both translation and cDNA hybridization techniques. Cyclic AMP causes a very rapid increase in nuclear PEPCK mRNA sequences, and, later on, an increase in PEPCK mRNAs in the cytosol (17). In these cells, insulin decreases translatable PEPCK mRNA activity and inhibits transcription of the PEPCK gene.

This results from a rapid decrease in the concentration of nuclear PEPCK transcripts which is followed by a proportional decline in cytoplasmic PEPCK mRNAs and enzyme synthesis (52). Moreover, addition of cAMP and dexamethasone to H4-II-E cells increase the transcription of the PEPCK gene, and insulin, added to either untreated cells or to cells pretreated with cAMP of dexamethasone, markedly decreases the rate of transcription of the gene coding for PEPCK mRNAs (134).

With an assay involving elongation of nascent RNA molecules synthesized from the engaged DNA-dependent RNA polymerases, the rate of transcription of PEPCK mRNAs by hepatic nuclei was shown to be increased during starvation or after injection of cAMP. Glucose feeding to fasted rats has the opposite effect (99, 103). Therefore, it has been concluded that cAMP stimulated PEPCK synthesis by specifically increasing the transcription of the PEPCK gene, and that a decrease in liver cAMP, which occurs during glucose refeeding due to a reduced plasma glucagon/insulin ratio, acutely depressed transcription (103).

Regulation by glucose

In addition to glycogen, glucose is another substrate for liver glycolysis and the inhibition of gluconeogenesis by glucose is mediated by the formation of fructose 2,6-bisphosphate. In hepatocytes from fasted rats, the stimulation of glycolysis by glucose occurs at relatively high concentrations of the hexose: the relationship between lactate production and the concentration of glucose is not linear and addition of 5 to 10 mM glucose has little effect whereas concentrations larger than 20 mM greatly stimulate lactate output (74). In addition, the relationship between fructose 2,6-bisphosphate concentration and lactate production is not linear: there are conditions under which an increase in fructose 2,6-bisphosphate is not related to a stimulation of lactate output (74). A similar situation is observed when hepatocytes are incubated with low concentrations of dihydroxyacetone or fructose (70). This lack of correlation might result from recycling of metabolites at the level of the fructose 6-phosphate cycle and/or from the binding of fructose 2,6-bisphosphate to cytosolic proteins. Experimental evidence supporting the two interpretations has been obtained (74). It therefore appears that the physiological significance of fructose 2,6-bisphosphate is best expressed at relatively high concentrations, when it allows the pathway to switch from gluconeogenesis to glycolysis, and *vice versa*.

Glycogen metabolism in the liver represents another system which is glucose sensitive with phosphorylase acting as a glucose sensor. Recent experiments have shown that the glucose sensitivity of the liver for glycolysis is not the same as that for glycogen synthesis (74). In fasted animals, the activation of glycogen synthase was more sensitive to glucose than the increase in fructose 2,6-bisphosphate concentration, whereas the opposite situation was observed in livers of fed mice. The physiological meaning of this observation is that, in the fasted state, the glycogen stores are first replenished, and it is only when an excess of glucose is given that it is glycolysed. When the liver capacity to synthesize glycogen is saturated, a glucose load can only be glycolysed or recycled. This difference in sensitivity should also be taken into consideration when discussing the fact, that after glucose administration to starved rats, liver glycogen is synthesized mainly from gluconeogenic precursors (84).

Regulation by fatty acids

Gluconeogenesis is an energy consuming process. The synthesis of 1 mole of glucose from pyruvate or lactate requires 6 moles of ATP. The metabolism of gluconeogenic amino acids such as alanine requires even more energy since 4 moles of ATP are needed to dispose of the nitrogen as urea. These values are probably underestimated since they are based on the assumption that glycolysis is virtually inhibited, which may not be the case under all circumstances (69, 166). When the liver is under gluconeogenic conditions as in the starved state, it is generally assumed that energy is provided by the oxidation of fatty acids which are transformed into ketone bodies for the benefit of extrahepatic tissues (97). The fatty acids oxidized in the liver are coming from adipose tissue. The question of the liver cell preference for endogenous fat as a source of energy rather than the supplied substrate, particularly when these substrates are amino acids, has not been elucidated.

The role of fatty acid oxidation in the regulation of gluconeogenesis has been a matter of controversy for a long time. The majority of investigators working with both the perfused rat liver (104, 131, 153, 172, 174) and with isolated hepatocytes (14, 23, 78) have reported that high concentrations of medium or long chain fatty acids stimulate hepatic gluconeogenesis from lactate, pyruvate or alanine. However, Exton and coworkers (37, 38) have shown that physiological levels of long chain fatty acids do not stimulate gluconeogenesis in perfused rat liver and they consider of doubtful physiological significance the enhanced gluconeogenesis by high concentrations of free fatty acids reported by other investigators. In other mammalian species, the situation is also confusing. It has been reported that medium chain fatty acids (octanoate, hexanoate) inhibited gluconeogenesis from lactate or alanine in perfused liver or in isolated hepatocytes from guinea pig, rabbit and cat (3, 79, 146, 183).

In contrast, it is clear that, in all the species studied, the inhibition of fatty acid oxidation produces a marked decrease in gluconeogenesis. In perfused liver or isolated hepatocytes from the rat and guinea pig, various inhibitors of fatty acid oxidation: tetradecylglycidic acid, POCA, MCHP (see next paragraph), pentenoic acid (156, 177), bromooctanoate (26, 122), (+)decanoylcarnitine (173, 175) and hypoglycin (137) inhibit gluconeogenesis.

Thus, it seems that fatty acid oxidation plays a permissive rather than a regulatory role on gluconeogenesis. A basal rate of fatty acid oxidation is necessary to provide the liver with the co-factors necessary for an efficient gluconeogenesis, ie acetyl-CoA for activation of pyruvate carboxylase, ATP for various enzymes involved in gluconeogenesis and cytosolic NADH for the reaction catalysed by glyceraldehyde-3-phosphate dehydrogenase. The crucial role of fatty acid oxidation for the regulation of gluconeogenesis has been demonstrated during the neonatal period in the rat (44, 45, 50).

Inhibitors

A number of compounds have been shown to be hypoglycaemic *in vivo* in starved or diabetic animals, ie in situations in which hepatic gluconeogenesis and ketogenesis are elevated. These compounds have been shown to inhibit hepatic gluconeogenesis at different levels in the gluconeogenic pathway.

ATP supply

Several enzymes involved in hepatic gluconeogenesis (pyruvate carboxylase, phosphoenolpyruvate carboxykinase, phosphoglycerate kinase) are dependent upon the provision of ATP or GTP. Thus, any compound that alters energy metabolism in liver should interfere with gluconeogenesis. Atractyloside, a specific inhibitor of the mitochondrial adenine nucleotide translocator, lowers cytosolic ATP and inhibits gluconeogenesis from lactate in isolated rat hepatocytes (128, 149). Diphenyleneiodonium (67) or dinitrophenol (128) inhibit ATP synthesis by the mitochondria and decrease gluconeogenesis from lactate.

Inhibitors of transaminases and of mitochondrial transport

Because of the intracellular localization of gluconeogenic enzymes, gluconeogenesis in the rat requires the transport of metabolites across the mitochondrial membranes. The use of compounds that alter the supply of pyruvate, aspartate or malate or their transport across the mitochondrial membrane has allowed one to establish the concept that, in rat liver, gluconeogenesis from lactate involves the translocation of aspartate across the mitochondrial membrane, whereas gluconeogenesis from pyruvate involves the translocation of malate to the cytosol to provide both carbons and reducing equivalents.

Inhibitors of transaminases. 1). *Aminooxyacetate.* Aminooxyacetate is an inhibitor of a variety of pyridoxal-dependent transaminases. In isolated hepatocytes from fasted rats aminooxyacetate inhibits alanine aminotransferase by 60% and aspartate aminotransferase by 90% (24). Aminooxyacetate strongly inhibits gluconeogenesis from lactate and alanine but not from pyruvate (129, 143).
2). *L-2-Amino-4-methoxy-trans-butenoic acid (AMB).* AMB is an irreversible inhibitor of aspartate aminotransferase which is inhibited by 90% at 0.25 mM AMB. Alanine aminotransferase is little affected at that concentration (24). Consistent with this effect, AMB strongly inhibits gluconeogenesis from lactate but not from alanine or pyruvate in isolated hepatocytes from fasted rats (24, 143).
3). *L-Cycloserine.* L-Cycloserine is a structural analogue of alanine. At 0.05 mM, it inhibits alanine aminotransferase by 90% and aspartate aminotransferase by less than 10% in isolated hepatocytes from fasted rats (24). Thus, it markedly inhibits gluconeogenesis from alanine but not from lactate or pyruvate (24).

Inhibitors of mitochondrial transport of metabolites. α-Cyano-4-hydroxycinnamate, an inhibitor of pyruvate transport into the mitochondria, strongly inhibits gluconeogenesis from pyruvate in isolated rat hepatocytes (27, 28). Glisoxepide, an inhibitor of aspartate/glutamate transport across the mitochondrial membrane, inhibits gluconeogenesis from lactate and alanine but not from pyruvate in isolated rat liver cells (144). Butylmalonate, a competitive inhibitor of malate transport across the mitochondrial membrane, inhibits gluconeogenesis from pyruvate in perfused rat liver (176).

Inhibitor of phosphoenolpyruvate carboxykinase

A number of compounds related in structure to quinolinic acid are hypoglycaemic. The most potent one is 3-mercaptopicolinic acid (3MPA). The hypoglycemic effect of 3MPA has been shown in starved and diabetic rats, starved guinea pigs, mice and new born rats, but not in fed animals (11, 29, 43). 3MPA inhibits gluconeogenesis from lactate, pyruvate and alanine but not from fructose dihydroxyacetone or glycerol in isolated liver preparation (29, 51, 80, 113, 127). In perfused guinea pig liver 3MPA inhibits gluconeogenesis from both lactate and glycerol (80). Metabolite crossover studies suggested that 3MPA inhibits gluconeogenesis at the level of PEPCK (11, 43, 51). This assumption was confirmed by kinetic studies with purified PEPCK from rat and guinea pig liver cytosols (80, 93). If 3MPA inhibits gluconeogenesis solely by acting at PEPCK, it is difficult to explain the inhibition of gluconeogenesis from glycerol in perfused guinea pig liver. In the guinea pig liver, a recycling of glycerol via mitochondrial PEPCK or a direct oxidation of glycerol in the citric acid cycle have been suggested (80).

2,5-Anhydro-D-mannitol

2,5-Anhydro-D-mannitol (AM), an analogue of fructose, decreases blood glucose in fasting or diabetic mice and rats by 20 to 60% (58). In hepatocytes from fasted rats, AM inhibits gluconeogenesis from substrates that enter the gluconeogenic pathway prior to fructose-1,6-bisphosphate (lactate, pyruvate, alanine, glycerol, dihydroxy-acetone, sorbitol, fructose) but not from xylitol that enter the pathway at fructose-6-phosphate level (58, 125, 128). The inhibition of gluconeogenesis by AM is accompanied by a stimulation of glycolysis (58, 125, 128). Furthermore, AM blocks the hormonal stimulation of gluconeogenesis and the inhibition of glycolysis (125, 128). Metabolite crossover studies indicate that the sites of inhibition of gluconeogenesis and enhancement of glycolysis by AM are consistent with an inhibition of fructose-1,6-bisphosphatase and an activation of pyruvate kinase (125, 126). AM decreases the cellular concentration of fructose-2,6-bisphosphate but does not change ATP concentrations. It is suggested that phosphorylation of AM and accumulation of 2,5-anhydro-D-mannitol-1-phosphate and -1,6-bisphosphate mimick the effects of fructose 2,6-bisphosphate in stimulating glycolysis and inhibiting gluconeogenesis (126).

Inhibitors of fatty acid oxidation

These compounds are inhibitors of the mitonchondrial carnitine acyltransferase system.

2-Tetradecylglycidic acid (TGDA) and its methyl ester produce a dose-dependent hypoglycaemia in fasted or diabetic rats, mice, guinea pigs, dogs and suckling newborn rats (158, 160, 163). It inhibits gluconeogenesis from pyruvate, lactate, dihydroxyacetone and fructose in hepatocytes from starved rats. In perfused guinea pig liver TDGA inhibits gluconeogenesis from lactate and pyruvate but not from glycerol or propionate (160).

TDGA inhibits the transport of long chain fatty acid into the mitochondria at the level of carnitine acyltransferase I (161, 162). In keeping with this, it has been shown that the inhibitory effect of TDGA on gluconeogenesis from pyruvate or lactate is relieved by addition of octanoate (45, 160, 161).

2-(Phenylalkyl)-oxirane-2-carboxylate (POCA) produces a dose-dependent hypo-glycaemic effect in fasted normal or diabetic rat, mouse, guinea pig, pig and dog (94, 179). It inhibits gluconeogenesis from lactate and pyruvate in perfused liver and isolated hepatocytes from fasted rats (136, 180). POCA is a potent inhibitor of carnitine acyltransferase I (159), and, as for TDGA, the inhibitory effect of POCA on gluconeogenesis from lactate and pyruvate is relieved by octanoate (136, 180).

2-(3-Methylcinnamylhydrazono)-propionate (MCHP) produces a dose dependent hypoglycaemia in starved guinea pigs (98). It inhibits gluconeogenesis from lactate, pyruvate, alanine, propionate, glutamine, dihydroxyacetone, glycerol and fructose in perfused liver or isolated hepatocytes from starved guinea pigs (98). MCHP is a potent inhibitor of the transfer of long chain fatty acids across the mitochondrial membrane; it inhibits ketogenesis from oleate, palmitoyl-CoA and palmitoyl-carnitine but not from octanoate in isolated mitochondria (26). This suggests that MCHP inhibits both carnitine acyltransferase I and II. The inhibitory effect of MCHP on gluconeogenesis from pyruvate in the perfused liver of starved guinea pig, is relieved by addition of octanoate (26).

Conclusions

During the last ten years, considerable progress has been accomplished in the understanding of the control mechanisms of gluconeogenesis. These include the interconversion of key glycolytic and gluconeogenic enzymes, the discovery of the fructose 2,6-bisphosphate system, and the regulation of gene expression. Many current efforts are aimed at unraveling the mechanisms of control of gene expression by hormones. One may expect a large number of studies on that subject, if not the ultimate answer. On the other hand, the hormonal regulation of the mitochondrial metabolism of pyruvate and, more generally, of the mitochondrial respiratory chain still requires an explanation. Finally, it is not excluded that mechanisms will be discovered that control the activity of the enzymes of the glucose/glucose 6-phosphate cycle, the only cycle in the pathway which still lacks refined control.

REFERENCES

1 Adam P. A., Haynes R. C. Jr: Control of hepatic mitochondrial CO_2 fixation by glucagon, epinephrine, and cortisol. *J. Biol. Chem.* 1969, **244**: 6444–6450.

2 Andreone T. L., Beale E. G., Bar R. S., Granner, D. K.: Insulin decreases phosphoenolpyruvate carboxykinase (GTP) mRNA activity by a receptor-mediated process. *J. Biol. Chem.* 1982, **257**: 35–38.

3 Arinze I. J., Hanson R. W.: Mitochondrial redox state and the regulation of gluconeogenesis in the isolated perfused cat liver. *FEBS Lett.* 1973, **31**: 280–282.

4 Barber E. F., Handlogten M. E., Vida T. A., Kilberg M. S.: Neutral amino acid transport in hepatocytes isolated from streptozotocin induced diabetic rats. *J. Biol. Chem.* 1982, **257**: 14960–14967.

5 Bartrons R., Hue L., Van Schaftingen E., Hers H. G.: Hormonal control of fructose 2,6-bisphosphate concentration in isolated hepatocytes. *Biochem. J.* 1983, **214**: 829–837.

6 Beale E. G., Katzen C. S., Granner D. K.: Regulation of rat liver phosphoenolpyruvate

carboxykinase (GTP) messenger ribonucleic acid activity by N6,O2-dibutyryl adenosine 3'-5'-phospate. *Biochemistry* 1981, **20**: 4878–4883.

7 Beale E. G., Hartley J. L., Granner D. K.: N6,O2,-dibutyryl cyclic AMP and glucose regulate the amount of messenger RNA coding for hepatic phosphoenolpyruvate carboxykinase (GTP). *J. Biol. Chem.* 1982, **257**: 2022–2028.

8 Beale E. G., Andreone T., Koch S., Granner M., Granner, D. : Insulin and glucagon regulate cytosolic phosphoenolpyruvate carboxykinase (GTP) mRNA in rat liver. *Diabetes* 1984, **33**: 328–332.

9 Berridge M. J.: Inositol trisphosphate and diacylglycerol as second messenger. *Biochem. J.* 1984, **220**: 345–360.

10 Berry M. N.: High yield preparation of morphologically intact isolated parenchymal cells from rat liver. *Methods in Enzymology* 1974, **32**: 625–632.

11 Blackshear P. J., Holloway P. A. H., Alberti K. G. M. M.: The effects of inhibition of gluconeogenesis on ketogenesis in starved and diabetic rats. *Biochem. J.* 1975, **148**: 353–362.

12 Blair J. B., James M. E., Foster J. L.: Adrenergic control of glucose output and adenosine 3',5'-monophosphate levels in hepatocytes from juvenile and adult rats. *J. Biol. Chem.* 1979, **254**: 7579–7584.

13 Blair J. B., James M. E., Foster J. L.: Adrenergic control of glycolysis and pyruvate kinase activity in hepatocytes from young and old rats. *J. Biol. Chem.* 1979, **254**: 7585–7590.

14 Brocks D. G., Siess E. A., Wieland O. H.: Distinctive roles of oleate and glucagon in gluconeogenesis. *Eur. J. Biochem.* 1980, **113**: 39–43.

15 Canivet B., Fehlmann M., Freychet P.: Glucocorticoid and catecholamine stimulation of amino acid transport in rat hepatocytes. Synthesis of a high-affinity component. *Molec. Cell Endocrinol.* 1980, **19**: 253–261.

16 Chan T. M., Exton J. H.: Studies on α-adrenergic activation of hepatic glucose output. Studies on α-adrenergic inhibition of hepatic pyruvate kinase and activation of gluconeogenesis. *J. Biol. Chem.* 1978, **253**: 6393–6400.

17 Chrapkiewick N. B., Beale E. G., Granner D. K.: Induction of the messenger ribonucleic acid coding for phosphoenolpyruvate carboxykinase in H4-II-E cells. Evidence for a nuclear effect of cyclic AMP. *J. Biol. Chem.* 1982, **257**: 14428–14432.

18 Christensen H. N.: Interorgan amino acid nutrition. *Physiol. Rev.* 1982, **62**: 1193–1233.

19 Cimbala M. A., Lamers W. H., Nelson K., Monahan J. E., Yoo-Warren H., Hanson R. W.: Rapid changes in the concentration of phosphoenolpyruvate carboxykinase mRNA in rat liver and kidney. Effects of insulin and cyclic AMP. *J. Biol. Chem.* 1982, **257**: 7629–7636.

20 Cladaras C., Cottam G. L.: Dietary alterations of translatable mRNA sequences coding for rat liver pyruvate kinase. *J. Biol. Chem.* 1980, **255**: 11499–11503.

21 Claus T. H., El-Maghrabi M. R., Pilkis S. J.: Modulation of the phosphorylation state of rat liver pyruvate kinase by allosteric effectors and insulin. *J. Biol. Chem.* 1979, **254**: 7855–7864.

22 Claus T. H., El-Maghrabi M. R., Regen D. M., Stewart H. B., McGrane M., Koutz P. D., Nyfeler F., Pilkis J., Pilkis S. J.: The role of fructose 2,6-bisphosphate in the regulation of carbohydrate metabolism. *Curr. Top. Cell Regul.* 1984, **23**: 57–86.

23 Cornell N. W., Lund P., Krebs H. A.: The effect of lysine on gluconeogenesis from lactate in rat hepatocytes. *Biochem. J.* 1974, **142**: 327–337.

24 Cornell N. W., Zuurendonk P. F., Kerich M. J., Straight C. B.: Selective inhibition of alanine aminotransferase and aspartate aminotransferase in rat hepatocytes. *Biochem. J.* 1984, **220**: 707–716.

25 Crettaz M., Kahn C. R., Fehlmann M.: Glucagon regulation of amino acid transport in hepatocytes: effect of cell enucleation. *J. Cell Physiol.* 1983, **115**: 186–190.

26 Deaciuc I. V., Kühnle H. F., Strauss K. M., Schmidt F. H.: Studies on the mechanism of action of the hypoglycemic agent, 2-(3-methylcinnamylhydrazono)-proprionate (BM 42.304). *Biochem. Pharmacol.* 1983, **32**: 3405–3412.

27 Demaugre F., Leroux J. P., Cartier P.: The effect of pyruvate concentration, dichloroacetate and α-cyano-4-hydroxycinnamate on gluconeogenesis, ketogenesis, and 3-hydroxybutyrate/3-oxobutyrate ratios in isolated rat hepatocytes. *Biochem. J.* 1978, **172**: 91–96.

28 Denton R. M., Halestrap A. P.: Regulation of pyruvate metabolism in mammalian tissues. *Essays in Biochemistry* 1979, **15**: 37–77.

29 Di Tullio N. W., Berkoff C. E., Blank B., Kostos E., Stack E. J., Saunders H. L.: 3-mercaptopicolinic acid, an inhibitor of gluconeogenesis. *Biochem. J.* 1974, **138**: 387–394.

30 Edmonson J. W., Lumeng L.: Biphasic stimulation of amino acid uptake by glucagon in hepatocytes. *Biochem. Biophys. Res. Commun.* 1980, **96**: 61–68.

31 Elliott K. R. F.: The preparation, characterization and use of isolated cells for metabolic studies. *In: Techniques in Metabolic Research*, Part I, Techniques in the Life Sciences, H. L. Korberg, J. C. Metcalfe, D. H. Northcote, C. I. Pogson, K. F. Tipton (Eds): Elsevier, Amsterdam, 1979, B204, pp 1–20.

32 Elliott K. R. F., Ash R., Pogson C. I., Smith S. A., Crisp D. K.: Comparative aspects of the preparation and biochemistry of liver cells from various species. *In: Use of Isolated Liver Cells and Kidney Tubules in Metabolic Studies*, J. M. Tager, H. D. Söling, J. R. Williamson (Eds): Elsevier North-Holland, 1976, pp 139–143.

33 Engström L.: The regulation of liver pyruvate kinase by phosphorylation-dephosphorylation. *Curr. Top. Cell. Regul.* 1978, **13**: 29–51.

34 Evans C., Miyanaga O., Cottam G. L.: The long-term effect of glucagon on pyruvate kinase activity in primary cultures of hepatocytes. *Arch. Biochem. Biophys.* 1984, **233**: 617–623.

35 Exton, J. H.: Molecular mechanisms involved in α-adrenergic responses. *Molec. Cell. Endocrinol.* 1981, **23**: 233–264.

36 Exton, J. H., Park, C. R.: Control of gluconeogenesis in liver. III. Effects of L-lactate, pyruvate, fructose, glucagon, epinephrine, and adenosine 3′,5′-monophosphate on gluconeogenic intermediates in the perfused rat liver. *J. Biol. Chem.* 1969, **244**: 1424–1433.

37 Exton, J. H., Corbin, J. G., Park, C. R.: Control of gluconeogenesis in liver. IV. Differential effects of fatty acids and glucagon on ketogenesis and gluconeogenesis in the perfused rat liver. *J. Biol. Chem.* 1969, **244**: 4095–4102.

38 Exton, J. H., Mallette, L. E., Jefferson, L. S., Wong, E. H. A., Friedmann, N., Miller, J. B., Park, C. R.: The hormonal control of hepatic gluconeogenesis. *Recent Prog. Horm. Res.* 1970, **26**: 411–461.

39 Fafournoux, P., Remesy, C., Demigne, C.: Stimulation of amino acid transport into liver cells from rats adapted to a high-protein diet. *Biochem. J.* 1982, **206**: 13–18.

40 Fehlmann, M., Le Cam, A., Kitabgi, P., Rey, J. F., Freychet, P.: Regulation of amino acid transport in the liver. Emergence of a high-affinity transport system in isolated hepatocytes from fasting rats. *J. Biol. Chem.* 1979, **254**: 401–407.

41 Fehlmann, M., Le Cam, A., Freychet, P.: Insulin and glucagon stimulation of amino acid transport in isolated rat hepatocytes. Synthesis of a high-affinity component of transport. *J. Biol. Chem.* 1979, **254**: 10431–10437.

42 Feliu, J. E., Hue, L., Hers, H. G.: Hormonal control of pyruvate kinase activity and of gluconeogenesis in isolated hepatocytes. *Proc. Natl. Acad. Sci.* 1976, **73**: 2762–2766.

43 Ferré P., Pégorier J. P., Girard J.: The effects of inhibition of gluconeogenesis in suckling newborn rats. *Biochem. J.* 1977, **162**: 209–212.

44 Ferré P., Pégorier J. P., Williamson D. H., Girard J.: *In vivo* interactions between oxidation of non-esterified fatty acids and gluconeogenesis in the newborn rat. *Biochem. J.* 1979, **182**: 593–598.

45 Ferré P., Satabin P., El-Manoubi L., Callikan S., Girard J.: Relationship between ketogenesis and gluconeogenesis in isolated hepatocytes from newborn rats. *Biochem. J.* 1981, **200**: 429–433.

46 Fleig W. E., Geerling I., Roben H., Ditschuneit H.: Effects of insulin, glucagon and dexamethasone on pyruvate kinase in cultured hepatocytes. *Biochem. Biophys. Acta* 1984, **805**: 165–173.

47 Garrison J. C., Haynes R. C. Jr: The hormonal control of gluconeogenesis by regulation of mitochondrial pyruvate carboxylation in isolated rat liver cells. *J. Biol. Chem.* 1975, **250**: 2769–2777.

48 Garrison J. C., Borland M. K.: Regulation of mitochondrial pyruvate carboxylation and gluconeogenesis in rat hepatocytes via an α-adrenergic, adenosine 3′:5′-monophosphate-independent mechanism. *J. Biol. Chem.* 1979, **254**: 1129–1133.

49 Garrison J. C., Johnsen D. E., Campanile C. P.: Evidence for the role of phosphorylase kinase, protein kinase C, and other Ca^{2+}-sensitive protein kinases in the response of hepatocytes to angiotensin II and vasopressin. *J. Biol. Chem.* 1984, **259**: 3283–3292.

50 Girard J. R.: Gluconeogenesis and the regulation of blood glucose concentration in the newborn.

In: Diabetes 1982, E. N. Mngola (Ed.): Excerpta Medica, Amsterdam, pp 417–421.

51 Goodman M. N.: Effect of 3-mercaptopicolinic acid on gluconeogenesis and gluconeogenic metabolite concentrations in the isolated perfused rat liver. *Biochem. J.* 1975, **150**: 137–139.

52 Granner D. K., Andreone T., Sazaki K., Belae E. G.: Inhibition of transcription of the phosphoenolpyruvate carboxykinase gene by insulin. *Nature* 1983, **350**: 549–551.

53 Groen A. K.: Quantification of control in studies on intermediary metabolism. PhD Thesis, University of Amsterdam, 1984, pp 1–148.

54 Groen A. K., Van der Meer R., Westerhoff H. V., Wanders R. J. A., Akerboom T. P. M., Tager J. M.: Control of metabolic fluxes. *In: Metabolic Compartmentation*, H. Sies (Ed.): Academic Press, New York, 1982, pp 9–37.

55 Groen A. K., Vervoorn R. C., Van der Meer R., Tager J. M.: Control of gluconeogenesis in rat liver cells. 1. Kinetics of the individual enzymes and the effect of glucagon. *J. Biol. Chem.* 1983, **258**: 14346–14353.

56 Halestrap A. P.: Hormonal control of mitochondrial respiratory chain activity. *In: Short-Term Regulation of Liver Metabolism*, L. Hue, G. van de Werve (Eds): Elsevier/North-Holland, Amsterdam, 1981, pp 389–409.

57 Halestrap A. P., Scott R. D., Thomas A. P.: Mitochondrial pyruvate transport and its hormonal regulation. *Int. J. Biochem.* 1980, **11**: 97–105.

58 Hanson R. L., Ho R. S., Wiseberg J. J., Simpson R., Younathan E. S., Blair J. B.: Inhibition of gluconeogenesis and glycogenolysis by 2,5-anhydro-D-mannitol. *J. Biol. Chem.* 1984, **259**: 218–223.

59 Harris R. A., Cornell N. W. (Eds): *Isolation, Characterization and Use of Hepatocytes*: Elsevier, New York, 1983, pp 1–624.

60 Heinrich R., Rapoport T. A.: A linear steady-state treatment of enzymatic chains. Critique of the crossover theorem and a general procedure to identify interaction sites with an effector. *Eur. J. Biochem.* 1974, **42**: 97–105.

61 Hems D. A., Whitton P. D.: Stimulation by vasopressin of glycogen breakdown and gluconeogenesis in the perfused rat liver. *Biochem. J.* 1973, **136**: 705–709.

62 Hems D. A., McCormack J. G., Denton R. M.: Rapid stimulation by vasopressin, oxytocin, and angiotensin II of glycogen degradation in hepatocyte suspensions. *Biochem. J.* 1978, **172**: 311–317.

63 Hers H. G.: The control of glycogen metabolism in the liver. *Ann. Rev. Biochem.* 1976, **45**: 167–189.

64 Hers H. G., Van Schaftingen E.: Fructose 2,6-bisphosphate 2 years after its discovery. *Biochem. J.* 1982, **206**: 1–12.

65 Hers H. G., Hue L.: Gluconeogenesis and related aspects of glycolysis. *Ann. Rev. Biochem.* 1983, **52**: 617–653.

66 Hetenyi G. Jr, Perez G., Vranic M.: Turnover and precursor-product relationships of non lipid metabolites. *Physiol. Rev.* 1983, **63**: 606–667.

67 Holland P. C., Clark M. G., Bloxham D. P., Lardy H. A.: Mechanism of action of the hypoglycemic agent diphenyleneiodonium. *J. Biol. Chem.* 1973, **248**: 6050–6056.

68 Hue L.: The role of futile cycles in the regulation of carbohydrate metabolism in the liver. *Adv. Enzymol.* 1981, **52**: 247–331.

69 Hue L.: Futile cycles and regulation of metabolism. *In: Metabolic Compartmentation*, H. Sies (Ed.): Academic Press, New York, 1982, pp 71–97.

70 Hue L., Bartrons, R.: Rôle of fructose 2,6-bisphosphate in the control by glucagon of gluconeogenesis from various precursors in isolated rat hepatocytes. *Biochem. J.* 1984, **218**: 165–170.

71 Hue L., Feliu J. E., Hers H. G.: Control of gluconeogenesis and of enzymes of glycogen metabolism in isolated rat hepatocytes. *Biochem. J.* 1978, **176**: 791–797 .

72 Hue L., Van Schaftingen E., Blackmore P. F.: Stimulation of glycolysis and accumulation of a stimulator of phosphofructokinase in hepatocytes incubated with vasopressin. *Biochem. J.* 1981, **194**: 1023–1026.

73 Hue L., Blackmore, P. F., Exton J. H.: Fructose 2,6-bisphosphate. Hormonal regulation and mechanism of its formation in liver. *J. Biol. Chem.* 1981, **256**: 8900–8903.

74 Hue L., Sorbino F., Bosca L.: Difference in glucose sensitivy of liver glycolysis and glycogen synthesis. Relationship between lactate production and fructose 2,6-bisphosphate concentration.

Biochem. J. 1984, **224**: 779–786.

75 Iynedjian P., Hanson R. W.: Increase in level of functional messenger RNA coding for phosphoenolpyruvate carboxykinase (GTP) during induction by cyclic 3′-5′-monophosphate. *J. Biol. Chem.* 1977, **252**: 655–662.

76 Iynedjian P. B., Salavert A.: Effects of glucagon, dexamethasone and triiodothyronine on phosphoenolpyruvate carboxykinase (GTP) synthesis and mRNA level in rat liver cells. *Eur. J. Biochem.* 1984, **145**: 489–497.

77 Jakob A., Diem S.: Metabolic responses of perfused rat livers to alpha- and beta-adrenergic agonists, glucagon and cyclic AMP. *Biochem. Biophys. Acta* 1975, **404**: 57–66.

78 Johnson M. E. M., Das N. W., Butcher F. R., Fain J. N.: The regulation of gluconeogenesis in isolated rat liver cells by glucagon, insulin, dibutyryl cyclic adenosine monophosphate and fatty acids. *J. Biol. Chem.* 1972, **247**: 3229–3235.

79 Jomain-Baum M., Hanson R. W.: Regulation of hepatic gluconeogenesis in the guinea pig by fatty acids and ammonia. *J. Biol. Chem.* 1975, **250**: 8978–8985.

80 Jomain-Baum M., Schramm V. L., Hanson R. W.: Mechanism of 3-mercaptopicolinic acid inhibition of hepatic phosphoenolpyruvate carboxykinase (GTP). *J. Biol. Chem.* 1976, **251**: 37–44.

81 Joseph S. K.: Inositol trisphosphate: an intracellular messenger produced by Ca^{2+} mobilizing hormones. *Trends Biochem. Sc.* 1984, **9**: 420–421.

82 Jungermann K., Probst I., Andersen B., Wölfle D.: Significance of substrates, hormones and hepatocyte heterogeneity for the regulation of hepatic glycolysis and gluconeogenesis. *In: Isolation, Characterization, and Use of Hepatocytes*, R. A. Harris, N. W. Cornell (Eds.): Elsevier Biomedical, 1983, pp 125–130.

83 Katz J., Rognstad R.: Futile cycles in the metabolism of glucose. *Curr. Top. Cell. Regul.* 1976, **10**: 237–289.

84 Katz J., McGarry J. D.: The glucose paradox: Is glucose a substrate for liver metabolism? *J. Clin. Invest.* 1984, **74**: 1901–1909.

85 Katz, J., Okajima F., Chenoweth M., Dunn A.: The determination of lactate turnover *in vivo* with ^3H and ^{14}C labelled lactate. The significance of sites of tracer administration and sampling. *Biochem. J.* 1981, **194**: 513–524.

86 Kelley, D. S., Evanson T., Van Potter R.: Calcium dependent hormonal regulation of amino acid transport and cyclic AMP accumulation in rat hepatocytes monolayer cultures. *Proc. Natl. Acad. Sci.* 1980, **77**: 5953–5957.

87 Kelley D. S., Campbell H. A., Van Potter R.: Effects of hormones and amino acid depletion on the kinetic parameters of amino acid uptake in monolayer cultures of rat hepatocytes. *J. Cell Physiol.* 1982, **112**: 67–75.

88 Kilberg M. S.: Amino acid transport in isolated rat hepatocytes. *J. Memb. Biol.* 1982, **69**: 1–12.

89 Kilberg M. S., Vida T. A., Barber E. F.: Regulation of neutral amino acid transport in hepatocytes from adrenalectomized rats. *J. Cell Physiol.* 1983, **114**: 45–52.

90 Kioussis D., Reshef L., Cohen A., Tilghman S. M., Iynedjian P. B., Ballard F. J., Hanson R. W.: Alterations in translatable messenger RNA coding for phosphoenolpyruvate carboxykinase (GTP) in rat liver cytosol during deinduction. *J. Biol. Chem.* 1978, **253**: 4327–4332.

91 Kacser H., Burns J. A.: Molecular democracy: who shares the control? *Biochem. Soc. Trans.* 1979, **7**: 1149–1160.

92 Kneer N. M., Wagner M. J., Lardy H. A.: Regulation by calcium of hormonal effects on gluconeogenesis. *J. Biol. Chem.* 1979, **254**: 12160–12168.

93 Kostos V., Di Tullio N. W., Rush J., Cieslinski L., Saunders H. L.: The effect of mercaptopicolinic acid on phosphoenolpyruvate carboxykinase (GTP) in the rat and guinea pig. *Arch. Biochem. Biophys.* 1975, **171**: 459–465.

94 Koundakjian P. P., Turnbull D. M., Bone A. J., Rogers M. P., Younan S. I. M., Sherratt H. S. A.: Metabolic changes in fed rats caused by chronic administration of ethyl 2-(5-(4-chlorophenyl)-pentyl)oxirane-2-carboxylate, a new hypoglycemic compound. *Biochem. Pharmacol.* 1984, **33**: 465–473.

95 Kraus-Friedmann N.: Hormonal regulation of hepatic gluconeogenesis. *Physiol. Rev.* 1984, **64**: 170–259.

96 Krebs H. A.: The Pasteur effect and the relations between respiration and fermentation. *Essays in*

Biochem. 1972, **8**: 1–34.

97 Krebs H. A.: Some aspects of the regulation of fuel supply in omnivorous animals. *Adv. Enz. Regul.* 1972, **10**: 397–420.

98 Kühnle H. F., Schmidt F. H., Deaciuc I. V.: *In vivo* and *in vitro* effects of a new hypoglycemic agent 2-(3-methylcinnamylhydrazono)propionate (BM 42,304) on glucose metabolism in guinea pigs. *Biochem. Pharmacol.* 1984, **33**: 1437–1444.

99 Lamers W. H., Hanson R. W., Meisner H. M.: cAMP stimulates transcription of the gene for cytosolic phosphoenolpyruvate carboxykinase in rat liver nuclei. *Proc. Natl. Acad. Sci.* 1982, **79**: 5137–5141.

100 Lardy H., Kneer N., Wernette M. E.: Regulation of gluconeogenesis by catecholamines, vasopressin and angiotensin. *In*: *Isolation, Characterization, and Use of Hepatocytes*, R. A. Harris, N. W. Cornell (Eds).: Elsevier Biomedical, 1983, pp 445–454.

101 Le Cam A., Freychet P.: Glucagon stimulates the A system for neutral amino acid transport in isolated hepatocytes of adult rats. *Biochem. Biophys. Res. Commun.* 1976, **72**: 893–901.

102 McGivan J. D., Ramsell J. C., Lacey, J. H.: Stimulation of alanine transport and metabolism by dibutyryl cyclic AMP in hepatocytes from fed rats. Assessment of transport as a potential rate-limiting step. *Biochem. Biophys. Acta* 1981, **644**: 295–304.

103 Meisner H. M., Lamers W. H., Hanson R. W.: Cyclic AMP and the synthesis of phosphoenol-pyruvate carboxykinase (GTP) mRNA. *Trends Biochem. Sci.* 1983, **8**: 165–167.

104 Menahan A., Wieland, O.: The role of endogenous lipid in gluconeogenesis and ketogenesis in perfused rat liver. *Eur. J. Biochem.* 1969, **9**: 182–188.

105 Miyanaga O., Nagano M., Cottam G. L.: Effect of insulin on liver pyruvate kinase *in vivo* and *in vitro. J. Biol. Chem.* 1982, **257**, 10617–10623.

106 Miyanaga O., Evans C., Cottam G. L.: The effect of dexamethasone on pyruvate kinase activity in primary culture of hepatocytes. *Biochim. Biophys. Acta* 1983, **758**: 42–48.

107 Munnich A., Marie J., Reach G., Vaulont S., Simon M. P., Kahn A.: *In vivo* hormonal control of L-type pyruvate kinase gene expression. Effects of glucagon, cyclic AMP, insulin, cortisol and thyroid hormones on the dietary induction of mRNAs in the liver. *J. Biol. Chem.* 1984, **259**: 10228–10231.

108 Nagano M., Ishibashi H., McCully V., Cottam G. L.: Epinephrine-stimulated phosphorylation of pyruvate kinase in hepatocytes. *Arch. Biochem. Biophys.* 1980, **203**: 271–281.

109 Nelson K., Cimbala M. A., Hanson R. W.: Regulation of phosphoenolpyruvate carboxykinase (GTP) mRNA turnover in rat liver. *J. Biol. Chem.* 1980, **255**: 8509–8515.

110 Nishizuka Y.: The role of protein kinase C in cell surface signal transduction and tumour promotion. *Nature* 1984, **308**: 693–698.

111 Noguchi T., Inoue H., Tanaka T.: Regulation of rat liver L-type pyruvate kinase mRNA by insulin and by fructose. *Eur. J. Biochem.* 1982, **128**: 583–588.

112 Noguchi T., Inoue H., Chen H. L., Matsubara K. I., Tanaka T.: Molecular cloning of DNA complementary to rat L-type pyruvate kinase mRNA. Nutritional and hormonal regulation of L-type pyruvate kinase mRNA concentration. *J. Biol. Chem.* 1983, **258**: 15220–15223.

113 Ochs R. S., Lardy H. A.: Catecholamine stimulation of hepatic gluconeogenesis at the site between pyruvate and phosphoenolpyruvate. *J. Biol. Chem.* 1983, **258**: 9956–9962.

114 Okajima F., Chenoweth M., Rognstad R., Dunn A., Katz J.: Metabolism of ^{3}H and ^{14}C-labelled lactate in starved rats. *Biochem. J.* 1981, **194**: 525–540.

115 Oliver I. T., Edwards A. M., Pitot H. L.: Hormonal regulation of phosphoenolpyruvate carboxykinase in primary cultures of adult rat liver parenchymal cells. *Eur. J. Biochem.* 1978, **87**: 221–227.

116 Pariza M. W., Butcher F. R., Kletzien R. F., Becker J. E., Van Potter R.: Induction and decay of glucagon-induced amino acid transport in primary cultures of adult rat liver cells: paradoxical effects of cycloheximide and puromycine. *Proc. Natl. Acad. Sci.* 1976, **73**: 4511–4515.

117 Pariza M. W., Butcher F. R., Becker J. E., Van Potter R.: 3′,5′-cyclic AMP: independent induction of amino acid transport by epinephrine, in primary cultures of adult rat liver cells. *Proc. Natl. Acad. Sci.* 1977, **74**: 234–237.

118 Pilkis S. J., Riou J. P., Claus T. H.: Hormonal control of (14C) glucose synthesis from (U-14C)dihydroxyacetone and glycerol in isolated rat hepatocytes. *J. Biol. Chem.* 1976, **251**: 7841–7842.

119 Pilkis S. J., Park C. R., Clause T. H.: Hormonal control of hepatic gluconeogenesis. *Vitam. Horm.* 1978, **36**: 383–460.

120 Prentki M., Crettaz M., Jeanrenaud B.: Role of microtubules in insulin and glucagon stimulation of amino acid transport in isolated rat hepatocytes. *J. Biol. Chem.* 1981, **256**: 4336–4340.

121 Probst I., Jungermann K.: The glucagon-insulin antagonism and glucagon-dexamethasone synergism in the induction of phosphoenolpyruvate carboxykinase in cultured rat hepatocytes. *Hoppe-Seyler's Z. Physiol. Chem.* 1983, **364**: 1739–1746.

122 Raaka B. M., Lowenstein J. M.: Inhibition of fatty acid oxidation by 2-bromooctanoate on ketogenesis and gluconeogenesis. *J. Biol. Chem.* 1979, **254**: 3303–3310.

123 Richards C. S., Yokoyama M., Furuya E., Uyeda K.: Reciprocal changes in fructose 6-phosphate,2-kinase and fructose 2,6-bisphosphatase activity in response to glucagon and epinephrine. *Biochem. Biophys. Res. Commun.* 1982, **104**: 1073–1079.

124 Richards, C. S., Uyeda K.: Hormonal regulation of fructose 6-P,2-kinase and fructose 2,6-P2 by two mechanisms. *J. Biol. Chem.* 1982, **257**: 8854–8861.

125 Riquelme P. T., Wernette-Hammond M. E., Kneer N. M., Lardy H. A.: Regulation of carbohydrate metabolism by 2,5-anhydro-D-mannitol. *Proc. Natl. Acad. Sci.* 1983, **80**: 4301–4305.

126 Riquelme P. T., Wernette-Hammond M. E., Kneer N. M., Lardy H. A.: Mechanism of action of 2,5-anhydro-D-mannitol in hepatocytes. Effect of phosphorylated metabolites on enzymes of carbohydrate metabolism. *J. Biol. Chem.* 1984, **259**: 5115–5123.

127 Rognstad R.: Rate-limiting steps in metabolic pathways. *J. Biol. Chem.* 1979, **254**: 1875–1878.

128 Rognstad R.: Effects of alterations in energy supply on gluconeogenesis from L-lactate. *Int. J. Biochem.* 1982, **14**: 765–770.

129 Rognstad R., Clark D. G.: Effects of aminooxyacetate on the metabolism of isolated liver cells. *Arch. Biochem. Biophys.* 1974, **111**: 638–646.

130 Ross B. D., Hems, R., Krebs H. A.: The rate of gluconeogenesis from various precursors in the perfused rat liver. *Biochem. J.* 1967, **102**: 942–951.

131 Ross B. D., Hems R., Freedland R. A., Krebs H. A.: Carbohydrate metabolism of the perfused rat liver. *Biochem. J.* 1967, **105**: 869–875.

132 Salavert A., Iynedjian P. B.: Regulation of phosphoenolpyruvate carboxykinase (GTP) synthesis in rat liver cells. Rapid introduction of specific mRNA by glucagon, or cyclic AMP and permissive effect of dexamethasone. *J. Biol. Chem.* 1981, **257**: 13404–13412.

133 Samson M., Fehlmann M., Morin O., Dolais-Kitabgi J., Freychet P.: Insulin and glucagon binding and stimulation of amino acid transport in isolated hepatocytes from streptozotocin-diabetic rats. *Metabolism* 1982, **31**: 766–772.

134 Sasaki K., Cripe T. P., Koch S. R., Andreone T. L., Petersen D. D., Beale E. G., Granner D. K.: Multihormonal regulation of phosphoenolpyruvate carboxykinase gene transcription. The dominant role of insulin. *J. Biol. Chem.* 1984, **259**: 15242–15251.

135 Schimassek H., Mitzkat H. J.: Uber eine spezifische Wirkung des Glucagon auf die Embden-Meyerhof-Kette in der Leber. *Biochem. Z.* 1963, **337**: 510–518.

136 Schudt C., Simon A.: Effects of sodium 2-(5-(4-chlorophenyl)-pentyl)-oxirane-2-carboxylate (POCA) on carbohydrate and fatty acid metabolism in liver and muscle. *Biochem. Pharmacol.* 1984, **33**: 3357–3362.

137 Sheratt H. S. A.: Inhibition of gluconeogenesis by non-hormonal hypoglycaemic compounds. *In: Short-term Regulation of Liver Metabolism*, L. Hue, G. van den Werve (Eds): Elsevier, New York, 1981, pp 199–227.

138 Shotwell M. A., Kilberg M. S., Oxender D. L.: The regulation of neutral amino acid transport in mammalian cells. *Biochim. Biophys. Acta* 1983, **737**: 267–284.

139 Siess E. A., Wieland O. H.: Early kinetics of glucagon action in isolated hepatocytes at the mitochondrial level. *Eur. J. Biochem.* 1980, **110**: 203–210.

140 Siess E. A., Fahimi F. M., Wieland O. H.: Evidence that glucagon stabilizes rather than activates mitochondrial functions in rat liver. *Hoppe-Seyler's Z. Physiol. Chem.* 1981, **362**: 1643–1651.

141 Siess E. A., Kientsch-Engel R. I., Fahimi F. M., Wieland O. H.: Possible role of Pi supply in mitochondrial action of glucagon. *Eur. J. Biochem.* 1984, **141**: 543–548.

142 Sips H. J., Goren A. K., Tager J. M.: Plasma membrane transport of alanine is rate-limiting for its metabolism in rat liver parenchymal cells. *FEBS Lett.* 1980, **119**: 271–274.

143 Smith S. B., Briggs S., Triebwasser K. L., Freedland R. A.: Re-evaluation of aminooxyacetate as an inhibitor. *Biochem. J.* 1977, **162**: 453–455.

144 Söling H. D., Seck A.: Precursor specific inhibition of hepatic gluconeogenesis by glisoxepide an inhibitor of the L-aspartate/L-glutamate antiport system. *FEBS Lett.* 1975, **51**: 52–59.

145 Söling H. D., Kleineke J.: Species dependent regulation of hepatic gluconeogenesis in higher animals. *In: Gluconeogenesis. Its Regulation in Mammalian Species*, R. W. Hanson, M. A. Mehlman (Eds): Wiley, New York, 1976, pp 369–462.

146 Söling H. D., Willms B., Kleineke J., Gehlhoff M.: Regulation of gluconeogenesis in the guinea pig liver. *Eur. J. Biochem.* 1970, **16**: 289–302.

147 Stalmans W.: The hepatic threshold to glucose. *Curr. Top. Cell. Regul.* 1976, **11**: 51–97.

148 Steiner K. E., Chan T. M., Claus T. H., Exton J. H., Pilkis S. J.: The role of phosphorylation in the α-adrenergic mediated inhibition of rat hepatic pyruvate kinase. *Biochem. Biophys. Acta* 1980, **632**: 366–374.

149 Stubbs M., Vignais P., Krebs H. A.: Is adenine nucleotide translocator rate limiting for oxidative phosphorylation? *Biochem. J.* 1978, **172**: 333–342.

150 Studer R. K., Borle A. B.: Differences between male and female rats in the regulation of hepatic glycogenolysis. The relative role of calcium and cAMP in phosphorylase activation by catecholamines. *J. Biol. Chem.* 1982, **257**: 7987–7993.

151 Süssmuth W., Höppner W., Seitz H. J.: Permissive action of thyroid hormones in the cAMP-mediated induction of phosphoenolpyruvate carboxykinase in hepatocytes in culture. *Eur. J. Biochem.* 1984, **143**: 607–611.

152 Tager J. M., Söling H. D., Williamson J. R. (Eds): *Use of Isolated Liver Cells and Kidney Tubules in Metabolic Studies*: Elsevier North-Holland, Amsterdam, 1976, pp 1–476.

153 Tuefel H., Menahan L. A., Shipp J. C., Boning S., Wieland O.: Effect of oleic acid on the oxidation and gluconeogenesis from $(1\text{-}^{14}C)$pyruvate in the perfused rat liver. *Eur. J. Biochem.* 1967, **2**: 182–186.

154 Thomas A. P., Halestrap A. P.: The role of mitochondrial pyruvate transport in the stimulation by glucagon and phenylephrine of gluconeogenesis from L-lactate in isolated rat hepatocytes. *Biochem. J.* 1981, **198**: 551–564.

155 Tilghman S. M., Hanson R. W., Ballard F. J.: Hormonal regulation of phosphoneolpyruvate carboxykinase (GTP) in mammalian tissues. *In: Gluconeogenesis: Its regulation in Mammalian Species*, R. W. Hanson, M. A. Mehlman (Eds): John Wiley, New York, 1976, pp 47–91.

156 Toews C. J., Lowry C., Ruderman N. B.: The regulation of gluconeogenesis. The effect of Pent-4-enoic acid on gluconeogenesis and on gluconeogenic metabolite concentrations of isolated perfused rat liver. *J. Biol. Chem.* 1970, **245**: 818–824.

157 Tolbert M. E. M., Butcher F. R., Fain J. N.: Lack of correlation between catecholamine effects on cyclic adenosine 3′:5′-monophosphate and gluconeogenesis in isolated rat liver cells. *J. Biol. Chem.* 1973, **248**: 5686–5692.

158 Turlan P., Ferré P., Girard J.: Effects of an inhibitor of long chain fatty acid oxidation: 2-tetradecylglycidic acid on glucose homoeostasis in suckling newborn rats. *Biol. Neonate* 1983, **43**: 103–108.

159 Turnbull D. M., Bartlett K., Younan S. I. M., Sherratt H. S. A.: The effect of 2-(5-(4-chlorophenyl)-pentyl)oxirane-2-carbonyl-CoA on mitochondrial oxidation. *Biochem. Pharmacol.* 1984, **33**: 475–481.

160 Tutwiler G. F., Brentzel H. J.: Relation of oxidation of long-chain fatty acids to gluconeogenesis in the perfused liver of the guinea pig: effect of 2-tetradecylglycidic acid (McN-3802). *Eur. J. Biochem.* 1982, **124**: 465–470.

161 Tutwiler G. F., Dellevigne P.: Action of the oral hypoglycemic agent 2-tetradecylglycidic acid on hepatic fatty acid oxidation and gluconeogenesis. *J. Biol. Chem.* 1979, **254**: 2935–2941.

162 Tutwiler G. F., Ryzlak M. T.: Inhibition of mitochondrial carnitine palmitoyltransferase by 2-tetradecylglycidic acid (McN-3802). *Life Sci.* 1980, **26**: 393–397.

163 Tutwiler G. F., Kirsch T., Mohrbacher R. J., Ho W.: Pharmacologic profile of methyl-2-tetradecylglycidate (McN-3716), an orally effective hypoglycemic agent. *Metabolism* 1978, **27**: 1539–1556.

164 Uyeda K., Furuya E., Richard C. S., Yokoyama M.: Fructose-2,6-P2, chemistry and biological function. *Molec. Cell. Endocrinol.* 1982, **48**: 97–120.

165 Van Den Berg G. B., Van Berkel T. J. C., Koster J.: The role of Ca^{2+} and cyclic AMP in the phosphorylation of rat liver soluble proteins by endogenous protein kinases. *Eur. J. Biochem.* 1980, **113**: 131–140.

166 Van Schaftingen E., Hue L., Hers H. G.: Control of the fructose 6-phosphate/fructose 1,6-bisphosphate cycle in isolated hepatocytes by glucose and glucagon. Rôle of a low molecular-weight stimulator of phosphofructokinase. *Biochem. J.* 1980, **192**: 887–895.

167 Van Schaftingen E., Hue L., Hers H. G.: Fructose 2,6-bisphosphate, the probable structure of the glucose- and glucagon-sensitive stimulator of phosphofructokinase. *Biochem. J.* 1980, **192**: 897–901.

168 Vaulont S., Munnich A., Marie J., Reach G., Pichard A. L., Simon M. P., Besmond C., Barbry P., Kahn A.: Cyclic AMP as a transcriptional inhibitor of upper eukariotic gene transcription. *Biochem. Biophys. Res. Commun.* 1984, **125**: 135–141.

169 Weber A., Marie J., Cottreau D., Simon M. P., Besmond C., Dreyfus J. C., Kahn A.: Dietary control of aldolase B and L-type pyruvate kinase mRNAs in rat. Study of translational activity and hybridization with cloned cDNA probes. *J. Biol. Chem.* 1984, **259**: 1798–1802.

170 Whitton P. D., Rodrigues L. M., Hems D. A.: Stimulation by vasopressin, angiotensin and oxytocin of gluconeogenesis in hepatocyte suspensions. *Biochem. J.* 1978, **176**: 893–898.

171 Williamson D. H., Ilic V., Tordoff .A. F. C., Ellington E. V.: Interactions between vasopressin and glucagon on ketogenesis and oleate metabolism in isolated hepatocytes from fed rats. *Biochem. J.* 1980, **186**: 621–624.

172 Williamson J. R., Kreisberg R. A., Felts P. W.: Mechanism for the stimulation of gluconeogenesis by fatty acids in perfused rat liver. *Proc. Natl. Acad. Sci.* 1966, **56**: 247–254.

173 Williamson J. R., Browning E. T., Scholz R., Kreisberg R. A., Fritz I. B.: Inhibition of fatty acid stimulation of gluconeogenesis by (+)-decanoylcarnitine in perfused rat liver. *Diabetes* 1968, **17**: 194–208.

174 Williamson J. R., Browning E. T., Scholz R.: Control mechanisms of gluconeogenesis and ketogenesis. 1. Effects of oleate on gluconeogenesis in perfused rat liver. *J. Biol. Chem.* 1969, **244**: 4607–4616.

175 Williamson J. R., Browning E. T., Thurman R. G., Scholz R.: Inhibition of glucagon effects in perfused rat liver by (+)-deaanoyl carnitine. *J. Biol. Chem.* 1969, **244**: 5055–5064.

176 Williamson J. R., Anderson J., Browning E. T.: Inhibition of gluconeogenesis by butylmalonate in perfused rat liver. *J. Biol. Chem.* 1970, **245**: 1717–1726.

177 Williamson J. R., Rostand S. G., Peterson M. J.: Control factors affecting gluconeogenesis in perfused rat liver. Effects of 4-pentenoic acid. *J. Biol. Chem.* 1970, **245**: 3242–3251.

178 Williamson J. R., Cooper R. H., Hoek J. B.: Role of calcium in the hormonal regulation of liver metabolism. *Biochem. Biophys. Acta* 1981, **639**: 243–295.

179 Wolf H. P. O., Eistetter K., Ludwig G.: Phenylalkyloxirane carboxylic acids a new class of hypoglycaemic substances: hypoglycaemic and hypoketonaemic effects of sodium 2-(5-(4-chlorophenyl)-pentyl)oxirane-2-carboxylate (B 807-27) in fasted animals. *Diabetologia* 1982, **22**: 456–463.

180 Wolf H. P. O., Engeel D. W.: Decrease of fatty acid oxidation, ketogenesis and gluconeogenesis in isolated perfused rat liver by phenylalkyl oxirane carboxylate (B 807–27) due to inhibition of CPT I (EC 2.3.1.21). *Eur. J. Biochem.* 1985, **146**: 359–363.

181 Yip B. P., Lardy H. A.: The role of calcium in the stimulation of gluconeogenesis by catecholamines. *Arch. Biochem. Biophys.* 1981, **212**: 370–377.

182 Yoo-Warren H., Cimbala M. A., Felz K., Monahan J. E., Leis J. P., Hanson R. W.: Identification of a DNA clone to phosphoenolpyruvate carboxykinase (GTP) from rat cytosol. Alterations in phosphoenolpyruvate carboxykinase RNA-levels detectable by hybridization. *J. Biol. Chem.* 1981, **256**: 10224–10227.

183 Zaleski J., Bryla J.: Effects of oleate, palmitate, and octanoate on gluconeogenesis in isolated rabbit liver cells. *Arch. Biochem. Biophys.* 1977, **183**: 553–562.

Research in *Isolated and cultured hepatocytes* A. Guillouzo & C. Guguen-Guillouzo eds. pp. 87–112.
© 1986 John Libbey Eurotext Ltd./INSERM.

5

Fatty acid oxidation and ketogenesis in isolated hepatocytes

Jean GIRARD and Marie-Irène MALEWIAK

Centre de Recherches sur la Nutrition du CNRS, 9 rue Jules Hetzel, 92190 Meudon-Bellevue (JG), and INSERM U177, Institut Biomédical des Cordeliers, 15–21 rue de l'Ecole de Médecine, 75006 Paris (M-IM), FRANCE (M-IM is Maître de Conferences at CNAM)

SUMMARY

The nutritional state and the endocrine environment markedly influence hepatic fatty acid oxidation and ketogenesis. The principal step affected is the partition of fatty acid between esterification and oxidation. Fasting, fat-feeding or diabetes enhance fatty acid oxidation and depress fatty acid esterification whereas carbohydrate-feeding or genetic obesity have the reverse effects. The regulation of partition of fatty acid between esterification and oxidation is exerted at the level of carnitine acyltransferase I (CAT I). This enzyme is markedly inhibited by malonyl-CoA the first commited intermediate of lipogenesis. When lipogenic rates and malonyl-CoA concentrations are elevated (carbohydrate-feeding, genetic obesity) CAT I is inhibited and fatty acid oxidation and ketogenesis are reduced. When lipogenic rates and malonyl-CoA concentrations are low (starvation, fat-feeding, diabetes), CAT I is very active and fatty acid oxidation and ketogenesis are enhanced. Glucagon seems to be the principal signal which turns on fatty acid and ketogenesis. This hormone, by inhibiting glycolysis at the level of pyruvate kinase and lipogenesis at the level of acetyl-CoA carboxylase, produces a marked fall in malonyl-CoA and thus derepresses CAT I. In addition, the sensitivity of CAT I to malonyl-CoA is decreased during starvation and diabetes, a mechanism which reinforces the inhibition of CAT I due to a decrease malonyl-CoA levels. Another site of regulation of ketogenesis exists in the mitochondria but it is quantitatively much less important than CAT I.

Introduction

The non-esterified fatty acids (NEFA) reaching the liver via the circulation are long-chain fatty acids derived from dietary and adipose tissue triacylglycerols. Only a very small proportion (less than 10 per cent) of dietary fat may escape esterification in the intestine and reach the liver via the portal vein in the form of NEFA (61). Most of the dietary fat is transported to the adipose tissue in the esterified form (chylomicrons) via the lymphatic system and is not directly available for hepatic metabolism. The medium- and short-chain fatty acids are mainly of exogenous origin. Ketogenic diets containing medium-chain triacylglycerols are used in certain clinical situations to provide a source of readily absorbable fat (51). Unlike long-chain fatty acids, medium-chain fatty acids are not esterified in the intestine and they are transported primarily to the liver via the portal vein (61). In certain conditions, long-chain fatty acids derived from the hydrolysis of liver triglycerides by a lysosomal acid lipase (37, 39) can contribute to hepatic fatty acid metabolism.

Long-chain fatty acids taken up by the liver undergo a partition between two pathways: 1) esterification to form triacylglycerol and phospholipids in the extramitochondrial compartment; and 2) oxidation to CO_2 and ketone bodies within the mitochondria (Fig. 1). Oxidation of fatty acids can also occur within the peroxisomes but this represents a quantitatively minor pathway (40) which will not be considered further in the present paper. The two major ketone bodies (acetoacetate and 3-hydroxybutyrate) produced by the liver are released in the bloodstream and serve as oxidative fuel, as lipogenic precursors and as regulators of metabolism in a number of extrahepatic tissues (116).

Several reviews on the regulation of various aspects of hepatic fatty acid metabolism have been published in recent years and have provided excellent overviews of the field (22, 23, 45, 49, 58, 89, 92, 118, 135, 136, 153, 154, 165, 169). The aim of the present paper is to provide the reader with a review of the current literature and especially to discuss recent data concerning the regulation of fatty acid

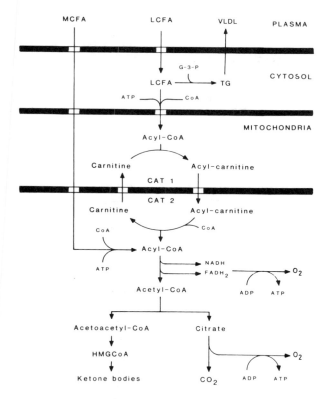

Fig. 1. Pathways of hepatic fatty acid esterification and oxidation. LCFA: long-chain fatty acids; MCFA: medium-chain fatty acids; TG: triglycerols; 3-GP: 3-glycerophosphate. Taken from reference 50.

oxidation and ketogenesis that have been obtained using isolated hepatocytes. As the developmental aspect of hepatic fatty acid oxidation and ketogenesis has been reviewed recently (50), it will not be discussed in the present paper.

Regulation of fatty acid uptake by the liver

NEFA are supplied to the liver from the plasma, where they are carried as the free acid bound to albumin (129). The uptake of NEFA by the liver appears to be an energy-independent process that functions to maintain an equilibrium between the plasma and the cellular pools of NEFA (129). Recent experiments using the perfused rat liver have suggested that the uptake of NEFA by the liver could be mediated by direct interaction of the albumin-NEFA complex with an albumin receptor on the hepatocyte surface (104). The uptake of NEFA by the liver is related to the concentration of NEFA in the plasma *in vivo* or in the medium perfusing the isolated liver *in vitro* (58). The uptake of NEFA by the liver *in vitro* can be modulated by the rate of perfusate flow (98) and by the ratio of NEFA to albumin in the medium (106,

126). Saturation of the rate of uptake of NEFA by the liver *in vitro* is approached only at concentrations exceeding 3 mM fatty acid (141), concentrations beyond those ordinarily seen in intact animals or man. The uptake of NEFA by the liver *in vitro* does not appear to be altered by starvation (72, 76, 106), diabetes (76, 141, 159, 160), pregnancy (143, 147), lactation (9, 147), thyroid state (60, 66, 130), glucagon (28, 57, 155), cyclic AMP (57), vasopressin (155) or insulin (138). However, the uptake of NEFA by isolated hepatocytes from female rats is greater than that from male rats (102, 127). Similarly, the uptake of NEFA by the perfused liver or isolated hepatocytes of rats treated with a hypolipidaemic drug, clofibrate, is higher than that from control rats (71). These differences have been related to the presence of higher amounts of fatty acid binding protein (FABP) in the cytosol of females or of males treated with clofibrate (102, 114). An increase in oleate uptake has been found in isolated hepatocytes from genetically obese Zucker rats (47, 70) which is in agreement with the enhanced activity of FABP in the liver of obese rats (99). After administration of a high fat diet to genetically obese rats, the hepatic uptake of oleate returns to the value observed in fat-fed lean littermates (70). As FABP is closely associated with hepatic fatty acid metabolism (25, 162), it remains to determine whether FABP is the mediator of sex and genetic differences and of clofibrate effects, or only a secondary response to enhanced liver fatty acid utilization.

From the above considerations, it is reasonable to postulate that *in vivo* the rate of uptake and metabolism of NEFA by the liver is primarily dependent upon the plasma concentrations of NEFA except in certain circumstances in which hepatic blood flow is decreased. For example, in short-term exercise in man there is a 40% decrease in splanchnic blood flow and hepatic ketone body production despite an increase in arterial concentration of NEFA (see reference 153). *In vivo*, the key factors which determine plasma NEFA concentrations are the amount of dietary lipids and the rate of fatty acid mobilization from adipose tissue. This latter process is primarily under hormonal and neural control (54). The extra-hepatic control of hepatic fatty acid oxidation and ketogenesis is beyond the scope of the present paper but a detailed discussion of this aspect can be found in recent reviews (78, 151, 153).

Partition of fatty acids between esterification and oxidation

On entry into the liver cells, fatty acids are immediately bound to a carrier, the fatty acid binding protein (FABP) a 12 000 dalton protein (103). Then, fatty acids of more than 12 carbon chain length are activated to their corresponding acyl-CoA in the cytosol by acyl-CoA synthetases located both in the microsomes and the outer mitochondrial membrane (118). The microsomal enzyme could be involved in providing acyl-CoA for esterification whereas the mitochondrial enzyme could provide acyl-CoA for oxidation. Whether these two enzymes share a single pool of long-chain fatty acids or whether incoming fatty acids are directed to either the microsomal or the mitochondrial enzyme depending on the physiological state is presently unknown. Moreover, as the activation of fatty acids is not rate limiting for either esterification (67) or oxidation (109), the significance of the presence of acyl-CoA synthetases in two locations in the extra-mitochondrial compartment remains obscure.

It has been suggested that FABP could be involved in directing long-chain fatty acids toward esterification since FABP enhances *in vitro* the activity of several enzymes of fatty acid esterification (26, 162). Recently it has also been reported that the binding of oleate to a cytosolic protein of 400 000 daltons was increased in starved and diabetic rats, while the binding to FABP was decreased (15). This was reversed by refeeding the starved rats or by giving insulin to diabetic rats (15). It is not known whether the 400 000 dalton protein has a specific role in directing fatty acids toward mitochondria for further oxidation. Obviously, further investigations are necessary to know the specific role of these fatty acid binding proteins in the regulation of partition of NEFA between microsomes or mitochondria.

Influence of nutritional and hormonal environment in vivo. The evidence that fatty acid oxidation and ketogenesis are tightly regulated by intrahepatic mechanisms has been obtained by using *in vitro* preparations such as the perfused liver or isolated hepatocytes in which the supply of exogenous fatty acids and regulatory factors can be accurately controlled.

When perfused or incubated (as hepatocytes) with the same concentration of oleate or palmitate, the liver of the fed rat converts a greater proportion of these long-chain fatty acids to triacylglycerol and a lesser proportion to ketone bodies than the liver of starved (9, 19, 72, 73, 76) or diabetic rats (76, 141) (Table 1). The time course of changes in blood ketone body concentration from the fed to the starved state is closely related to the rates of ketogenesis in isolated livers perfused *in vitro* with a constant concentration of oleate (80). When rats are fed a high-fat carbohydrate-free diet for 8 days, the rate of ketogenesis from oleate in isolated perfused liver was 300% higher than that of rats fed a high carbohydrate diet, and 50% higher than that of rats starved for 48 hours (65). Similar results have been obtained using isolated hepatocytes, that show that the liver of rats fed a high fat diet for 18 days converts a greater proportion of oleate to ketone bodies and a lesser proportion to triacylglycerols (Table 1). In perfused liver from pregnant rats, oleate is channelled preferentially into esterified products rather than in CO_2 or ketone bodies (143, 144). This redirection of fatty acid metabolism, however, has not been found in isolated hepatocytes from late pregnant rats (147). At peak lactation, ketogenesis from oleate was decreased whereas esterification was increased (9, 147).

It has been also demonstrated that the hormonal environment to which the liver was exposed *in vivo* influenced fatty acid metabolism *in vitro*. Livers isolated from fed rats injected or infused with anti-insulin serum (AIS) showed a decrease in triacylglycerol production and an increase in ketone body production when perfused *in vitro* with oleate (83, 159, 160). When insulin was administered to AIS-treated rats the rate of production of triacylglycerol and ketone bodies were restored *in vitro* (159, 160). Furthermore, when fed rats are infused *in vivo* for three hours with glucagon, this treatment results in an increased ketogenic capacity *in vitro*, as assessed by measuring ketone body production from constant level of oleate (83). Since these two treatments were associated *in vivo* with high plasma glucagon but with very different plasma insulin levels (low with AIS but high with glucagon infusion), this led McGarry (83) to conclude that glucagon was the principal hormonal signal to switch liver metabolism to the ketogenic mode. Other hormones such as thyroid hormones,

Table 1. Partition of [1-^{14}C] oleate taken up by hepatocytes isolated from rats in different physiological conditions between pathways of esterification and oxidation.

Physiological conditions		% distribution in			Reference
		Esterified fats	CO_2	Ketone bodies	
Males	Fed	65.9± 2.2	6.7±0.8	27.5± 1.7	106
	Fasted	30.1± 1.1	6.6±0.4	63.3± 1.1	
Males	Fed high carbohydrate diet	58.4± 3.2	3.2±0.2	38.4± 3.4	Griglio & Malewiak (unpublished data)
	Fed high fat diet	37.0± 2.6	3.0±0.3	60.0± 2.9	
Females	Virgin Fed	71.7± 7.0	10.8±2.0	17.4± 6.6	147
	Pregnant (18–21 days) Fed	57.8±10.6	9.5±2.1	32.6±10.7	
	Lactating (10–17 days) Fed	85.4± 5.6	8.3±2.9	6.3± 3.7	

glucocorticoids and sex hormones may influence hepatic fatty acid partitioning. Livers from hypothyroid rats display decreased rates of oxidation and increased rates of triacylglycerol synthesis, while livers from hyperthyroid rats show the opposite picture (5, 60, 66, 100, 105, 130, 132). Although adrenalectomy does not affect liver fatty acid metabolism *in vitro*, dexamethasone treatment induces an increased capacity for esterification and a decreased capacity for oxidation and ketogenesis (30). Livers from female rats oxidize less and esterify more fatty acids taken up than livers from male rats (102, 127) and differences become larger upon treatment of females with estradiol (146). In the perfused liver or isolated hepatocytes from genetically obese and hyperinsulinemic Zucker rats (see reference 18 for a review), long chain fatty acids are preferentially directed into the esterification pathway at the expense of oxidation (3, 4, 47, 70). After administration of a high fat diet to obese rats, the partition of fatty acids between esterification and oxidation becomes comparable to that of fat-fed lean littermates (70). Thus, in a large number of physiological situations there is a reciprocal relationship between fatty acid esterification and oxidation in the liver. One notable exception is the liver from clofibrate-treated rats that esterifies fatty acids as much as the control livers, but oxidizes fatty acids at a rate 3–4 fold greater than in controls (71).

Direct hormonal effects in vitro. Several hormones have been shown to have a direct effect on hepatic fatty acid metabolism *in vitro*. Glucagon stimulates the oxidation and decreases the esterification of long-chain fatty acids in the perfused liver (57) and in isolated hepatocytes (9, 28, 29, 88, 90, 125, 161) from rats fed or refed a high carbohydrate diet. The effects of glucagon are particularly evident at low concentration of fatty acids in the medium (91) and when rats are meal fed a high sucrose, fat free diet (88, 90). Glucagon is without effect on fatty acid oxidation and esterification in the liver of fasted rats. Vasopressin and angiotensin II inhibit ketogenesis by 20–25% and stimulate esterification of oleate or palmitate in isolated hepatocytes from fed rats (1, 122, 155). In addition, vasopressin and angiotensin II increase the conversion of oleate to CO_2 and this effect accounts for 40–50% of the decrease in ketone body formation (122, 133, 137). There are few reports on the direct effects of catecholamines on hepatic ketogenesis. Slight stimulation of ketogenesis by adrenaline was observed using the perfused rat liver (62) but no effect or a slight inhibition (15–20%) of ketogenesis from oleate by adrenaline or noradrenaline were found using isolated hepatocytes from fed rats (122, 137).

Evidence for direct effects of insulin on hepatic fatty acid metabolism *in vitro* is scanty. Insulin has been reported to inhibit ketogenesis and to stimulate the esterification of oleate by livers from fed rats perfused with homologous whole blood (6, 138). In contrast, insulin has marginal effects on the metabolism of oleate in hepatocytes isolated from meal fed rats (12) or has no effect on isolated hepatocytes from fed, starved or diabetic rats (157, 161). The reason for insulin insensitivity in most *in vitro* liver preparations is unknown. In contrast, insulin is capable to antagonize the ketogenic effects of submaximal concentrations of glucagon in isolated hepatocytes from fed rats (56, 157, 161) and in cultured hepatocytes (56). This has led to a postulate that the acute effects of insulin on liver metabolism in vitro are exclusively exerted through its ability to offset the catabolic effects of glucagon (12).

Mechanisms involved in the regulation of partition of fatty acids between esterification and oxidation

From a theoretical standpoint there are a number of possible ways of regulating the partitioning of long-chain fatty acyl-CoA between the pathways of esterification and oxidation. These include a change in the activity of the rate limiting enzymes either by allosteric effectors or by substrate and cofactor availability (short-term control) or by the actual amount of enzyme (long-term control). In addition, since regulation is being exerted at a branch-point it can either be exerted on one of the two pathways or in a reciprocal manner on both pathways simultaneously. The two pathways will be analysed successively.

Fatty acid esterification. At least two mechanisms could be involved in the regulation of liver fatty acid esterification: 1) the alteration in the activity of one or several enzymes implied in the pathway of triacylglycerol synthesis; and, 2) the availability of glycerol-3-phosphate.

In the liver, triacylglycerol synthesis is initiated by glycerol phosphate acyltransferase (GPAT) which is located in both the microsomal and the mitochondrial membranes (23, 118). The microsomal and mitochondrial enzymes have different properties and are different proteins. Since mitochondria lack the enzymes required for further metabolism of phosphatidate, this intermediate must be transferred to the microsomes where triglyceride synthesis is completed. Phosphatidate is first converted to diacylglycerol by phosphatidate phosphohydrolase (PAP) and diacylglycerol is converted to triacylglycerol by diacylglycerol acyltransferase (DGAT) (for reviews see references 23 and 118).

Starvation and diabetes have been shown to decrease the activity of mitochondrial GPAT but not of microsomal GPAT (7), and to increase the activity of PAP (23). In addition, the activity of GPAT and PAP is under short-term regulation by several hormones. Insulin increases mitochondrial GPAT in perfused rat liver (6, 8). Glucagon or cyclic AMP decreases GPAT (128, 134) and DGAT (53) activities in perfused liver or isolated hepatocytes. Vasopressin increases the activity of microsomal and mitochondrial GPAT (134) and of PAP (112) in isolated rat hepatocytes. It was recently demonstrated that oleic acid promotes the activation and the translocation of PAP from the cytosol to particulate fractions of isolated rat hepatocytes (26), thus facilitating the increased synthesis of triacylglycerol in the liver when it is presented with an increased supply of fatty acids (26). However, the changes in enzyme activities mentioned above are not always correlated with changes in triacylglycerol synthesis (for example the activity of PAP increases during starvation whereas fatty acid esterification decreases) and they are generally of small magnitude (± 20–30%).

The possibility that the availability of glycerol-3-phosphate (G-3-P) could determine the rate of triacylglycerol synthesis was first proposed by Fritz (46) who postulated that the enhanced rate of hepatic fatty acid oxidation seen in ketotic states was secondary to a diminished esterification capacity resulting from a fall in glycerol-3-phosphate (due to decreased glycolysis and increased gluconeogenesis).

Several recent observations seem to support this hypothesis. First, in glycogen-depleted hepatocytes from fed rats the concentration of G-3-P was very low as well as the rate of palmitate esterification (41, 42). Raising the G-3-P concentration by addition of precursors to the cells resulted in a marked stimulation of palmitate esterification (41, 42). Secondly, glucagon which stimulated fatty acid oxidation and inhibited esterification also decreased G-3-P concentration in isolated rat hepatocytes (10, 29, 38, 41, 42, 69). Addition of glycerol into the incubation medium prevented the fall in liver G-3-P and restored a high rate of fatty acid esterification (41, 42, 69). Thirdly, decreased G-3-P concentration and diminished rate of triacylglycerol synthesis have also been found in the perfused liver of hyperthyroid rats (105). Infusion of glycerol raised the G-3-P levels in the liver and enhanced triacylglycerol synthesis (105). All these data suggest that G-3-P can be rate limiting for fatty acid esterification when its concentration falls below 0.5 μmol/g. However, it is doubtful that G-3-P concentration in the liver *in vivo* falls below this value under conditions where active lipolysis occurs in adipose tissue since the amount of glycerol released is made available to the liver to synthesize G-3-P. The fall in cellular G-3-P may thus be peculiar to the conditions which occur in isolated hepatocytes *in vitro* (eg glycogen depletion, absence of glycerol).

A number of observations, however, are not consistent with the hypothesis that G-3-P could determine the rate of triglyceride synthesis. First, there is a lack of correlation between the ability of various compounds to reverse starvation ketosis in the rat and their effects on liver glycerol-3-phosphate concentration (150). Secondly, liver glycerol-3-phosphate concentration is increased during starvation (72) and nevertheless the rate of fatty acid esterification is depressed. Thirdly, time course studies during the development of diabetic ketoacidosis in rats revealed that hyperketonaemia preceded the accumulation of triacylglycerol in the liver (94).

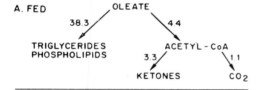

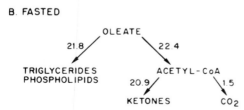

Fig. 2.
Metabolism of oleate in perfused livers from fed and fasted rats. Values refer to the flux of oleate through various pathways and, for simplicity, are expressed in arbitrary units. (+)-Decanoylcarnitine was used to inhibit the carnitine acyltransferase reaction. Reproduced from references 76 & 80.

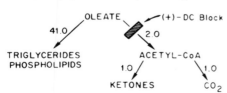

Altogether, these data suggest that enhanced triglyceride synthesis represented a 'spillover' of fatty acids from a saturated oxidation pathway (92). Fourthly, when the oxidation of oleate in liver from fasted or diabetic rats was inhibited by (+)-decanoylcarnitine (79, 80), (+)-octanoylcarnitine (82) or tetradecylglycydic acid (59), oleate taken up by the liver was entirely converted to esterified products (Fig. 2), indicating that the esterification capacity was intact and functional in the ketotic states.

Thus, limitation of fatty acid esterification does not appear to be a major factor in the regulation of ketogenesis in starvation and diabetes.

Fatty acid oxidation. As the inner mitochondrial membrane is impermeable to CoA and acyl-CoA, a specific transport system is required for the transfer of long-chain acyl-CoA into the mitochondria for subsequent β-oxidation (Fig. 1). This transfer involves the sequential actions of two carnitine acyltransferases (reviews are available in references 21 and 46). Carnitine acyltransferase I (CAT I), located on the outer side of the inner mitochondrial membrane, catalyses the synthesis of acylcarnitine esters which are then translocated through the inner mitochondrial membrane into the matrix by carnitine acylcarnitine translocase (see reviews in references 21 and 22). Carnitine acyltransferase II (CAT II), located on the inside surface of the inner mitochondrial membrane, converts acylcarnitine esters into their corresponding acyl-CoA which are oxidized in two stages by specific enzymes located in the mitochondrial matrix. In the first stage, acyl-CoA undergoes β-oxidation which generates acetyl-CoA, NADH and $FADH_2$. In the second stage, a part of acetyl-CoA is oxidized via the citric cycle to yield CO_2, H_2O and further NADH and $FADH_2$ and the other part is used for ketone body synthesis. The reduced equivalents (NADH and $FADH_2$) may enter the respiratory chain to yield ATP (Fig. 1).

In contrast to long-chain fatty acids (oleate, palmitate), the short-chain (butyrate) or medium-chain (octanoate) fatty acids readily traverse the mitochondrial membranes and are activated to their corresponding acyl-CoA by the short- or medium-chain acyl-CoA synthetases located in the mitochondrial matrix (Fig. 1). Short- or medium-chain acyl-CoA then undergo β-oxidation as do long-chain acyl-CoA. Thus, octanoate and butyrate are routinely used in comparison with oleate or palmitate to distinguish between metabolic regulation occurring before or after the carnitine-dependent steps of fatty acid oxidation. The rates of oxidation and ketogenesis from short-chain (butyrate) or medium-chain (octanoate) fatty acids are slightly higher in the liver of starved and diabetic rats than in the liver of fed rats (64, 72, 147). Similarly, rats fed a high fat diet have a higher rate of ketogenesis from octanoate than rats fed a high carbohydrate diet (64). However, the differences in the rates of oxidation and ketogenesis are considerably less marked than with long-chain fatty acids (Table 2). This suggested that the principal site of control of fatty acid oxidation and ketogenesis was located at the level of the carnitine acyltransferase complex.

How is the activity of CAT complex regulated? There are at least three possibilities: 1) an increase in maximal activity of CAT I, of carnitine acylcarnitine translocase or of CAT II; 2) an alteration in the concentration of their substrates: carnitine, acyl-CoA and acylcarnitine; and, 3) the variation in the concentration of an allosteric effector of those enzymes.

Table 2. Comparison of the rates of ketogenesis from oleate, octanoate or butyrate by perfused liver or isolated hepatocytes from rats in different physiological conditions.

Physiological conditions	Rates of ketogenesis (μmol/hour/g wet weight)				Reference
	Endogenous	Oleate	Octanoate	Butyrate	
Perfused liver					
Females					
Fed	5±1	33± 4	57± 5	54± 3	64 & 65
Fasted 48 hours	30±3	98± 5	128± 7	94±14	
Fed high fat diet	44±4	146± 8	145± 8	—	
Isolated hepatocytes					
Females					
Fed	2±1	23± 9	—	73±17	147
Fasted 24 hours	33±9	95±16	—	139±20	
Males					
Fed high carbohydrate diet	3±1	33± 3	69±11	—	Griglio & Malewiak
Fed high fat diet	7±2	88±12	141±19	—	(unpublished data)

1) Control of carnitine acylhandsferase complex. The activity of CAT I, but not of CAT II has been reported to increase by 50–100% on starvation, in diabetes, in hyperthyroid states and during the feeding of a high-fat diet (2, 20, 55, 119, 120, 121, 131), but other workers have not found any difference in the total activity of CAT between fed and starved states, in diabetes or after feeding a high fat diet (14, 44, 86). A slight increase in carnitine-acylcarnitine translocase activity has been found in the mitochondria of ketotic rats (110) which could account for the 70–100% increase in (−)-octanoylcarnitine oxidation in mitochondria from starved rats (163). Indeed, this precursor requires only carnitine-acylcarnitine translocase and CAT II for its entry into β-oxidation. Initial studies showing that the rate of ketogenesis from (−)-octanoylcarnitine was increased in the perfused liver of starved or diabetic rats (81) have not been confirmed by experiments performed with isolated hepatocytes (92). It has been suggested that the differences seen in perfused liver could have reflected changes in permeability of the tissue towards (−)-octanoylcarnitine rather than alterations in the activity of translocase or CAT II; such differences not being expressed in isolated hepatocytes (92). Nevertheless, even if changes in maximal activity of CAT I, or of carnitine acylcarnitine translocase occur in the expected direction to enable an increased rate of fatty acid oxidation, they are of too small a magnitude to explain the enhanced rate of fatty acid oxidation seen in starved or diabetic rats. On the other hand, fatty acid oxidation by hepatocytes from genetically obese rats is decreased (70, 140) while the oxidative capacity of hepatic mitochondria from these rats is unchanged (13) as well as the activity of CAT I (13, 101).

This explains why McGarry and his collaborators chose to examine whether alterations in the availability of a substrate or of an effector of the carnitine acyltransferase system could be responsible for the activation of the rate of transfer of long-chain acyl-CoA into the mitochondria in ketotic states. This aspect has been described in detail in recent reviews (45, 89, 92) and it will be only summarized briefly here.

2) Availability of carnitine. It has been found that the concentration of hepatic carnitine was increased *in vivo* in a number of situations associated with an enhanced rate of ketogenesis *in vitro*: starvation, uncontrolled diabetes, injection of fed rats with glucagon or anti-insulin serum (83, 84, 117). McGarry and his collaborators have proposed two hypotheses to explain the increase in liver carnitine: 1) *de novo* synthesis within the liver or; 2) transport from peripheral tissue and increased uptake by the liver. However, recent experiments suggest that the rise in hepatic carnitine concentration during starvation could be entirely accounted for by the decrease in liver mass secondary to water and glycogen mobilization. Moreover, the relation between ketogenesis and liver carnitine concentration does not always hold. Indeed, the liver of fed early-lactating rats has a 2–3-fold higher concentration of carnitine than the liver of non-lactating rats, yet on perfusion *in vitro*, the rates of ketogenesis from added oleate are similar (117). A clue to this paradox might lie in an unique feature of the liver of the fed lactating rat that is simultaneously rich in both carnitine and glycogen (see the paragraphs on malonyl-CoA levels). Studies with perfused liver (84) or isolated hepatocytes (27, 152) from fed rats have also shown that exogenously added carnitine increases ketogenesis from oleate and decreases the proportion of the fatty acid esterified, but that the absolute increase in ketogenesis is

50% less than that observed in hepatocytes from starved rats. Furthermore, administration of carnitine to fed rats to achieve hepatic concentrations found in starvation did not increase circulating ketone bodies (16). Likewise, addition of carnitine does not fully restore the ketogenic capacity of hepatocytes obtained from obese Zucker rats (140). Finally, carnitine does not increase the rate of oxidation of palmitoylcarnitine by isolated rat liver mitochondria which suggests that the activity of carnitine acylcarnitine translocase plus CAT II is not limited by the availability of carnitine (17). This suggests that other factors, in addition to carnitine, are involved in the regulation of hepatic fatty acid oxidation and ketogenesis.

3) Malonyl-CoA levels. In the rat, a temporal relationship between hepatic glycogen content *in vivo* and the rate of ketogenesis *in vitro* has been demonstrated during the transition from the fed to the starved state (80) and after administration of anti-insulin serum or glucagon to fed animals (83).

If it is accepted that the major physiological role of ketone bodies is to supply an alternative substrate to glucose for the brain, it clearly would be of a considerable advantage if there was a regulatory link not only between the blood concentrations of glucose and ketone bodies but also between the carbohydrate status of the liver and the rate of ketogenesis. In this context the term carbohydrate status includes not only the availability of glycogen and concentrations of glycolytic intermediates within the liver, but also the predominant direction of carbon flux, ie glycogenolysis, glycolysis and lipogenesis versus gluconeogenesis.

Indirect evidence suggests that it is not the molecule of glycogen *per se* which influences the rate of ketogenesis. Overnight fasting hyperketonaemia is observed both in infants in whom hepatic glycogen is virtually absent (glycogen synthetase deficiency) or who are incapable of mobilizing their large liver glycogen stores (glycogen phosphorylase or amylo-1,6-glucosidase deficiencies) (see reference 153 for a review). In contrast, infants with glucose-6-phosphatase or fructose-1,6-diphosphatase deficiencies have a lower ketonaemia but a higher triglyceridaemia in response to an overnight fast (a review is in reference 153). Moreover, experiments performed with the perfused liver of fed rats have shown that a part of glycogen which is degraded provides acetyl-CoA to sustain hepatic lipogenesis (142, 158). This suggests that the glycolytic or lipogenic fluxes, or the availability of glycolytic or lipogenic intermediates may provide a link between carbohydrate status of the liver and its ketogenic capacity.

Possible mechanisms whereby alterations in the rates of glycolysis and lipogenesis could contribute to the regulation of hepatic ketone body production are also discussed in a recent review (92) and will be only briefly summarized here. It has long been known that the opposing sequences of fatty acid synthesis and fatty acid oxidation in liver were reciprocally related; with carbohydrate feeding (low glucagon:insulin ratio in plasma) the capacity of the liver to oxidize NEFA is limited and its ability to synthetize fat from carbohydrate is high. Conversely, in starvation or uncontrolled diabetes (high glucagon:insulin ratio in plasma) hepatic fatty acid synthesis is abolished with concomitant activation of fatty acid oxidation. Furthermore, just as glucagon administration activates ketogenesis in the liver, it was also known that glucagon suppressed hepatic fatty acid synthesis (31, 49, 88, 90). This raised the possibility that some intermediates involved in fatty acid synthesis from carbohydrates might act as an inhibitor of fatty acid oxidation (Fig. 3). Among the various intermediates of glycolysis, citric acid cycle and lipogenesis tested for their capacity to block oleate oxidation *in vitro*, only one compound was effective: malonyl-CoA (85). Malonyl-CoA is the first committed intermediate in the conversion of carbohydrate to fat and its concentration in liver fluctuates in parallel with the rate of fatty acid synthesis (31, 52, 87). The property to inhibit fatty acid oxidation was specific for malonyl-CoA, since it could not be duplicated by a number of other CoA derivatives and was reversible (85). The site of action of malonyl-CoA is the CAT I, the first reaction specific of fatty acid oxidation (86). Malonyl-CoA inhibits the oxidation of oleate, palmitate and palmitoyl-CoA, all of which require CAT I plus CAT II to enter the β-oxidation sequence, but malonyl-CoA does not inhibit the oxidation of octanoate, octanoylcarnitine or palmitoylcarnitine which bypass CAT I (86). Malonyl-CoA is an extremely potent inhibitor of CAT I, with a K_i of 1–2 μM, whereas CAT II is insensitive to malonyl-CoA (86). The inhibition was initially thought to be competitive with long-chain acyl-CoA but recent kinetic studies suggest that carnitine and acyl-CoA are bound to a catalytic sub-unit, while malonyl-CoA binds to a regulatory sub-unit (36, 95, 96). Thus, under condition of carbohydrate feeding, the conversion of glucose into fat is enhanced, malonyl-CoA levels are elevated and inhibit CAT I; consequently, fatty acid oxidation is shut down. In contrast, in ketotic states the conversion of glucose to fat is suppressed, malonyl-CoA levels are very low and CAT I becomes derepressed; and, consequently, fatty acid oxidation and ketogenesis are enhanced. The acute stimulatory

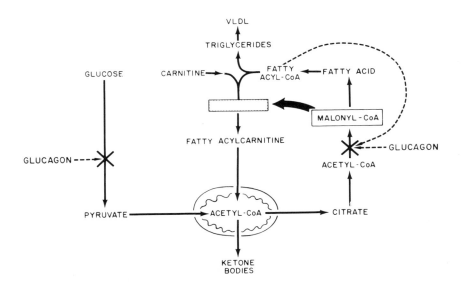

Fig. 3. Regulatory interactions between the pathways of fatty acid synthesis and oxidation in liver. In the fed state, malonyl-CoA levels are high, assuring rapid fatty acid synthesis and suppression of fatty acid oxidation (through inhibition of carnitine acyltransferase I). Malonyl-CoA concentrations may be lowered by glucagon excess or high tissue levels of fatty acyl-CoA. In both cases, the net result is cessation of lipogenesis and activation of fatty acid oxidation and ketogenesis (see text for details). Reproduced from reference 92.

effect of glucagon on hepatic fatty acid oxidation and ketogenesis could result from its capacity to inhibit two key enzymes of glycolysis and lipogenesis: pyruvate kinase and acetyl-CoA carboxylase, thus decreasing hepatic malonyl-CoA concentrations (reviews in references 49 and 92). More prolonged exposure of the liver to conditions of insulin deficiency and glucagon excess, such as during starvation and diabetes, presumably leads to a major decrease in the amount of pyruvate kinase and acetyl-CoA carboxylase (reviews in references 49 and 92).

The validity of this hypothesis has been tested in isolated rat hepatocytes in a variety of conditions where the concentration of malonyl-CoA and the rate of fatty acid synthesis were altered over a wide range. When hepatocytes from meal fed rats were incubated in the presence of glucose, lactate and pyruvate, the rate of lipogenesis as well as the malonyl-CoA levels were very high whereas oleate oxidation was very low (Fig. 4). The exposure of these hepatocytes to a combination of glucagon and 5-(tetradecyloxy)-2-furoic acid (RMI 14,514, an inhibitor of lipogenesis) produced a fall of malonyl-CoA and of lipogenesis, and a 5- and 12-fold increase of fatty acid oxidation and ketogenesis (Fig. 4). The further addition of carnitine had no effect on malonyl-CoA or lipogenesis but enhanced fatty acid oxidation and ketogenesis, 7- and 19-fold respectively (88, 90). In the obese Zucker rat, abnormally high rates of hepatic lipogenesis have been reported (70a, 139) which can be depressed by feeding a high fat diet (70a). High malonyl-CoA concentrations could explain the low rate of hepatic fatty acid oxidation in the obese rat. Fat feeding by lowering hepatic malonyl-CoA levels could restore a high rate of hepatic fatty acid

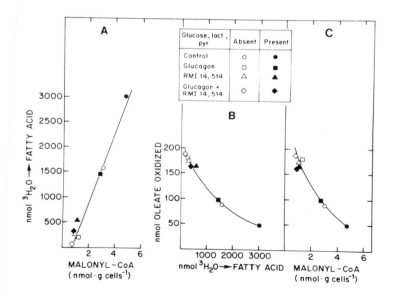

Fig. 4. Relationship between fatty acid synthesis, fatty acid oxidation and malonyl-CoA levels in hepatocytes from fed rats. Hepatocytes were incubated with 0.4 mM sodium oleate (labelled or unlabelled) bound to albumin in the absence or presence of the agents indicated. Glucose, lactate, pyruvate, RMI 14,514 and glucagon were used in concentrations of 10 mM, 1 mM, 1 mM, 0.2 mM and 4 μg per ml, respectively. Reproduced from reference 92.

oxidation. This is supported by the fact that fat feeding does not affect fatty acid oxidation in isolated mitochondria (14). However, it has been suggested that the reciprocal relationship between fatty acid synthesis and oxidation in liver, while related to the control of ketogenesis, could not account for the huge increase in hepatic ketogenic capacity caused by fasting or diabetes (9). Indeed, the depression of lipogenesis in the liver of fed rats by increased concentration of non-esterified fatty acids (74, 91), by inhibition of citrate cleavage enzyme with (-)hydroxycitrate (24), by inhibition of acetyl-CoA carboxylase with 5-(tetradecyloxy)-2-furoic acid (9, 32, 48) or by acute depletion of glycolytic intermediates (152) does not result in the same large rise of ketogenesis as that observed in starved or diabetic rats. This suggests that if changes in malonyl-CoA concentration obviously represent an important mechanism for controlling fatty acid oxidation and ketogenesis, some other mechanisms must also exist to fully explain the transition from fed to starved or diabetic states.

Several groups of investigators have shown that the sensitivity of CAT I to inhibition by malonyl-CoA is much greater in fed than in the fasted (20, 33, 34, 107, 116, 119, 120, 121) or diabetic rats (35). However, McGarry & Foster (93) have claimed that the difference in CAT I sensitivity to malonyl-CoA was of minor importance to explain the changes in fatty acid oxidation in the transition from the fed to starved state. They report their data to an equivalent amount of cells by equating 1 g cells from fed rats to 0.625 g cells from starved rats, assuming a 37.5% decrease in cell weight with starvation. Under these conditions, the high rates of fatty acid oxidation observed in hepatocytes from starved rats must be accounted for by the fall in hepatic malonyl-CoA (88, 90). Since it is the concentration of malonyl-CoA and not its total cell content which affects CAT I activity, it has been proposed that malonyl-CoA concentration should be compared per an equivalent water space, ie per g of cell (108). In these conditions, fatty acid oxidation was increased by 2.5-fold in hepatocytes from starved rats whereas malonyl-CoA was decreased by only 16% (108). This suggests that fatty acid oxidation in hepatocytes from starved rats is less sensitive to malonyl-CoA inhibition than fatty acid oxidation in hepatocytes from refed rats.

A decreased sensitivity to malonyl-CoA could theoretically result from several factors including an enhanced CAT I activity, an increased K_m for acyl-CoA or K_i for malonyl-CoA. Recent studies have shown that the apparent K_m of CAT I for acyl-CoA was not altered by starvation (36). In contrast, the K_i of CAT I for malonyl-CoA was increased 10-fold during starvation, so that the affinity of the enzyme for malonyl-CoA was greatly reduced (36).

Subsequently, it was shown that the relative sensitivity of CAT I activity to malonyl-CoA inhibition in rat liver mitochondria isolated from animals in various physiological states was proportional to the hepatic malonyl-CoA concentration *in vivo* (116). More recently it was shown that CAT I in rat liver mitochondria preincubated with malonyl-CoA was more sensitive to inhibition by malonyl-CoA than was the enzyme in mitochondria preincubated in the absence of malonyl-CoA (166). This effect was rapid and reversible and resulted in a transition from a state of low affinity of CAT I for malonyl-CoA to a state of high affinity for malonyl-CoA (167, 168).

So, the bulk of evidence suggests that the increase in long-chain fatty acid oxidation which occurs in ketotic states results primarily from both a decrease in hepatic malonyl-CoA concentration and a lowered sensitivity of CAT I to malonyl-CoA.

Mitochondrial β-oxidation

There is evidence that once acyl-CoA have reached the mitochondrial matrix the rate of β-oxidation is turned on and is not influenced by nutritional or hormonal factors. This has been clearly demonstrated by measuring the metabolic rates of $[1-^{14}C]$-octanoate in perfused liver from fed, fasted and diabetic rats (Table 3). $[1-^{14}C]$-octanoate was oxidized to acetyl-CoA at identical rates in livers from fed, fasted and diabetic rats (290, 293 and 302 μmol/hour/100 g body wt, calculated from the total recovery of isotope into ketones, CO_2 and fatty acids) (77). Thus the rate of conversion of acyl-CoA to acetyl-CoA in the mitochondria is identical in non-ketotic and in ketotic states.

Table 3. The incorporation of $[1-^{14}C]$-octanoate into CO_2, fatty acids and ketone bodies in perfused livers from fed, fasted and diabetic rats. From McGarry & Foster (77).

Condition	Labelled C units incorporated into (μmol/hour/100 g body wt)		
	Ketones	CO_2	Fatty acids
Fed	111± 4	87±6	92±13
Fasted	243±11	41±3	9± 1
Diabetic	273±18	18±1	11± 1

Partition of acetyl-CoA between citrate synthesis and acetoacetyl-CoA synthesis

From the data presented in Table 3 it is clear that the partition of acetyl-CoA between citrate synthesis and ketogenesis is controlled. The underutilization of acetyl-CoA in citric acid cycle and in lipogenesis accounts for the 2.5-fold increase in ketogenesis in fasted and diabetic rats (Table 3). This is in agreement with the calculations of Williamson *et al.* (156) indicating that a depression of citric acid cycle is not required for accelerated rates of ketogenesis to occur in fasted rats and with the assessment made by Regen & Terrell (113) that underutilization of acetyl-CoA for lipogenesis contributes to enhanced ketogenesis during starvation. In fasted rats, the defect in lipogenesis is primarily responsible for the diversion of acetyl-CoA into the ketogenic pathway whereas in diabetic rats a decrease in citric acid cycle contributes also to direct acetyl-CoA to ketogenic pathway (Table 3).

It has been postulated that a primary factor responsible for the diversion of acetyl-CoA from citrate synthesis to ketone body formation was an oxaloacetate deficiency. The fall in hepatic oxaloacetate concentration could result from its diversion to malate because of the increased redox state during fatty acid oxidation (148) or PEP because of the enhanced rate of gluconeogenesis (63). *In vivo*, the administration of 3-mercaptopicolinate (a specific inhibitor of phosphoenolpyruvate carboxykinase and of gluconeogenesis) to fasted, diabetic or medium-chain triglyceride fed rats produced an increase in hepatic oxaloacetate concentration and a fall in blood ketone bodies (11, 145). In isolated hepatocytes from starved rats the rate of ketogenesis from oleate has been found to be inversely correlated with free mitochondrial oxaloacetate concentration (123, 124). According to these authors, the decrease in hepatic oxaloacetate concentration could only explain 25–30% of the increase in ketone body production in starved animals. More recently it has been shown that 3-mercaptopicolinate inhibited ketogenesis from oleate and octanoate in hepatocytes from fasted rats (43) incubated in the presence of lactate and pyruvate (Table 4). In primary chick liver cell culture, cAMP activates ketogenesis from octanoate or acetate as a result in a fall of mitochondrial oxaloacetate concentration (97). The stimulatory effect of cAMP on ketogenesis from acetate is reversed by lactate secondarily to an increase in mitochondrial oxaloacetate concentration (97). Thus, it is clear that ketogenesis is controlled at the mitochondrial branch point of acetyl-CoA metabolism but, from a quantitative point of view, this regulatory step is far less important than CAT I.

Table 4. Rates of ketogenesis from oleate or octanoate by hepatocytes from fasted rats incubated in the presence or the absence of 3-mercaptopicolinate, an inhibitor of gluconeogenesis.

Condition	Rates of ketogenesis from ($\mu mol/50\ min/10^9\ hepatocytes$)	
	Oleate	Octanoate
None	33 ± 3	214 ± 28
3 MPA	33 ± 3	194 ± 19
Lactate + pyruvate	26 ± 2	204 ± 31
Lactate + pyruvate + 3 MPA	19 ± 1*	139 ± 21*

Rats were fasted 48 hours. Hepatocytes were incubated either in the presence of oleate 0.35 mM or octanoate 0.78 mM. When added, lactate and pyruvate concentrations were 0.75 and 0.075 mM and 3 MPA concentration was 0.1 mM. * Difference significant ($P<0.01$) from control values. From reference 43.

Conversion of acetoacetyl-CoA to ketone bodies

The major route of formation of ketone bodies in the liver mitochondria is via hydroxymethylglutaryl-CoA (HMG-CoA) (149, 151). HMG-CoA synthase is thought to be the rate limiting enzyme for ketogenesis from acetyl-CoA (149, 151). The hepatic activities of the enzymes of the HMG-CoA pathway in the rat liver do not change during starvation (75, 149) but increase slightly after fat feeding or induction of diabetes (149). This minor fluctuation in the activities of hepatic enzymes responsible for ketogenesis cannot account for the dramatic increase in ketosis associated with diabetes or starvation (a review is in reference 92).

Conclusions

The data described above strongly suggest that the principal mechanism involved in the regulation of fatty acid oxidation and ketogenesis is the inhibition or activation of CAT I. Other sites of regulation exist at the level of esterification and of partition of acetyl-CoA between citric acid cycle and ketogenesis but they are quantitatively of minor importance. However, it must be recalled that all the data on the regulation of fatty acid oxidation and ketogenesis have been collected in a single species: the rat. To what extent the mechanisms involved in the regulation of fatty acid oxidation and ketogenesis in the rat can be extrapolated to other species and particularly to man needs further investigation. For example, in ruminants and the pig the rates of hepatic lipogenesis are very low both in fed and starved animals and it is not unreasonable to question the importance of malonyl-CoA in the regulation of fatty acid oxidation in these species (68, 111). Furthermore, if the pig has been shown that more than 90 per cent of oleate taken up by the liver cells was esterified whatever the nutritional status (111). This clearly underlines the necessity to collect more information in different species before accepting the idea that changes in malonyl-CoA levels represent the only mechanism to turn on hepatic fatty acid oxidation and ketogenesis.

REFERENCES

1 Almas I., Singh B., Borreback B.: The action of vasopressin and calcium on palmitate metabolism in hepatocytes and isolated mitochondria from rat liver. *Arch. Biochem. Biophys.* 1983, **222**: 370–379.

2 Amatruda J. M., Lockwood D. H., Margolis S., Kiesow L. A.: [^{14}C] Palmitate uptake in isolated rat liver mitochondria: effects of fasting, diabetes mellitus, and inhibitors of carnitine acyltransferase. *J. Lipid Res.* 1978, **19**: 688–694.

3 Azain M. J., Martin R. J.: Effect of genetic obesity on the regulation of hepatic fatty acid metabolism. *Am. J. Physiol.* 1983, **244**: R400–R406.

4 Azain M. J., Martin R. J.: Hepatic palmitate metabolism in fasting Zucker rats: effect of lactate on partitioning. *Am. J. Physiol.* 1984, **246**: R1011–R1014.

5 Bartels P. D., Sestoft L.: Thyroid hormone-induced changes in gluconeogenesis and ketogenesis in perfused rat liver. *Biochim. Biophys. Acta* 1980, **633**: 56–57.

6 Bates E. J., Topping D. L., Sooranna S. R., Saggerson D., Mayes P.: Acute effects of insulin on glycerol phosphate acyltransferase activity, ketogenesis and serum free fatty acid concentration in perfused rat liver. *FEBS Lett.* 1977, **84**: 225–228.

7 Bates E. J., Saggerson D.: A selective decrease in mitochondrial glycerol phosphate acyltransferase activity in livers from streptozotocin-diabetic rats. *FEBS Lett.* 1977, **84**: 229–232.

8 Bates E. J., Saggerson E. D.: A study of the glycerol phosphate acyltransferase and dihydroxyacetone phosphate acyltransferase activities in rat liver mitochondria and microsomal fractions. *Biochem. J.* 1979, **182**: 751–762.

9 Benito M., Williamson D. H.: Evidence for a reciprocal relationship between lipogenesis and ketogenesis in hepatocytes from fed virgin and lactating rats. *Biochem. J.* 1978, **176**: 331–334.

10 Beynen A. C., Vaartjes W. J., Geelen M. J. M.: Acute effects of insulin on fatty acid metabolism in isolated rat hepatocytes. *Horm. Metab. Res.* 1980, **12**: 425–430.

11 Blackshear P. J., Holloway P. A. H., Alberti K. G. M. M.: The effects of inhibition of gluconeogenesis on ketogenesis in starved and diabetic rats. *Biochem. J.* 1975, **148**: 353–362.

12 Boyd M. E., Albright E. B., Foster D. W., McGarry J. D.: *In vitro* reversal of the fasting state of liver metabolism in the rat. Reevaluation of the roles of insulin and glucose. *J. Clin. Invest.* 1981, **68**: 142–152.

13 Brady L. J., Hoppel C. L.: Hepatic mitochondrial function in lean and obese Zucker rats. *Am. J. Physiol.* 1983, **245**: E239–E245.

14 Brady L. J., Hoppel C. L.: Effect of diet and starvation on hepatic mitochondrial function in the rat. *J. Nutr.* 1983, **113**: 2129–2137.

15 Brandes R., Arad R.: Liver cytosolic fatty acid binding proteins. Effect of diabetes and starvation. *Biochim. Biophys. Acta* 1983, **750**: 334–339.

16 Brass E. P., Hoppel C. L.: Disassociation between acid-insoluble acylcarnitines and ketogenesis following carnitine administration *in vivo. J. Biol. Chem.* 1978, **253**: 5274–5276.

17 Brass E. P., Hoppel C. L.: Effect of carnitine on mitochondrial oxidation of palmitoylcarnitine. *Biochem. J.* 1980, **188**: 451–458.

18 Bray G. A., York D. A.: Hypothalamic and genetic obesity in experimental animals: an anatomic and endocrine hypothesis. *Physiol. Rev.* 1979, **59**: 719–809.

19 Bremer J., Christiansen R. Z., Borreback B.: Regulation of partition of free fatty acids between triglyceride synthesis and β-oxidation in liver. In: *Regulatory Mechanisms of Carbohydrate Metabolism*, V. Esmann (Ed.): Pergamon Press, Oxford, 1978, pp 161–170.

20 Bremer J.: The effect of fasting on the activity of liver carnitine palmitoyltransferase and its inhibition by malonyl-CoA. *Biochim. Biophys. Acta* 1981, **665**: 628–631.

21 Bremer J.: Carnitine. Metabolism and functions. *Physiol. Rev.* 1983, **63**: 1420–1480.

22 Bremer J., Osmundsen H.: Fatty acid oxidation and its regulation. In: *Fatty Acid Metabolism and its Regulation*, S. Numa (Ed.): Elsevier, Amsterdam, 1984, pp 113–154.

23 Brindley D. N., Lawson N.: Control of triglyceride synthesis. In: *The Adipocyte and Obesity: Cellular and Molecular Mechanisms*, A. Angel, C. H. Hollenberg, D. A. K. Roncari (Eds): Raven Press, New York, 1983, pp 155–164.

24 Brunengraber H., Bautry M., Lowenstein J. M.: Fatty acid, 3-β-hydroxysterol and ketone synthesis in the perfused rat liver. Effects of (-)hydroxycitrate and oleate. *Eur. J. Biochem.* 1978, **82**: 373–384.

25 Burnett D. A. Lysenko L., Manning J. A., Ockner R. K.: Utilization of long chain fatty acids by rat liver: studies of the role of fatty acid binding protein. *Gastroenterology* 1979, **77**: 241–249.

26 Cascales C., Mangiapane E. H., Brindley D. N.: Oleic acid promotes the activation and translocation of phosphatidate phosphoydrolase from the cytosol to particulate fractions of isolated rat hepatocytes. *Biochem. J.* 1984, **219**: 911–916.

27 Christiansen R., Borreback B., Bremer J.: Effect of (-)carnitine on the metabolism of palmitate in liver cells isolated from fasted and refed rats. *FEBS Lett.* 1976, **62**: 313–317.

28 Christiansen R. Z.: Regulation of palmitate metabolism by carnitine and glucagon in hepatocytes isolated from fasted and carbohydrate refed rats. *Biochim. Biophys. Acta* 1977, **488**: 249–262.

29 Christiansen R. Z.: The effects of antiketogenic agents and pyruvate on the oxidation of palmitate in isolated hepatocytes. *FEBS Lett.* 1979, **103**: 89–92.

30 Cole T. G., Wilcox H. G., Heimberg M.: Effects of adrenalectomy and dexamethasone on hepatic lipid metabolism. *J. Lipid Res.* 1982, **23**: 81–91.

31 Cook G. A., Nielsen R. C., Hawkins R. A., Mehlman M. A., Lakshmanan M. R., Veech R. L.: Effect of glucagon on hepatic malonyl-CoA concentration and on lipid synthesis. *J. Biol. Chem.* 1977, **252**: 4421–4424.

32 Cook G. A., King M. T., Veech R. L.: Ketogenesis and malonyl coenzyme A content of isolated rat hepatocytes. *J. Biol. Chem.* 1978, **253**: 2529–2531.

33 Cook G. A., Otto D. A., Cornell N. W.: Differential inhibition of ketogenesis by malonyl-CoA in mitochondria from fed and starved rats. *Biochem. J.* 1980, **192**: 955–958.

34 Cook G. A., Otto D. A., Cornell N. W.: Malonyl-CoA inhibition of carnitine palmitoyltransferase: interpretation of I_{50} and Ki values. *Biochem. J.* 1983, **212**: 525–527.

35 Cook G. A., Stephens T. W., Harris R. A.: Altered sensitivity of carnitine palmitoyltransferase to inhibition by malonyl-CoA in ketotic diabetic rats. *Biochem J.* 1984, **219**: 337–339.

36 Cook G. A.: Differences in the sensitivity of carnitine palmitoyltransferase to inhibition by malonyl-CoA are due to differences in Ki values. *J. Biol. Chem.* 1984, **259**: 12030–12033.

37 Debeer L. J., Thomas J., De Schepper P. J., Mannaerts G. P.: Lysosomal triacylglycerol lipase and lipolysis in isolated rat hepatocytes. *J. Biol. Chem.* 1979, **254**: 8841–8846.

38 Debeer L. J., Declercq P. E., Mannaerts G. P.: Glycerol-3-phosphate content and triacylglycerol synthesis in isolated hepatocytes from fed and starved rats. *FEBS Lett.* 1981, **124**: 31–34.

39 Debeer L. J., Beynen A. C., Mannaerts G. P., Geelen M. J. H.: Lipolysis of hepatic triacylglycerol stores. *FEBS Lett.* 1982, **140**: 159–164.

40 Debeer L. J., Mannaerts P.: The mitochondrial and peroxisomal pathways of fatty acid oxidation in rat liver. *Diabete et Metabolisme* 1983, **9**: 134–140.

41 Declercq P. E., Debeer L., Mannaerts G. P.: Glucagon inhibits triacylglycerol synthesis in isolated hepatocytes by lowering their glycerol-3-phosphate content. *Biochem. J.* 1982, **202**: 803–806.

42 Declercq P. E., Debeer L., Mannaerts G. P.: Role of glycerol 3-phosphate and glycerophosphate acyltransferase in the nutritional control of hepatic triacylglycerol synthesis. *Biochem. J.* 1982, **204**: 247–256.

43 Demaugre F., Buc H., Girard J., Leroux J. P.: Role of the mitochondrial metabolism of pyruvate on the regulation of ketogenesis in rat hepatocytes. *Metabolism* 1982, **32**: 40–48.

44 Di Marco J. P., Hoppel C.: Hepatic mitochondrial function in ketogenic states: Diabetes, starvation and after growth hormone administration. *J. Clin. Invest.* 1975, **55**: 1237–1244.

45 Foster D. W.: From glycogen to ketones and back. *Diabetes* 1984, **33**: 1188–1199.

46 Fritz I. B.: Factors influencing the rates of long chain fatty acid oxidation and synthesis in mammalian systems. *Physiol. Rev.* 1961, **41**: 51–129.

47 Fukuda N., Azain M. J., Ontko J. A.: Altered hepatic metabolism of free fatty acids underlying hypersecretion of very low density lipoproteins in the genetically obese Zucker rat. *J. Biol. Chem.* 1982, **257**: 14066–14072.

48 Fukuda N., Ontko J. A.: Interactions between fatty acid synthesis, oxidation and esterification in the production of triglyceride-rich lipoproteins by the liver. *J. Lipid Res.* 1984, **25**: 831–842.

49 Geelen M. J. H., Harris H. A., Beynen A. C., McCune S. A.: Short-term hormonal control of hepatic lipogenesis. *Diabetes* 1980, **29**: 1006–1022.

50 Girard J., Duee P. H., Ferre P., Pegorier J. P., Escriva F., Decaux J-F.: Fatty acid oxidation and ketogenesis during development. *Reprod. Nutr. Develop.* 1985, **25**: 303–319.

51 Greenberger N. J., Skillman T. G.: Medium chain triglycerides: physiologic considerations and clinical implications. *New Engl. J. Med.* 1969, **280**: 1045–1058.

52 Guynn R. W., Veloso D., Veech R. L.: The concentration of malonyl-CoA and the control of fatty acid synthesis *in vivo*. *J. Biol. Chem.* 1972, **247**: 7325–7331.

53 Haagsman H. P., De Haas G. G. M., Geelen M. J. H., Van Golde L. M. G.: Regulation of triacylglycerols synthesis in the liver. A decrease in diacylglycerol acyltransferase activity after treatment of isolated rat hepatocytes with glucagon. *Biochim. Biophys. Acta* 1981, **664**: 74–81.

54 Hales C. N., Luzio J. P., Siddle K.: Hormonal control of adipose tissue lipolysis. *Biochem. Soc. Symp.* 1978, **43**: 97–135.

55 Harano Y., Kowal J., Yamazaki R., Lavine L., Miller M.: Carnitine palmitoyltransferase activities (1 and 2) and the rate of palmitate oxidation in liver mitochondria from diabetic rats. *Arch. Biochem. Biophys.* 1972, **153**: 426–437.

56 Harano Y., Kosugi K., Kashiwagi A., Nakano T., Hidaka H., Shigeta Y.: Regulatory mechanism of ketogenesis by glucagon and insulin in iolated and cultured hepatocytes. *J. Biochem.* 1982, **91**: 1739–1748.

57 Heimberg M., Weinstein I., Kohout M.: The effects of glucagon, dibutyryl cyclic adenosine 3',5'-monophosphate and concentration of free fatty acid on hepatic lipid metabolism. *J. Biol. Chem.* 1969, **244**: 5131–5139.

58 Heimberg M., Goh E. H., Klausner H. A., Soler-Argilaga C., Weinstein I., Wilcox H. G.: Regulation of hepatic metabolism of free fatty acids: interrelationships among secretionof very-low density lipoproteins, ketogenesis and cholesterogenesis. *In: Disturbances in Lipid and Lipoprotein Metabolism*, J. M. Dietschy, A. M. Gotto Jr., J. A. Ontko (Eds): American Physiol. Society, Bethesda, 1978, pp 251–267.

59 Ide T., Ontko J. A.: Increased secretion of very low density lipoprotein triglyceride following inhibition of long chain fatty acid oxidation in isolated rat liver. *J. Biol. Chem.* 1981, **256**: 10247–10255.

60 Keyes W. G., Heimberg M.: Influence of thyroid status on lipid metabolism in the perfused rat liver. *J. Clin. Invest.* 1979, **64**: 182–190.

61 Kiyasu J. Y., Bloom B., Chaikoff I. L.: The portal transport of absorbed fatty acids. *J. Biol. Chem.* 1952, **199**: 415–419.

62 Kosugi K., Harano Y., Nakano T., Suzuki M., Kashiwagi A., Shigeta Y.: Mechanism of adrenergic stimulation of hepatic ketogenesis. *Metabolism* 1983, **32**: 1081–1087.

63 Krebs H. A.: The regulation of the release of ketone bodies by the liver. *Adv. Enzyme Regul.* 1966, **4**: 339–353.

64 Krebs H. A., Wallace P. G., Hems R., Freedland R. A.: Rates of ketone body formation in the perfused rat liver. *Biochem. J.* 1969, **112**: 595–600.

65 Krebs H. A., Hems R.: Fatty acid metabolism in the perfused rat liver. *Biochem. J.* **119**: 525–533.

66 Laker M. E., Mayes P. A.: Effect of hyperthyroidism on lipid and carbohydrate metabolism of the perfused rat liver. *Biochem. J.* 1981, **196**: 247–255.

67 Lloyd-Davies K. A., Brindley D. N.: Palmitate activation and esterification in microsomal fractions of rat liver. *Biochem. J.* 1975, **152**: 39–49.

68 Lomax M. A., Donaldson I. A., Pogson C. I.: The control of fatty acid metabolism in liver cells from fed and starved sheep. *Biochem. J.* 1983, **214**: 553–560.

69 Lund H., Borreback B., Bremer J.: Regulation of palmitate esterification/oxidation by glucagon in isolated hepatocytes. The role of 3-glycerophosphate concentration. *Biochim. Biophys. Acta* 1980, **620**: 364–371.

70 Malewiak M. I., Griglio S., Kalopissis A. D., Le Liepvre X.: Oleate metabolism in isolated hepatocytes from lean and obese Zucker rats. Influence of a high-fat diet and *in vitro* response to glucagon. *Metabolism* 1983, **32**: 661–668.

70a Malewiak M. I., Griglio S., Le Liepvre X.: Relationship between lipogenesis, ketogenesis and malonyl-CoA content in isolated hepatocytes from the obese Zucker rat adapted to a high-fat diet. *Metabolism* 1985, **4**: 604–611.

71 Mannaerts G. P., Thomas J., Debeer L. J., McGarry J. D., Foster D. W.: Hepatic fatty acid oxidation and ketogenesis after clofibrate treatment. *Biochim. Biophys. Acta* 1978, **529**: 201–211.

72 Mayes P. A., Felts J. M.: Regulation of fat metabolism in the liver. *Nature* 1967, **215**: 716–718.

73 Mayes P. A.: Studies on the major pathways of hepatic lipid metabolism using the perfused liver. *In*: *Adipose Tissue*, B. Jeanrenaud, D. Hepp. (Eds): Georg Thieme Verlag, Stuttgart, 1970, pp 186–195.

74 Mayes P. A., Topping D. L.: Regulation of hepatic lipogenesis by plasma free fatty acids: simultaneous studies on lipoprotein secretion, cholesterol synthesis, ketogenesis and gluconeogenesis. *Biochem. J.* 1974, **140**: 111–114.

75 McGarry J. D., Foster D. W.: Ketogenesis *in vitro*. *Biochim. Biophys. Acta* 1969, **177**: 35–41.

76 McGarry J. D., Foster D. W.: The regulation of ketogenesis from oelic acid and the influence of antiketogenic agents. *J. Biol. Chem.* 1971, **246**: 6247–6253.

77 McGarry J. D., Foster D. W.: The regulation of ketogenesis from octanoic acid. The role of the tricarboxylic acid cycle and fatty acid synthesis. *J. Biol. Chem.* 1971, **246**: 1149–1159.

78 McGarry J. D., Foster D. W.: Regulation of ketogenesis and clinical aspects of the ketotic state. *Metabolism* 1972, **21**: 471–489.

79 McGarry J. D., Foster D. W.: Acute reversal of experimental diabetic ketoacidosis in the rat with (+) decanoylcarnitine. *J. Clin. Invest.* 1973, **52**: 877–884.

80 McGarry J. D., Meier J. M., Foster D. W.: The effects of starvation and refeeding on carbohydrate and lipid metabolism *in vivo* and in the perfused rat liver. The relationship between fatty acid oxidation and esterification in the regulation of ketogenesis. *J. Biol. Chem.* 1973, **248**: 270–278.

81 McGarry J. D., Foster D. W.: The metabolism of (−) octanoylcarnitine in perfused livers from fed and fasted rats. *J. Biol. Chem.* 1974, **249**: 7984–7990.

82 McGarry J. D., Foster D. W.: Studies with (+) octanoylcarnitine in experimental diabetic ketoacidosis. *Diabetes* 1974, **23**: 485–493.

83 McGarry J. D., Wright P. H., Foster D. W.: Hormonal control of ketogenesis. Rapid activation of hepatic ketogenic capacity in fed rats by anti-insulin serum and glucagon. *J. Clin. Invest.* 1975, **55**: 1202–1209.

84 McGarry J. D., Robles-Valdes C., Foster D. W.: Role of carnitine in hepatic ketogenesis. *Proc. Natl. Acad. Sci.* 1975, **72**: 4385–4388.

85 McGarry J. D., Mannaerts G. P., Foster D. W.: A possible role for malonyl-CoA in the regulation of hepatic fatty acid oxidation and ketogenesis. *J. Clin. Invest.* 1977, **60**: 265–270.

86 McGarry J. D., Leatherman G. F., Foster D. W.: Carnitine palmitoyltransferase I. The site of inhibition of hepatic fatty acid oxidation by malonyl-CoA. *J. Biol. Chem.* 1978, **253**: 4128–4136.

87 McGarry J. D., Stark M. J., Foster D. W.: Hepatic malonyl-CoA levels of fed, fasted and diabetic rats as measured using a simple radioisotopic assay. *J. Biol. Chem.* 1978, **253**: 8291–8293.

88 McGarry J. D., Takabayashi Y., Foster D. W.: The role of malonyl-CoA in the coordination of fatty acid synthesis and oxidation in isolated rat hepatocytes. *J. Biol. Chem.* 1978, **253**: 8294–8300.

89 McGarry J. D.: New perspectives in the regulation of ketogenesis. *Diabetes* 1979, **28**: 517–523.

90 McGarry J. D., Foster D. W.: In support of the roles of malonyl-CoA and carnitine acyltransferase

I in the regulation of hepatic fatty acid oxidation and ketogenesis. *J. Biol. Chem.* **1979, 254**: 8163–8168.

91 McGarry J. D., Foster D. W.: Effects of exogenous fatty acid concentration on glucagon-induced changes in hepatic fatty acid metabolism. *Diabetes* 1980, **29**: 236–240.

92 McGarry J. D., Foster D. W.: Regulation of hepatic fatty acid oxidation and ketone body production. *Ann. Rev. Biochem.* 1980, **49**: 395–420.

93 McGarry J. D., Foster D. W.: Importance of experimental conditions in evaluating the malonyl-CoA sensitivity of liver carnitine acyltransferase. Studies with fed and starved rats. *Biochem. J.* 1981, **200**: 217–223.

94 Meier J. M., McGarry J. D., Faloona G. R., Unger R. H., Foster D. W.: Studies on the development of diabetic ketosis in the rat. *J. Lipid Res.* 1972, **13**: 228–233.

95 Mills S. E., Foster D. W., McGarry J. D.: Interaction of malonyl-CoA and related compounds with mitochondria from different rat tissues. Relationship between ligand binding and inhibition of carnitine palmitoyltransferase I. *Biochem. J.* 1983, **214**: 83–91.

96 Mills S. E., Foster D. W., McGarry J. D.: Effects of pH on the interaction of substrates and malonyl-CoA with mitochondrial carnitine palmitoyltransferase I. *Biochem. J.* 1984, **219**: 601–608.

97 Mooney R. A., Lane M. D.: Control of ketogenesis and fatty acid synthesis at the mitochondrial branch-point for acetyl-CoA in the chick liver cell: Effect of adenosine 3′,5′-monophosphate. *Eur. J. Biochem.* 1982, **121**: 281–287.

98 Morris B.: Some factors affecting the metabolism of free fatty acids and chylomicron triglycerides by the perfused rats' liver. *J. Physiol.* 1968, **168**: 584–598.

99 Morrow F. D., Allen C. E., Martin R. J.: Intracellular fatty acid binding protein: hepatic levels in lean and obese rats. *Fed. Proc.* 1979, **38**: 280. (Abstract.)

100 Muller M. J., Koster H., Seitz H. J.: Effect of thyroid state on ketogenic capacity of the isolated perfused liver of starved rats. *Biochim. Biophys. Acta* 1981, **666**: 475–481.

101 Nosadini R., Ursini F., Tessari P., Tiengo A., Gregolin C.: Perfused liver carnitine palmitoyltransferase activity and ketogenesis in streptotocin treated and genetic hyperinsulinemic rats. Effect of glucagon. *Horm. Metab. Res.* 1979, **11**: 661–664.

102 Ockner R. K., Burnett D. A., Lysenko L., Manning J. A.: Sex differences in long chain fatty acid utilization and fatty acid binding protein concentration in rat liver. *J. Clin. Invest.* 1979, **64**: 172–181.

103 Ockner R. K., Manning J. A., Poppenhausen R. B., Ho W. K. L.: A binding protein for fatty acids in cytosol of intestinal mucosa, liver, myocardium and other tissues. *Science* 1972, **177**: 56–58.

104 Ockner R. K., Weisiger R. A., Gollan J. L.: Hepatic uptake of albumin-bound substances: albumin receptor concept. *Am. J. Physiol.* 1983, **245**: G13–G18.

105 Olubadewo J., Wilcox H. G., Heimberg M.: Modulation by glycerol of hepatic glycerol-3 phosphate concentration, ketogenesis and output of triglyceride and glucose in perfused livers from hyperthydroid rats. *J. Biol. Chem.* 1984, **259**: 8857–8862.

106 Ontko J. A.: Metabolism of free fatty acids in isolated liver cells. Factors affecting the partition between esterification and oxidation. *J. Biol. Chem.* 1972, **247**: 1788–1800.

107 Ontko J. A., Johns M. L.: Evaluation of malonyl-CoA in the regulation of long-chain fatty acid oxidation in the liver. *Biochem. J.* 1980, **192**: 959–962.

108 Otto D. A., Cook G. A., Reiss P. D.: Parameters for comparing rates of fatty acid oxidation and malonyl-CoA concentrations in hepatocytes from starved and fed rats. *In: Isolation, Characterization and Use of Hepatocytes*, R. A. Harris, N. W. Cornell (Eds): Elsevier Biomedical, New York, 1983, pp 41–48.

109 Pande S. V.: On rate-controlling factors of long chain fatty acid oxidation. *J. Biol. Chem.* 1971, **246**: 5384–5390.

110 Parvin R., Pande S. V.: Enhancement of mitochondrial carnitine and carnitine acylcarnitine translocase-mediated transport of fatty acids into liver mitochondria under ketogenic conditions. *J. Biol. Chem.* 1979, **254**: 5423–5429.

111 Pegorier J. P., Duee P. H., Girard J., Peret J.: Metabolic rate of non-esterified fatty acids in isolated hepatocytes from newborn and young pigs. Evidence for a limited capacity for oxidation and increased capacity for esterification. *Biochem. J.* 1983, **212**: 93–97.

112 Pollard A. D., Brindley D. N.: Effects of vasopressin and corticosterone on fatty acid metabolism and on the activities of glycerol phosphate acyltransferase and phosphatidate phosphohydrolase in rat hepatocytes. *Biochem. J.* 1984, **217**: 461–469.

113 Regen D. M., Terrell E. B.: Effects of glucagon and fasting on acetate metabolism in perfused rat liver. *Biochim. Biophys. Acta* 1968, **170**: 95–111.

114 Renaud G., Foliot A., Infante R.: Increased uptake of fatty acids by isolated rat liver raising the fatty acid binding protein concentration with clofibrate. *Biochem. Biophys. Res. Com.* 1978, **80**: 327–334.

115 Robinson A. M., Williamson D. H.: Physiological roles of ketone bodies as substrates and signals in mammalian tissues. *Physiol. Rev.* 1980, **60**: 143–187.

116 Robinson I. N., Zammit V. A.: Sensitivity of carnitine acyltransferase I to malonyl-CoA inhibition in isolated rat liver mitochondria is quantitatively related to hepatic malonyl-CoA concentration *in vivo*. *Biochem. J.* 1982, **206**: 177–179.

117 Robles-Valdes C., McGarry J. D., Foster D. W.: Maternal-fetal carnitine relationship and neonatal ketosis in the rat. *J. Biol. Chem.* 1976, **251**: 6007–6012.

118 Saggerson E. D., Bates E. J.: Regulation of glycerolipid synthesis. *In: Short Term Regulation of Liver Metabolism*, L. Hue, G. Van de Werve (Eds): Elsevier, Amsterdam, 1981, pp 247–262.

119 Saggerson E. D., Carpenter C. A.: Effects of fasting, adrenalectomy and streptozotocin-diabetes on sensitivity of hepatic carnitine acyltransferase to malonyl-CoA. *FEBS Lett.* 1982, **129**: 225–228.

120 Saggerson E. D., Carpenter C. A.: Response to starvation of hepatic carnitine palmitoyltransferase activity and its regulation by malonyl-CoA. Sex differences and effects of pregnancy. *Biochem. J.* 1982, **208**: 673–678.

121 Saggerson E. D., Carpenter C. A., Tselentis B. S.: Effects of thyroidectomy and starvation on the activity and properties of hepatic carnitine palmitoyltransferase. *Biochem. J.* 1982, **208**: 667–672.

122 Schofield P. S., Kirk C. J. C., Sugden M. C.: Hormonal regulation of ketogenesis in hepatocytes from fed rats before and after glycogen depletion. *Biochem. Int.* 1984, **9**: 611–620.

123 Siess E. A., Kientsch-Engel R. I., Wieland O. H.: Role of free oxaloacetate in ketogenesis. Derivation from the direct measurement of mitochondrial [3-hydroxybutyrate]/[acetoacetate] ratio in hepatocytes. *Eur. J. Biochem.* 1982, **121**: 493–499.

124 Siess E. A., Kientsch-Engel R. I., Wieland O. H.: Concentration of free oxaloacetate in the mitochondrial compartment of isolated liver cells. *Biochem. J.* 1984, **218**: 171–176.

125 Singh B., Osmundsen H., Borreback B.: The time course of glucagon action on the utilization of [1-^{14}C] palmitate by isolated hepatocytes. *Arch. Biochem. Biophys.* 1982, **217**: 244–250.

126 Soler-Argilaga C., Infante R., Renaud G., Polonovski J.: Factors influencing free fatty acid uptake by the isolated perfused rat liver. *Biochimie* 1974, **56**: 757–761.

127 Soler-Argilaga C., Heimberg M.: Comparison of metabolism of free fatty acids by isolated perfused livers from male and female rats. *J. Lipid Res.* 1976, **17**: 605–615.

128 Soler-Argilaga C., Russell R. L., Heimberg M.: Enzymatic aspects of the reduction of microsomal glycerolipid biosynthesis after perfusion of the liver with dibutyryl adenosine -3′,5′-monophosphate. *Arch. Biochem. Biophys.* 1978, **190**: 367–372.

129 Spector A. A.: Metabolism of free fatty acids. *Progr. Biochem. Pharmacol.* 1971, **6**: 130–176.

130 Stakkestad J. A., Bremer J.: The metabolism of fatty acids in hepatocytes isolated from triiodothyronine-treated rats. *Biochem. Biophys. Acta* 1982, **711**: 90–100.

131 Stakkestad J. A., Bremer J.: The outer carnitine palmitoyltransferase and regulation of fatty acid metabolism in rat liver in different thyroid states. *Biochim. Biophys. Acta* 1983, **750**: 244–252.

132 Stakkestad J. A., Lund H.: The effect of nutritional and thyroid state on the distribution of fatty acids between oxidation and esterification in isolated rat hepatocytes. *Biochim. Biophys. Acta* 1984, **793**: 1–9.

133 Sugden M. C., Ball A. J., Ilic V., Williamson D. H.: Stimulation of [1-^{14}C] oleate oxidation to $^{14}CO_2$ in isolated rat hepatocytes by vasopressin: effects of Ca^{2+}. *FEBS Lett.* 1980, **116**: 37–40.

134 Sugden M. C., Williamson D. H., Sugden P. H.: Effects of vasopression, glucagon and dibutyryl cyclic AMP on the activities of enzymes of fatty acid esterification in rat hepatocytes. *FEBS Lett.* 1980, **119**: 312–316.

135 Sugden M. C., Williamson D. H.: Short-term hormonal control of ketogenesis. *In: Short-Term Regulation of Liver Metabolism*, L. Hue, G. Van de Werve (Eds): Elsevier, Amsterdam, 1981, pp 291–309.

136 Sugden M. C., Williamson D. H.: Fatty acid metabolism and ketogenesis. *In: Metabolic Compartmentation*, H. Sies (Ed.): Academic Press, New York, 1982, pp 287–315.

137 Sugden M. C., Watts D. I.: Stimulation of [1-^{14}C] oleate oxidation to ^{14}CO$_2$ in isolated rat hepatocytes by the catecholamines, vasopressin and angiotensin. *Biochem. J.* 1983, **212**: 85–91.

138 Topping D. L., Mayes P. A.: The immediate effects of insulin and fructose on the metabolism of the perfused liver. Changes in lipoprotein secretion, fatty acid oxidation and esterification, lipogenesis and carbohydrate metabolism. *Biochem. J.* 1972, **126**: 295–311.

139 Triscari J., Greenwood M. R. C., Sullivan A. C.: Regulation of lipid synthesis in hepatocytes from lean and obese Zucker Rat. *Metabolism* 1981, **30**: 1135–1142.

140 Triscari J., Greenwood M. R. C., Sullivan A. C.: Oxidation and ketogenesis in hepatocytes of lean and obese Zucker rats. *Metabolism* 1982, **31**: 223–228.

141 Van Harken D. R., Dixon C. W., Heimberg M.: Hepatic metabolism in experimental diabetes. V. The effect of concentration of oleate on metabolism of triglycerides and on ketogenesis. *J. Biol. Chem.* 1969, **244**: 2278–2285.

142 Walli R. A.: Interrelation of aerobic glycolysis and lipogenesis in isolated perfused liver of well-fed rats. *Biochim. Biophys. Acta* 1978, **539**: 62–80.

143 Wasfi I., Weinstein I., Heimberg M.: Hepatic metabolism of [1-^{14}C] oleate in pregnancy. *Biochim. Biophys. Acta* 1980, **619**: 471–481.

144 Wasfi I., Weinstein I., Heimberg M.: Increased formation of triglyceride from oleate in perfused livers from pregnant rats. *Endocrinology* 1980, **107**: 584–590.

145 Watts D. I., Sugden M. C.: Role of free oxaloacetate in ketogenesis. *Biochem. Int.* 1982, **4**: 255–261.

146 Weinstein I., Soler-Argilaga C., Werner H. V., Heimberg M.: Effects of ethynyloestradiol on the metabolism of [1-^{14}C] oleate by perfused livers and hepatocytes from female rats. *Biochem. J.* 1979, **180**: 265–271.

147 Whitelaw E., Williamson D. H.: Effects of lactation on ketogenesis from oleate or butyrate in rat hepatocytes. *Biochem. J.* 1977, **164**: 521–528.

148 Wieland O. H. Ketogenesis and its regulation. *Adv. Metab. Dis.* 1968, **3**: 1–47.

149 Williamson D. H., Bates M. W., Krebs H. A.: Activity and intracellular distribution of enzymes of ketone-body metabolism in rat liver. *Biochem. J.* 1968, **108**: 353–361.

150 Williamson D. H., Veloso D., Ellington E. V., Krebs H. A.: Changes in the concentrations of hepatic metabolites on administration of dihydroxyacetone or glycerol to starved rats and their relationship to control of ketogenesis. *Biochem. J.* 1969, **114**: 575–584.

151 Williamson D. H., Hems R.: Metabolism and function of ketone bodies. *In: Assays in Cell Metabolism*, W. Bartley, J. R. Quayle, H. L. Kornberg (Eds): Wiley, London, 1970, pp 257–281.

152 Williamson D. H., Whitelaw E.: Interactions between ketogenesis and carbohydrate metabolism in rat liver. *In: Regulatory Mechanisms of Carbohydrate Metabolism*, V. Esmann (Ed.): Pergamon Press, Oxford, 1978, pp 151–160.

153 Williamson D. H., Whitelaw E.: Physiological aspects of the regulation of ketogenesis. *Biochem. Soc. Symp.* 1978, **43**: 137–161.

154 Williamson D. H.: Recent developments in ketone body metabolism. *Biochem. Soc. Transac.* 1979, **7**: 1313–1321.

155 Williamson D. H., Ilic V., Tordoff F. C., Ellington E. V.: Interactions between vasopressin and glucagon on ketogenesis and oleate metabolism in isolated hepatocytes from fed rats. *Biochem. J.* 1980, **186**: 621–624.

156 Williamson J. R., Scholz R., Browning E. T.: Control of gluconeogenesis and ketogenesis. II. Interactions between fatty acid oxidation and the citric acid cycle in perfused rat liver. *J. Biol. Chem.* 1969, **244**: 4617–4627.

157 Witters L. A., Trasko C. S.: Regulation of hepatic free fatty acid metabolism by glucagon and insulin. *Am. J. Physiol.* 1979, **237**: E23–E29.

158 Woods H. F., Krebs H. A.: Lactate production in the perfused liver. *Biochem. J.* 1971, **125**: 129–139.

159 Woodside W. F., Heimberg M.: Effect of anti-insulin serum, insulin and glucose on output of triglyceride and on ketogenesis by the perfused rat liver. *J. Biol. Chem.* 1976, **251**: 13–23.

160 Woodside W. F., Heimberg M.: The metabolism of oleic acid by the perfused rat liver in experimental diabetes induced by anti-insulin serum. *Metabolism* 1978, **27**: 1763–1776.

161 Woodside W. F.: Influence of insulin and glucagon on ketogenesis by isolated rat hepatocytes. *In: Hormones and Energy Metabolism*, D. M. Klachko, R. R. Anderson, M. Heimberg (Eds): Plenum Press, New York, 1979, pp 97–101.

162 Wu-Rideout M. Y. C., Elson C., Shrago E.: The role of fatty acid binding protein on the metabolism of fatty acids in isolated rat hepatocytes. *Biochem. Biophys. Res. Comm.* 1976, **71**: 809–816.

163 Zammit V. A.: The effect of glucagon treatment and starvation of virgin and lactating rats on the rats of oxidation of octanoyl-L-carnitine and octanoate by isolated liver mitochondria. *Biochem. J.* 1980, **190**: 293–300.

164 Zammit V. A.: Regulation of hepatic fatty acid metabolism. *Biochem. J.* 1981, **198**: 75–83.

165 Zammit V. A.: Regulation of hepatic fatty acid oxidation and ketogenesis. *Proc. Nutr.Soc.* 1983, **42**: 289–302.

166 Zammi V A.: Increased sensitivity of carnitine palmitoyltransferase I activity to malonyl-CoA inhibition after preincubation of intact rat liver mitochondria with micromolar concentrations of malonyl-CoA *in vitro*. *Biochem. J.*, 1983, **210**: 953–956.

167 Zammit V. A.: Reversible sensitization and desensitization of carnitine palmitoyltransferase I to inhibition by malonyl-CoA in isolated rat liver mitochondria. *Biochem. J.* 1983, **214**: 1027–1030.

168 Zammit V. A.: Time-dependence of inhibition of carnitine palmitoyltransferase I by malonyl-CoA in mitochondria isolated from livers of fed or starved rats. *Biochem. J.* 1984, **218**: 379–386.

169 Zammit V. A.: Mechanisms of regulation of the partition of fatty acids between oxidation and esterification in the liver. *Prog. Lipid Res.* 1984, **23**: 39–67.

Research in *Isolated and cultured hepatocytes* A. Guillouzo & C. Guguen-Guillouzo eds, pp. 113–134
© 1986 John Libbey Eurotext Ltd./INSERM.

6

Lipoprotein metabolism in isolated and cultured hepatocytes

Part 1: HEPATIC VLDL SYNTHESIS AND SECRETION

Athina-Despina KALOPISSIS

Laboratoire de Physiopathologie de la Nutrition, INSERM U177, Institut Biomédical des Cordeliers, 15 rue de l'Ecole de Médecine, 75270 Paris Cedex 06, FRANCE

SUMMARY

Very low density lipoproteins (VLDL) are spherical pseudomicelles consisting of a hydrophobic core (composed mainly of triacylglycerol) and a hydrophilic surface monolayer. They are formed by sequential, multistep assembly of lipids, apoproteins and glucides. Lipids, synthesized in the smooth endoplasmic reticulum (ER) and apoproteins, synthesized in the rough ER, are assembled at the rough-smooth ER junctions and form nascent VLDL particles. After transit through the Golgi apparatus VLDL are packaged inside secretory vesicles, transported to the plasma membrane and secreted in the space of Disse. The entire biosynthetic process requires 15 to 20 minutes. Hepatic VLDL carry apoprotein (apo-) B, apo-E and apo-C. Apo-B is necessary for VLDL assembly and stability, apo-E is involved in cholesterol metabolism and apo-C regulates plasma VLDL catabolism. VLDL formation is under nutritional and hormonal control. Fasting and fat-feeding decreases and sucrose ingestion increases VLDL-triacylglycerol and apoprotein output, whereas fatty acids only increase VLDL-triacylglycerol secretion. Lipid and apoprotein storage allows continuous VLDL production, while apoprotein ability to assemble with variable amounts of lipids permits rapid, short-term modulations of VLDL secretion in response to external challenges. Finally, VLDL biogenesis is stimulated by oestrogens and thyroid hormone and inhibited by glucagon; however, the direct role of insulin is still controversial.

Introduction

One of the principal functions of hepatic parenchymal cells (hepatocytes) is the synthesis and secretion of lipoproteins of very low density (VLDL), low density (LDL) and high density (HDL). Apart from the liver, lipoproteins are also produced by the intestine, an organ of the same embryological origin. When the diet contains lipids, the intestine, but not the liver, can secrete a fourth lipoprotein class — the chylomicrons.

The physiological importance of lipoproteins as lipid carriers through the vascular compartment has long been recognized. Disorders in lipoprotein metabolism, whether in their production rate or their plasma catabolism, are thought to bring about or aggravate several metabolic diseases such as atherosclerosis, diabetes, renal failure or obesity.

What are lipoproteins?

Lipoproteins are spherical pseudomicellar particles formed by the association of lipids, proteins and glucides in such a way, that their hydrophobic components (apolar lipids: triacylglycerols and cholesterol esters) are placed at the core and their hydrophilic components (polar lipids: phospholipids and free cholesterol; proteins and glucides) at the periphery of the particles. Thus, lipoproteins are soluble in the aqueous environment of the blood (for a review see reference 26).

Many differences exist between the four lipoprotein classes, especially as regards the nature and the amount of lipids and proteins they carry. So, lipoproteins are classified as triacylglycerol-rich ones (namely chylomicrons and VLDL) or cholesterol-rich ones (namely LDL and HDL). Since the lipoprotein size is proportional to their triacylglycerol content, it decreases in the order: chylomicrons, VLDL, LDL and HDL. The opposite occurs for their hydrated density (d) which is related to the amount of proteins and increases in the order: chylomicrons (d=0.97 g/ml), VLDL (d=1.006 g/ml), LDL (d=1.063 g/ml) and HDL (d=1.21 g/ml). The protein constituents are called apolipoproteins or apoproteins by analogy to the prosthetic group of enzymes. Apoproteins are of primary importance for the assembly, secretion, stability and metabolic fate of lipoproteins. Several apoproteins differing in molecular weight and metabolic properties have been identified to date and the list is probably not exhaustive. Their classification in alphabetical 'families' (A, B, C . . . H) has greatly simplified research in this field (2). Each family consists either of different peptides (ie apo-AI, AII, AIV; apo-B_{100}, B_{48}; apo-CI, CII, CIII etc) or of isoforms of the same peptide differing in isoelectric point (ie apo-E with a molecular weight of 35 kDa: apo E_1, . . . E_5).

The present discussion will develop current concepts on hepatic VLDL synthesis and secretion. HDL appears to follow a similar pathway, but their metabolic regulation is different and their production about 5 to 10-times lower than that of VLDL (46). A controversy exists as regards LDL formation. According to some authors, LDL are solely a catabolic product of VLDL, whereas according to others they are secreted by the liver. Finally, intestinal lipoproteins are formed by a similar sequence of events. Nevertheless, many differences exist between intestinal and hepatic lipoproteins, essentially because intestine and liver possess a specificity in apoprotein synthesis, ie the intestine produces only apo-B_{48}, whereas the liver produces apo-B_{100} and apo-B_{48}; apo-E and apo-C are synthesized almost exclusively in the liver; apo-AI and apo-AIV are mainly secreted in the intestine (74, 75).

The VLDL synthetic and secretory pathway

During the last 20 years various experimental approaches have been used for the study of VLDL biogenesis, such as autoradiographic or immunocytochemical techniques coupled with electron microscopy, isolation of subcellular organelles or time course studies using labelled precursors of VLDL constituents. Certain drugs inhibiting specific steps of VLDL formation or secretion were very useful in elucidating the factors required for a normal VLDL production. Now, it is well established that VLDL are synthesized by sequential, multi-step assembly of apoproteins, lipids and glucides, each step occurring at a specific hepatocyte compartment and requiring a definite time.

Topography and function of intrahepatic organelles implicated in VLDL production

Five hepatocyte compartments are involved in VLDL production (synthesis and secretion): smooth endoplasmic reticulum (ER), rough ER, Golgi apparatus, GERL and microtubules. When isolated from liver homogenates, smooth and rough ER fractions are referred to as microsomes.

Smooth endoplasmic reticulum. The smooth ER is the site of lipid synthesis and esterification (7). These reactions are catalysed by specific enzymes located at the cytoplasmic surface of smooth ER membranes. The fate of the synthesized lipids depends on the hepatic metabolic status of the moment. Here we will consider the fate of triacylglycerols, since they are the major VLDL constituent. Part of the triacylglycerols formed enters immediately the VLDL synthetic pathway for export, while the remainder is stored temporarily in the cytoplasm. It is presumed that storage triacylglycerols form the cytoplasmic electron-dense 'lipid droplets' of variable diameters (0.5–2 μm) as they appear in electron microscopy (23). Mooney & Lane (42), using chick hepatocytes in monolayer culture, demonstrated that these lipid droplets are membrane-coated vesicles containing almost exclusively triacylglycerols (>95%) and some phospholipids. The size and the number of lipid droplets presumably depends on the amount of cell triacylglycerols that cannot be immediately incorporated in VLDL.

Thus, the hepatocyte contains at least two triacylglycerol pools. One, located on the membranes of the smooth ER, is the immediate precursor of VLDL and has a rapid turn-over rate. The second pool, located in the cytoplasm, probably serves a storage function and has a slow turn-over rate; it appears to correspond to the 'floating fat' fraction isolated from liver homogenates (5). The existence of these two pools has been suggested by many investigators (5, 21, 42, 62).

Rough endoplasmic reticulum. In the rough ER apoproteins are synthesized on membrane-bound rather than on free ribosomes, a feature that appears to be characteristic of secretory proteins (53, 54). As most apoproteins are glycoproteins, they acquire their primary or core glycosyl residues (mannose and N-acetylglucosamine) during translation. Then the completed polypeptide chains are extruded from the membranes into the lumen of the rough ER.

Different times are required for the synthesis of each apoprotein, depending on molecular size. Siuta-Mangano *et al.* (59) using chick liver cells in culture reported that the low molecular weight (MW) avian apoprotein II (MW=9.5 kDa) was synthesized in 0.2 minutes. However, about 10 minutes were necessary for translation, core glycosylation and extrusion into the rough ER lumen of the high molecular weight apoprotein B (MW=350 kDa).

Although it has not been directly demonstrated, it is probable that apoproteins can be stored temporarily in rough ER cisternae before incorporation into lipoproteins. Apoprotein storage is suggested by several lines of evidence: VLDL secretion continues for 50–60 minutes after inhibition of protein synthesis by cycloheximide (6); after perfusion of the liver with antibodies against apo-B or antibodies against total VLDL apoproteins, there is an accumulation of immunoprecipitate within rough ER cisternae (4).

Golgi apparatus. The Golgi apparatus is a complex organelle whose structure and multiple roles are not fully understood to date. The classical view of the Golgi apparatus resulted from cross sections in which the Golgi cisternae appear as narrow, elongated saccules tightly arranged in parallel and surrounded by small Golgi vesicles. The face of the cisternae which is the functional continuity of the smooth ER is called proximal, forming or cis face. The other face, terminated by expanded, bulbous tubules, is called distal, secretory or trans face. When these bulbous expansions are filled with lipoprotein particles, they become detached from the end of the cisternae and form the 'secretory vesicles' which will transport the lipoproteins to the hepatocyte membrane for secretion.

Hepatocyte Golgi complexes are not highly polarized as in typical secretory cells (ie exocrine pancreatic cells) where they occupy a definite position between the nucleus and the excretory regions. Nevertheless, liver individual Golgi complexes possess an intrinsic polarity in that they are always found at right angles with the lamellae of a corresponding rough ER stack. Between the rough ER and the Golgi cisternae is interposed a more or less abundant smooth ER in the form of a tubular network (11). As VLDL particles appear in electron microscopic images to pass intact from the ER to the Golgi apparatus, a functional-structural continuity is suggested between these three subcellular organelles: the smooth-surfaced ends of the rough ER appear to fuse with smooth ER tubules → smooth ER network fuses in turn with the forming face of the Golgi apparatus and this transitional structure has the appearance of a fenestrated plate (11).

However, while the existence of a structural continuity between smooth ER and Golgi is not disputed, the nature of the intermediary structure remains unclear. Morré & Ovtracht (43), studying either purified preparations of isolated Golgi apparatus or tangential sections of liver tissue by electron microscopy, proposed the existence of the 'boulevard périphérique', namely a specialized smooth ER of the Golgi apparatus zone. In their theoretical model the Golgi cisternæ are not simple saccules but consist of a saccular region about 0.5 μm in diameter with a fenestrated periphery to which 30–50 nm tubules are attached. These small-diameter tubules are extensions of the fenestrated cisternal peripheries and are connected with the 'boulevard périphérique'.

As regards metabolic activities, the Golgi apparatus does not appear to possess enzymes for glycerolipid or protein synthesis with the possible exception of some phospholipid synthetic activity (29). However, it is the site of terminal glycosylation of proteins. Here, apoproteins acquire their terminal glycosyl residues, namely galactose, N-acetylglucosamine and sialic acid (16, 54).

GERL. The acronym GERL was given to a region of smooth ER which is located at the trans face of the *G*olgi apparatus and appears to produce various types of lysosomes (47). Electron microscopic images of GERL-derived lysosomes resemble closely Golgi-derived secretory vesicles inasmuch as both types of vesicles are situated at the trans face of the Golgi apparatus and are filled with VLDL particles. However, GERL structures are identified by staining with the lysosomal marker enzyme acid phosphatase, whereas Golgi ones are marked by thiamine pyrophosphatase. Whether or not GERL derives from the Golgi apparatus itself remains an open question.

The role of GERL in VLDL synthesis and/or secretion is uncertain. GERL is present in normal rat liver and in fatty liver induced by orotic acid-feeding which completely inhibits VLDL secretion while little affecting HDL secretion (47). The orotic acid-induced fatty liver can be prevented or even reversed by administration of ethylchlorophenoxyisobutyrate (CPIB) which restores a normal VLDL secretion and causes a great proliferation of GERL (48). In CPIB-treated rats the greatest part of the VLDL-filled vesicles that were accumulating in the trans face of the Golgi apparatus are apparently hydrolysed by lysosomal enzymes derived from GERL; at the same time, part of the VLDL particles are secreted in the space of Disse. The observation that GERL appears inactive when VLDL secretion is inhibited but very abundant and active after CPIB addition which restores VLDL secretion, raises the possibility that GERL, apart from/or concomitantly with, its degradative role, could also be implicated in some final step of the VLDL synthetic pathway. For instance, one cannot exclude the possibility that a proteic, lipidic or glucidic VLDL component should need lysosomal cleavage before secretion.

Microtubules. Microtubules are assembled from the dimeric protein sub-unit tubulin, a reaction requiring GTP. An intact microtubular system is necessary for the final steps of secretion of secretory granules (64), but their exact mode of action is not fully elucidated. Microtubules may act as guidelines for the movement of secretory vesicles towards the plasma membrane (37). They could also be essential for the maintainance of the specific organization or mobility of membrane components which permit fusion of the membranes of secretory vesicles with selective sites of the plasma membrane (76).

Sequence of VLDL formation, intracellular transport and secretion

VLDL transport route through the Golgi apparatus. As apoproteins and lipids are synthesized in separate compartments, either apoproteins or lipids must 'travel' to a specific site in the cell to form a lipoprotein particle. Alexander *et al.* (4) suggested that the assembly of VLDL constituents occurs at the smooth-surfaced junctions between rough and smooth ER (Fig. 1). This is supported by several time sequence studies with or without electron microscopy (21, 23, 30, 63). In these studies, VLDL were labelled in their lipid moieties by administration of radioactive free fatty acids or glycerol either *in vivo* (by IV injection) or *in vitro* (by liver perfusion), in order to follow their formation and transport route through the hepatocyte.

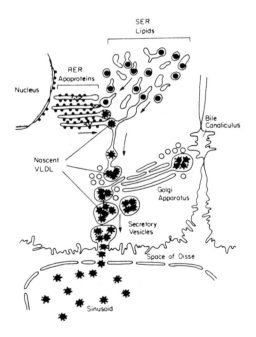

Fig. 1.
Sequence for the biosynthesis of VLDL in the hepatocyte, as proposed by Alexander, Hamilton & Havel. Reproduced from *The Journal of Cell Biology* 1976, Vol. 69, pp 241–263, by copyright permission of the Rockefeller University Press.

VLDL formation is a rapid process: already by 2 minutes after administration of the precursor, newly synthesized VLDL are most prominent in the smooth-surfaced terminal ends of the cisternae of the rough ER and within the lumen of the smooth ER. The greater part of the label is incorporated in triacylglycerols, the remainder being found essentially in phospholipids (21, 63). Nascent VLDL appear as electron-dense osmiophilic granules, their electron-opacity increasing when the liver is perfused with a highly unsaturated (and therefore osmiophilic) fatty acid like linoleate (30). In the tubular channels of the smooth ER, VLDL are invariably seen singly or in rows, but never in clusters. As a rule, they do not come into contact with the profile of the smooth ER tubule, but are held back in the centre of the lumen by a distance of about 80 Å (11). Nascent VLDL are never seen within cisternae of the rough ER.

After 5 minutes of perfusion, many VLDL particles are present in the Golgi area (23, 30). They first appear at the cis or forming face and then pass to the trans or secretory face. The maximal concentration of VLDL in the Golgi apparatus is observed between 10 to 15 minutes. Inside the Golgi structures, VLDL appear in clusters unlike in the smooth ER tubules where they appear singly. VLDL are seen only rarely in the central, plate-like portions of the flat Golgi cisternae. Instead, they are always visualized at the periphery of the Golgi apparatus, in the bulbous, terminal extensions and most often at those of the trans face. When these terminal extensions, filled with VLDL, attain a certain size, they appear to detach themselves from the main body of the Golgi cisternae and form closed vesicles. These vesicles are called 'secretory vesicles' because of their function to transport secretory products across the cytoplasm to the plasma membrane for export. The VLDL inside the secretory vesicles are closely packed and relatively homogeneous in size. Their diameter appears to be dependent on the experimental conditions and especially on the nutritional state of the liver prior to the perfusion. In the literature, the reported diameters for VLDL vary between 300–600 Å, 400–600 Å and 300–800 Å. At this stage, they are considered as 'mature' VLDL, although the possibility of some further transformations cannot be excluded (ie exchange of constituents between VLDL particles or between VLDL and the membrane of the secretory vesicles.).

From 15 minutes onwards, the final step of VLDL secretion takes place at the hepatocyte sinusoidal border. There, the membrane of the secretory vesicles fuses with the cell membrane and VLDL are discharged in the space of Disse by exocytosis (23). Newly synthesized VLDL can be measured in the circulation 15–20 minutes after administration of a lipid precursor (21, 27).

Biochemical studies have established the identity of hepatic VLDL with plasma VLDL. Schlunk & Lombardi (55) were the first to isolate and purify from the ER VLDL granules, then called 'liposomes'. They showed by chemical analyses that their main constituent were triacylglycerols (61%) while phospholipids and cholesterol esters accounted for 4 and 2.6% respectively and protein for 20%.

Mahley *et al.* (39) analysed VLDL particles from a purified Golgi apparatus fraction. Golgi VLDL floated at d=1.006 g/ml in the ultracentrifuge, like plasma VLDL. Their diameters ranged from 300 to 1000 Å. The lipid composition of Golgi VLDL was similar to that of plasma VLDL and they both contained about 10% protein. Furthermore, Golgi VLDL formed lines of identity with plasma VLDL during immunodiffusion against antiserum to plasma VLDL. On paper electrophoresis, however, only a few Golgi VLDL migrated to the pre-β position like plasma VLDL, but the bulk remained near the origin. This latter observation suggests that nascent VLDL are subjected to some further transformation(s) after transit through the Golgi apparatus.

Alternative pathway for VLDL secretion. Morré (44) presented morphological evidence for a second export route for VLDL particles synthesized in the rat liver. This second pathway seems to be more rapid and direct in that it bypasses the Golgi apparatus and proceeds exclusively via smooth ER → secretory vesicles → plasma membrane.

After formation in the smooth ER, single, large VLDL particles (600–1000 Å) were seen enclosed in smooth ER vesicles which migrated to the plasma membrane, coalesced with it and discharged their VLDL particle in the space of Disse (68). Single VLDL particles were observed in the space of Disse within 5 minutes of their appearance in the smooth ER network, whereas at that time point other VLDL had not reached the secretory face of the Golgi apparatus. The smooth ER-vesicles containing single VLDL granules reached a maximal concentration in the perisinusoidal cytoplasm at 15 minutes after the start of liver perfusion with free fatty acids.

More experimental evidence is needed to establish the role of this second pathway of VLDL biogenesis. An important question that arises from the eventual existence of two different VLDL synthetic pathways is whether these pathways provide the same or different VLDL particles. According to Morré (44), VLDL transiting within smooth ER vesicles are considerably larger (600–1000 Å) than Golgi VLDL (400–600 Å). This suggests that smooth ER-derived VLDL contain more triacylglycerols than Golgi-derived VLDL and that they may form a discreet VLDL subpopulation, eventually with a distinct apoprotein content and metabolic role. On the other hand, several recent studies in rat and rabbit reported the existence of a cholesterol ester-rich VLDL subclass, called β-VLDL, which is also enriched in apo-E; β-VLDL are formed after adaptation of the animals to a hypercholesterolemic diet. Swift *et al.* (65) demonstrated in the rat that these cholesterol ester-rich VLDL particles originate from the liver and pass through the Golgi apparatus.

It would be interesting to investigate if genetic or nutritional factors stimulate specifically one or the other VLDL synthetic pathway. If this were the case, it could partially explain the great heterogeneity of plasma VLDL.

Apoprotein composition of nascent VLDL

Hepatic VLDL contain essentially three apoproteins: apo-B, apo-E and apo-C (12, 22, 34, 36). In this section, current knowledge on the properties, metabolic role and site of incorporation of these apoproteins into nascent VLDL will be briefly discussed.

Apo-B

Apo-B is a very hydrophobic glycoprotein with a high molecular weight. In mammals there are at least two apo-B forms: a high molecular weight apo-B (350 to 550 kDa according to the species studied and presumably also to the different isolation and solubilization procedures used) and a lower molecular weight apo-B (~240–260 kDa). Apo-B studies were simplified by the use of the centile system proposed by Kane *et al.* (33), whereby the high molecular weight apoprotein was termed arbitrarily apo-B_{100} and the low molecular weight one apo-B_{48}. Two more apo-B forms occurring frequently in man appear to be apo-B_{74} and apo-B_{26} (33).

Rat hepatocytes secrete both apo-B_{100} and apo-B_{48} (8, 61, 75), whereas rat enterocytes produce only apo-B_{48} (71, 75). In man, apo-B_{100} originates probably only from liver and apo-B_{48} only from the intestine (33). In the chicken, only the high molecular weight form exists (350 kDa, reference 59).

As shown in cultured chick hepatocytes, apo-B has multiple glycosylation sites (59). The core glycosylation occurs during translation of the apoprotein on the polysomes attached to the rough ER membranes in, at least, two stages. The first glycosyl residues are added when the nascent chain achieves a molecular weight of ~120 kDa and the second when it achieves a molecular weight of ~280 kDa. The terminal glycosylation takes place in the Golgi apparatus. At present, the metabolic function of the glycosyl moieties remains unknown. They do not, however, play a role either in apo-B formation or in its assembly with lipids to form nascent VLDL particles or even in the subsequent VLDL secretion in the plasma, as was demonstrated after inhibition of glycosylation by tunicamycin (60). Apo-B_{48} but not apo-B_{100} is also phosphorylated and contains phosphoserine (15).

Apo-B is essential for the assembly, stability and secretion of triacylglycerol-rich lipoproteins (VLDL and chylomicrons) as evidenced by the fact that VLDL and chylomicrons are absent from the circulation in the case of abetalipoproteinemia, a rare disease with a genetic defect of apo-B. Thus, apo-B assembly with triacylglycerols, phospholipids and presumably also cholesterol results in the formation of nascent VLDL particles at the junctions between rough and smooth ER (4, 27). An intriguing possibility as to the physiological role of the different apo-B peptides was suggested by studies with cultured chick hepatocytes (27, 58). It appears that even incomplete apo-B chains artificially produced, with molecular weights ranging from 300 to as low as 66 kDa retain their ability to bind triacylglycerols and to form VLDL that are subsequently secreted in the incubation medium. It is not yet known, however, if these incomplete apo-B peptides are normally metabolized in the circulation.

A major difference between apo-B and the other apoproteins is that apo-B cannot exchange between lipoprotein particles in the plasma, probably because of its high hydrophobicity. Thus, apo-B has the same turnover rate as the lipoproteins on which it is secreted and serves as a reliable index for the metabolic transformations of these lipoproteins in the plasma compartment. Furthermore, apo-B is specifically recognized by the extrahepatic LDL apo (B, E) receptor as well as by the hepatic apo (B, E) receptor (see the second part of this chapter by Griglio).

Apo-E

Apo-E has a molecular weight of 35 kDa and originates almost exclusively from the liver (74). When analysed by isoelectric focusing, at least five apo-E isoforms appear. Apo-E polymorphism is under genetic control (69). Recently, it was established that apo-E is closely implicated in cholesterol metabolism and serves as a recognition signal for the extrahepatic (B, E) LDL receptor and the hepatic apo (E) remnant receptor (for details see the second part of this chapter).

Dashti *et al.* (12) reported that 65% of the total apo-E secreted by rat hepatocytes in monolayer culture was isolated in the d:1.23 g/ml fraction. Gel filtration chromatography of the lipoproteins secreted by rat hepatocytes in suspension showed that only 25% of the total secreted apo-E was associated with VLDL while the remaining 75% was associated with lipoproteins of smaller diameters (36). This latter apo-E (Lp-E according to reference 2) was almost equally distributed in two peaks corresponding to a particle size of ~100 Å and a molecular weight of ~60 kDa. Thus, the normal rat hepatocyte appears to secrete a significant proportion of apo-E as a low molecular weight, essentially lipid-free form. Conversely, these authors demonstrated with hepatocytes prepared from hypercholesterolemic rats that only 35% (instead of 75%) of apo-E was found in small Lp-E particles with the remainder becoming associated with the larger VLDL particles. These results suggest that the distribution of apo-E between lipoprotein classes is largely dependent on the amount of cholesterol to be secreted by the liver cell, which in turn appears to be regulated by nutritional factors (ie hypercholesterolemic diet).

The exact site of apo-E incorporation into nascent lipoproteins has not been established. Lipoproteins isolated from the Golgi apparatus already contain apo-E (39, 65). It would be interesting to investigate if apo-E becomes attached to VLDL at a pre-Golgi stage, possibly even at the assembly point.

Apo-C

The apo-C family comprises low molecular weight peptides differing widely in metabolic properties (for a review see reference 26). Apo-CII (MW = 12.5 kDa) has a very important physiological function as the activator of lipoprotein lipase (18, 70). Apo-CIII, a glycoprotein, is glycosylated in the Golgi apparatus during transition from the cis to the trans face (16). Human apo-CIII (MW = 8.24 kDa) has three isoforms: $CIII_0$, $CIII_1$ and $CIII_2$ containing 0, 1 or 2 sialic acid molecules at the terminal position of the carbohydrate chain. Rat apo-CIII is larger (MW = 10 kDa) and has two isoforms: $CIII_0$ possessing no sialic acid or hexosamine and $CIII_3$, the major form, containing 1 galactosamine and 3 sialic acid residues per molecule.

Apo-CIII glycosylation appears to depend on metabolic or nutritional conditions. The major part of apo-C peptides originates from the liver (74). Apo-Cs are very mobile peptides, exchanging freely between triacylglycerol-rich lipoproteins and HDL (24).

The intrahepatic site at which nascent VLDL acquire their apo-C complement remains unclear. VLDL isolated from purified Golgi apparatus fractions contain little or no apo-C peptides (28, 45). Nevertheless, VLDL secreted by the perfused rat liver contain apo-C in similar amounts as plasma VLDL (46). On the other hand, VLDL produced by isolated or cultured rat hepatocytes carry very small amounts of apo-C (13, 22, 34, 36). A plausible explanation that could account for these contradictory results is that VLDL acquire apo-C after passage through the Golgi apparatus, either inside the secretory vesicles or in the space of Disse after secretion. Thus, apo-C could be secreted by the hepatocyte either as part of HDL or as free peptides and then transfer to VLDL in the circulation. The reasons why apo-C should apparently become attached to VLDL at the post-secretory stage have not been elucidated to date.

Metabolic regulation of VLDL production

Advantages of studies on isolated or cultured hepatocytes

Isolated or cultured hepatocytes have proven a very useful tool for studying metabolic factors regulating VLDL production. VLDL studies *in vivo* are complicated by two facts: first, the presence in the plasma compartment of lipoproteins originating from liver and intestine; secondly, the rapid catabolism of VLDL by the action of the enzyme lipoprotein lipase (LPL). Thus, at a given moment, circulating VLDL levels result from the hepatic and intestinal secretory rates and from the rate of catabolism depending on LPL activity. Moreover, plasma VLDL have a very different composition compared to nascent VLDL, these qualitative and quantitative changes occurring immediately after secretion. For instance, nascent VLDL contain more triacylglycerols and free cholesterol than plasma VLDL; after secretion, their triacylglycerols are hydrolysed by LPL and their free cholesterol is partly esterified by the enzyme lecithin-cholesterol-acyl-transferase (LCAT). This is not to mention the action of circulating transfer-proteins which facilitate the transfer of all lipid classes between the four lipoprotein populations, with the net result of decreasing VLDL-triacylglycerols and phospholipids and increasing VLDL-cholesterol esters. As regards apoprotein composition, nascent hepatic VLDL contain apo-B, apo-E and probably very little apo-C. Once secreted, VLDL particles retain the same apo-B content (as apo-Bs cannot transfer between lipoproteins) and acquire apo-Cs and more apo-E.

This brief description of the multiple and rapid transformations of nascent VLDL in the plasma compartment illustrates the necessity to use an *in vitro* system in order to study VLDL synthesis and secretion under various metabolic conditions. The perfused rat liver was used successfully in studies of lipoprotein production. It is, however, incovenient to use for comparing different nutritional or hormonal effects, because at least two livers should be perfused in parallel. The isolated hepatocyte model has the advantage over the perfused liver by allowing the simultaneous testing of several metabolic factors on cells originating from the same liver. Furthermore, the investigator can study the metabolic behaviour of hepatocytes only, as the other two liver cell types (endothelial and Küpffer cells) are eliminated during the preparation procedure.

Isolated or cultured hepatocytes are particularly suited for studying the production of VLDL or HDL in their nascent form, as their potential interaction with other lipoprotein fractions within the space of Disse is avoided. For instance, it could be established with isolated hepatocytes that VLDL are secreted without apo-C but acquire them in the space of Disse (see the section on Apo-C).

Lastly, freshly isolated hepatocytes in suspension are capable of synthesizing and secreting appreciable amounts of VLDL, at rates about 50% of those measured *in vivo* after Triton WR-1339 administration (Kalopissis, unpublished results). Furthermore, isolated hepatocytes retain the metabolic characteristics of the donor liver for several hours. Davis *et al.* (13) reported that the nutritional status of the donor rats was manifest in cultured hepatocytes for as long as three days, but these cells have much lower VLDL secretion rates. Both isolated and cultured hepatocytes can be used successfully to investigate substrate and hormonal effects. Isolated rat hepatocytes were first used for VLDL studies by Jeejeebhoy *et al.* (28).

Regulatory factors of VLDL production

VLDL synthesis and secretion appear to be finely regulated by a variety of nutritional and hormonal factors. The observation that VLDL secretion rates do not undergo important variations in physiological conditions (they can be reduced by half or stimulated 2- to 3-fold) suggests that VLDL production is under strict metabolic control.

VLDL biogenesis requires energy in the form of ATP (20), the presence of apoprotein but not an ongoing protein synthesis (6, 27) and an intact microtubular system (64) among others. Although our knowledge on this subject has greatly advanced in recent years, we still have no inkling as to the rate-limiting step(s) of the complex VLDL synthesizing and secretory process.

Nutritional factors. We consider as normal the VLDL secretion of animals fed a standard pellet diet (chow) *ad libitum.* Fasting lowers hepatic VLDL secretion and apo-B_{48} synthesis (40). Even a 4-hour food deprivation of the rats caused a 20% decrease in VLDL-triacylglycerol secretion as measured *in vivo* after Triton WR-1339 injection, which blocks plasma catabolism of VLDL by LPL (31). Electron microscopic images of hepatocytes obtained from 48-hour fasted rats showed very few VLDL particles, whereas 10 to 20 minutes after the start of refeeding the rats with chow containing sesame oil, numerous VLDL particles appeared in the perisinusoidal cytoplasm (68).

Perfusion of liver or incubation of hepatocytes with free fatty acids resulted in a 2- to 3-fold enhanced VLDL production from 20 minutes onwards (the lag time required for synthesis and secretion of VLDL particles — see the section on VLDL transport route through the Golgi apparatus), indicating that the liver rapidly incorporated exogenous fatty acids into VLDL and re-exported them in the circulation (1, 14, 23, 30, 50).

VLDL-triacylglycerol secretion appears to be modulated by the concentration as well as by the nature of the fatty acids added in the medium. Thus, fatty acids at concentrations of 0.25 to 0.75 mM stimulated VLDL-triacylglycerol production by isolated hepatocytes 3 times (1). All fatty acids tested in these experiments (laurate, myristate, stearate, palmitoleate, oleate) stimulated VLDL-triacylglycerol secretion, small differences existing between the various fatty acids. VLDL secretion tended to increase with acyl chain length but no influence of unsaturation could be observed. To obviate differences due to other metabolic effects of each fatty acid (like a different uptake or oxidation), a better estimation of VLDL enhancement was obtained by calculating the ratio: medium triacylglycerols/cell triacylglycerols, than by the value of medium triacylglycerols alone.

Nevertheless, this stimulatory effect is apparent only on the triacylglycerol moiety of the VLDL particles, their apoprotein content (apo-B, apo-E and apo-C) remaining unchanged (14, 50). Thus, the short-term effect of fatty acids is not a true increase of hepatic VLDL secretion, which would imply an increased apoprotein synthesis as well. Instead, in the presence of fatty acids, the liver secretes larger VLDL particles, enriched in triacylglycerols. This is corroborated by electron microscopic studies, where VLDL particles formed in the hepatocytes have diameters from 300 to 600 Å. After liver perfusion with fatty acids, nascent VLDL appearing along the synthetic and secretory pathway have diameters ranging between 600 and 1000 Å (23).

These results suggest the following. First, that triacylglycerol and apoprotein synthesis are not tightly coupled (as also demonstrated by reference 27). Secondly, that apoproteins have the ability to interact with variable amounts of cellular lipids.

In our laboratory, we investigated the long-term effect of dietary fatty acids. We used Wistar rats adapted to a high fat diet for three weeks which results in elevated plasma non-esterified fatty acid levels during the greater part of the 24-hour cycle, especially during the nocturnal spontaneous feeding period. These animals had a 40% decreased total (hepatic and intestinal) post-Triton VLDL secretion in the plasma (31). Moreover, post-Triton VLDL secretion measured at 08, 14 and 20 h was not correlated with the corresponding plasma non-esterified fatty acid concentrations either with the control or with the high-fat diet. The decreased VLDL production was solely attributable to the liver, as isolated hepatocytes of fat-fed rats secreted 50% less VLDL-triacylglycerols and incorporated 70% less 1–^{14}C oleate in VLDL-triacylglycerol as compared to cells prepared from control rats (32). Fat feeding also induces a mild steatosis of rat liver which appears to be proportional to the amount of dietary fat and to the duration of ingestion of this diet (Kalopissis, unpublished observations). This observation is a further indication that triacylglycerols tend to accumulate in the liver with this diet and are much less exported in the circulation in the form of VLDL-triacylglycerols.

Coupled together, short- and long-term fatty acid studies point out that exogenous fatty acids can rapidly modulate hepatic VLDL-triacylglycerol production but are probably not the prime determinant regulating this pathway.

Conversely, a diet rich in sucrose induced a 2- to 3-fold increased VLDL formation, an effect mediated by the fructose molecule (67). This stimulation concerned both the triacylglycerol and the apoprotein components of VLDL, reflecting an increased number of VLDL particles and not just an enrichment of VLDL in triacylglycerols (51). When challenged with the same fatty acid loads as hepatocytes from control rats, hepatocytes of sucrose-fed animals can thus respond by increasing their VLDL-triacyglycerol and apoprotein production 2-times more (14, 57). Electron microscopic studies corroborated these findings (47, 48).

At the same time, a sucrose-rich diet greatly enhances *de novo* fatty acid synthesis (lipogenesis). As a close parallelism appears to exist between lipogenesis and VLDL secretion in many physiological situations, the concept arose that these two metabolic pathways could be causally related (73). Nevertheless, it was never verified experimentally.

We tested this hypothesis in our laboratory by first trying to evaluate the amount of fatty acids synthesized *de novo* that was secreted as VLDL-triacylglycerols or phospholipids (32). Under standard nutritional conditions, fatty acids synthesized by the lipogenic pathway could account at most for 13% of the total VLDL-triacylglycerols and only for traces of the VLDL-phospholipids secreted by isolated hepatocytes after a 2-hour incubation. We then inhibited lipogenesis *in vitro* by incubating hepatocytes with a long-chain fatty acid (oleate, at a concentration of 1 mM). VLDL secretion by hepatocytes in which lipogenesis was inhibited by 75%

was identical with the secretion of control cells (without oleate) where lipogenesis was operative. These results argue against a causal relationship between lipogenesis and VLDL production. More recently, Pullinger & Gibbons (52) studying VLDL-triacylglycerol and cholesterol secretion by isolated hepatocytes under two different nutritional conditions (just before the animals had access to food and 6 hours after the start of the feeding period) also observed that VLDL secretion was not necessarily coupled to the liver lipogenic rate.

In order to identify all the possible hepatic precursors of VLDL-triacylglycerols (which are the major VLDL component accounting for 60 to 70% of their mass), we focused our attention on the two metabolically distinct triacylglycerols pools, the small, active pool located on the smooth ER-membranes and the large, inactive storage pool located in the cytoplasm (see the section on smooth ER). Experimental evidence (5) suggests that the cytoplasmic triacylglycerol pool represents in fact the third precursor of hepatic VLDL-triacylglycerols which has not always been recognized as such, most authors investigating the exogenous or endogenous origin of the VLDL-triacylglycerol-fatty acids. From a quantitative point of view, this precursor appears to account for approximately one-half the VLDL-triacylglycerols secreted by isolated hepatocytes obtained from rats fed a standard diet (32). Here again, electron microscopy is very useful as it illustrates, how under conditions of

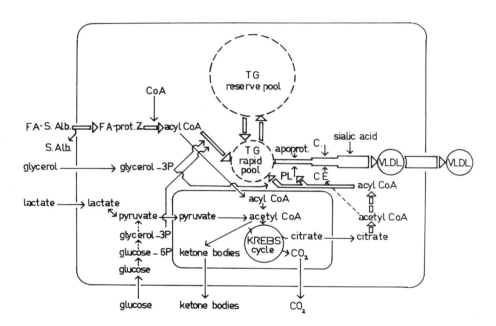

Fig. 2. Pathway of incorporation of fatty acids into VLDL-triacylglycerols (TG) in the hepatocyte. The 'TG rapid pool', located on the membranes of the smooth ER, and the 'TG reserve pool', located in the cytoplasm, are in dynamic equilibrium. It is proposed that, independently of an exogenous or endogenous origin, the 'TG rapid pool' is the immediate precursor of VLDL-triacylglycerols; the passage of triacylglycerols from the 'TG reserve pool' to the 'TG rapid pool' could involve a lysosomal hydrolysis step. FA: fatty acids; S. Alb.: serum albumin; prot. Z: protein Z; apoprot.: apoproteins.

hepatic triacyglycerol mobilization, the membrane-rimmed cytoplasmic lipid droplets progressively disappear, while at the same time their labelled triacylglycerols are partly secreted in the medium as VLDL-triacylglycerols (42).

In Fig. 2, we represent the three precursors of VLDL-triacylglycerols in the hepatocytes, namely: 1) exogenous (plasma) fatty acids; 2) endogenous (synthesized *de novo*) fatty acids, and 3) fatty acids originating from triacylglycerols previously stored in the cytoplasm. The following pathway of incorporation of fatty acids into nascent VLDL-triacylglycerols is proposed.

Independently of their exogenous or endogenous origin, the major part of the fatty acids present inside the hepatocytes is rapidly esterified to triacylglycerols on the membranes of the smooth ER which possess the necessary enzymatic equipment (7). This membrane-pool represents the small active pool of triacylglycerols (62). Part of these triacylglycerols is immediately assembled with apo-B (and eventually other apoproteins) at the junctions between smooth and rough ER, thus forming nascent VLDL particles. The amount of triacylglycerols that will be incorporated in VLDL depends apparently on apoprotein availability; in other words, it depends on the size of the apoprotein storage pool in the rough ER lumen (see section on rough ER). The remaining triacylglycerols are stored temporarily inside vesicles which could be formed, at least in some cases (ie fatty liver), by direct vesiculation of the smooth ER. A dynamic equilibrium appears to exist between the two hepatocyte triacylglycerol pools, equilibration occurring in 2 hours (62). It was proposed that the reverse pathway, namely the passage of stored triacylglycerols from the cytoplasm to the membranes of the smooth ER, could involve prior hydrolysis, probably in the lysosomes (5). Mooney & Lane (42) showed that this was actually the case in cultured chick hepatocytes. Using isolated rat hepatocytes in which lysosomal activity was inhibited by chloroquine we obtained a 30 to 50% inhibition of VLDL-triacylglycerol secretion after 1 hour (Francone & Kalopissis, published in abstract form in *Diabète et Métabolisme* (Paris) 1984, **10**: 339–350). Thus, available experimental evidence suggests that triacylglycerols stored in the cytoplasm are first subjected to lysosomal hydrolysis and then re-esterified on the smooth ER membranes and targeted near the vicinity of apoproteins to form nascent VLDL particles.

In this text we will not include hypercholesterolemic diets, since these diets are artificial and designed to mimic in animal models the lipoprotein profile of humans with genetic forms of hypercholesterolemia.

Summarizing the effects of nutritional factors on hepatocyte VLDL production, it would appear that neither exogenous nor endogenous fatty acid supply *per se* exercises a regulatory role on this metabolic process. The capability of the liver to synthesize and secrete VLDL is probably best reflected in the size of its apoprotein storage pool. This apoprotein pool and the ability of the apoproteins to assemble with variable amounts of apolar lipids are probably the basis for the rapid, short-term responses of hepatocytes to external challenges that modulate VLDL production rates. To our knowledge, the mechanism by which the size of the apoprotein storage pool is regulated remains unknown.

Hormonal factors. The VLDL synthetic and secretory pathway is also under hormonal control. In this section we will briefly discuss the role of oestrogens, thyroid hormone, glucagon and insulin.

The role of estrogens in VLDL production is well established. Wilcox *et al.* (72) were among the first investigators to show that perfused livers from female rats secreted more VLDL than livers obtained from male rats. Moreover, this phenomenon was measured over a wide range of concentrations of infused oleic acid (between 0 and 1.5 mM). Female rat livers secreted larger VLDL particles containing proportionately more triacylglycerol than phospholipid and cholesterol.

The influence of estrogens on VLDL production is even more clearcut in chick liver cells. In this species, VLDL originate only from liver and their synthesis appears to be exclusively under estrogen control. Chickens treated with 17-β-estradiol display very high plasma VLDL levels. Cultured hepatocytes obtained from estrogenized chicks secreted 5-times more VLDL than hepatocytes of untreated chicks (66). Estradiol treatment resulted also in a 4.2-fold increased apo-B synthesis without affecting secretion of apo-AI and other VLDL apoproteins (41). Furthermore, this hormone specifically induces the production of apo-II, a major VLDL apoprotein in the avian species, which is not synthesized prior to estradiol treatment. This unique apoprotein of small molecular weight (MW=9.5 kDa) shares with apo-B the characteristic to bind very tightly to VLDL lipids and to remain attached to VLDL particles after their secretion in plasma without being transferred to other lipoproteins (41).

Alterations in the circulating levels of thyroid hormone in man are associated with varying concentrations of plasma triacylglycerols. Therefore, the direct influence of the thyroid status on hepatic VLDL production was investigated *in vitro*, using perfused rat livers (35). Compared to euthyroid animals, rats rendered hyperthyroid after a 7-day treatment with triidothyronine (T_3) displayed a 60% decreased VLDL-triacylglycerol secretion as well as a 60% decreased incorporation of an exogenous fatty acid into VLDL-triacylglycerols, while at the same time hepatic ketogenesis increased. Conversely, livers from hypothyroid rats (treated during 7 days with propyl-thiouracyl) tended to increase their VLDL-triacylglycerol secretion and the incorporation of the infused fatty acid in this fraction. However, the thyroid status did not alter fatty acid uptake by the liver. In keeping with its inhibitory effect on hepatic fatty acid esterification and VLDL-triacylglycerol output, hyperthyroidism produced smaller VLDL particles having a higher proportion of surface lipids (phospholipids and cholesterol) relative to core lipid (triacylglycerols).

Glucagon exercises an inhibitory effect on hepatic VLDL secretion, which is consistent with low plasma triacylglycerol levels measured *in vivo* when gluca-gonemia is elevated (ie during fasting). Heimberg *et al.* (25) demonstrated that glucagon decreased by half triacylglycerol output from perfused rat livers. The same 50% VLDL decrease was measured with or without infusion of fatty acids. In these experiments, glucagon inhibited triacylglycerol secretion without affecting fatty acid uptake by the liver. The hormone also had a marked ketogenic effect when infused in the presence of fatty acids up to a concentration of 1 mM.

The role of glucagon was also tested in isolated hepatocytes obtained from rats in two nutritional conditions: 1) just before the start of the feeding period, and; 2) 6 hours after the animals began to eat (52). In both cases glucagon inhibited VLDL-triacylglycerol secretion by 75 and 65% respectively, while at the same time it virtually abolished lipogenesis. The effect of glucagon was further tested with hepatocytes incubated with pyruvate which induced a 2-fold stimulation of lipogenesis and VLDL production. Here again glucagon inhibited the stimulated VLDL output, but only by ~30%. Thus, the stimulatory effect of pyruvate prevailed, the VLDL secretion remaining higher than that of control liver cells.

The same inhibitory effect of glucagon and cAMP on VLDL production was obtained with cultured chick hepatocytes (42). This study also clarified the mechanism of action of cAMP on hepatic triacylglycerol metabolism. It appears that cAMP decreased considerably the cytoplasmic triacylglycerol storage pool by activating, directly or indirectly, triacylglycerol hydrolysis presumably via a lysosomal lipase (see section on nutritional factors and Fig. 2). The resulting fatty acids entered preferentially in the mitochondria and were oxidized to ketone bodies. The passage of fatty acids in the mitochondria was further enhanced by addition of carnitine. The authors also showed that cAMP did not affect 'en bloc' triacylglycerol secretion, ie without prior lipolysis. Their 'en bloc' triacylglycerol secretion may correspond to triacylglycerols located on the smooth ER (small, active pool) which are immediately assembled with apoproteins to form nascent VLDL for export. It would be interesting to establish if cAMP exerts the same mechanism of action in mammalian livers.

A great controversy exists in the literature regarding the direct role of insulin on hepatic VLDL production. In a study *in vivo*, Alcindor *et al.* (3) reported a 30% inhibition of post-Triton VLDL secretion following a single insulin injection into the rats. Addition of insulin to cultured rat hepatocytes ellicited small decreases in VLDL-triacylglycerol secretion which were proportional to the hormonal concentration (17). At physiological insulin concentrations (15 to 30 μU/ml for the rat) VLDL production was not altered; it began to decrease from concentrations $\geqslant$50 μU/ml. Thus, triacylglycerol output was lowered by 12, 20 or 45% in the presence of insulin at 50, 100 or 200 μU/ml respectively. As regards VLDL apoproteins, only apo-B synthesis was diminished by 20% upon addition of insulin (at 50 or 200 μU/ml) whereas apo-E and apo-CIII$_3$ production was unaffected by the hormone (49). An interesting observation was the decreased proportion of these three apoproteins in the VLDL fraction when insulin was present (49). In another study, using isolated hepatocytes prepared in two nutritional conditions (see preceding paragraph and reference 52), a 20% lower VLDL-triacylglycerol output was obtained in the presence of insulin (1000 μU/ml). However, when VLDL production was stimulated 2-fold by pyruvate, insulin provoked a pronounced inhibition of this pathway (by 70 to 80%). Thus, the stimulation of VLDL secretion by pyruvate was abolished in the presence of insulin and VLDL output returned to control levels.

On the contrary, the Mayes' laboratory (38, 67) reported 30% increased VLDL secretion rates by rat livers perfused with insulin. Tarlow *et al.* (66) using cultured chick hepatocytes obtained a 2- to 3-fold increased VLDL-apoprotein secretion in the presence of insulin and attributed it to a non-specific effect of the hormone on total protein synthesis.

Indirect evidence for a positive effect of insulin in VLDL production is provided by two different experimental models: 1) the genetically obese Zucker rat where hyperinsulinemia is associated with a 2.5-fold increased hepatic VLDL secretion (56), and 2) the streptozotocin-diabetic rat which has a very decreased hepatic VLDL secretion, the various VLDL constituents being inhibited in different degrees, ie triacylglycerols by 60%, cholesterol by 70%, apoprotein by 40% (10). Experimental diabetes further induces qualitative alterations in apoprotein synthesis, the most intriguing being the virtual disappearance of apo-E (10).

Thus, while the negative effects of thyroid hormone and glucagon and the positive effect of estradiol on hepatic VLDL production appear well established, the role of insulin on this process remains unclear. A direct effect of insulin on VLDL formation is not yet proven, as only very elevated doses of the hormone could ellicit small changes (either decreases or increases) of VLDL secretion.

REFERENCES

1 Åkesson B.: Effect of different fatty acids on triacylglycerol secretion in isolated rat hepatocytes. *Lipids* 1980, **15**: 677–681.

2 Alaupovic P., Lee D. M., McConathy W.: Studies on the composition and structure of plasma lipoproteins. Distribution of lipoprotein families in major density classes of normal human plasma lipoproteins. *Biochim. Biophys. Acta* 1972, **260**: 689–707.

3 Alcindor L. G., Infante R., Soler-Argilaga C., Polonovski J.: Effect of a single insulin administration on the hepatic release of triglycerides into the plasma. *Biochim. Biophys. Acta* 1973, **306**: 347–352.

4 Alexander C. A., Hamilton R. L., Havel R. J.: Subcellular localization of B apoprotein of plasma lipoproteins in rat liver. *J. Cell Biol.* 1976, **69**: 241–263.

5 Bar-On H., Roheim P. S., Stein O., Stein Y.: Contribution of floating fat triglyceride and of lecithin towards formation of secretory triglyceride in perfused rat liver. *Biochim. Biophys. Acta* 1971, **248**: 1–11.

6 Bar-On H., Kook A. I., Stein O., Stein Y.: Assembly and secretion of VLDL by rat liver following inhibition of protein synthesis with cycloheximide. *Biochim. Biophys. Acta* 1973, **306**: 106–114.

7 Bell R. M., Coleman R. A.: Enzymes of glycerolipid synthesis in eukaryotes. *Ann. Rev. Biochem.* 1980, **49**: 459–487.

8 Bell-Quint J., Forte T., Graham P.: Synthesis of two forms of apolipoprotein B by cultured rat hepatocytes. *Biochem. Biophys. Res. Commun.* 1981, **99**: 700–706.

9 Bell-Quint J., Forte T., Graham P.: Glycosylation of apolipoproteins by cultured rat hepatocytes. *Biochem. J.* 1981, **200**: 409–414.

10 Berry E. M., Ziv E., Bar-On H.: Lipoprotein secretion by isolated perfused livers from streptozotocin-diabetic rats. *Diabetologia* 1981, **21**: 402–408.

11 Claude A.: Growth and differentiation of cytoplasmic membranes in the course of lipoprotein granule synthesis in the hepatic cell. I. Elaboration of elements of the Golgi complex. *J. Cell Biol.* 1970, **47**: 745–766.

12 Dashti N., McConathy W. J., Ontko J. A.: Production of apolipoproteins E and A-I by rat hepatocytes in primary culture. *Biochim. Biophys. Acta* 1980, **618**: 347–358.

13 Davis R. A., Engelhorn S. C., Pangburn S. H., Weinstein D. B., Steinberg D.: Very low density lipoprotein synthesis and secretion by cultured rat hepatocytes. *J. Biol. Chem.* 1979, **254**: 2010–2016.

14 Davis R. A., Boogaerts J. R.: Intrahepatic assembly of very low density lipoproteins. Effect of fatty acids on triacylglycerol and apolipoprotein sythesis. *J. Biol. Chem.* 1982, **257**: 10908–10913.

15 Davis R. A., Clinton G. M., Borchardt R. A., Malone-McNeal M., Tan T., Lattier, G. R.: Intrahepatic assembly of very low density lipoproteins. Phosphorylation of small molecular weight apolipoprotein. B. *J. Biol. Chem.* 1984, **259**: 3383–3386.

16 Dolphin P. J., Rubinstein D.: Glycosylation of apoproteins of rat very low density lipoproteins during transit through the hepatic Golgi apparatus. *Can. J. Biochem.* 1976, **55**: 83–90.

17 Durrington P. N., Newton R. S., Weinstein D. B., Steinberg D.: Effects of insulin and glucose on very low density lipoprotein triglyceride secretion by cultured rat hepatocytes. *J. Clin. Invest.* 1982, **70**: 63–73.

18 Ekman R., Nilsson-Ehle P.: Effects of apolipoproteins on lipoprotein lipase activity of human

adipose tissue. *Clin. Chim. Acta* 1975, **63**: 29–35.

19 Eisenberg S., Bilheimer D. W., Levy R. I., Lindgren F. T.: On the metabolic conversion of human plasma very low density lipoprotein to low density lipoprotein. *Biochim. Biophys. Acta* 1973, **326**: 361–377.

20 Farber E.: Ethionine fatty liver. *Adv. Lipid Res.* 1967, **5**: 119–183.

21 Glaumann H., Bergstrand A., Ericsson J. L. E.: Studies on the synthesis and intracellular transport of lipoprotein particles in rat liver. *J. Cell Biol.* 1975, **64**: 356–377.

22 Haagsman H. P., van Golde L. M. G.: Synthesis and secretion of very low density lipoproteins by isolated rat hepatocytes in suspension: role of diacylglycerol acyltransferase. *Arch. Biochem. Biophys.* 1981, **208**: 395–402.

23 Hamilton R. L., Regen D. M., Gray M. E., Lequire V. S.: Lipid transport in rat liver 1. Electron microscopic identification of very low density lipoproteins in perfused rat liver. *Lab. Invest.* 1967, **16**: 305–319.

24 Havel R. J., Kane J. P., Kashyap M. L.: Interchange of apolipoproteins between chylomicrons and high density lipoproteins during alimentary lipemia in man. *J. Clin. Invest.* 1973, **52**: 32–38.

25 Heimberg M., Weinstein I., Kohout M.: The effects of glucagon, dibutyryl cyclic adenosine 3′,5′-monophosphate and concentration of free fatty acid on hepatic lipid metabolism. *J. Biol. Chem.* 1969, **244**: 5131–5139.

26 Jackson R. L., Morrisett J. D., Gotto A. M. Jr: Lipoprotein structure and metabolism. *Physiol. Rev.* 1976, **56**: 259–316.

27 Janero D. R., Lane M. D.: Sequential assembly of very low density lipoprotein apolipoproteins, triacylglycerol and phosphoglycerides by the intact liver cell. *J. Biol. Chem.* 1983, **258**: 14496–14504.

28 Jeejeebhoy K. N., Ho J., Breckenridge C., Bruce-Robertson A., Steiner G., Jeejeebhoy J.: Synthesis of VLDL by isolated rat hepatocytes in suspension. *Biochem. Biophys. Res. Comm.* 1975, **66**: 1147–1153.

29 Jelsema C. L., Morré D. J.: Distribution of phospholipid biosynthetic enzymes among cell components of rat liver. *J. Biol. Chem.* 1978, **253**: 7960–7971.

30 Jones A. L., Ruderman N. B., Herrera M. G.: Electron microscopic and biochemical study of lipoprotein synthesis in the isolated perfused rat liver. *J. Lipid Res.* 1967, **8**: 429–446.

31 Kalopissis A. D., Griglio S., Malewiak M. I., Rozen R.: Effect of a high-fat diet on rat very low density lipoprotein secretion. *Biochim. Biophys. Acta* 1980, **620**: 111–119.

32 Kalopissis A. D., Griglio S., Malewiak M. I., Rozen R., Le Liepvre X.: Very-low-density-lipoprotein secretion by isolated hepatocytes of fat-fed rats. *Biochem. J.* 1981, **198**: 373–377.

33 Kane J. P., Hardman D. A., Paulus H. E.: Heterogeneity of apolipoprotein B: Isolation of a new species from human chylomicrons. *Proc. Natl. Acad. Sci.* 1980, **77**: 2465–2469.

34 Kempen H. J. M.: Lipoprotein secretion by isolated rat hepatocytes: characterization of the lipid-carrying particles and modulation of their release. *J. Lipid Res.* 1980, **21**: 671–680.

35 Keyes W. G., Wilcox H. G., Heimberg M.: Formation of the very low density lipoprotein and metabolism of 1–^{14}C oleate by perfused livers from rats treated with triiodothyronine or propylthiouracil. *Metabolism* 1981, **30**: 135–146.

36 Krul E. S., Dolphin P. J. Rubinstein D.: Secretion of nascent lipoproteins by isolated rat hepatocytes. *Can. J. Biochem.* 1981, **59**: 676–686.

37 Lacy P. E., Howell S. L., Young D. A., Fink C. J.: New hypothesis of insulin secretion. *Nature* 1968, **219**: 1177–1179.

38 Laker M. E., Mayes P. A.: Investigations into the direct effects of insulin on hepatic ketogenesis, lipoprotein secretion and pyruvate dehydrogenase activity. *Biochim. Biophys. Acta* 1984, **795**: 427–430.

39 Mahley R. W., Hamilton R. L., Lequire V. S.: Characterization of lipoprotein particles isolated from the Golgi apparatus of rat liver. *J. Lipid Res.* 1969, **10**: 433–439.

40 Marsh J. B., Sparks C. E.: The effect of fasting on the secretion of lipoproteins and two forms of apo-B by perfused rat liver. *Proc. Soc. Exp. Biol. Med.* 1982, **170**: 178–181.

41 Miller K. W., Lane M. D.: Estradiol-induced alteration of very-low-density-lipoprotein assembly. *J. Biol. Chem.* 1984, **259**: 15277–15286.

42 Mooney R. A., Lane M. D.: Formation and turnover of triglyceride-rich vesicles in the chick liver cell. Effects of cAMP and carnitine on triglyceride mobilization and conversion to ketones. *J. Biol.*

Chem. 1981, **256**: 11724–11733.

43 Morré D. J., Ovtracht L.: Structure of rat liver Golgi apparatus: relationship to lipoprotein secretion. *J. Ultrastructure Res.* 1981, **74**: 284–295.

44 Morré D. J.: An alternative pathway for secretion of lipoprotein particles in rat liver. *Europ. J. Cell Biol.* 1981, **26**: 21–25.

45 Nestruck A. C., Rubinstein D.: The synthesis of apoproteins of very low density lipoproteins isolated from the Golgi apparatus of rat liver. *Can. J. Biochem.* 1976, **54**: 617–628.

46 Noel S. P., Rubinstein D.: Secretion of apolipoproteins in very low density and high density lipoproteins by perfused rat liver. *J. Lipid Res.* 1974, **15**: 301–308.

47 Novikoff P. M., Roheim P. S., Novikoff A. B., Edelstein D.: Production and prevettion of fatty liver in rats fed clofibrate and orotic acid diets containing sucrose. *Lab. Invest.* 1974, **30**: 732–750.

48 Novikoff P. M., Yam A.: The cytochemical demonstration of GERL in rat hepatocytes during lipoprotein mobilization. *J. Histochem. Cytochem.* 1978, **26**: 1–13.

49 Patsch W., Franz S., Schonfeld G.: Role of insulin in lipoprotein secretion by cultured rat hepatocytes. *J. Clin. Invest.* 1983, **71**: 1161–1174.

50 Patsch W., Tamai T., Schonfeld G.: Effect of fatty acids on lipid and apoprotein secretion and association in hepatocyte cultures. *J. Clin. Invest.* 1983, **72**: 371–378.

51 Petersburg S. J., Madeley A., Robinson D. .S: A study of the interrelationship between the triacylglycerol and protein components of very-low-density lipoproteins using the perfused rat liver. *Biochem. J.* 1975, **150**: 315–321.

52 Pullinger C. R., Gibbons G. F. Effects of hormones and pyruvate on the rates of secretion of very-low density lipoprotein triacylglycerol and cholesterol by rat hepatocytes. *Biochim. Biophys. Acta* 1985, **833**: 44–51.

53 Redman C. M.: The synthesis of serum proteins on attached rather than free ribosomes of rat liver. *Biochem. Biophys. Res. Commun.* 1968, **31**: 845–850.

54 Redman C. M., Cherian M. G.: The secretory pathways of rat serum glycoproteins and albumin. Localization of newly formed proteins within the endoplasmic reticulum. *J. Cell Biol.* 1972, **52**: 231–245.

55 Schlunk F. F., Lombardi B.: Liver liposomes. I. Isolation and chemical characterization. *Lab. Invest.* 1967, **17**: 30–38.

56 Schonfeld G., Pfleger B.: Overproduction of very low-density lipoproteins by livers of genetically obese rats. *Am. J. Physiol.* 1971, **220**: 1178–1182.

57 Schonfeld G., Pfleger B.: Utilization of exogenous free fatty acids for the production of very low density lipoprotein triglyceride by livers of carbohydrate-fed rats. *J. Lipid Res.* 1971, **12**: 614–621.

58 Siuta-Mangano P., Lane M. D.: Very low density lipoprotein synthesis and secretion. Extrusion of apoprotein B nascent chains through the membrane of the endoplasmic reticulum without protein synthesis. *J. Biol. Chem.* 1981, **256**: 2094–2097.

59 Siuta-Mangano P., Howard S. C., Lennarz W. J., Lane M. D.: Synthesis, processing and secretion of apolipoprotein B by the chick liver cell. *J. Biol. Chem.* 1982, **257**: 4292–4300.

60 Siuta-Mangano P., Janero D. R., Lane M. D.: Association and assembly of triglyceride and phospholipid with glycosylated and unglycosylated apoproteins of very low density lipoprotein in the intact liver cell. *J. Biol. Chem.* 1982, **257**: 11463–11467.

61 Sparks C. E., Marsh J. B.: Metabolic heterogeneity of apolipoprotein B in the rat. *J. Lipid Res.* 1981, **22**: 519–527.

62 Stein Y., Shapiro B.: Assimilation and dissimilation of fatty acids by the rat liver. *Am. J. Physiol.* 1959, **196**: 1238–1241.

63 Stein O., Stein Y.: Lipid synthesis intracellular transport, storage and secretion. I. Electron microscopic radioautographic study of liver after injection of tritiated palmitate or glycerol in fasted and ethanol-treated rats. *J. Cell Biol.* 1967, **33**: 319–339.

64 Stein O., Sanger L., Stein Y.: Colchicine-induced inhibition of lipoprotein and protein secretion into the serum and lack of interference with secretion of biliary phospholipids and cholesterol by rat liver *in vivo. J. Cell Biol.* 1974, **62**: 90–103.

65 Swift L. L., Soulé P. D., Lequire V. S.: Hepatic Golgi lipoproteins: precursors to plasma lipoproteins in hypercholesterolemic rats. *J. Lipid Res.* 1982, **23**: 962–971.

66 Tarlow D. M., Watkins P. A., Reed R. E., Miller R. S., Zwergel E. E., Lane M. D.: Lipogenesis and the synthesis and secretion of very low density lipoprotein by avian liver cells in

nonproliferating monolayer culture. *J. Cell Biol.* 1977, **73**: 332–353.

67 Topping D. L., Mayes P. A.: The immediate effects of insulin and fructose on the metabolism of the perfused liver. Changes in lipoprotein secretion, fatty acid oxidation and esterification, lipogenesis and carbohydrate metabolism. *Biochem. J.* 1972, **126**: 295–311.

68 Twaddle M. L., Jersild R. A., Dileepan K. N., Morre D. J.: Kinetics of appearance of lipoprotein particles in perisinusoidal cisternae of smooth endplasmic reticulum of isolated rat livers perfused with free fatty acids. *Europ. J. Cell Biol.* 1981, **26**: 26–34.

69 Utermann G., Langenbeck U., Beisiegel U., Weber U.: Genetics of the apolipoprotein E system in man. *Am. J. Hum. Genet.* 1980, **32**: 339–347.

70 Vainio P., Virtanen J. A., Sparrow J. T., Gotto A. M. Jr, Kinnunen, P. K. V.: Esterase-type of activity possessed by human plasma apolipoprotein CII and its synthetic fragments. *Chem. Phys. Lipids* 1983, **33**: 21–32.

71 Van't Hooft F. M., Hardman D. A., Kane J. P., Havel R. J.: Apolipoprotein B (B-48) of rat chylomicrons is not a precursor of the apolipoprotein of low density lipoproteins. *Proc. Natl. Acad. Sci.* 1982, **79**: 179–182.

72 Wilcox H. G., Woodside W. F., Breen K. J., Knapp H. R. Jr, Heimberg M.: The effect of sex on certain properties of the very low density lipoprotein secreted by the liver. *Biochem. Biophys. Res. Comm.* 1974, **58**: 919–926.

73 Windmueller H. G., Spaeth A. E.: *De novo* synthesis of fatty acid in perfused rat liver as a determinant of plasma lipoprotein production. *Arch. Biochem. Biophys.* 1967, **122**: 362–369.

74 Wu A. L., Windmueller H. G.: Relative contribution by liver and intestine to individual plasma apolipoprotein in the rat. *J. Biol. Chem.* 1979, **254**: 7316–7322.

75 Wu A. L., Windmueller H. G.: Variant forms of plasma apolipoprotein B. Hepatic and intestinal biosynthesis and heterogeneous metabolism in the rat. *J. Biol. Chem.* 1981, **256**: 3615–3618.

76 Wunderlich F., Mueller R., Speth V.: Direct evidence for a colchicine-induced impairment in the mobility of membrane components. *Science* 1973, **182**: 1136–1138.

Research in *Isolated and cultured hepatocytes* A. Guillouzo & C. Guguen-Guillouzo eds. pp. 135–154.
© 1986 John Libbey Eurotext Ltd./INSERM.

6

Lipoprotein metabolism in isolated and cultured hepatocytes

Part 2: LIPOPROTEIN CATABOLISM BY LIVER CELLS

Sabine GRIGLIO

Laboratoire de Physiopathologie de la Nutrition, INSERM U177, Institut Biomédical des Cordeliers, 15, rue de l'Ecole de Médecine, 75270 Paris Cedex 06, FRANCE

SUMMARY

In vivo clearance studies and *in vitro* experiments with perfused livers, isolated hepatocytes and sinusoidal cells have allowed a comprehensive view of hepatic lipoprotein metabolism. *In vivo*, triglyceride-rich lipoproteins are first degraded into remnants which are taken up avidly by the liver and catabolized through a receptor-mediated process. Thus 70% of chylomicron remnants are recognized by the remnant apoprotein (apo-E) receptor, 70% of very low density lipoproteins (VLDL) remnants — both by remnant and low density lipoproteins (LDL) (apo-B, -E) receptors. Suspended hepatocytes and monolayers bind these remnants with high affinity, but only cultured cells degrade appreciably both their protein and lipid moieties. Apo-E is the determinant of binding to the remnant receptor while apo-CIII is an inhibitor of this process. Lipogenesis and cholesterol synthesis are inhibited in the perfused liver by triglyceride-rich lipoproteins and their remnants. However, inhibition of cholesterol synthesis in suspended hepatocytes has not been clearly demonstrated. LDL are also catabolized by the liver by means of both a receptor-dependent and a receptor-independent process. The LDL (apo-B, -E) receptor can be measured in cultured hepatocytes of adult rabbits, in hepatic plasma membranes from young dogs and from human fetuses and also in hepatocytes of neonatal pigs. Few LDL receptors are detected in hepatocytes of adult rats, but LDL binding to these cells is greatly enhanced after oestrogen treatment of the animals. HDL are bound and degraded *in vivo* by the liver and *in vitro* by either suspended or cultured hepatocytes through a receptor-mediated process. Apo-A–I is the ligand for this receptor. It is not yet clearly established how high density lipoproteins (HDL) are degraded, inasmuch as their cholesteryl ester is catabolized to a much larger extent than their apoproteins. Freshly prepared hepatocytes bind remnants, LDL and HDL but a defect in the lysosomal degradation pathway has been repeatedly reported suggesting that a step subsequent to binding needs to be restored after the isolation of the cells with collagenase. Finally, a metabolic cooperation between hepatocytes and non-parenchymal cells has been suggested by Van Berkel, which could ensure *in vivo* the high capacity of the liver to degrade the triglyceride-rich lipoprotein remnants.

Introduction

The liver plays an important role in lipoprotein catabolism and as such has received an increasing amount of interest over the past decade. An overview of lipoprotein structure and metabolism is given by Kalopissis in the first part of this chapter. It has been demonstrated using *in vivo* experiments with several animal species that it is the major site, but not the unique one, for the degradation of lipoprotein components: apoproteins of VLDL (66) and of HDL (19), cholesterol of the cholesteryl ester-rich particles like 'remnant particles' (20, 46, 48) and also cholesteryl ester present in LDL and HDL.

In vivo clearance studies with radio-labelled lipoproteins have enabled some comprehension of the physiological processes but are not sufficient to understand the precise mechanism of the catabolism of lipoproteins in the liver. The reasons for this are the following: first, the different components of the lipoproteins are exchanged between lipoprotein classes in lymph and then in the plasma so that the native particles are modified before reaching the liver; secondly, many other organs like muscles and the heart, adipose tissue and cells like macrophages, endothelial cells and fibroblasts participate in lipoprotein catabolism; thirdly, the liver is not an homogeneous tissue and contains hepatocytes and non-parenchymal cells (NPC), consisting of endothelial, Kupffer, fat storing and pit cells. The presence and the relative concentrations of receptors, and also of enzymes in these cell populations, will determine the uptake and catabolism of lipoproteins by the liver. Thus, the use of hepatocytes, either freshly isolated or as monolayers, has become necessary to further investigate the mechanism of lipoprotein degradation, and has brought additional insights into this important metabolic aspect.

The catabolism of both chylomicrons and VLDL proceeds in two steps. First, an extrahepatic degradation is accomplished by the lipoprotein lipases (LPL) which are essentially localized at the surface of the capillary endothelial cells of the heart, muscle and adipose tissue. These lipases hydrolyse a large fraction of the lipoprotein triglycerides. The resulting particles, called remnants for chylomicrons and by some authors intermediate density lipoproteins (IDL) for VLDL catabolic products, also lose some of their surface phospholipids, most of their apo-C, and in the case of chylomicrons most of their apo A–I and apo A–IV, by exchange with the HDL in the plasma. In contrast, remnants get enriched in apo-E and apo-B. Both types of remnants are in their majority removed by the liver as intact particles. About one-half of the LDL are degraded in the liver, while the hepatic catabolism of HDL is still not entirely elucidated, since HDL may deliver cholesterol without uptake of the whole particle.

Uptake of chylomicrons, VLDL and their respective remnants

Role of initial hydrolysis by lipoprotein lipase

It has been established that the initial lipolysis of chylomicron and VLDL triglycerides by the extrahepatic LPL is essential for their efficient catabolism (21). Intact chylomicrons are taken up rather slowly by the perfused liver whereas chylomicron and VLDL remnants (15, 68) are metabolized to a large extent that can reach 30 to 40% in 5 min (78). Uptake and degradation of cholesteryl ester labelled chylomicron remnants also were ensured much more efficiently by rat hepatocyte monolayers as reported by Floren & Nilsson (22). It was shown that an initial hydrolysis of 10% of the triglycerides was sufficient to produce VLDL-remnants that were taken up at the same rate by the perfused liver than smaller particles obtained after 80% hydrolysis (78). The increased catabolism apparently does not depend on the size of the lipoprotein but rather on the modification of a surface component of the particle. However, the question of size has not received a clear-cut response. Indeed *in vivo* very large chylomicrons cannot diffuse into the liver through the endothelial fenestrae which sieve particles of less than 0.1 μm, but *in vitro* small chylomicrons (sf <400) were taken up faster than the larger ones (sf >400) by hepatocyte monolayers (48). Thus, size may still influence the uptake of the chylomicron and VLDL remnants when these particles reach the space of Disse.

Role of phospholipids

The problem of size is, in fact, linked to the surface components (phospholipids and apoproteins) carried by the lipoprotein particles. The possibility that binding of intact chylomicrons to the liver cells is inhibited by phospholipids has been suggested by Borensztajn *et al.* (6). Eighty per cent radioactivity was recovered in the liver when cholesterol-labelled remnants and phospholipid-depleted chylomicrons were injected while only 10% was measured with intact chylomicrons. Phospho-lipid-depleted chylomicrons were recognized and internalized in the isolated 5 min after their addition to the liver perfusate (6). When these lipoproteins were double-labelled with [³H] cholesterol and [¹⁴C] palmitic acid, the [³H]/[¹⁴C] ratio in the liver was similar to the perfusate which strongly suggests that these chylomicrons were taken up as whole particles.

Because one of the major transformation that occurs during the catabolism of chylomicrons into remnants is the loss of phospholipids, Borensztajn suggested that a rearrangement of the apoproteins may occur on the lipoprotein surface, and thus make them more accessible to the liver cell receptors.

Hepatic LDL and HDL uptake

It is now accepted that LDL are taken up by the liver. When LDL were labelled with [¹⁴C] sucrose, which was not catabolized inside the cells, it was possible to demonstrate that 40% of the injected LDL were recovered in the liver of the pig (57) and 24% in the rat (5). This proportion could be increased up to 45% after estradiol treatment of the rats. These LDL were taken up by the different hepatic cell types and have been shown to be degraded through receptor-dependent and receptor-independent pathways. The latter has been demonstrated *in vivo* with methylated LDL which are catabolized only by a receptor-independent pathway (12) because methylation blocks recognition by the receptors. In the rat, 67% of hepatic uptake is attributable to the LDL receptors.

HDL cholesterol is transported back to the liver by two mechanisms: an indirect one by transfer of the esterified cholesterol to the triglyceride-rich lipoproteins (chylomicrons and VLDL) in the plasma and a direct one through uptake by the liver.

In vivo [¹²⁵I]-HDL injection studies showed that the liver is the major site of catabolism of HDL. About 10% of the injected HDL was found in the liver within 10 min (45). Using radioautographic techniques, Rachmilewitz *et al.* (59) observed a high concentration of radioactivity associated with lysosomes, mostly in hepatocytes, while only few radioautographic grains were found on non-parenchymal cells. Following uptake of HDL containing both cholesteryl-ether and an apo A–I with covalently linked [¹²⁵I]-labelled tyramine-cellobiose, Glass *et al.* (25) showed that cholesteryl ether accumulated predominantly in the liver but that apo A–I was much less trapped, suggesting that perhaps cholesterol molecules rather than the whole HDL were taken up. After a partial hepatectomy the removal of radioactive cholesteryl esters and also phospholipids of injected HDL was clearly decreased (74), while the degradation rate of apo-A and apo-C was not modified.

These findings suggest that the lipid and protein moieties of HDL follow different metabolic pathways in the liver.

Hepatic lipoprotein receptors

During the last decade, a large number of laboratories have established the central role for lipoprotein receptors in regulating plasma cholesterol and triglyceride turnover (for reviews see references 9, 51 and 61). A pioneer work was the discovery by Brown & Goldstein of the receptor-mediated endocytosis of LDL by human cultured fibroblasts. These cells possess high affinity, saturable and Ca⁺⁺-dependent binding sites for LDL. The lipoprotein binds primarily at 'coated pit'

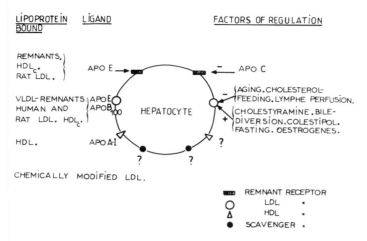

Fig. 1. Scheme of the hepatocyte with its lipoprotein receptors, their identified ligands and the factors regulating the binding properties of lipoproteins.

regions of the plasma membrane and is internalized in endocytotic vesicles, then degraded in secondary lysosomes. After hydrolysis of both lipid and protein moieties, the lipoprotein-derived cholesterol that leaves the lysosomes for the cellular compartment, regulates the endogenous sterol metabolism by: 1) down-regulating hydroxy-methyl-glutaryl-coenzyme A (HMG-CoA) reductase; and, 2) activating acyl-CoA, cholesterol acyltransferase (ACAT). This cholesterol was shown also to down-regulate the number of LDL receptors.

The so-called LDL pathway functions in a great number of cells: human skin fibroblasts, smooth muscle cells, lymphocytes, endothelial cells, HeLa cells, adrenal cortical cells and probably also adipocytes.

In the liver, two main types of lipoprotein receptors have been described: a remnant receptor responsible for most uptake of chylomicron and VLDL remnants, and a LDL receptor that is immunologically and genetically identical to the fibroblast receptor. The remnant receptor recognizes all lipoproteins containing apo-E while the LDL receptor bind all lipoproteins containing apo-E and/or apo-B. HDL are also bound to hepatocytes by a saturable mechanism but VLDL and LDL compete for this binding, thus showing that its specificity was not very high. It is the reason why Ose (55) proposed the general term of 'lipoprotein-binding site' for HDL binding. Other receptors have been identified in the liver. Thus, hepatic uptake of chemically modified LDL like acetyl LDL, *in vivo* as well as *in vitro* by hepatocytes and NPC cells, lead to the definition of an acetyl-LDL receptor or scavenger receptor that allows the degradation of abnormal lipoproteins. Figure 1 shows a scheme of the known hepatic lipoprotein receptors with their identified ligands and their factors of regulation.

Hepatic remnant (apo-E) receptor.

The liver plays a major role in the clearance of chylomicron and VLDL remnants. Parenchymal cells account for nearly 70% of this uptake *in vivo* (72) and perhaps even for the totality according to very recent observations (36). These remnants are taken up by absorptive endocytosis and several studies indicate the following. First, microtubules are involved in their transport and in the formation of endocytotic vesicles. Indeed remnant catabolism was inhibited by microtubular inhibitors such as colchicine and vinblastine *in vivo* (46), in suspended hepatocytes (47) and hepatocyte monolayers (23). Secondly, remnant degradation may take place in the lysosomes as shown by the inhibition of cholesteryl-ester degradation by chloroquine (an inhibitor of lysosomal hydrolases) in liver post-nuclear supernatant (67) or in rat hepatocyte monolayers (22, 23). Thirdly, remnant uptake proceeds through a high affinity saturable process mediated by a receptor that specifically recognizes apo-E as determinant. The remnant receptor is also called 'apo-E receptor'.

It has been clearly established by Mahley *et al.* (43) that apo-E is indeed the recognition signal. HDL_c, which are HDL obtained from dogs or rats fed either a high cholesterol diet or an atherogenic diet, have the characteristic of containing only apo-E. In binding studies, these HDL_c behave exactly like remnants and are often used to measure remnant receptors (63).

When chylomicron remnants were depleted of apo-E, they were removed at one-third the amount of the non-depleted remnants by the perfused liver (2). Thus, two-thirds of the chylomicron remnant uptake appear to be receptor dependent. VLDL remnants are also removed in the same proportions by an apo-E receptor-dependent process, but their removal has some different properties. Indeed, VLDL remnant uptake was stimulated 2- to 3-fold after oestradiol treatment, known to specifically induce the LDL receptor, whereas VLDL remnant uptake was reduced by 70% after cholesterol feeding of the rats (2). Under these conditions uptake of chylomicron remnants remained unchanged. Thus, part of the hepatic uptake of VLDL remnants is regulated by the same factors that control LDL removal. Recently, Hui *et al.* (33) studied the binding of β-VLDL isolated from Type III hyperlipoproteinaemic subjects (β-VLDL result from partial hydrolysis of chylomicrons and of hepatic VLDL enriched in cholesterol). With monoclonal antibodies, these authors not only demonstrated that apo-E was the binding determinant but they showed also that apo-B_{100} (and not apo-B_{48}) may somehow help the binding of β-VLDL to the LDL receptor. On the other hand, it has been evidenced by Borensztajn *et al.* (7) that apo-B has no effect on chylomicron remnant uptake. Indeed, chylomicrons that were first depleted of all their apoproteins by a pronase treatment, then incubated with serum to reassociate all their apoproteins except apo-B, were cleared *in vivo* at the same rate as intact chylomicrons.

Since hepatic remnant (apo-E) receptors resemble the LDL receptors in many aspects and since remnants bind to both type of receptors, the question arose: are these two receptors different? In fact, the specificity of the remnant (apo-E) receptor was shown by the following findings: 1) binding of particles containing apo-E (HDL_c, remnants, β-VLDL) was not inhibited by an excess of human LDL that contained only apo-B; 2) hepatic membranes of adult animals (rat, swine, dog) and humans, which bound only negligible amounts of LDL, were able to bind HDL_c, chylomicron and VLDL remnants; 3) many physiological conditions inducing or repressing the LDL receptor (such as fasting, lymph infusion, cholestyramine treatment) did not modify the binding of HDL_c (1). Thus, the remnant receptor is a site distinct from the LDL receptor.

Binding of $[^{125}I]$-chylomicron and VLDL remnants to rat plasma membranes was shown by Cooper *et al.* (16) to be saturable, with high affinity, moderately inhibited by 10 mM EDTA (thus, poorly Ca^{++} dependent) and competitively inhibited by rat HDL_c as well as by purified apo-E included in phospholipid vesicles. This receptor is very similar to the one described for dog membranes, except that Ca^{++}-dependence was demonstrated for the latter (32). This may be a species difference or, alternatively, be linked to binding conditions, since Hui *et al.* utilized higher concentrations of EDTA (30 mM).

Isolated hepatocytes have also been used to study binding of $[^{125}I]$-lipoprotein remnants. A VLDL remnant receptor with high affinity binding has been described by Van Berkel *et al.* (71) in suspended hepatocytes. This binding could be inhibited competitively by rat LDL and HDL but not by human LDL (which contains only apo-B) even in a 200-fold excess, indicating that apo-B was not involved in this binding.

Binding of VLDL remnants to rat hepatocytes was followed by a small degradation, and the greater part of the iodinated lipoprotein (70 to 80%) remained bound on the external surface of the cell. After a 3 hour incubation, only 4 to 8% of the cell associated $[^{125}I]$-labelled VLDL remnants were degraded. With hepatocyte monolayers, cultivated for 24 hours and then incubated for up to 4 hours, Floren & Nilsson (24) also observed an uptake of chylomicron remnants by a saturable process. The apparent V_{max} for binding was 300 ng remnant protein/h/mg cell protein and the apparent Km was 7.7 μg remnant protein/mg cell protein. These values were close to those obtained for VLDL remnants in suspended freshly isolated hepatocytes (V_{max}=628 ng, Km=2.65 μg) as calculated from values in reference 71. The hydrolysis of the protein moiety was also relatively low (1.4%) in the hepatocyte monolayers compared to total uptake (16.2%) (24) but here, the hydrolysis occurred inside the cell and was inhibited by colchicine, concanavalin A, chloroquine and ammonia. At a concentration of 25 μM, chloroquine inhibited protein degradation by 32%. When chylomicron remnants were labelled in their cholesteryl ester moiety, hydrolysis was found to be much higher and reached 25% after a 4-h incubation. This hydrolysis was inhibited by colchicine and chloroquine by more than 50% (23).

Chylomicron remnant binding and degradation were also shown to be specific and saturable in human hepatoma cell line H-35 (69). Competition studies demonstrated that this receptor was different from the receptors binding LDL and HDL_c.

If binding of remnant lipoproteins by a specific receptor was well demonstrated in cultured and suspended hepatocytes some differences were still observed between both types of cell preparation. The fact that degradation of remnants in hepatocytes monolayers is inhibited by colchicine and chloroquine reveals that fusion of the endocytotic vesicles with the primary lysosomes and subsequent lysosomal hydrolysis take place, as in fibroblasts. In freshly suspended hepatocytes no effect of chloroquine on cholesteryl ester hydrolysis or on protein degradation could be observed (71). However, uptake and hydrolysis of chylomicron remnants has been shown to be improved after a preincubation of the cells for 2 hours before adding the lipoproteins (47). The presence of cycloheximide during the preincubation, inhibited the remnant uptake, indicating that active protein synthesis was required. These data suggest that during collagenase cell isolation a rate limiting cellular change occurs which could possibly be restored either after 2 hours of preincubation for suspended cells or after 24 hours of culture for hepatocyte monolayers. With freshly isolated hepatocytes, Van Berkel *et al.* (71) pointed also to the low degradation of the protein moiety of VLDL remnants, which suggests a defect in the intracellular transport of the lipoprotein to the degradation sites. Now it has been shown by Capuzzi *et al.* (11) that some collagenase remained attached to the hepatocytes even after 5 successive washes and this constitutes a serious contamination together with impurities, such as various proteases, found in commercial preparations of collagenase.

Thus, if binding properties seem to be preserved in suspended hepatocytes, the steps beyond binding need to be further investigated with cells prepared without collagenase contamination.

Effects of apoproteins on remnant binding and uptake

Studies on perfused rat liver showed that the removal of hepatic VLDL and small chylomicrons was greatly depressed when these lipoproteins were first enriched with apo-C (by preincubation with a VLDL-free plasma) (77). In contrast, the removal of remnants which are depleted of apo-C during their vascular synthesis is greatly enhanced. *In vitro* addition of several isoforms of apo-C (apo-C-II, -C-III-O, -C-III-3) to rat hepatic VLDL, reduced their uptake whereas addition of apo-E to apo-E-devoid chylomicrons, had the opposite effect (77). Thus hepatic remnant uptake is regulated by both apo-C and apo-E. The same conclusions were drawn in non-recycling rat liver perfusion, using triglyceride emulsions loaded with purified human apo-C and apo-E (62). Studies on hepatocyte monolayers with the same emulsions revealed identical properties (58). Apo-C-III-2 had the most inhibitory effect on triglyceride association with the cells whether apo-E was present in the emulsion or not. Addition of egg phosphatidyl choline decreased the uptake of triglyceride emulsions by hepatocyte monolayers but surprisingly, it partially antagonized the inhibition produced by apo-C-III-2.

These experiments point to the complexity of the mechanism involved. Quarfordt *et al.* (58) suggested that apo-C-III could be sequestered in the phospholipids and become relatively unable to inhibit triglyceride uptake. An inhibitory effect of apo-C-III on triglyceride cell association was also reported in suspended hepatocytes by Van Berkel *et al.* (73) who used chylomicrons originally devoid of apo-C and apo-E, then enriched *in vitro* with the same purified, iodinated apoproteins.

Recently, an important progress in understanding apoprotein structure and binding properties was achieved regarding the apo-E domain. When devoid of lipids, this apoprotein does not bind to plasma membranes but it acquires an enhanced binding affinity combined with phospholipids. Furthermore, it has been shown that apo-E_3 was the isoform which interacted with the LDL and the remnant receptors, at least for human lipoproteins (33).

Little is known concerning the regulatory effect of the other apoproteins on remnant binding. A role for apo-B_{100} has been proposed as favouring the binding of remnants and β-VLDL to the LDL receptor (2, 33) while apo-B_{48} would have no effect or would rather prevent chylomicron binding to the LDL receptor. This has yet to be demonstrated, and is presently difficult to conciliate with the *in vivo* higher clearance of apo-B_{48}-rich-VLDL as compared with apo-B_{100}-rich VLDL (65).

The effect of other apoproteins (either carried on lipoproteins or circulating free in the plasma), such as apo-A-IV, have not been studied on the receptor mediated uptake of remnants. To our knowledge, only one study attempted to show an effect of apo-A-I depletion on chylomicron and remnant uptake by rat hepatocyte monolayers. The uptake of the former was decreased and that of the latter was increased (48).

Effect of remnant uptake on hepatic cholesterol metabolism

The receptor mediated uptake of LDL by fibroblasts is followed by an inhibition of HMG-CoA reductase and by an activation of ACAT. Does remnant uptake mediate the same kind of regulation? A lipoprotein isolated from the plasma of cholesterol- fed rats and showing many characteristics of remnant particles, was shown to inhibit HMG-CoA reductase when incubated for 24 hours with hepatocyte monolayers whereas VLDL and HDL stimulated the enzyme and human LDL had no effect (8). A regulation of HMG-CoA reductase by remnant lipoproteins has been reported in the perfused rat liver (76) that depends on the lipid composition of the particles: cholesterol-rich particles suppressed and triglyceride-rich ones stimulated the enzyme activity. Cholesteryl ester-rich β-VLDL isolated from a patient with Type III hyperlipoproteinaemia also reduced sterol synthesis in rat hepatocyte monolayers (10).

With freshly isolated hepatocytes more divergent effects have been observed. Indeed, a very efficient inhibition of cholesterol synthesis was reported with increasing amounts of chylomicron remnants (39). However, when preparing the remnants by an *in vivo* procedure (with functionally hepatectomized rats) instead of the *in vitro* incubation with LPL as used in (39), Nomura *et al.* (50) showed that there was no inhibition of cholesterol synthesis. These authors attributed the difference observed to a contamination of the *in vitro* prepared remnants by LPL which further hydrolysed the remnant triglycerides during incubation with the hepatocytes. The inhibition could then be attributed to the LPL released free fatty acids. To circumvent this artefact, remnants were prepared by Lakshmanan *et al.* (40) by retrograde perfusion of isolated rat heart. Unfortunately, cholesterol synthesis was not measured in this experiment; yet, lymph VLDL, chylomicron and VLDL remnants were shown to inhibit lipogenesis by 10–20% and remnants devoid of apo-C after pre-incubation with HDL, lead to a concentration dependent inhibition increasing up to 70%. While these experiments show that triglyceride-rich lipoproteins and their remnants exert metabolic effects on isolated hepatocytes, the involved mechanism is not yet clearly explained, since freshly isolated hepatocytes have a defect at the level of intracellular transport of the lipoprotein. Considering the high concentrations of lipoprotein tested (40) some particles may have entered by a receptor independent pathway. However, the permissive effect of remnant apo-C depletion suggest that internalization of the particles is also receptor mediated.

The LDL (apo-B, -E) receptor

The presence in the liver of an LDL receptor distinct from the remnant receptor has been well documented. It was called (apo-B, -E) receptor by Mahley because it could bind apo-B-containing lipoproteins, such as human LDL, as well as apo-E-containing lipoproteins, such as remnants and HDL_c (1, 32). This receptor has the same binding properties as the LDL receptor of fibroblasts. Moreover, in contrast with the remnant receptor, expression of the LDL-receptor is highly dependent on the age, the nutritional state and the animal species.

Several laboratories have reported that cultured rabbit hepatocytes (4, 64) bind LDL. The specific receptor could be induced in the adult animal after hepatocytes have been first cultured for 20 hours and then pre-incubated for 12 to 16 hours in a lipoprotein-free medium. Binding and degradation of $[^{125}I]$-LDL were shown to be saturable and of high affinity. Their degradation was prevented by colchicine and chloroquine and HMG-CoA reductase activity was decreased in their presence. A particular model for studying LDL catabolism is given by the Watanabe rabbit which displays a spontaneous hypercholesterolemia. No LDL receptor was found on their fibroblasts nor on their hepatocytes in culture (4, 37). However, hepatocytes of the Watanabe rabbit still degraded LDL. This degradation was not saturable and was not inhibited by an excess of unlabelled LDL, neither by chloroquine nor colchicine. The activity of HMG-CoA reductase was not suppressed. Therefore Attie *et al.* (4) suggested that a 'non-specific' receptor-independent pathway exists in these cells, similar to the receptor-independent degradation of human LDL described in rat hepatocytes (3).

In the pig, the presence of a LDL receptor could only be demonstrated in the hepatocytes of the neonatal animals (56). It presented all the characteristics of a high affinity binding, and was associated with inhibition of HMG-CoA reductase. When lysine residues of LDL were modified by reductive methylation (lysine is required for binding to the LDL receptor) LDL uptake was reduced.

In the dog, Mahley *et al.* (43) showed that the LDL receptor was only present on hepatic plasma membranes of immature growing animals, but not in adult ones. As for the above described species, binding of $[^{125}I]$-LDL was saturable, competitively inhibited by unlabelled LDL as well as by human LDL and dog HDL_c. Interestingly, cholesterol feeding suppressed this hepatic LDL receptor in the immature dogs while fasting, treatment with cholestyramine and colestipol (acting as bile acid sequestrants) or biliary diversion induced expression of the LDL receptor in adult dogs. The short time down-regulation of this receptor was shown by its repression after a 6-hour infusion of taurocholate or of dog intestinal lymph into immature or cholestyramine-treated dogs (1). Moreover, a decrease of LDL binding was reported with increasing age in hepatic membranes from immature dogs (43).

An LDL receptor was also found on liver membranes from human fetuses aged 16–20 weeks, whereas membranes from adults did not bind LDL significantly (43).

Thus, the hepatic LDL receptor appears to be rapidly induced in response to increased needs for cholesterol as in the developing liver of young animals and to be repressed when the need is fulfilled.

In the rat, the existence of a LDL receptor was difficult to demonstrate because, as in other species, the adult animal has a low LDL-binding capacity. LDL were cleared slowly by cultured hepatocytes through a non-saturable, low-affinity and Ca^{++}-independent mechanism. Chloroquine had only a small inhibitory effect and colchicine was without effect on human LDL uptake and degradation in this species. HMG-CoA reductase activity and cholesterol esterification were not modified by these LDL (3). In contrast, marked effects were observed in the same hepatocytes with lactosylated LDL which are recognized by a galactose specific receptor and catabolized through the lysosomal pathway. It was concluded that LDL were degraded by a non-specific mechanism, at least in the cultured hepatocytes. However, in the rat *in vivo*, two-thirds of the hepatic LDL degradation is receptor-dependent (12). This discrepancy is at present not clearly explained.

Rat hepatocytes in suspension were able to bind LDL (54, 70, 71), but the major part of these lipoproteins remained bound to the external surface of the cell. After isopycnic centrifugation of hepatocyte homogenates in sucrose gradients, Ose *et al.* (54) showed that the [^{125}I]-LDL remained in the fraction enriched with the plasma membrane marker 5'-nucleotidase. Other reports (27) described a high affinity receptor in freshly isolated hepatocytes which interacts with apo-B and/or apo-E-containing lipoproteins, but the binding was insufficient to measure the degradation rates. After injection of 17α-ethinylestradiol to rats, it was nevertheless possible to observe a 16-fold increase in the LDL association to freshly isolated hepatocytes (30). This oestrogen-induced receptor was analogous to the fibroblast LDL receptor in that: 1) lipoprotein containing apo-B and/or apo-E, bound with high affinity; 2) binding was Ca^{++}-dependent; 3) lysine and arginine were essential for recognition of human LDL; and 4) LDL were degraded to a significant extent and choloroquine inhibited this degradation by 30%. This effect of chloroquine was observed in the hepatocytes after the [^{125}I]-LDL were injected to intact rats, the cells isolated 10 min later and subsequently incubated with the drug. Hence, it appears that in the rat, the LDL receptor became functional (or accurately measurable) following the estrogen treatment, as previously observed with plasma membranes (38) which is in agreement with the increased LDL uptake measured *in vivo* (31) or in the perfused liver (79) under the same conditions.

With human HEp G_2 hepatoma cells, a receptor dependent binding of human LDL has been reported (17) which shared many of the properties of the LDL receptor of fibroblasts: 1) the binding has a high affinity component, and was Ca^{++}-dependent; 2) cholesterol synthesis was inhibited and esterification stimulated by LDL; and, 3) chloroquine inhibited LDL degradation. Moreover the capacity of the HEp G_2 cells for LDL degradation was well in the range of the *in vivo* values. Therefore, these cells constitute a good model for studying the catabolism of human lipoproteins.

Rat hepatoma cells of the H-35 line were also studied (69). They were able to bind LDL by a Ca^{++}-dependent receptor with specific and saturable properties. Lipoproteins containing apo-B and apo-E were bound at the same rate.

Thus, the hepatic recognition and uptake of LDL in several animal species appears as more complex than it was initially observed for extrahepatic sites. The classical LDL pathway could not be clearly evidenced in hepatocytes from all adult mammals, but could be induced by several treatments of the animals and was well measured in human and rat hepatoma cells.

Hepatic HDL receptors

Studies with perfused livers and isolated liver cells have confirmed that the liver was an important site of HDL catabolism. [^{125}I]-HDL were shown to be bound both with low and high affinity by a saturable process, then endocytosed and degraded by suspended rat hepatocytes (45, 55, 70). Chloroquine inhibited the proteolysis, but only at a very high concentration (5 mM) thus questioning a role of lysosomal degradation under these conditions. The subcellular distribution of [^{125}I]-HDL, after injection *in vivo*, corresponded to the lysosomal fraction, but *in vitro* [^{125}I]-HDL accumulated in the plasma membrane fraction of the isolated hepatocytes (53, 54) as was observed for LDL. Moreover, the HDL degradation process was rather slow: 5.8% was degraded after 2 hours of incubation (45). A low extent of degradation was also reported in hepatocytes by Van Berkel *et al.* (70) and by Ose *et al.* (53). HDL binding studies showed that this process was not Ca^{++}-dependent or competitively inhibited by VLDL and LDL, thus showing a low specificity (55, 70). It was also demonstrated that apo-E did not compete for HDL binding confirming that the binding site was different from the LDL (apo-B, -E) and the remnant (apo-E) receptors. Pronase treatment, known to modify the receptors located on the plasma membranes, reduced the cell association of HDL. The number of binding sites was estimated to be 2.2×10^6 sites per cell, with an association constant of 8.2×10^6 (mol/l)$^{-1}$ (55).

In accordance with the *in vivo* clearance studies (25, 74), rabbit (52) and rat (41) hepatocyte monolayers incubated with homologous HDL showed a selective uptake of the cholesterol moiety compared to the protein, suggesting again that the HDL are not taken up as a whole particle. Thus, after a 3-hour incubation of rabbit hepatocytes in culture, an 8-fold selective uptake for [^{14}C]-cholesterol was observed compared with the [^{125}I] marker of the added HDL (52) while in suspended rat cells, binding for both was identical (55).

With hepatoma cells H-35 (69), competition studies showed separate receptors for LDL, remnants and HDL. In particular it was reported that the HDL fraction devoid of apo-E, bound to a receptor different from that of the apo-E-containing lipoproteins. Thus, apo-E seems not to be involved in the HDL uptake process (41). In fact, apo-A–I has been proposed to be the cellular recognition molecule for rat HDL$_2$ (69) and HDL$_3$ (45). Indeed, very recently, a specific binding to rat liver plasma membranes with high affinity and saturation characteristics has been reported for [^{125}I]-HDL$_3$, which was competitively inhibited by phospholipid complexes containing apo-A–I (13). Moreover, apo-E-deficient rat HDL were shown to bind to hepatocytes and to be competed for by excess HDL and by dimyristoyl phosphatidylcholine (DMPC)-apo-A–I complexes (60). DMPC-apo-A–I complexes also bound to suspended hepatocytes, thus suggesting that apo-A–I might be the ligand for the specific HDL receptor.

Role of hepatic non-parenchymal cells

It is now known and accepted that the non-parenchymal cells (NPC) of the liver can bind, take up and degrade all the main lipoproteins (18, 26, 30, 42, 53, 54, 70, 71, 72, 75). When both types of cell population were isolated 30 min after the injection of chylomicron or VLDL remnants, 25 to 35% of the label taken up by the liver was recovered in the NPC (26, 75). If results were expressed per mg of cell protein, NPC compared to hepatocytes contained 4.7, 4.9, 6.1 and 5.3 times the amount of labelled iodine for VLDL, VLDL remnants, LDL and HDL respectively (75). *In vitro*, binding of these lipoproteins to NPC was also found to be 5- to 8-fold higher when expressed per mg of cell protein. Similar results were obtained for LDL and HDL with hepatocytes and NPC in suspension, whether the lipoproteins were iodinated or cholesteryl-ester labelled (18).

Competition binding experiments showed that the receptor for VLDL remnants interacts with rat LDL and HDL and not human LDL; it may be equivalent to the remnant (apo-E) receptor of hepatocytes (71, 72). Nevertheless, the extent of internalization of the particle was low and corresponded to less than 30% of the cell-associated lipoprotein, chloroquine and ammonia had no effect on the degradation, and binding did not require Ca^{++} (54).

Another receptor could be identified that shows the characteristics of the LDL (apo-B, -E) receptor. Human LDL injected into rats, bound to the NPC isolated 30 min later and represented 57% of the receptor-mediated LDL binding to the liver (28). A high affinity binding was observed together with a degradation which was inhibited by about 50% by chloroquine (100 μM) when after LDL injection, NPC were separated and incubated with the lysosomal inhibitor (30). It has been shown that the lysine residues of apo-B from human LDL were important for the LDL cell association (30). Moreover, [^{14}C] sucrose labelled LDL used to study the receptor dependent catabolism, revealed that in the liver, the Kupffer cells were the main cell type that catabolized LDL by way of the LDL (apo-B, -E) receptor-mediated uptake (29).

A third type of receptor, that was found in NPC and named the scavenger receptor, was shown to bind chemically modified LDL (ie acetyl-LDL) (44). This receptor does not interact with rat LDL or HDL, or human LDL. The binding was very efficient, especially in endothelial cells which have been isolated after the injection of acetylated LDL. *In vitro* incubation revealed both a binding and degradation capacity of these endothelial cells that was 4- to 5-times greater than for Kupffer cells. Chloroquine (50 μM) and ammonia (10 mM) inhibited the high affinity degradation by more than 90% *in vitro*, thus showing that the lysosomal functions were preserved in the endothelial cells (44).

The overall importance of NPC in lipoprotein catabolism has been a subject of controversy. Autoradiographic localization studies indicated that injected lipoproteins: rat chylomicrons, VLDL and their remnants as well as LDL and HDL (14, 36, 59, 66) measured as grain densities, accumulated predominantly over the parenchymal cells, thus questioning the role of NPC. Nevertheless, an important part of hepatic LDL degradation by means of an apo-B, -E receptor was shown to be accomplished by the Kupffer cells (29), whereas endothelial cells appeared to be specialized in acetyl-LDL degradation (44). The question of remnant degradation by NPC has not so far received an unequivocal answer. An apo-E receptor has been measured on these cells. Moreover, if the different cell types were fractionated after the injection of chylomicrons or VLDL to rats (26, 75) or if these lipoproteins were added to a perfused liver (42), up to 35% of the radioactivity taken up by the liver was recovered in the NPC. Yet, to date, no study has demonstrated that the remnants were degraded by an endocytotic receptor-mediated pathway in these cells.

Conclusions

The first puzzling observation is that with *in vivo* techniques and also in the isolated perfused liver, lipoprotein degradation rates are always greater than when studied in isolated hepatocytes and in non-parenchymal cells. For instance, chylomicron remnants are avidly taken up by the perfused liver (40 per cent uptake after 5 minutes) and so are VLDL remnants (40 per cent uptake in 30 minutes) (78), while in cultured hepatocytes only 25% of the former were taken up after a 4-hour incubation (23). The amount of cells could be one explanation of the difference in the metabolic efficacity of these two models, bearing in mind that a liver contains about 1 to 1.5×10^9 hepatocytes and that the *in vitro* studies are usually done with 0.5 to 10×10^6 cells per incubation flask. Also, the quantities of lipoproteins tested were different in each case. For instance, Arbeeny *et al.* (2) used 200 μg of chylomicron remnant-protein in a liver perfusion experiment whereas Floren & Nilsson (23) used 30 μg of protein with cultured hepatocytes, thus creating a large difference in substrate availability per cell, which might partly explain the better metabolic efficacity of the perfused liver.

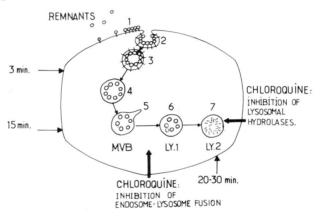

Fig. 2. Scheme illustrating the binding and the processing of chylomicron or VLDL remnants in the hepatocyte. The sites of action of chloroquine are indicated by the arrows. The time course of the processing of lipoproteins after *in vivo* injection is taken from electron microscopic radioautography observations made by Jones *et al.* (36). The steps are the following: 1) binding of the remnants and clustering of the receptors in the coated-pit regions of the plasma membrane. 2) Coated vesicle formation. 3) & 4) Endocytotic vesicles processing following internalization. 5) MVB: multivesicular bodies in the Golgi region (they still contain the receptor-ligand complexes). 6) Primary lysosomes. 7) Secondary lysosomes.

The second observation concerns the ability of chloroquine to block the lysosomal degradation of lipoproteins which is specific of a receptor-mediated process. Figure 2 schematizes this degradation in the case of remnants, as it may be deduced from the autoradiographic images obtained by Jones *et al.* (36). These images are indistinguishable from those achieved for LDL in livers from control and estradiol-treated rats (31) and the scheme is analogous to the Brown & Goldstein's LDL degradation pathway. The inhibitory effect of chloroquine has been shown *in vivo* after injection of chylomicron and VLDL-remnants (36) or of LDL (31) and *in vitro* after addition of remnants (22, 23, 24, 48) or LDL (4, 56, 64) to cultured hepatocytes.

In suspended hepatocytes, no marked effect of chloroquine could be observed as we mentioned before in this chapter, thus failing to demonstrate a lysosomal degradation of either remnants, LDL or HDL. As previously suggested, a step at the binding level or beyond the binding of lipoproteins seems to be disturbed at the

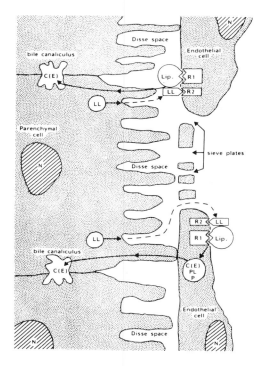

Fig. 3.
Concept of metabolic cooperation between parenchymal and endothelial liver cells. (Reproduced from reference 72, by permission of the authors and of Elsevier Biomedical Press BV Amsterdam). Lip: lipoprotein; LL: liver lipase; C(E): cholesterol(ester); R_1: remnant (apo-E) receptor; R_2: liver lipase receptor; PL: phospholipids; P: protein.

early stages following collagenase isolation of the cells. Such a putative lability seems to be a particularity of lipoprotein receptors inasmuch as asialofetuin receptors in hepatocytes are not damaged under the same conditions.

Finally, the great difference between the capacity for metabolizing lipoprotein remnants observed with *in vivo* models and perfused liver on one hand, and with isolated hepatocytes on the other hand, may result from a metabolic cooperation between the different cell types in the intact organ, as suggested by Van Berkel *et al.* (72). The mechanism(s) whereby these different cells may contribute to remnant degradation remains unknown; however, several possible pathways have been proposed (Fig. 3). The remnants reaching the space of Disse bind to their receptors located on the endothelial cells or on the hepatocytes. A hepatic triglyceride lipase (HTGL), secreted by the hepatocytes (34) and which ensures the hydrolysis of both triglycerides and phospholipids also binds to the endothelial cells (35). The first pathway suggested for remnant catabolism is that HTGL attacks the lipoprotein (possibly by means of its phospholipase activity (72)). The various components of the particle enter the endothelial cell, the cholesteryl ester is subsequently hydrolysed within the lysosomes, then re-esterified and transported into the hepatocyte. The existence of such a pathway is not sustained by the electron microscopy studies (36). According to a second hypothesis, the lipoprotein remains outside the endothelial cell, fixed on the apo-E receptor of the hepatocyte and close to the binding site of the HTGL, which may then attack the remnant particle. The latter will finally enter the hepatocyte and migrate towards the lysosomes which contain the acid lipase, the cholesterol esterase and cathepsin D required for the ultimate lipoprotein catabolism.

Such a metabolic coordination between hepatocytes and endothelial cells is very attractive and could be operative considering: 1) the anatomical proximity of both cell populations in the space of Disse and, 2) the existence of receptors for remnant particles and for HTGL on these different cell types. Nevertheless, such a cooperation remains highly speculative. Very recently, strong autoradiographic evidence was provided that the majority of lipoprotein remnants were processed through a receptor-mediated endocytosis in the hepatocyte (36). The question arises, then, as to whether HTGL is actually involved in this degradation. If this is the case, does this enzyme act prior to the binding of the remnant particle to its receptor, subsequently to this binding and through what mechanism does it act? It is reasonable to think that further experiments with functional freshly isolated hepatocytes will help to answer these questions.

To conclude, it should be stressed that together with the *in vivo* approaches, the use of hepatocytes either freshly isolated or in monolayer culture is a valuable tool for advance in our knowledge of lipoprotein metabolism. If conclusions should be drawn with caution inasmuch as artifacts may be introduced by the isolation procedure or the culture conditions, isolated cells nevertheless offer the possibility of testing the numerous factors that interfere in the complex mechanisms of uptake and degradation of lipoproteins by the liver.

REFERENCES

1 Angelin B., Raviola C. A., Innerarity T. L., Mahley R. W.: Regulation of hepatic lipoprotein receptors in the dog. Rapid regulation of apolipoprotein B, E receptors but not of apolipoprotein E receptors, by intestinal lipoproteins and bile acids. *J. Clin. Invest.* 1983, **71**: 816–831.

2 Arbeeny C. M., Rifici V. A.: The uptake of chylomicron remnants and very low density lipoprotein remnants by the perfused rat liver. *J. Biol. Chem.* 1984, **259**: 9662–9666.

3 Attie A. D., Pittman R. C., Steinberg D.: Metabolism of native and of lactosylated human low density lipoprotein: Evidence of two pathways for catabolism of exogenous proteins in rat hepatocytes. *Proc. Natl. Acad. Sci* 1980, **77**: 5923–5927.

4 Attie A. D., Pittman R. C., Watanabe Y., Steinberg D.: Low density lipoprotein receptor deficiency in cultured hepatocytes of the WHHL rabbit. *J. Biol. Chem.* 1981, **256**: 9789–9792.

5 Bhattacharya S., Balasubramaniam S., Simons L. A.: The role of the liver in low-density lipoprotein catabolism in the rat. *Biochem. J.* 1984, **220**: 333–336.

6 Borensztajn J., Kostlar T. J.: Hepatic uptake of phospholipid-depleted chylomicrons *in vivo*. *Biochem. J.* 1981, **200**: 547–553.

7 Borensztajn J., Getz G. S., Padley R. J., Kotlar T. J.: The apoprotein B-independent hepatic uptake of chylomicron remnants. *Biochem J.* 1982, **204**: 609–612.

8 Breslow J. L., Lothrop D. A., Clowes A. W., Lux S. E.: Lipoprotein regulation of 3-hydroxy-3-methylglutaryl coenzyme A reductase activity in rat liver cell cultures. *J. Biol. Chem* 1977, **252**: 2726–2733.

9 Brown M. S., Goldstein J. L.: How LDL receptors influence cholesterol and atherosclerosis. *Sci. Am.* 1984, **251**: 52–60.

10 Calandra S., Tarugi P., Battistini N., Ferrari R.: Cholesterol synthesis in isolated rat hepatocytes: effect of homologous and heterologous serum lipoproteins. *Metabolism* 1979, **28**: 843–850.

11 Capuzzi D. M., Sparks C. E., Dehoff J. L.: Effect of residual enzymes on degradation of radioiodinated VLDL by collagenase dispersed hepatocytes. *Biochem. Biophys. Res. Commun.* 1979, **90**: 587–595.

12 Carew T. E., Pittman R. C., Steinberg D.: Tissue sites of degradation of native and reductively methylated [^{14}C] sucrose labeled low density lipoprotein in rats. Contribution of receptor-dependent and recetor independent pathways. *J. Biol. Chem.* 1982, **257**: 8001–8008.

13 Chacko G. K.: Characterization of high density lipoprotein binding sites in rat liver and testis membranes. *Biochim. Biophys. Acta* 1984, **795**: 417–426.

14 Chao Y. S., Jones A. L., Hradek G. T., Windler E. E. T., Havel R. J.: Autoradiographic localization of the site of uptake, cellular transport and catabolism of low density lipoproteins in the liver of normal and oestrogen-treated rats. *Proc. Natl. Acad. Sci.* 1981, **78**: 597–601.

15 Cooper A. D.: The metabolism of chylomicron remnants by isolated perfused rat liver. *Biochim. Biophys. Acta.* 1977, **488**: 646–464.

16 Cooper A. D., Ericksson S. K., Nutik R., Shewsbury M. A.: Characterization of chylomicron remnant binding to rat liver membranes. *J. Lipid Res.* 1982, **23**: 42–52.

17 Dashti N., Wolfbauer G., Koren E., Knowles B., Alaupovic P.: Catabolism of human low density lipoproteins by human hepatoma cell line HepG$_2$. *Biochim. Biophys. Acta* 1984, **794**: 373–384.

18 Drevon C. A., Berg T., Norum K. R.: Uptake and degradation of cholesterol ester-labelled rat plasma lipoproteins in purified rat hepatocytes and non parenchymal liver cells. *Biochim. Biophys. Acta* 1977, **487**: 122–136.

19 Eisenberg S.: High density lipoprotein metabolism. *J. Lipid Res.* 1984, **25**: 1017–1056.

20 Faergeman O.: Metabolism of plasma lipoproteins. *Acta Med. Scand.* (Suppl) 1977, **614**: 1–29.

21 Felts J. M., Berry M. N.: The metabolism of free fatty acids and chylomicron triglyceride fatty acids by isolated rat liver cells. *Biochem. Biophys. Acta* 1970, **231**: 1–7.

22 Florén C. H., Nilsson Å.: Degradation of chylomicron remnant cholesteryl ester by rat hepatocyte monolayers. Inhibition by chloroquine and colchicine. *Biochem. Biophys. Res. Commun.* 1977, **74**: 520–528.

23 Florén C. H., Nilsson Å.: Binding, interiorization and degradation of cholesteryl ester-labelled chylomicron remnant particles by rat hepatocyte monolayers. *Biochem J.* 1977, **168**: 483–494.

24 Florén C. L., Nilsson Å.: Uptake and degradation of iodine labelled chylomicron remnant particles by monolayers of rat hepatocytes. *Biochem J.* 1978, **174**: 827–838.

25 Glass C., Pittman R. C., Weinstein D. B., Steinberg D.: Dissociation of tissue uptake of cholesterol ester from that of apoprotein AI of rat plasma high density lipoprotein: Selective delivery of cholesterol ester to liver, adrenal, and gonad. *Proc. Natl. Acad. Sci.* 1983, **80**: 5435–5439.

26 Groot P. H. E., Van Berkel T. J. C., Van Tol A.: Relative contributions of parenchymal and non-parenchymal sinusoidal liver cells in the uptake of chylomicrons remnants. *Metabolism* 1981, **30**: 792–797.

27 Harkes L., Van Berkel T. J. C.: A saturable, high affinity binding site for human low density lipoprotein on freshly isolated rat hepatocytes. *Biochem. Biophys. Acta* 1982, **712**: 677–683.

28 Harkes L., Van Berkel T. J. C.: Cellular localization of the receptor-dependent and receptor-independent uptake of human LDL in the liver of normal and 17α-ethinyl oestradiol rats. *FEBS Lett.* 1983, **154**: 75–80.

29 Harkes L., Van Berkel T. J. C.: Quantitative role of parenchymal and non-parenchymal liver cells in the uptake of [^{14}C] sucrose-labelled low-density lipoprotein *in vivo*. *Biochem. J.* 1984, **224**: 21–27.

30 Harkes L., Van Berkel T. J. C.: *In vivo* characteristics of a specific recognition site for LDL on non-parenchymal rat liver cells which differs from the 17α-ethinyl oestradiol-induced LDL receptor on parenchymal liver cells. *Biochem. Biophys. Acta* 1984, **794**. 340–347.

31 Hornick G. A., Jones A. L., Renaud G., Hradek G., Havel R. J.: Effect of chloroquine on low-density lipoprotein catabolic pathway in rat hepatocytes. *Am. J. Physiol.* 1984, **246**: G187–G194.

32 Hui D. Y., Innerarity T. L., Mahley R. W.: Lipoprotein binding to canine hepatic membranes metabolically distinct apo E and apo B, E receptors. *J. Biol. Chem.* 1981, **256**: 5646–5655.

33 Hui D. Y., Innerarity T. L., Mahley R. W.: Defective hepatic lipoprotein receptor binding of β-very low density lipoproteins from type III hyperlipoproteinemic patients. Importance of apoprotein E. *J. Biol. Chem.* 1984, **259**: 860–869.

34 Jansen H., Kalkman C., Zonneveld A. J., Hulsmann W. C.: Secretion of triacylglycerol hydrolase activity by isolated parenchymal rat liver cells. *FEBS Lett.* 1979, **98**: 299–302.

35 Jansen H., Van Berkel T. J. C., Hulsmann W. C.: Properties of binding of lipases to non-parenchymal rat liver cells. *Biochem. Biophys. Acta* 1980, **619**: 119–128.

36 Jones A. L., Hradek G. T., Hornick C., Renaud G., Windler E. E. T., Havel R. J.: Uptake and processing of remnants of chylomicrons and very low density lipoproteins by rat liver. *J. Lipid Res.* 1984, **25**: 1151–1158.

37 Kita T., Golstein J. L., Brown M. S., Watanabe Y., Hornick C. A., Havel R. J.: Hepatic uptake of chylomicron remnants in WHHL rabbits: a mechanism genetically distinct from the low density lipoprotein receptor. *Proc. Natl. Acad. Sci.* 1982, **79**: 3623–3627.

38 Kovanen P. T., Brown M. S., Goldstein J. L.: Increased binding of low density lipoprotein to liver membranes from rats treated with 17α-ethinyl estradiol. *J. Biol. Chem.* 1979, **254**: 11367–11373.

39 Lakshmanan M. R., Muesing R. A., La Rosa J. C.: Regulation of cholesterol biosynthesis and 3-hydroxy-3-methylglutaryl coenzyme A reductase activity by chylomicron remnants in isolated hepatocytes and perfused liver. *J. Biol. Chem.* 1981, **256**: 3037–3043.

40 Lakshmanan M. R., Vander Matten M., Muesing R. A., O'Looney P., Vahouny G. V.: The role of high density lipoproteins in regulation of hepatic fatty acid synthesis by chylomicron and very low density lipoprotein remnants. *J. Biol. Chem.* 1983, **258**: 4746–4749.

41 Leitersdorf E., Stein O., Eisenberg S., Stein Y.: Uptake of rat plasma HDL subfractions labelled with [^{3}H] cholesteryl linoleyl ether or with [^{125}I] by cultured rat hepatocytes and adrenal cells. *Biochim. Biophys. Acta* 1984, **796**: 72–82.

42 Lippiello P. M., Dijkstra J., Van Galen M., Scherphof G., Waite B. M.: The uptake and metabolism of chylmicron-remnant lipids by non-parenchymal cells in perfused liver and by Kupffer cells in culture. *J. Biol. Chem.* 1981, **256**: 7454–7460.

43 Mahley R. W., Hui D. Y., Innerarity T. L.: Two independent lipoprotein receptors on hepatic membranes of dog, swine and man. Apo B, E and apo E receptors. *J. Clin. Invest.* 1981, **68**: 1197–1206.

44 Nagelkerke J. F., Barto K. P., Van Berkel T. J. C.: *In vivo* and *in vitro* uptake and degradation of acetylated low density lipoprotein by rat liver endothelial, Kupffer and parenchymal cells. *J. Biol. Chem.* 1983, **258**: 12221–12227.

45 Nakai T., Otto P. S., Kennedy D. L., Whayne T. F.: Rat high density lipoprotein subfraction (HDL$_3$) uptake and catabolism by isolated rat liver parenchymal cells *J. Biol. Chem.* 1976, **251**: 4914–4921.

46 Nilsson Å.: Antimicrotubular agents inhibit the degradation of chyle cholesterol ester *in vivo*. *Biochem. Biophys. Res. Commun.* 1975, **66**: 60–66.

47 Nilsson Å.: Effects of anti-microtubular agents and cycloheximide on the metabolism of chylomicron cholesteryl esters by hepatocyte suspensions. *Biochem. J.* 1977, **162**: 367–377.

48 Nilsson Å., Enholm C., Floren C. H.: Uptake and degradation of rat chylomicron remnants, produced *in vivo* and *in vitro*, in rat hepatocyte monolayers. *Biochem. Biophys. Acta* 1981, **663**: 408–420.

49 Noël S. P., Dupras R.: The kinetic parameters of the uptake of very-low density lipoprotein remnant cholesteryl esters by perfused rat livers. *Biochem. Biophys. Acta* 1983, **754**: 117–125.

50 Nomura T., Irving E. A., Harris R. A.: Comparison of the metabolic effects of chylomicrons and their remnants on isolated hepatocytes. *Arch. Biochem. Biophys.* 1981, **211**: 211–221.

51 Norum K. R., Berg T., Helgerud P., Drevon C. A.: Transport of cholesterol. *Physiol. Rev.* 1983, **63**: 506–520.

52 O'Malley J. P., Soltys P. A., Portman O. W.: Interaction of free cholesterol and apoproteins of low and high density lipoproteins with isolated rabbit hepatocytes. *J. Lipid Res.* 1981, **22**: 1214–1224.

53 Ose L., Ose T., Norum K. R., Berg T.: Uptake and degradation of [^{125}I] labelled high density lipoproteins in rat liver cells *in vivo* and *in vitro*. *Biochem. Biophys. Acta* 1979, **574**: 521–586.

54 Ose T., Berg T., Norum K. R., Ose L.: Catabolism of [^{125}I] low density lipoproteins in isolated rat liver cells. *Biochem. Biophys. Res. Commun.* 1980, **97**: 192–199.

55 Ose L., Røken I., Norum K. R., Drevon C. A., Berg T.: The binding of high density lipoproteins to isolated rat hepatocytes. *Scand. J. Clin. Lab. Invest.* 1981, **41**: 63–73.

56 Pangburn S. H., Newton R. S., Chang C. M.: Receptor-mediated catabolism of homologous low density lipoproteins in cultured pig hepatocytes. *J. Biol. Chem.* 1981, **256**: 3340–3347.

57 Pittman R. C., Attie A. D., Carew T. E., Steinberg D.: Tissue sites of degradation of low density lipoprotein: application of a method for determining the fate of plasma proteins. *Proc. Natl. Acad. Sci.* 1979, **76**: 5345–5349.

58 Quarford S. H., Michalopoulos G., Schirmer B.: The effect of human C apolipoproteins on the *in vitro* hepatic metabolism of triglyceride emulsions. *J. Biol. Chem.* 1982, **257**: 14642–14647.

59 Rachmilewitz D., Stein O., Roheim P. S., Stein Y.: Metabolism of iodinated high density lipoproteins in the rat. II Autoradiographic localization in the liver. *Biochem. Biophys. Acta* 1972,

270: 414–425.

60 Rifici V. A., Eder H. A.: A hepatocyte receptor for high-density lipoproteins specific for apolipoprotein A–I. *J. Biol. Chem.* 1984, **259**: 13814–13818.

61 Schonfeld G.: Disorders of lipid transport uptake 1983. *Prog. Cardiovasc. Dis.* 1983, **26**: 89–108.

62 Shelburne F., Hanks J., Meyers W., Quarfordt S.: Effect of apoproteins on hepatic uptake of triglyceride emulsions in the rat. *J. Clin. Invest.* 1980, **65**: 652–658.

63 Sherril B. C., Innerarity T. L., Mahley R. W.: Rapid hepatic clearance of the canine lipoproteins containing only the E apoprotein by a high affinity receptor. Identity with the chylomicron remnant transport process. *J. Biol. Chem.* 1980, **255**: 1804–1807.

64 Soltys P. A., Portman O. W.: Low density lipoprotein receptors and catabolism in primary cultures of rabbit hepatocytes. *Biochem. Biophys. Acta* 1979, **574**: 505–520.

65 Sparks C. E., Marsh J. B.: Metabolic heterogeneity of apolipoprotein B in the rat. *J. Lipid Res.* 1981, **22**: 519–527.

66 Stein O., Rachmilewitz D., Sanger L., Eisenberg S., Stein Y.: Metabolism of iodinated very low density lipoprotein in the rat. Autoradiographic localization in the liver. *Biochim. Biophys. Acta* 1974, **360**: 205–216.

67 Stein Y., Ebin V., Bar-On H., Stein O.: Chloroquine induced interference with degradation of serum lipoproteins in rat liver, studied *in vivo* and *in vitro*. *Biochim. Biophys. Acta* 1977, **486**: 286–297.

68 Suri B. S., Targ M. E., Robinson D. S.: The removal of partially metabolized very-low density lipoproteins by the perfused rat liver. *Biochem. J.* 1981, **196**: 787–794.

69 Tamai T., Patsch W., Lock D., Schonfeld G.: Receptors for homologous plasma lipoproteins on a rat hepatoma cell line. *J. Lipid Res.* 1983, **24**: 1568–1577.

70 Van Berkel T. J. C., Kruijt J. K., Van Gent T., Van Tol A.: Saturable high affinity binding of low density and of high density lipoprotein by parenchymal and non-parenchymal cells from rat liver. *Biochem. Biophys. Res. Commun.* 1980, **92**: 1002–1008.

71 Van Berkel T. J. C., Kruijt J. K., Van Gent T., Van Tol A.: Saturable high affinity binding, uptake and degradation of rat plasma lipoproteins by isolated parenchymal and non-parenchymal cells from rat liver. *Biochim. Biophys. Acta* 1981, **665**: 22–33.

72 Van Berkel T. J. C., Nagelkerke J. F., Harkes L.: Liver sinusoidal cells and lipoprotein metabolism (1982). *In: Sinusoidal Liver Cells*, D. L. Knook, E. Wisse (Eds): Elsevier Biochemical Press, 1982, pp 305–318.

73 Van Berkel T. J. C., Kruijt J. K., Scheek L. M., Groot P. H. E.: Effect of apolipoproteins E and C-III on the interaction of chylomicrons with parenchymal and non-parenchymal cells from rat liver. *Biochem J.* 1983, **216**: 71–80.

74 Van't Hooft F. M., Van Gent T., Van Tol A.: Turnover and uptake by organs of radioactive serum high-density lipoprotein cholesteryl esters and phospholipids in the rat *in vivo*. *Biochem. J.* 1981, **196**: 877–885.

75 Van Tol A., Van Berkel T. J. C.: Uptake and degradation of rat and human very low density (remnant) apolipoproteins by parenchymal and non-parenchymal rat liver cells. *Biochem. Biophys. Acta* 1980, **619**: 156–166.

76 Van Zuiden P. E. A., Erickson S. K., Cooper A. D.: Effect of removal of lipoproteins of different composition on hepatic 3-hydroxy-3-methylglutaryl coenzyme A reductase activity and hepatic very low density lipoprotein secretion. *J. Lip. Res.* 1983, **24**: 418–428.

77 Windler E., Chao Y. S., Havel R. J.: Regulation of the hepatic uptake of triglyceride-rich lipoproteins in the rat. Opposing effects of homologous apolipoprotein E and individual C apoproteins. *J. Biol. Chem.* 1980, **255**: 8303–8307.

78 Windler E., Chao Y. S., Havel R. J.: Determinants of hepatic uptake of triglyceride-rich lipoproteins and their remnants in the rat. *J. Biol. Chem.* 1980, **255**: 5475–5480.

79 Windler E. E. T., Kovanen P. T., Chao Y. S., Brown M. S., Havel R. J., Golstein J. L.: The oestradiol-stimulated lipoprotein receptor of rat-liver. A binding site that mediates the uptake of rat lipoproteins containing apoproteins B and E. *J. Biol. Chem.* 1980, **255**: 10464–10471.

Research in *Isolated and cultured hepatocytes* A. Guillouzo & C. Guguen-Guillouzo eds, pp. 155–170
© John Libbey Eurotext Ltd./INSERM.

7

Plasma protein production by cultured adult hepatocytes

André GUILLOUZO

*Unité de Recherches Hépatologiques INSERM U49, Hôpital Ponchaillou,
35033 Rennes Cédex, FRANCE*

SUMMARY

Adult hepatocytes continue to synthesize and secrete plasma proteins *in vitro*. Synthesis rates and their maintenance are dependent upon the protein tested, the species, the composition of the medium and the nature of the support. When the cells are cultured in standard conditions, a rapid decrease in protein synthesis is observed preceded by that of specific mRNAs. These mRNAs can be temporarily stabilized by using a serum-free hormonally defined medium. Although not phenotypically stable in pure culture, adult hepatocytes retain a broad response to exogenous signals, particularly hormones and factors secreted following inflammation. The long-term culture of adult hepatocytes secreting high levels of various plasma proteins and maintaining the capacity to transcribe specific genes is now possible by co-culturing these cells with another liver epithelial cell type. Hepatocyte cultures are also useful for the study of the different steps of the secretory process of plasma proteins.

Introduction

Most plasma proteins with the exception of immunoglobulins are produced by the liver. Biochemical and morphological studies have clearly demonstrated that their synthesis is a relatively specialized function of hepatocytes (21). In common with other export proteins, liver plasma proteins are synthesized on bound ribosomes, then conveyed via the endoplasmic reticulum and Golgi apparatus towards the extracellular space (25, 34, 54). Most of them are glycosylated during their transport within the cell. Immunohistochemical analyses suggest that there are no specialized hepatocytes engaged in the formation of one or more plasma proteins in the normal liver. All parenchymal cells can be involved in the production of one or several proteins at the same time (32, 46, 80). However, when the synthesis of some proteins is increased under certain conditions this increase may not be observed simultaneously in all of the cells. Thus, during acute phase response following injection of inflammatory compounds, perilobular hepatocytes are the first to exhibit an increased production of acute phase proteins (15, 43).

The production of plasma proteins by the liver is regulated by a variety of endogenous and exogenous factors. In order to understand these regulating factors and particularly their mode of action, a number of investigators have turned to metabolically simpler liver systems and during the last decade have increasingly used freshly isolated or cultured hepatocytes. This article reviews various studies concerning plasma proteins using isolated and cultured hepatocytes and underlines the major findings. Studies concerning lipoproteins are considered in chapter 6.

Evidence for production of plasma proteins by isolated and cultured hepatocytes

Hepatocytes continue to synthesize and secrete plasma proteins after isolation, but usually synthesis rates decrease more or less abruptly within a few days of culture. However, these rates are dependent on the protein tested, culture conditions and species. Thus, while albumin production rapidly declines in adult rat hepatocyte cultures, it increases during the first 6–8 days before declining in cultures of adult human hepatocytes (12, 29). As in the intact liver, all cells freshly isolated or in short-term culture stain for various proteins by immunoenzymatic methods (Fig. 1). The proteins are distributed heterogeneously in the cytoplasm in structures which at the ultrastructural level appear to be the rough and smooth endoplasmic reticulum and Golgi apparatus (32, 47, 76). The staining is more intense in cells located in small rather than large colonies suggesting that synthesis rates can be related to cell density.

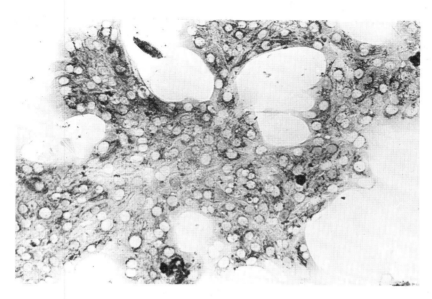

Fig. 1. Immunolocalization of albumin in cultured rat hepatocytes. All the hepatocytes were stained for the protein. Day 2 of culture. Fixation: paraformaldehyde 4%–0.2% glutaraldehyde followed by membrane permeabilization with saponin. Immunoperoxidase method. Magnification×150 (from reference 32).

The reverse haemolytic plaque assay has been used to demonstrate plasma protein secretion at the cell level as well as to determine the percentage of cells actively secreting a given protein. This technique involves complement-mediated lysis of sheep erythrocytes coated with specific antibodies. Recently, Bernuau *et al.* (9) found that 74, 82 and 98% of hepatocytes isolated from normal rats secreted albumin after 1, 2 and 4 h of incubation respectively.

The simultaneous production of the same protein by all the hepatocytes can also be shown by *in situ* hybridization. Recently, using albumin cDNA probes we were able to detect albumin mRNA molecules in all rat hepatocytes after 24 h of culture (Fig. 2) (Clément *et al.*, unpublished observations).

To determine whether all parenchymal cells can synthesize proteins at the same rate, albumin production has been measured in diploid and tetraploid hepatocyte subpopulations separated by elutriation. Le Rumeur *et al.* (47, 48) reported that in both suspension and short-term culture diploid cells secreted two-fold less albumin than tetraploid cells (see Table 1). A similar difference was found for total protein synthesis after incorporation of [^{3}H]-leucine or [^{35}S]-methionine (48).

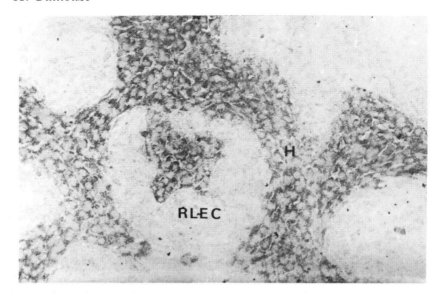

Fig. 2. Localization of albumin mRNAs in rat hepatocytes co-cultured with rat liver epithelial cells. Specific mRNA were demonstrated by *in situ* hybridization with an albumin cDNA probe in 4 days co-culture. Cells were fixed in ethanol/acetic acid 3:1 (vol/vol) for 20 min. Numerous silver grains are visible over all hepatocytes (H) and absent on rat liver epithelial cells (RLEC). Magnification×100.

Table 1. Secretion of albumin by diploid and tetraploid rat hepatocytes cultured on different supports.

	Support	
	Plastic	*Fibronectin*
2n	32.9±4.0 (8)	37.0±4.0 (5)
4n	58.3±7.2 (8)	66.8±2.2 (5)
4n:2n	1.8:1.0	1.8:1.0

Albumin accumulated in the medium between the 4th and the 22nd after cell seeding was expressed in µg per 10^6 attached cells (mean±sd). The number of experiments is in parentheses.

Influence of experimental conditions on the rate of protein synthesis

Environmental factors can greatly influence the rate of protein synthesis. Comparison of the results obtained by different laboratories is often difficult because of the variety of media and supports used. Nevertheless, freshly isolated and cultured hepatocytes generally synthesize lower rates of plasma proteins than the intact liver. Freshly isolated cells incubated in a medium enriched with vitamins, hormones and serum produce albumin at a rate 40 to 80% of the *in vivo* rate of 3 µg/h/10^6 cells (16, 20, 40). However, when calculating the amount of secreted proteins per cell it is important to take into account *in vivo* pretreatment (see following section) and the age of the animals. Albumin synthesis decreases with age in hepatocytes obtained from 3 to 24-month-old rats and increases sharply in cells isolated from older animals (75).

Synthesis of plasma proteins is constant for the first few hours, this period depending on the protein. Weigand *et al.* (77) found that albumin and angiotensinogen, which play an important role in the regulation of blood pressure, were synthesized at a constant rate for 5 h. Jeejeebhoy *et al.* (39) showed that in rat hepatocyte suspensions, the rate of hemopexin synthesis was linear for 48 h while that of albumin and fibrinogen was close to linear for only 12 h after which it decreased continuously.

Influence of the medium

A number of studies have been undertaken to define nutritional requirements of adult hepatocytes *in vitro*. Freshly isolated cells incubated in an amino acid-free medium, are in a strongly negative nitrogen balance, due to the rate of protein synthesis which is 10 times lower than that of protein degradation (64). This situation is maintained throughout the first 24 h of culture in a medium without proteins but supplemented with amino acid concentrations approximating normal plasma levels (62). However, later on degradation of proteins gradually diminished, resulting in a strongly reduced loss of protein (4%/h to 1%/h). This was not correlated to protein synthesis, the rate of which also decreased but to a lesser extent. Crane & Miller (17) came to similar conclusions by showing that in 48 h hepatocytes catabolized 10–15% of their own protein. Protein loss was partially prevented by leupeptin, an inhibitor of lysosomal proteases (62).

In an extensive study, Seglen *et al.* (65) found that amino acids influenced both the protein degradation rate and the rate of total protein synthesis in cultured hepatocytes. A balanced mixture of amino acids could maintain hepatocytes in a protein anabolic state while, when added individually, these amino acids had various effects on protein synthesis, some being stimulatory, some inhibitory. Alanine was the most effective. Addition of energy substrates, particularly pyruvate at an optimal concentration (20 mM), reduced the effects of all the individually active amino acids. However, in the presence of 10×normal concentrations of amino acids the addition of 20 mM pyruvate resulted in a net increase of protein synthesis. Similar observations were made with hepatocytes in suspension as well as in 4-day culture (63). On the basis of their results these authors defined a new incubation medium to maintain hepatocytes in an anabolic state. This medium contained the following mixture of amino acids: 5 mM asparagine and glutamine, 2.5 mM leucine, 2 mM phenylalanine and tyrosine, 1 mM histidine plus all the other amino acids found to be optimal for protein synthesis (63, 65). Twenty millimolar pyruvate was found to be the most effective energy source (63). The critical role of amino acids has been stressed by others. Synthesis of albumin and angiotensinogen diminished by 40% in hepatocyte suspensions incubated in a medium lacking amino acids, for 5 h (77). Tanaka *et al.* (72) reported that after 3 days in a medium containing bovine serum and 10^{-5}M dexamethasone, rat hepatocytes became anabolic and consumed amino acids in the presence of levels of amino acids between 0.5 mM and 1.0 mM while they were catabolic and lost amino acids when incubated with lower levels.

The above studies indicate that protein synthesis rate in cultured hepatocytes depends upon the level of endogenous amino acids generated primarily by the lysosomal pathway particularly when the level of exogenous amino acids is low. Other studies have underlined the influence of certain hormones upon the protein synthesis rate. Thus, insulin and glucagon can affect lysosomal protein degradation, the levels depending on the concentration of amino acids. Insulin at low and high concentrations inhibits only slightly protein degradation but is much more effective at intermediate concentrations (57). Since the hormone was used at extraphysiological concentrations, it is possible that the responses seen were not specific (18). Stimulation of protein degradation by glucagon is also strongly amino acid dependent and is largely reduced when optimal levels of amino acids are present (57).

Hormone supplementation does not affect synthesis of all plasma proteins equally. In hormone-free medium the initial rates of hemopexin, albumin and fibrinogen synthesis measured by radioimmunoassay in rat hepatocyte suspensions were respectively 0.17, 0.30 and 0.081 mg/g of hepatocyte/h during the first 48 h (39). When the cells were cultured in a hormone-supplemented medium, which included insulin, cortisol, glucagon, triiodothyronine and growth hormone, between 6 and 48 h after plating, the synthesis rate of hemopexin was not affected whereas that of albumin and fibrinogen increased from 22% and 123% respectively. Hooper *et al.* (37) obtained a 70% increase in leucine incorporation into haptoglobin relative to albumin in rat hepatocyte cultures after an 18 h incubation in a medium containing a mixture of hormones including hydrocortisone, insulin, glucagon, somatotropin and triiodothyronine.

The importance of amino acid levels and hormones in protein synthesis has also been demonstrated by analysing polyribosome profiles. Dickson & Pogson (19) reported that $10 \times$ normal rat plasma levels of amino acids had to be added to the perfusate for isolating polyribosomes in the aggregated state. Following cell isolation, disaggregation is constantly observed (70, 73) whatever the composition of the medium (presence or absence of serum and amino acids) and the support (plastic or collagen). Insulin, which favours protein synthesis, prevented extensive disaggregation of polysomes (70).

A number of studies have included serum in the incubating medium because it favours cell attachment and survival. However, serum contains factors which influence the synthesis of various proteins. It enhances 3- to 5-fold albumin, fibrinogen and α-1-globulin-M and to a lesser extent other proteins in chick embryonic hepatocyte cultures (56). The stimulatory activity of serum showed no developmental or species specificity, thereby suggesting that protein synthesis is controlled by ubiquitous but uncharacterized components of the serum.

Osmolarity also affects protein synthesis. A hypertonic medium (approximately 400 mosM), obtained by addition of extra NaCl is required to provide optimal conditions in the presence of high levels of amino acids (63).

Influence of the support

When hepatocytes are cultured on natural substrates, their survival and certain functions are improved. Such substrata include rat tail collagens, fibronectin, connective liver tissue biomatrix and the extracellular material secreted by bovine corneal endothelial cells. On these substrata, plating efficiency is higher and cell spreading is often more rapid than on plastic (31). Hepatocytes cultured on these substrata continue to secrete plasma proteins but at a low rate (31, 50, 59). Moreover, the synthesis rate was found to drop earlier in cells which showed more rapid spreading than on plastic (31). In contrast, parenchymal cells which were cultured on floating collagen, retained a cuboidal morphology and secreted higher amounts of albumin, transferrin and α_1-acid-glycoprotein (67).

Influence of other cells

Hepatocytes plated onto feeder cells such as 3H/10T1/2 mouse embryo cells (44) or normal human fibroblasts (51) also survive longer and, as on organic substrata, exhibit rapid phenotypic changes resulting in a strong decrease in the level of their specific functions. In contrast, when co-cultured with rat liver epithelial cells, parenchymal cells were found not only to survive for several weeks but also to express various specific functions at high levels. These functions included production of various plasma proteins such as albumin (12, 30), haptoglobin and hemopexin (33). Active production of plasma proteins was maintained for several weeks even in a serum-free medium (Fig. 3). At least during the first weeks, albumin was detected in all the hepatocytes, mainly in structures corresponding to Golgi complexes located near bile canaliculi with the immunoperoxidase method. This indicates that in this system, hepatocytes remain polarized (12). The influence of cell-cell interactions on the expression of specific functions, including plasma protein production, in co-cultured hepatocytes is discussed in detail in another chapter.

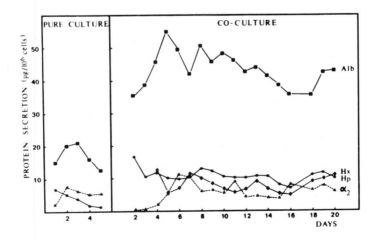

Fig. 3. Secretion of plasma proteins in the medium of pure and mixed cultures of adult rat hepatocytes. Amounts of albumin, haptoglobin, α_2-macroglobulin and hemopexin were determined by an electroimmunoassay. The values are expressed in $\mu g/day/10^6$ hepatocytes and are means of two independent experiments performed in duplicate. The number of attached hepatocytes was evaluated by measuring the intracellular lactic dehydrogenase content before addition of rat liver epithelial cells. Cultures were maintained in serum-free medium (Taken from reference 33).

Influence of *in vivo* pretreatment on the rate of plasma protein secretion

As underlined by Crane & Miller (18), isolated hepatocytes 'enter the culture medium with a prior history or memory of signals to which they are responding'. The previous endocrine state controls the rate of protein synthesis during the first two days of culture. Thus, glucocorticosteroids and epinephrine markedly increase fibrinogen in hepatocytes from adrenalectomized animals whereas normal cells have variable responses (17). Chen & Feigelson (14) measured production of α_2u-globulin by hepatocytes from normal, ovariectomized or castrated rats, or estradiol-treated or adrenalectomized males. The level of α_2u-globulin, an androgen-inducible estrogen-repressible protein, was consistent with the endocrine state from which the cells were derived.

Hepatocytes from injured animals also continue to secrete specific proteins at relatively linear rates for 1 or 2 days (10, 45, 61). The group of proteins which appear following inflammation are termed 'acute phase reactants'. Whereas some of these proteins have well-defined functions, eg fibrinogen and haptoglobin, others including C-reactive protein, serum amyloid A protein (SAA) and serum amyloid P component (SAP) are poorly defined. Thus, rabbit hepatocytes isolated 18–24 hr after turpentine administration continue to secrete C-reactive protein for at least 48 h in culture. During the first 24 h, the average of C-reactive protein synthesis to total secreted protein synthesis determined by incorporation of a [^{3}H]-labelled-L-amino acid mixture was found to be 10 times higher in hepatocytes from inflamed animals than in cells from normal rabbits (61). Fibrinogen, another acute phase reactant protein, was also found to be secreted by rat hepatocytes in higher levels during the first 4 hours following isolation 24 h after injection of turpentine (9). Similar observations were made for the secretion of SAP by hepatocytes from thio-glycolatte-treated mice (45) and for that of SAA by cells from casein-treated mice (10).

Regulation of specific plasma protein synthesis by hormones and factors secreted during inflammation

Hormones and factors secreted during inflammation which stimulate synthesis of acute phase reactant proteins, have been the compounds most widely studied as regulators of plasma protein production.

Hormones either alone or in a mixture may strongly influence synthesis of certain plasma proteins. In particular, corticosteroids have been reported to modulate production of various proteins. They mainly affect acute phase proteins but do so to various extents (5). Thus, 10^{-7}M dexamethasone induced production of α_2-macroglobulin, a protein actively synthesized in fetal liver but not in normal adults, and increased α_1-acid glycoprotein 3.5-fold and α_1-proteinase inhibitor 1.4-fold after an 18 h incubation in adult rat hepatocyte cultures. After a lag-phase of 3 h, the synthesis of both proteins showed a steady increase during 2 days (26). The early increase of α_2-macroglobulin secretion that we found in pure cultures and in co-cultures of rat hepatocytes could also be attributed to glucocorticoids since the cultures were continuously maintained in the presence of hydrocortisone hemisuccinate after the first removal of medium (33). Stimulation of acute phase proteins by adrenal corticosteroids is consistent with *in vivo* observations showing that these hormones increase (71) and are essential for the induction of α_2-macroglobulin (36) during experimental inflammation. Fibrinogen was also increased about 3 times after 10 hours in the presence of cortisol (17). In contrast, synthesis of acute phase proteins was not modified in mouse hepatocytes cultured in the presence of dexamethasone (6, 7).

Glucocorticoids also stimulate synthesis of α_2u-globulin in hepatocytes isolated from castrated male rats. This protein which is the major protein in adult rat male urine, was selectively increased 2-fold in the presence of 0.1 μM dexamethasone (13). In contrast, these hormones do not seem to directly influence albumin synthesis. Indeed, the rates of albumin synthesis in hepatocytes isolated from adrenalectomized rats were not significantly lower than those in cells from normal animals (17). The synthesis rate remained unchanged in rat hepatocytes cultured in the presence of 10^{-7}M dexamethasone for 2 days (26, 79). However, Weigand *et al.* (77) reported a slight increase in albumin synthesis in rat hepatocytes treated with high doses of hydrocortisone (10^{-4}M). In culture, higher levels of albumin synthesis in the presence of corticosteroids have been reported by several authors (3, 30, 41, 42). This increase could result from the beneficial effect of these hormones on cell survival and various functions in hepatocyte cultures (see reference 28). A similar explanation could be advanced for the modest increase of ceruloplasmin in rat hepatocyte cultures after an 18 h incubation in the presence of dexamethasone (78) and for the increased albumin secretion by rat hepatocytes co-cultured with rat liver epithelial cells in the presence of hydrocortisone (3, 30).

Other hormones may also influence production of plasma proteins. Insulin was found to enhance albumin production in isolated rat hepatocytes (17) and in cultured amphibian hepatocyte cultures (70). Growth hormone partially restores albumin synthesis in cultured hepatocytes from hypophysectomized rats. In these animals, the decrease in albumin relative to total protein is 30–50% (20). Addition of 17β-estradiol to the medium of female frog hepatocyte cultures resulted in the increase of the egg yolk precursor vitellin synthesis relative to other secreted proteins. This protein was the major one exported after 6 days of treatment (69).

As seen in the preceding section, hepatocytes isolated from inflamed animals, retain the ability to secrete high levels of acute phase proteins for at least 24 h (10, 45, 61). Substances inducing an inflammatory response are not themselves involved in the induction of these acute phase proteins but require a mediator. A number of *in vivo* studies suggest that factors synthesized by macrophages are involved. Hepatocyte cultures offer a unique approach to characterize inducers that recruit hepatocytes for the production of acute phase proteins.

Using isolated hepatocytes from liposaccharide (LPS) non-responder mice, Selinger *et al.* (66) have shown that culture supernatants from LPS-stimulated macrophages caused parenchymal cells to give a SAA response. Le & Mortensen (45) found stimulation of SAP in cultured mouse hepatocytes incubated with inter-leukin-1 (IL-1), a factor isolated from induced macrophages, or with thio-glycolatte-elicited macrophages not producing IL-1. Since an additive effect on SAP production was observed when IL-1 was added to these macrophages, the participation of other factors (cytokines) was probable. However, another group only observed induction of SAA upon addition of IL-1 containing macrophage supernatants to cultured mouse hepatocytes (74). Although these apparently contradictory results could be attributed to the different culture conditions used, they were most probably related to the presence of inhibitory protein(s) in IL-1 preparations. A factor secreted by leucocytes also appears to be involved in the regulation of fibrinogen synthesis by plasmin-derived fragments of fibrinogen and fibrin. Ritchie et al. (58) showed that either fibrinogen or fibrin fragment D or E had no effect on the synthesis and secretion of fibrinogen in rat hepatocyte cultures. However, if the fragments were incubated with isolated peripheral blood leucocytes, they caused these cells to release a factor that increased fibrinogen synthesis in hepatocyte cultures 4- to 6-fold over controls.

Recent work suggests that several factors may be involved in stimulation of plasma protein synthesis by hepatocytes during the acute phase reaction (8). The authors compared the effect of conditioned media from squamous carcinoma COLO-16 cells, normal epidermal cells and activated peripheral monocytes on the synthesis of specific acute-phase proteins in primary cultures of rat and mouse hepatocytes and in human hepatoma cells (HepG$_2$ cells). Conditioned media from the three cell types studied enhanced synthesis of various proteins in the different hepatic cells. However, the effect of the different conditioned media and the response of hepatic cells from the three species were different. The following proteins were found to be stimulated: α_1-antichymotrypsin in HepG$_2$; α_1-antichymotrypsin, α_1-acid glycoprotein, α_1-acute-phase protein and α_2-macroglobulin in rat hepatocytes; and, α_1-acid glycoprotein, haptoglobin and hemopexin in mouse hepatocytes.

Koj et al. (42) have provided further evidence that acute phase proteins could also be induced by heterogenous cytokines. They showed that human cytokines obtained from endotoxin stimulated monocytes or unstimulated human COLO-16 cells consistently increased synthesis of α_2-macroglobulin and α_1-acute-phase protein. In contrast, albumin production was found to be decreased in the presence of cytokines (8, 42).

The role of glucocorticoids in the stimulation of acute phase proteins during the inflammatory response has been well documented in rat hepatocytes. A partially purified human leukocyte pyrogen in the presence of cortisol caused a 70% increase in leucine incorporation in haptoglobin relative to albumin during a 48 h period (37). A crude extract of leukocytes from inflamed animals increased fibrinogen synthesis 5-fold during 24 h but only when cortisol or hydrocortisone was added to the medium (60). Similarly, the 4-fold increase of α_2-macroglobulin 10–12 h after addition of medium from LPS-stimulated rat Kupffer cell cultures to cultured rat hepatocytes was dependent upon the presence of low concentrations of dexamethasone (10^{-9}M) (4). Conditioned media from COLO-16 cells and monocytes enhanced the synthesis of acute phase proteins in the presence of dexamethasone (8). However, the effect was found only in rat hepatocytes. Its absence in mouse hepatocytes and HepG$_2$ cells suggests that species differences exist in the capability of liver cells to respond to inducers.

Control mechanisms of plasma protein secretion

The rate of plasma protein production by isolated and cultured hepatocytes can be controlled at the transcriptional level, or by stabilization of mRNA or by translational or post-translational events. Clayton & Darnell (11) analysed liver specific mRNA sequences by Northern blots in mouse hepatocytes cultured in a medium containing hydrocortisone, insulin and 10% fetal calf serum. They found little change in various liver specific mRNA sequences including albumin and α_1-antitrypsin mRNA during the first 24 h. A gradual decrease occurred during the following 3 days and the specific sequences became virtually undetectable by day 7. Transcription rates of specific genes were greatly diminished during the first day. Similar observations were made with rat hepatocytes cultured in a medium supplemented with serum (38). In contrast, when the cells were cultured in a serum-free hormonally defined medium, albumin and α_1-antitrypsin mRNA sequences remained high during the first 5 days although the transcription rate was again low. These observations suggest that, in the particular medium used, the abundance of mRNAs was regulated by a post-transcriptional mechanism involving mRNA stabilization. Addition of serum to this culture medium resulted in a dramatic alteration of liver specific mRNA sequences. In support to these findings a dramatic decline in albumin mRNA within 24 h in chick embryo hepatocytes cultured in serum-free medium was partially reversed in the presence of insulin (55). Moreover, in this study transferrin mRNA remained constant during 3 days indicating that mRNA sequences of different proteins are regulated differently. Consequently, culture conditions are critical for the maintenance of gene transcription and for mRNA stabilization. Recently, Fraslin *et al.* (22) have shown that the transcription rate of specific genes was 2-fold higher after 4 days and maintained for at least 12 days in rat hepatoctyes co-cultured with rat liver epithelial cells compared to pure hepatocyte cultures. These results are extensively discussed in the chapter dealing with the influence of cell-cell interactions on the expression of liver functions in cultured hepatocytes (chapter 12).

Levels of mRNA are increased in cultured hepatocytes during stimulation of plasma proteins by hormones or factors secreted by induced macrophages or other cells. It has not yet been established whether this increase involves transcription or stabilization of specific RNAs, or both.

Intracellular processing of plasma proteins in cultured hepatocytes

Hepatocytes in culture are a suitable system to study in more detail the different steps of the secretory process in order to better understand the molecular basis of the mechanisms involved in intracellular transport of proteins.

Many secretory proteins are formed as larger molecular weight precursors (pro-forms) and processed to their final mature forms by post-translational proteolysis. Rat hepatocyte cultures have been used by several authors to distinguish intracellular forms of various proteins by electrophoresis in sodium dodecyl sulfate poly-acrylamide gels (27). Andus *et al.* (1, 2) identified two forms for α_2-macroglobulin, transferrin, α_1-acid glycoprotein and α_1-proteinase inhibitor. The following molecular weights were estimated for intracellular precursors and the secreted forms: α_2-macroglobulin 176 000 and 182 000, transferrin 84 000 and 86 000, α_1-acid glycoprotein 39 000 and 43 000–60 000, α_1-proteinase inhibitor 49 000 and

54 000. Different intracellular and secreted forms have also been demonstrated for α_2u-globulin (35). These different forms are not sensitive to the same enzymes. Thus, only the intracellular forms of α_2-macroglobulin, transferrin, α_1-acid glycoprotein and α_1-proteinase inhibitor were sensitive to endoglucosaminidase H which cleaves only high mannose oligosaccharides. The secreted forms are sensitive to sialidase (2).

Drugs that affect intracellular processing of proteins at distinct sites are very useful for analysing the different steps of secretion and of the glycosylation process. The most widely used drugs are tunicamycin, monensin, colchicine and taxol. Tunicamycin, which inhibits glycosylation by blocking the transfer of glycosamine from UDP glycosamine to a dolichol acceptor, did not affect the secretion of the unglycosylated form of α_2u-globulin weighing 20 000 daltons. Only the secretion of two glycosylated higher molecular weight species was inhibited (35). This drug also affects secretion of other glycoproteins, including α_2-macroglobulin, transferrin, α_1-acid glycoprotein and α_1-proteinase inhibitor. Transferrin was the least affected (2). Since unglycosylated α_2u-globulin (35, 68) and α_1-antitrypsin (24, 27) were found in the medium of tunicamycin-treated cells, it may be concluded that the carbohydrate moiety is not essential for the secretion of proteins. This is supported by the findings with monensin, a carboxylic ionophore for monovalent cations. This drug inhibits intracellular transport and maturation of proteins in the Golgi apparatus. In monensin-treated cultured hepatocytes, most of the newly synthesized α_1-proteinase inhibitor and albumin were not processed to the final mature forms, resulting in accumulation of the two 51 000 forms and proalbumin respectively. However, proalbumin and the endoglycosidase-H-resistant α_1-protease inhibitor were finally secreted (53). In contrast to proalbumin, processing of the haptoglobin proform was not blocked in monensin-treated cells, indicating that the haptoglobin proform is cleaved before entering the Golgi apparatus (52). Secretion of plasma proteins by cultured hepatocytes is also inhibited either with colchicine, which depolymerizes microtubules, or with taxol, which promotes polymerization of tubulin, resulting in the formation of dysfunctional microtubules. Unprocessed, partially processed or processed proteins accumulated within the cells and only mature proteins were finally secreted into the medium. The results with albumin and α_1-protease inhibitor indicated that the site of blockade of intracellular transport by these drugs was after proteolysis (albumin) or processing of oligosaccharide chains (α_1-protease inhibitor) (53).

Cultured hepatocytes have also been used to determine the time-course for the intracellular transport of serum albumin by pulse-chase experiments. Albumin was found to appear earlier than glycoproteins in the culture medium (30 min versus about 60 min) (2). The transport rate for proteins from the endoplasmic reticulum to the Golgi apparatus varied greatly ($t\frac{1}{2}$=14–137 min) while it was about the same value for all proteins from the Golgi apparatus to the medium ($t\frac{1}{2}$=15 min) (23). Similar results were obtained with hepatoma cells (49). On the basis of these observations it was proposed that the transport of plasma proteins from the endoplasmic reticulum to the Golgi apparatus might be mediated by membrane-bound receptors (23).

ACKNOWLEDGEMENTS

The author thanks B. Clément, J. M. Fraslin and G. Lescoat for the critical reading of the manuscript and is indebted to A. Vannier for typing. Personal research was supported by INSERM, MRT and Fondation pour la Recherche Médicale.

REFERENCES

1   Andus T., Gross V., Tran-Thi T. A., Heinrich P. C.: Synthesis of α_2-macroglobulin in rat hepatocytes and in cell-free system. *FEBS Lett.* 1983, **151**: 10–14.
2   Andus T., Gross V., Tran-Thi T. A., Schreiber G., Nagashima M., Heinrich P. C.: The biosynthesis of acute-phase proteins in primary cultures of rat hepatocytes. *Eur. J. Biochem.* 1983, **133**: 561–571.
3   Baffet G., Clement B., Glaise D., Guillouzo A., Guguen-Guillouzo C.: Hydrocortisone modulates the production of extracellular material and albumin in long-term co-cultures of adult rat hepatocytes with other liver epithelial cells. *Biochem. Biophys. Res. Commun.* 1982, **109**: 507–512.
4   Bauer J., Birmelin M., Northoff G. H., Northemann W., Tran-Thi T. A., Ueberberg H., Decker K., Heinrich P. C.: Induction of rat α_2-macroglobulin *in vivo* and in hepatocyte primary cultures: synergistic action of glucocorticoids and a Kupffer cell-derived factor. *FEBS Lett.* 1984, **177**: 89–94.
5   Baumann H., Firestone G. L., Burgess T. L., Gross K. W., Yamamoto K. R., Held W. A.: Dexamethasone regulation of α_1-acid glycoprotein and other acute phase reactants in rat liver and hepatoma cells. *J. Biol. Chem.* 1983, **258**: 563–570.
6   Baumann H., Jahreis G. P.: Regulation of mouse haptoglobin synthesis. *J. Cell Biol.* 1983, **97**: 728–736.
7   Baumann H., Jahreis G. P., Gaines K. C.: Synthesis and regulation of acute phase plasma proteins in primary cultures of mouse hepatocytes. *J. Cell Biol* 1983, **97**: 866–876.
8   Baumann H., Jahreis G. P., Sander D. N., Koj A.: Human keratinocytes and monocytes release factors which regulate the synthesis of major acute phase plasma proteins in hepatic cells from man, rat and mouse. *J. Biol. Chem.* 1984, **259**: 7331–7342.
9   Bernuau D., Rogier E., Feldmann G.: Decreased albumin and increased fibrinogen secretion by single hepatocytes from rats with acute inflammatory reaction. *Hepatology* 1983, **3**: 29–33.
10 Berson M. D., Kleiner E.: Synthesis and secretion of serum amyloid A (SAA) by hepatocytes in mice treated with casein. *J. Immunol.* 1980, **124**: 495–499.
11 Clayton D. F., Darnell J. E. Jr: Changes in liver-specific compared to common gene transcription during primary culture of mouse hepatocytes. *Molec. Cell. Biol.* 1983, **3**: 1552–1561.
12 Clement B., Guguen-Guillouzo C., Campion J. P., Glaise D., Bourel M., Guillouzo A.: Long-term co-cultures of adult human hepatocytes with rat liver epithelial cells: modulation of albumin secretion and accumulation of extracellular material. *Hepatology* 1984, **4**: 373–380.
13 Chen C. L. C., Feigelson P.: Glucocorticoid induction of alpha 2 u-globulin protein synthesis and its RNA in rat hepatocytes *in vitro*. *J. Biol. Chem.* 1978, **253**: 7880–7885.
14 Chen C. L. C., Feigelson P.: Hormonal control of α_2u-globulin synthesis and its mRNA in isolated hepatocytes. *Ann. N.Y. Acad. Sci.* 1980, **349**: 28–45.
15 Courtoy P. J., Lombart C., Feldmann G., Moguilevski N., Rogier E.: Synchronous increase of four acute phase proteins synthesized by the same hepatocytes during the inflammatory reaction. A combined biochemical and morphological kinetics study in the rat. *Lab. Invest.* 1981, **44**: 105–115.
16 Crane L. J., Miller D. L.: Synthesis and secretion of fibrinogen and albumin by isolated rat hepatocytes. *Biochem. Biophys. Res. Commun.* 1974, **60**: 1269–1277.
17 Crane L. J., Miller D. L.: Plasma protein synthesis by isolated hepatocytes. *J. Cell Biol.* 1977, **72**: 11–25.
18 Crane L. J., Miller D. L.: Plasma protein induction by isolated hepatocytes. *Molec. Cell. Biochem.* 1983, **148**: 466–477.
19 Dickson A. J., Pogson C. I.: Polyribosomes in isolated liver cells. Preparative procedures, effects of incubation and correlation with protein synthesis. *Biochem. J.* 1980, **186**: 35–45.
20 Feldhoff R. C., Taylor J. M., Jefferson L. S.: Synthesis and secretion of rat albumin *in vivo*, in

perfused liver and in isolated hepatocytes. *J. Biol. Chem.* 1977, **252**: 3611–3616.

21 Feldmann G.: Morphological aspects of hepatic synthesis and secretion of plasma proteins. *In*: *Progress in Liver Diseases*, H. Popper, F. Schaffner (Eds): Grune & Stratton, New York, 1979, Vol. VI, pp 23–41.

22 Fraslin J. M., Kneip B., Vaulont S., Glaise D., Munnich A., Guguen-Guillouzo C.: Dependence of hepatocyte specific gene expression on cell-cell interactions during primary culture. *EMBO J.* 1985, **4**: 2487–2491.

23 Fries E., Gustafsson L., Peterson P. A.: Four secretory proteins synthesized by hepatocytes are transported from endoplasmic reticulum to Golgi complex at different rates. *EMBO J.* 1984, **3**: 147–152.

24 Geiger T., Northemann W., Schmelzer E., Gross V., Gauthier F., Heinrich P. C.: Synthesis of α_1-antitrypsin in rat-liver hepatocytes and in a cell-free system. *Eur. J. Biochem.* 1982, **126**: 189–195.

25 Glaumann H., Ericsson J. L. E.: Evidence for the participation of the Golgi apparatus in the intracellular transport of nascent albumin in the liver cell. *J. Cell Biol.* 1971, **47**: 555–567.

26 Gross V., Andus T., Tran-Thi T. A., Bauer J., Decker K., Heinrich P. C.: Induction of acute-phase proteins by dexamethasone in rat hepatocyte primary cultures. *Exp. Cell Res.* 1984, **157**: 46–54.

27 Gross V., Geiger T., Tran-Thi T. A., Gauthier F., Heinrich P. C.: Biosynthesis and secretion of α_1-antitrypsin in primary cultures of rat hepatocytes. *Eur. J. Biochem.* 1982, **129**: 317–323.

28 Guguen-Guillouzo C., Guillouzo A.: Modulation of functional activities in cultured rat hepatocytes. *Molec. Cell. Biochem.* 1983, **53/54**: 35–56.

29 Guguen-Guillouzo C., Baffet G., Clement B., Begue J. M., Glaise D., Guillouzo A.: Human adult hepatocytes: isolation and maintenance at high levels of specific functions in a co-culture system. *In*: *Isolation, Characterization and Use of Hepatocytes*, R. A. Harris, N. W. Cornell (Eds): Elsevier, New York, 1983, pp 105–110.

30 Guguen-Guillouzo C., Clement B., Baffet G., Beaumont C., Morel-Chany E., Glaise D., Guillouzo A.: Maintenance and reversibility of active albumin secretion by adult rat hepatocytes co-cultured with another liver epithelial cell type. *Exp. Cell Res.* 1983, **143**: 47–54.

31 Guguen-Guillouzo C., Seignoux D., Courtois Y., Brissot P., Marceau N., Glaise D., Guillouzo A.: Amplified phenotypic changes in adult rat and baboon hepatocytes cultured on a complex biomatrix. *Biol. Cell* 1982, **46**: 11–20.

32 Guillouzo A., Beaumont C., Le Rumeur E., Rissel M., Latinier M. F., Guguen-Guillouzo C., Bourel M.: New findings on immunolocalization of albumin in rat hepatocytes. *Biol. Cell* 1982, **43**: 163–172.

33 Guillouzo A., Delers F., Clement B., Bernard N., Engler R.: Long term production of acute-phase proteins by adult rat hepatocytes co-cultured with another liver cell type in serum-free medium. *Biochem. Biophys. Res. Commun.* 1984, **120**: 311–317.

34 Guillouzo A., Feldmann G., Maurice M., Sapin C., Benhamou J. P.: Ultrastructural distribution of albumin in rat hepatocytes during postnatal development. *J. Microscopie Biol. Cell.* 1976, **26**: 35–41.

35 Haars L. J., Pitot H. C.: α_2u-globulin in the rat. The regulation of the appearance of multiple forms *in vivo* and in primary cultures of adult hepatocytes. *J. Biol. Chem.* 1979, **254**: 9401–9407.

36 Heim W. G., Ellenson S. R.: Adrenal cortical control of the appearance of rat slow alpha-2-globulin. *Nature* 1967, **213**: 1260–1261.

37 Hooper D. C., Steer C. J., Dinardello C. A., Peacock A. C.: Haptoglobin and albumin synthesis in isolated rat hepatocytes. Response to potential mediators of the acute-phase reaction. *Biochem. Biophys. Acta* 1981, **653**: 118–129.

38 Jefferson D. M., Clayton D. F., Darnell J. E. Jr, Reid L. M.: Posttranscriptional modulation of gene expression by media conditions in cultured rat hepatocytes. *Molec. Cell. Biol.* 1984, **4**: 1929–1934.

39 Jeejeebhoy K. N., Bruce-Robertson A., Ho J., Kida S., Muller-Eberhard U.: Synthesis of hemopexin with and without hormonal supplementation in rat hepatocyte suspensions: comparison with that of albumin and fibrinogen. *Can. J. Biochem.* 1976, **54**: 74–78.

40 Jeejeebhoy K. N., Ho J., Greenberg G. R., Phillips M. J., Bruce-Robertson A., Stodkte U.: Albumin, fibrinogen and transferrin synthesis in isolated rat hepatocyte suspensions. *Biochem. J.* 1975, **146**: 141–155.

41 Kawahara A., Sato K., Amano M.: Regulation of protein synthesis by estradiol 17β, dexamethasone and insulin in primary cultured *Xenopus* hepatocytes. *Exp. Cell Res.* 1983, **148**: 423–436.

42 Koj A., Gauldie J., Regoeczi E., Sauder D. N., Sweeney G. D.: The acute-phase response of cultured rat hepatocytes. *Biochem. J.* 1984, **224**: 505–514.

43 Kushner I., Feldmann G.: Control of the acute phase response. Demonstration of C-reactive protein synthesis and secretion by hepatocytes during acute inflammation in the rabbit. *J. Exp. Med.* 1978, **148**: 466–477.

44 Langenbach R., Malick L., Kuszynski C., Freed M., Huberman E.: Maintenance of adult rat hepatocytes on C3H/10 T 1/2 cells. *Cancer Res.* 1979, **39**: 3509–3514.

45 Le P. T., Mortensen R. F.: *In vitro* induction of hepatocyte synthesis of the acute phase reactant mouse serum amyloid P-component by macrophages and IL1. *J. Leuk. Biol.* 1984, **35**: 587–604.

46 Le Bouton A. V., Peters Masse J.: A random arrangement of albumin-containing hepatocytes seen with histo-immunologic methods. II. Conditions that produce the artefact. *Anat. Rec.* 1980, **197**: 195–203.

47 Le Rumeur E., Beaumont C., Guillouzo C., Rissel M., Bourel M., Guillouzo A.: All normal rat hepatocytes produce albumin at a rate related to their degree of ploidy. *Biochem. Biophys. Res. Commun.* 1981, **101**: 1038–1046.

48 Le Rumeur E., Guguen-Guillouzo C., Beaumont C., Saunier A., Guillouzo A.: Albumin secretion and protein synthesis by cultured diploid and tetraploid rat hepatocytes separated by elutriation. *Exp. Cell Res.* 1983, **147**: 247–254.

49 Lodish M. F., Kong N., Snider M., Strous G. J. A. M.: Hepatoma secretory proteins migrate from rough endoplasmic reticulum to Golgi at characteristic rates. *Nature* 1983, **304**: 80–83.

50 Michalopoulos G., Pitot H. C.: Primary culture of parenchymal cells on collagen membrane: morphological and biochemical observations. *Exp. Cell Res.* 1975, **94**: 70–78.

51 Michalopoulos G., Russell G., Biles C.: Primary cultures of hepatocytes on human fibroblasts. *In Vitro* 1979, **15**: 796–806.

52 Misumi Y., Tanaka Y., Ikehara Y.: Biosynthesis, intracellular processing and secretion of haptoglobin in cultured rat hepatocytes. *Biochem. Biophys. Res. Commun.* 1983, **114**: 729–736.

53 Oda K., Misumi Y., Ikehara Y.: Disparate effects of monensin and colchicine on intracellular processing of secretory proteins in cultured rat hepatocytes. *Eur. J. Biochem.* 1983, **135**: 209–216.

54 Peters T. Jr: The biosynthesis of rat serum albumin. I. Properties of rat albumin and its occurrence in liver cell fractions. *J. Biol. Chem.* 1962, **237**: 1181–1185.

55 Plant P. W., Deeley R. G., Grieninger G.: Selective block of albumin gene expression in chick embryo hepatocytes cultured without hormones and its partial reversal by insulin. *J. Biol. Chem.* 1983, **258**: 13355–13360.

56 Plant P. W., Liang T. J., Pindyck J., Grieninger G.: Serum stimulation of plasma protein synthesis in culture is selective and rapidly reversible. *Biochim. Biophys. Acta* 1981, **655**: 407–422.

57 Poli A., Gordon P. B., Schwarze P. E., Grinde B., Seglen P. O.: Effects of insulin and anchorage on hepatocytic protein metabolism and amino acid transport. *J. Cell Sci.* 1981, **48**: 1–8.

58 Ritchie D. G., Levy B. A., Adams M. A., Fuller G. M.: Regulation of fibrinogen synthesis by plasma-derived fragments of fibrinogen and fibrin: An indirect feedback pathway. *Proc. Natl. Acad. Sci.* 1982, **79**: 1530–1544.

59 Rojkind M., Gatmaitan Z., Mackensen S., Giambrone M. N., Ponce P., Reid L. M.: Connective tissue biomatrix. Its isolation and utilisation for long-term cultures of normal rat hepatocytes. *J. Cell Biol.* 1980, **87**: 255–263.

60 Rupp R. G., Fuller G. M.: Comparison of albumin and fibrinogen biosynthesis in stimulated rats and cultured fetal rat hepatocytes. *Biochem. Biophys. Res. Commun.* 1979, **88**: 327–334.

61 Schultz D., Macintyre S., Kushner I.: Studies of C-reactive protein synthesis by primary cultures of rabbit hepatocytes. *Ann. N.Y. Acad. Sci.* 1980, **349**: 387–388.

62 Schwarze P. E., Seglen P. O.: Protein metabolism and survival of rat hepatocytes in early culture. *Exp. Cell Res.* 1980, **130**: 185–190.

63 Schwarze P. E., Solheim A. E., Seglen P. O.: Amino acid and energy requirements for rat hepatocytes in primary culture. *In Vitro* 1982, **18**: 43–54.

64 Seglen P. O.: Protein-catabolic state of isolated rat hepatocytes. *Biochem. Biophys. Acta* 1977, **496**: 182–191.

65   Seglen P. O., Solheim A. E., Grinde B., Gordon P. B., Schwarze P. E., Gjessing R., Poli A.: Amino acid control of protein synthesis and degradation in isolated rat hepatocytes. *Ann. N.Y. Acad. Sci.* 1980, **349**: 1–7.

66   Selinger M. J., McAdam K. P. N. J., Kaplan M. M., Sipe J. A., Vogel S. A., Rosentreich D. L.: Monokine-induced synthesis of serum amyloid A protein by hepatocytes. *Nature* 1980, **285**: 498–500.

67   Sirica A. E., Richards W., Tsukada C., Sattler C., Pitot H. C.: Fetal phenotypic expression by adult rat hepatocytes on collagen gel/nylon meshes. *Proc. Natl. Acad. Sci.* 1979, **76**: 283–287.

68   Spence J. T., Haars L., Edwards A., Bosh A., Pitot H. C.: Regulation of gene expession in primary cultures of adult rat hepatocytes on collagen gels. *Ann. N.Y. Acad. Sci.* 1980, **349**: 99–110.

69   Stanchfield J. E., Yager J. D.: An estrogen responsive primary amphibian liver cell culture system. *Exp. Cell Res.* 1978, **116**: 239–252.

70   Stanchfield J. E., Yager J. D.: Insulin effects on protein synthesis and secretion in primary cultures of amphibian hepatocytes. *J. Cell Physiol.* 1979, **100**: 279–290.

71   Szafarczyk A., Moretti J. M., Boissin J., Assenmacher I.: Effects of time on administration of an inflammatory agent on plasma corticosterone and haptoglobin levels in the rat. *Endocrinology* 1974, **94**: 284–287.

72   Tanaka K., Kishi K., Ichihara A.: Biochemical studies on liver functions in primary cultured hepatocytes of adult rats. II Regulation of protein and amino-acid metabolism. *J. Biochem.* 1979, **86**: 863–870.

73   Tanaka K., Sato M., Tomita Y., Ichihara A.: Biochemical studies on liver functions in primary cultured hepatocytes of adult rats. I Hormonal effects on cell viability and protein synthesis. *J. Biochem.* 1978, **84**: 937–946.

74   Tatsuta E., Slipe J. D., Shirahama T., Skinner M., Cohen A. S.: Different regulatory mechanisms for serum amyloid A and serum amyloid P synthesis by cultured mouse hepatocytes. *J. Biol. Chem.* 1983, **258**: 5414–5418.

75   Van Bezooijen C. F. A., Grell T., Knook D. L.: Albumin synthesis by liver parenchymal cells isolated from young adult and old rats. *Biochem. Biophys. Res. Commun.* 1976, **71**: 513–519.

76   Vassy J., Rissel M., Kraemer M., Foucrier J., Guillouzo A.: Ultrastructural indirect immuno-localization of transferrin in cultured rat hepatocytes permeabilized with saponin. *J. Histochem. Cytochem.* 1984, **32**: 538–540.

77   Weigand K., Wernze H., Falge C.: Synthesis of angiotensinogen by isolated rat liver cells and its regulation in comparison to serum-albumin. *Biochem. Biophys. Res. Commun.* 1977, **75**: 102–110.

78   Weiner A. L., Cousins R. J.: Hormonally produced changes in caeruloplasmin synthesis and secretion in primary cultured rat hepatocytes. *Biochem. J.* 1983, **212**: 297–304.

79   Yamada S., Otto P. S., Kennedy D. L., Wayne T. F.: The effects of dexamethasone on metabolic activity of hepatocytes in primary monolayer culture. *In Vitro* 1980, **16**: 559–570.

80   Yokota S., Fahimi H. D.: Immunocytochemical localization of albumin in the secretory apparatus of rat liver parenchymal cells. *Proc. Natl. Acad. Sci.* 1981, **78**: 4970–4974.

Research in *Isolated and cultured hepatocytes* A. Guillouzo & C. Guguen-Guillouzo eds. pp. 171–186.
© 1986 John Libbey Eurotext Ltd./INSERM.

8

Enzymes and plasma proteins in cultures of fetal hepatocytes

George YEOH

Department of Physiology, University of Western Australia, Nedlands,
WESTERN AUSTRALIA 6009

SUMMARY

The fetal hepatocyte culture model offers many advantages for studying liver function. The cells retain differentiated properties over a much longer period than adult hepatocytes. Furthermore, in several instances, during culture, the cells have been shown to acquire features of their more mature counterparts when cells from early gestation fetuses are used for study. This permits one to investigate the changes which occur during hepatocyte differentiation under conditions which can be manipulated in a reproducible manner. The hormonal responses of the cells have been shown to reflect the pattern observed *in vivo* thereby rendering them potentially useful for studies of enzyme regulation and the humoral control of plasma protein synthesis.

Introduction

Since other chapters in this book will deal with isolated hepatocytes as well as drug metabolism in liver cells, this review will exclude enzymes concerned with drug detoxification and studies involving isolated hepatocytes. It will be concerned only with fetal hepatocyte studies on cells maintained in primary culture in which the production of plasma proteins or enzymes, especially those that are liver specific, is reported.

Methods for isolating fetal hepatocytes for culture

Invariably, the starting material for these studies consists of finely divided pieces of fetal liver which have been chopped, minced, sliced, diced or cubed using a scalpel, razor blade or fine scissors. The pieces are then incubated with a buffered salts solution containing trypsin, collagenase, a combination of trypsin and collagenase or collagenase and hyaluronidase. For human liver, both trypsin (3, 20) and collagenase (8) have been used successfully, whereas for embryonic chick liver, trypsin is used exclusively (5, 7, 22, 26). In contrast, collagenase is the dissociating agent of choice for the isolation of hepatocytes from rat liver (13, 15, 31), although trypsin has been used successfully by Plas *et al.* (22, 23) to isolate hepatocytes from rats of 15-day gestation. Collagenase has also been used in combination with hyaluronidase for isolating fetal rat hepatocytes for culture (17). In our experience, trypsin is unsuitable for preparation of rat liver cells, especially from late gestation animals. When trypsin is used, by the end of the incubation period a gelatinous viscous cell-free mixture is all that remains of the original tissue. However, we have used the same concentration of trypsin (0.1–0.25%) to isolate hepatocytes from embryonic chick for culture. Collagenase (0.4–0.5 mg/ml) can also be used with chick liver but in our experience, the yield is inferior to that achieved with trypsin.

Figure 1 summarizes the method used by this laboratory for preparing fetal hepatocytes from rats of gestational age 17-days or older. A collection of about ten livers previously dissected free of connective tissue is placed on the stage of a Mickle chopper housed in a laminar flow cabinet, as illustrated in Fig. 2. The livers are chopped using two passes of the stage set at right angles to each other.

The micrometer gauge is set at 0.1 mm, and the force of the blade and speed is regulated so as not to slice the Whatman's filter paper on which the livers rest. As many as 100 livers can be chopped and pooled for treatment with collagenase. The

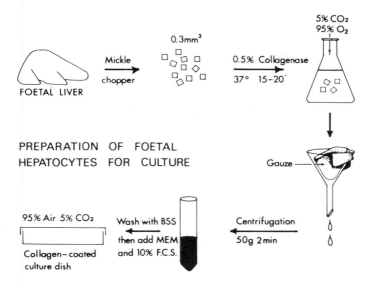

Fig. 1. Summary of the procedure for preparation of fetal rat hepatocytes for culture.

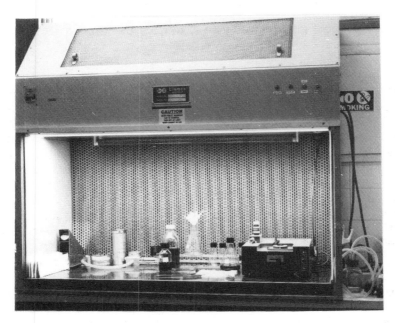

Fig. 2. Laminar flow cabinet housing equipment for preparing fetal rat hepatocytes for culture. The Mickle chopper is housed on the left of the cabinet and chopped liver is transferred to the conical flask fitted with a screw-cap lid on the left of the unit. Collagenase is added to the flask to a final concentration of 0.5%. After incubation, the mixture is filtered through nylon gauze supported in a filter funnel directly into round-bottom glass centrifuge tubes (25 ml Kimax) which are visible behind the flask.

174   *G. Yeoh*

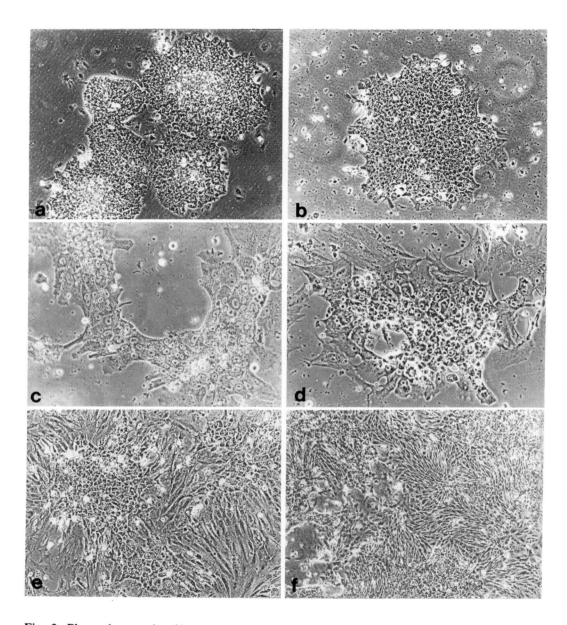

Fig. 3. Photomicrographs of hepatocyte cultures derived from 19-day gestation rats viewed under phase microscopy. (*a*) Showing attached aggregates of cells on day 1, magnification ×55. (*b*) Group of cells which have spread sufficiently for all cells to be visible by day 2, magnification ×55. (*c*) By day 3, the majority of cells are distinctly hepatocytes and few round erythroid cells are evident, magnification ×110. (*d*) Note 'epithelial' cells which emerge from the groups which proliferate and occupy the space between the groups, magnification ×110. (*e*) By day 6, a significant proportion of the cells are 'epitheloid' in morphology, with only the centre of the original groups displaying distinct hepatocyte characteristics, magnification ×55. (*f*) Beyond a week of culture, cells with a fibroblast morphology are observed, magnification ×20.

'diced' pieces are transferred to a conical flask containing Hanks balanced salts solution (BSS) (10) and collagenase (Boehringer) is added to give a final concentration of 0.5 mg/ml. The flask is aerated with a mixture of oxygen and carbon dioxide (95%, O_2; 5%, CO_2), stoppered and incubated at 37°C for 45 min with shaking in a water bath. The contents are filtered through nylon gauze and the filtrate pelleted by centrifugation at 50 g for 2 min, washed twice with BSS and finally resuspended in the culture medium of Eagle's minimal essential medium supplemented with 10% fetal bovine serum, penicillin, streptomycin and fungizone. The cells are plated out into culture dishes coated with collagen extracted from rat tails (19) and maintained at 37°C in a humidified atmosphere of 5% CO_2. The cells adhere within five hours after which groups of hepatocytes begin to spread out. It is worth noting that it is our experience that the hepatocytes aggregate as soon as the isolated cells are placed in culture medium. Very few individual cells survive, and it is only the aggregates which attach and spread. Generally, ten litters from rats of 19-day gestation, which represents about 100 fetuses, yield 150 ml of inoculum of which 1 ml, 3 ml and 10 ml are dispensed into 35 mm, 60 mm and 90 mm culture dishes respectively.

Cells are isolated from fetuses which are of 16-days gestation or earlier by dissociating the tissue suspended in BSS by aspiration through a wide bore Pasteur pipette. After about ten aspirations, the dissociated material is transferred to a second conical centrifuge tube while the larger pieces are aspirated further. The aspirated samples are combined and processed as for the cells isolated from older fetuses without filtration through nylon gauze.

Characteristics of the cells

Morphology

Figure 3 shows the morphology of the cells derived from 19-day gestation liver during culture. Initially, the cells attach and by day 1 the edges of the aggregates have flattened sufficiently to be observed by phase contrast microscopy (Fig. 3*a*). Some cells which remain rounded up are most likely to be early erythroid cells. These are removed when the medium is replaced after 5 hours of plating or on the following day. If cultures which are relatively free of erythroid cells are required the following day, then the medium is replaced after 5 hours. However, this procedure does reduce the yield of the cells on day 1. Should the experimental design necessitate a maximum yield, then the cultures are given fresh medium the following day. Generally, by this time more cells have attached to the substrate but so too have some of the erythroid cells.

By day 2, the groups of hepatocytes are flattened so that the cells in the centre are no longer refractive and the cells at the edges begin to spread (Fig. 3*b*). Day 3 cultures are usually optimal for our studies because they are completely free of immature cells of the erythroid lineage and there are few clear epitheloid cells (Fig. 3*c*). After 4 days culture, there is evidence of some clear epitheloid cells which begin to fill up the space between the hepatocyte groups (Fig. 3*d*). Pulse labelling with tritiated thymidine followed by autoradiography shows that this is the area of greatest cell proliferation (Fig. 4*a* & *b*) although hepatocytes also incorporate the label (Fig. 4*c* & *d*). By day 5, most of the space between the hepatocyte groups is covered by the clear epithelial cells and the relative number of cells which are distinctly hepatocytes is less, possibly due to spreading of hepatocytes at the edges (Fig. 3e). Eventually, the hepatocyte groups flatten out to an extent which alters the morphology of the individual cells so that they no longer look like typical liver cells, with the exception of small clusters in the centre of the groups (Fig. 3f). Even at this stage, albumin, transferrin (33) and alpha-fetoprotein (AFP) secretion (unpublished results) can be measured in such cultures and tyrosine aminotransferase is inducible by dexamethasone (34). After a week of culture, cells with a fibroblast morphology are evident (Fig. 3f). In cultures plated at a high density their numbers are few; however, if the initial density of the culture is low, they are more plentiful.

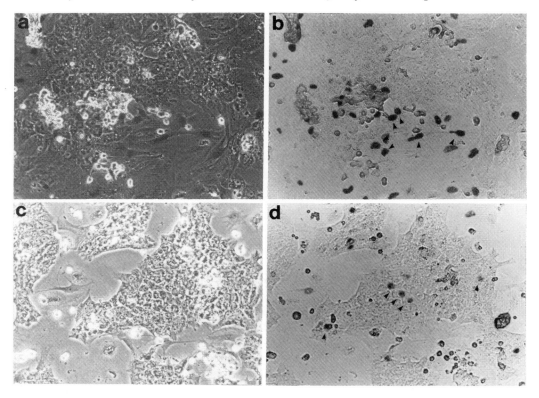

Fig. 4. Autoradiograph of a day 4 culture of hepatocytes showing uptake of tritiated thymidine by cells at the edge of the hepatocyte clusters and between clusters (a & b) and within clusters in cells with a distinct liver morphology (c & d). The morphology of the cells can be seen in the respective phase photomicrographs (a & c) and the labelled cells indicated by arrows are more easily seen in the corresponding bright-field photomicrographs (b & d). Magnification ×110.

Cell division

Growth can be assessed in two ways and care has to be taken when interpreting the results. First, it is possible to measure the DNA content of the cultures. This shows a gradual increase in cultures derived from fetuses of 15-day gestation because there are practically no erythroid cells to complicate matters (Fig. 5). However, with cultures established from rats of 19-day gestation, unless precautions are taken to minimize red cell contamination, the amount of DNA in the culture as a function of time remains essentially the same (Fig. 5). This is especially true if the cells are plated out at a high density and are not washed with BSS and given fresh medium after 5 hours of inoculation. Changes in DNA content of the culture dish is the net result of the loss of cells which do not adhere to the substrate, especially erythroid cells which are lost during the first two days of culture, and increase due to proliferation of hepatocytes.

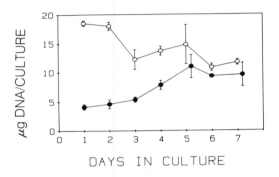

DAYS IN CULTURE

Fig. 5.
DNA content of cultures derived from (●—●) 15- day and (○—○) 19-day gestation rat liver. On each day of culture, cells were removed using a teflon policeman, pelleted by centrifugation and DNA extracted by incubation in 5% TCA for 90 min at 90°C. Aliquots were then taken for DNA estimation by fluorometry. The results are expressed as μg DNA/35 mm culture dish.

The other method of assessing growth is by determining the extent of uptake of tritiated thymidine on each day of culture. This rises steadily in both 15-day and 19-day gestation cultures, and plateaus at about day 4 or 5 (Fig. 6). It is difficult to interpret these results because one cannot be certain that the population is homogeneous. As seen previously (Fig. 4a–c), autoradiographs show that thymidine is incorporated into cells which are distinctly hepatocytes as well as the clear epitheloid cells which have a tendency to accumulate between the hepatocyte groups. The labelling of these cells is most apparent in cultures 4 days and older. Therefore, whether the clear cells are deemed to be liver parenchymal cells has a bearing on the interpretation of these results. That fibroblasts eventually overgrow such cultures is beyond doubt, for they have a distinct elongated form and line up alongside each other (Fig. 3f). They are plentiful in cultures maintained beyond a week, hence they complicate the interpretation of data in such long-term studies. However, the clear cells which are seen in 3 and 4 day-old cultures may be derived from parenchymal cells which have altered their morphology and probably their pattern of gene expression due to the culture conditions and by virtue of their position at the edge of the hepatocyte group. This proposal is supported by time-lapse studies (unpublished observations) which show this change occurring progressively in the cells at the extremity of the hepatocyte clusters. Furthermore, such cells stain immunocytochemically, albeit weakly, for the plasma proteins transferrin and albumin (unpublished observations), and when only such cells and fibroblasts are present, as is the case with week-old cultures, albumin and transferrin secretion is still demonstrable (33).

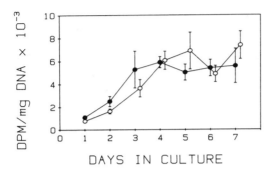

Fig. 6.
Tritiated thymidine incorporation in cultures derived from (●—●) 15-day and (○—○) 19-day gestation rat liver. Cells were exposed to 1 μCi of tritiated thymidine for 4 hours on each day of culture, harvested and washed four times with BSS. DNA was extracted by incubation in 5% TCA for 90 min at 90°C and aliquots taken for DNA estimation and determination of radioactivity by liquid scintillation counting. The results are expressed as dpm/mg DNA.

Workers from other laboratories have determined that growth of fetal rat hepatocyte cultures requires serum factors and is sensitive to the level of ornithine or arginine in the medium (4, 14). Growth also depends on the basement membrane matrix on which the hepatocytes attach. Hirata *et al.* (11) have reported that laminin is superior to Type IV collagen or fibronectin in this regard in studies using mouse fetal liver.

Plasma proteins

By far the most extensively studied property of cultured fetal hepatocytes has been their ability to synthesize and secrete plasma proteins. This is a feature of liver parenchymal cells, and continued production of plasma proteins would be a reliable indicator of maintenance of the differentiated state of the cells. It is also an advantage to study plasma proteins which are secreted into the culture medium, for it is possible to follow the daily production of such protein(s) for a given preparation of cells for a protracted period. Generally, the level of production is sufficiently high to permit the use of conventional assays such as immunodiffusion, fluorescent-immunoassay or ELISA. A further advantage in measuring plasma protein production is that, with few exceptions, it is a property which is peculiar to liver cells. Particularly in the case of fetal hepatocytes, AFP is especially useful because it is only synthesized in significant amounts by fetal and neonatal liver and is virtually absent in the adult. Therefore, the ability of a culture of fetal hepatocytes to sustain production of a plasma protein or proteins is a reliable index of maintenance of the differentiated state of the culture. However it is worth noting that changes in a particular plasma protein may be quite different from that of another in a given set of conditions. For instance, Grieninger & Granick (7) have shown that while embryonic chick hepatocytes cease albumin synthesis after 3 days of culture, other plasma proteins (not specified) continue to be produced.

Leffert & Paul (13) reported that albumin secretion could be detected in primary cultures of fetal liver cells even after eleven days of culture. From a more detailed study, Sell *et al.* (28) proposed that synthesis of some plasma proteins such as AFP and hemopexin was related to the growth state of the cells, whereas albumin and haptoglobin synthesis was independent of cell proliferation. In the case of AFP, Guillouzo *et al.* (9) conclude from a study combining the techniques of ^{3}H-thymidine pulse labelling and localization of the protein by immunocytochemistry, that AFP is primarily synthesized in the G1 phase of the cell cycle. It is clear that with fetal hepatocyte cultures maintained under normal conditions albumin secretion is not sustained. This has been reported by Hirata *et al.* (11) for fetal cells derived from mouse liver and by Grieninger & Granick (7) for embryonic chick liver cells. However, albumin secretion can be maintained if the hepatocytes are cultured on an appropriate substrate such as laminin (11) or if the medium is supplemented with dexamethasone, as reported by this laboratory (33).

In this study, albumin secretion was monitored in cultures of fetal rat liver maintained in the presence of dexamethasone which was added in order to maximize the production of tyrosine aminotransferase. After 7 days of culture, albumin could still be detected and quantitated by radial immunodiffusion in the media of cultures treated with the steroid analogue. The level of albumin production was about 50 μg/million cells/24 h which is close to the *in vivo* levels reported for adult liver cells. We have since shown that if dexamethasone is omitted from the culture medium, albumin secretion reaches undetectable levels after 7 days culture (unpublished data). In this context, Baffet *et al.* (1) have shown that hydrocortisone will elevate the level of albumin secretion by adult rat hepatocytes in culture. Steroid and steroid analogues have also been shown to produce a significant increase in fibrinogen production in cultures of chick embryonic liver parenchymal cells (21). Other hormones have also been shown to influence plasma protein production by cultured fetal hepatocytes. When added to chicken cells, insulin has a differential effect on the synthesis of specific plasma proteins as assessed by electroimmunoassay (7). Further analysis by Liang & Grieninger (16) has revealed that insulin has a biphasic response in this system. Initially, albumin and alpha 1-globulin increase and it is only after a prolonged exposure that synthesis of fibrinogen and lipoproteins is elevated. In contrast, transferrin remains unaltered. The synthesis of fibrinogen by embryonic chick hepatocytes has also been demonstrated by Pindyck *et al.* (21) in a study which showed that cortisol was able to significantly increase the level of its synthesis and secretion. Using a fetal rat hepatocyte culture model, Rupp & Fuller (25) have investigated the control of fibrinogen synthesis by leucocytic and serum factors. Fibrinogen is a positive acute phase protein in common with other plasma proteins such as alpha 1-acid glycoprotein and alpha 2-macroglobulin which are elevated in response to tissue injury or inflammation. Presently, the humoral mediator(s) of this response remain undefined and the liver culture model is potentially useful in determining the factors which may be responsible for this phenomenon. This has been underlined by the demonstration by Rupp & Fuller (25) that fetal rat hepatocytes will synthesize fibrinogen and furthermore will mimic the *in vivo* response when treated with leucocytic extracts or serum of rats in acute phase response.

Enzymes

The hepatocyte culture model is most useful for studying various aspects of enzyme regulation because it provides a system in which the environment is simplified and can be manipulated in a reproducible fashion. In the whole animal, it is often not possible to avoid an interplay of different factors. For example, in our attempts to investigate the effects of insulin on tyrosine aminotransferase in neonatal rats, we found that its administration to surgically delivered pups resulted in a hypoglycemia which in turn stimulated glucagon release from the adrenals. Since glucagon is a known inducer of tyrosine aminotransferase the interpretation of data from this experiment is equivocal. In culture, it is possible to have the medium completely lacking in a particular factor or hormone; for instance, insulin. Such a condition would be unattainable *in vivo*. Therefore, this model lends itself admirably to experiments designed to study the hormonal regulation of enzyme activity and synthesis.

Glycogen synthesis

The effect of cortisol on the development of glycogen storage by Plas *et al.* (22, 23) represents one of the earliest reports of such a study on cultured fetal hepatocytes. These investigators demonstrated two important properties of their model which was based on hepatocytes derived from rats of 15-day gestation. First, the cells were able to acquire the ability to produce glycogen from glucose, a feature of more mature hepatocytes; and, secondly, the cells were responsive to cortisol at physiological concentrations, without which glycogen synthesis could not be sustained in culture. This study showed that enzyme or enzymes which were rate limiting to glycogen synthesis from glucose were acquired during culture and the synthesis of these enzymes was dependent upon the presence of cortisol.

Tyrosine aminotransferase

This laboratory has investigated the regulation of the hepatocyte-specific enzyme tyrosine aminotransferase (TAT) in cultured fetal rat hepatocytes. First, we wished to know when liver cells capable of synthesizing the enzyme were present in the developing rat liver, and, secondly, what hormones were involved in the regulation of its activity. Although TAT is normally found postnatally (6), two lines of evidence suggest that hepatocytes which are competent to synthesize this enzyme are already present before birth. First, TAT can be induced by administration of cyclic AMP (35) or glucagon (12) *in utero* or it can be prematurely induced by surgically delivering rat fetuses (12). Secondly, fetal liver explants will begin to produce the enzyme (29). To answer the first question, ie when does the liver possess cells which are able to synthesize TAT, cells were taken from animals of various gestational age, cultured and assayed for enzyme. The reason for using a culture system to address this question was to ensure that the environment was constant for all cells. Differences between the cells would then reflect inherent differences and not be due to the hormonal status of the fetus. These experiments revealed that tyrosine aminotransferase could be detected in cultures of hepatocytes derived from fetuses of 16 days gestation or older (31), thus confirming that the conditions of culture were favourable for TAT expression if the cells were competent. What was even more interesting was the finding that when cells taken from rats of 15-day gestation were cultured, although TAT was not detected after 24 hours of culture, it could be reproducibly detected and quantitated after 72 hours. Variable results were obtained at 48 hours and this is probably due to inaccuracies in determining the exact age of the animals. In our view, cells derived from the liver of 15-day gestation rats are capable of undergoing differentiation in culture; whether we use the criteria of Plas *et al.* (22) based upon glycogenolysis or the acquisition of TAT according to our findings (31). This is especially significant because it is in contrast with the behaviour of adult hepatocytes in culture. It is commonly reported that adult hepatocytes 'de-differentiate' and thereby lose their phenotypic properties.

Pyruvate kinase isoenzymes

More recently, we have analysed the transition of pyruvate kinase isoenzymes in such cultures and reached a similar conclusion, ie fetal rat hepatocytes are capable of differentiating in culture. In these studies, expression of the M2 isoenzyme, an embryonic form, was compared with the definitive liver form, the L isoenzyme. When 19-day gestation hepatocytes were placed in culture, the expression of both isoenzymes was demonstrable (27). However, initially with cultures derived from 15-day gestation hepatocytes only M2 form was present. It was only after 4 days culture that the L form of pyruvate kinase was detectable (Fig. 7). Once again, this evidence supports the proposal that the immature cells are able to differentiate during culture so that they are able to express a gene which they were unable to express at the beginning of culture. Pyruvate kinase isoenzymes have also been analysed in cultures of fetal human hepatocytes by Guguen-Guillouzo *et al.* (8) in a

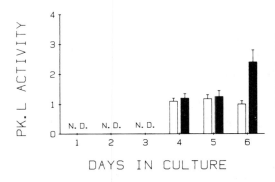

Fig. 7.
The appearance of the L isoenzyme of pyruvate kinase in cultures derived from 15-day gestation rat liver maintained in the absence (□) and presence of fructose (2 mM) and insulin (0.1 μM) (■).

study which showed that cells derived from a 4-month old fetus could synthesize both the M2 and L forms of the enzyme. During culture, the M2 form increased, which reflected an increase in the fibroblast population, and although the L form appeared to decrease during culture, it was still detectable after 10 days culture.

Effect of hormones

Clearly, the hormonal status of the culture will influence the level of expression of a particular enzyme. Since TAT is affected by both steroid and cyclic AMP, the presence of cortisol, dexamethasone, glucagon etc. will determine the level of TAT which is obtained. Similarly, the L isoenzyme of pyruvate kinase is influenced by insulin and fructose (27) and the yield of this enzyme in cultured hepatocytes is maximized when these factors are present. It is, therefore, possible to modulate the level of expression for a given gene product between extremes under appropriate conditions. Figure 8 shows TAT levels in fetal hepatocytes maintained in a standard (MEM) medium supplemented with 10% bovine calf serum then switched to the same medium supplemented with 10% bovine calf serum previously treated with activated charcoal and finally the latter medium supplemented with 10 nM dexamethasone. The level of enzyme oscillates between high levels to near undetectable levels and then reaches very high induced levels. These results show that it is important to know the best conditions to permit expression of a particular gene product. However, this is often not possible. We have carried out preliminary studies on the expression of the aldolase isoenzymes in cultured fetal hepatocytes. Initially, although the cells express both the liver and muscle isoenzymes, **the** liver isoenzyme is rapidly lost during culture (unpublished results). Our attempts to retain this isoenzyme in cultures derived from 19-day gestation hepatocytes by supplementing the medium with cyclic AMP or dexamethasone or a combination of both have only resulted in a slowing of the rate of loss of liver specific aldolase. Since these cells retain the L isoenzyme of pyruvate kinase and TAT over the same period

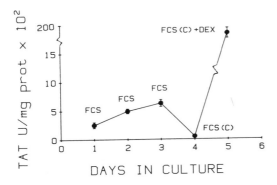

Fig. 8.
Tyrosine aminotransferase level in a culture of fetal hepatocytes derived from 19-day gestation liver maintained firstly in MEM+10% FCS, then transferred to MEM+10% FCS (pretreated with charcoal to remove endogenous steroids) and finally in the latter medium supplemented with 10 nM dexamethasone.

of culture, it must be concluded that other as yet unidentified factors responsible for maintaining liver aldolase are missing from our culture medium.

Collectively our experiments suggest that while hormones may be important in regulating the level of a particular enzyme, they may not be the primary event which renders the hepatocytes capable of producing that enzyme. For instance, while TAT is very sensitive to the level of steroid in the culture medium (see Fig. 8), we have shown that in 15-day gestation hepatocytes, which do not produce the enzyme on day 1 of culture, it has no effect. However on day 3, when TAT is measurable, dexamethasone is a strong inducer of the enzyme. Similarly, while fructose and insulin are capable of inducing pyruvate kinase (L form) in cultured hepatocytes (27), neither agent can hasten the appearance of this enzyme in cultures derived from 15-day gestation liver (27). It is our view that first the respective genes become available for transcription during culture of the immature hepatocytes and, subsequently, their activities can be modulated by hormones or other factors.

Other enzymes

Rupniak & Paul (24) have studied the induction of ornithine decarboxylase in cultures of fetal rat liver and concluded that prostaglandin E1 and cyclic AMP will induce this enzyme. Other enzymes which have been measured in cultured fetal rat hepatocytes include phosphoenolpyruvate carboxykinase (2), glucose-6-phosphatase (32), serine dehydratase (18) and aspartate aminotransferase (31). In most instances, the known *in vivo* hormonal inducers have been shown to be effective at near physiological levels in inducing the respective enzymes. Therefore, the liver culture model appears to be satisfactory for studying the mechanisms associated with hormonal regulation of enzyme synthesis.

ACKNOWLEDGEMENTS

The studies by this laboratory were supported by grants from the National Health and Medical Research Council of Australia and the Raine Centre for the Study of Perinatal and Developmental Biology. I wish to record my appreciation of significant contributions by the technical staff and research students of the Departments of Physiology and Biochemistry who have worked in this laboratory. Special thanks to Robyn Dixon and the Apple II+ for the preparation of this manuscript.

REFERENCES

1 Baffet G., Clement B., Glaise D., Guillouzo A., Guguen-Guillouzo, C.: Hydrocortisone modulates the production of extracellular material and albumin in long-term cocultures of adult rat hepatocytes with other liver epithelial cells. *Biochem. Biophys. Res. Comm.* 1982, **109**: 507–512.
2 Bulanyi G. S., Steele J. G., McGrath M. C., Yeoh G. C. T., Oliver I. T.: Hormonal regulation of phosphoenolpyruvate carboxykinase in cultured foetal hepatocytes from the rat. *Eur. J. Biochem.* 1979, **102**: 93–100.
3 Congote L. F., Stern D. M., Solomon S.: Hormone control of heme synthesis in cultures of human fetal liver cells. *Biochemistry*, 1974, **13**: 4255–4263.
4 Dieter P., Walter S.: Initiation of DNA synthesis in primary fetal rat. *Proc. Soc. Exp. Biol. Med.* 1974, **145**: 456–460.

5 Granick S., Sinclair P., Sassa S., Grienlinger G.: Effects of heme, insulin, and serum albumin on heme and protein synthesis in chick embryo liver cells cultured in a chemically defined medium, and a spectrofluorometric assay for porphyrin composition. *J. Biol. Chem.* 1975, **250**: 9215–9225.

6 Greengard O.: The developmental formation of enzymes in rat liver. *In: Biochemical Action of Hormones*, Vol. 1, G. Litwack (Ed.): Academic Press, New York & London, 1970, pp 53–87.

7 Grieninger G., Granick S.: Synthesis and differentiation of plasma proteins in cultured embryonic chicken liver cells: A system for study of regulation of protein synthesis. *Proc. Nat. Acad. Sci.* 1975, **72**: 5007–5011.

8 Guguen-Guillouzo C., Marie J., Cottreau D., Pasdeloup N., Kahn A.: Isoenzyme shift in cultured fetal human hepatocytes: a study of pyruvate kinase and phosphofructokinase. *Biochem. Biophys. Res. Comm.* 1980, **93**: 528–534.

9 Guillouzo A., Boisnard-Rissel M., Belanger L., Bourel M.: Alpha-fetoprotein production during the hepatocyte growth cycle of developing rat liver. *Biochem. Biophys. Res. Comm.* 1979, **91**: 327–331.

10 Hanks J. H., Wallace R. E.: Relation of oxygen and temperature in the preservation of tissues by refrigeration. *Proc. Soc. Exp. Biol.* 1949, **71**: 196–200.

11 Hirata K., Usui T., Koshiba H., Maruyama Y., Oikawa I., Freeman A. E., Shiramatsu K., Hayasaka H.: Effects of basement membrane matrix on the culture of fetal mouse hepatocytes. *Gann* 1983, **74**: 687–692.

12 Holt P. G., Oliver I. T.: Factors affecting the premature induction of tyrosine aminotransferase in foetal rat liver. *Biochem. J.* 1968, **108**: 333–338.

13 Leffert H. L., Paul D.: Studies on primary cultures of differentiated fetal liver cells. *J. Cell Biol.* 1972, **52**: 559–568.

14 Leffert H. L., Paul D.: Serum dependent growth of primary cultured differentiated fetal rat hepatocytes in arginine-deficient medium. *J. Cell. Physiol.* 1972, **81**: 113–123.

15 Leffert H. L., Koch K. S., Moran T., Williams M.: Liver Cells. *Meth. Enzymol.* 1979, **58**: 536–544.

16 Liang T. J., Grieninger G.: Direct effect of insulin on the synthesis of specific plasma proteins: Biphasic response of hepatocytes cultured in serum- and hormone-free medium. *Proc. Natl. Acad. Sci.* 1981, **78**: 6972–6976.

17 Murison G. L.: Growth of fetal rat liver cells in response to hydrocortisone. *Exp. Cell Res.* 1976, **100**: 439–443.

18 Oliver I. T., Martin R. L., Fisher C. J., Yeoh G. C. T.: Enzymic differentiation in cultured foetal hepatocytes of the rat: Induction of serine dehydratase activity by dexamethasone and dibutyryl cyclic AMP. *Differentiation* 1983, **24**: 234–238.

19 Paul J.: *Cell and Tissue Culture*, 5th Edn. Churchill Livingstone, Edinburgh, London & New York, 1975.

20 Pelkonen O., Korhonen P., Jouppila P., Karki N.: Induction of aryl hydrocarbon hydroxylase in human fetal liver cell and fibroblast cultures by polycyclic hydrocarbons. *Life Sci.* 1975, **16**: 1403–1410.

21 Pindyck J., Mosesson M. W., Roomi M. W., Levere R. D.: Steroid effects on fibrinogen synthesis by cultured embryonic chicken hepatocytes. *Biochem. Med.* 1975, **12**: 22–31.

22 Plas C., Nunez J.: Role of cortisol on the glycogenolytic effect of glucagon and on the glycogenic response to insulin in fetal hepatocyte culture. *J. Biol. Chem.* 1976, **254**: 1431–1437.

23 Plas C., Chapeville F., Jacquot R.: Development of glycogen storage ability under cortisol control in primary cultures of rat fetal hepatocytes. *Dev. Biol.* 1973, **32**: 82–91.

24 Rupniak H. T., Paul D.: Factors regulating the induction of ornithine decarboxylase in fetal rat liver cells in culture. *Biochim. Biophys. Acta* 1978, **543**: 10–15.

25 Rupp R. G., Fuller G. M.: The effects of leucocytic and serum factors on fibrinogen biosynthesis in cultured hepatocytes. *Exp. Cell Res.* 1979, **118**: 23–30.

26 Schoenfeld N., Epstein O., Atsmon A.: Inhibitory effect of some membrane active drugs on RNA and DNA synthesis in cultured chick embryo liver cels. *Biochem. Biophys. Res. Comm.* 1977, **76**: 460–468.

27 Scott R. J., Yeoh G. C. T.: Appearance of the liver form of pyruvate kinase in differentiating cultured foetal hepatocytes. *Differentiation* 1983, **25**: 64–69.

28 Sell S., Skelly H., Leffert H. L., Muller-Eberhard U., Kida S.: Relationship of the biosynthesis of

alpha-fetoprotein, albumin, hemopexin, and haptoglobin to the growth state of fetal rat hepatocyte cultures. *Ann. N.Y. Acad. Sci.* 1975, **259**: 45–58.
29 Sereni F., Sereni F. P.: Spontaneous development of tyrosine aminotransferase activity in fetal liver cultures. *Adv. Enz. Regul.* 1970, **8**: 253–267.
30 Tanaka T., Harano Y., Morimura H., Mori R.: Evidence for the presence of two types of pyruvate kinase in rat liver. *Biochem. Biophys. Res. Comm.* 1965, **21**: 55–60.
31 Yeoh G. C. T., Bennett F. A., Oliver I. T.: Hepatocyte differentiation in culture: Appearance of tyrosine aminotransferase. *Biochem. J.* 1979, **180**: 153–160.
32 Yeoh G. C. T.: The effect of 3′-methyl-4-dimethyl-aminoazobenzene on foetal rat hepatocytes in culture. *Eur. J. Canc. Clin. Oncol.* 1981, **17**: 743–752.
33 Yeoh G. C. T., Wassenburg J. A., Edkins E., Oliver I. T.: Synthesis and secretion of albumin and transferrin by foetal rat hepatocyte cultures. *Biochem. Biophys. Acta* 1979, **565**: 347–355.
34 Yeoh G. C. T., Oliver I. T.: The effect of cytosine arabinoside and bromodeoxyuridine on the appearance of tyrosine aminotransferase in cultured foetal hepatocytes of the rat. *Biochem. J.* 1980, **188**: 929–932.
35 Yeung Y. G, Yeung D.: Prenatal induction of tyrosine aminotransferase in rat liver. *Int. J. Biochem.* 1976, **7**: 153–157.

Research in *Isolated and cultured hepatocytes* A. Guillouzo & C. Guguen-Guillouzo eds., pp. 187–208
© 1986 John Libbey Eurotext Ltd./INSERM.

9

Control of enzyme expression deduced from studies on primary cultures of hepatocytes

Akira ICHIHARA, Toshikazu NAKAMURA, Chiseko NODA and Keiji TANAKA

Institute for Enzyme Research, School of Medicine, University of Tokushima, Tokushima 770, JAPAN

SUMMARY

Hormonal regulation of enzyme activity in liver can be studied most easily in primary cultures of hepatocytes, because results on these cells are not complicated by the many other factors present *in vivo*. We found that the activities of serine dehydratase, tyrosine aminotransferase and tryptophan oxygenase, which are all liver specific enzymes, are induced by glucocorticoid and glucagon and suppressed by insulin and catecholamine (alpha action). Results showed that changes in these enzyme activities by these hormones were due to changes in the mRNA activities for these enzymes and so in the amounts of enzymes. Therefore, these hormones act on the sites regulating the genes for these enzymes. The effects of the hormones are regulated through their receptors on hepatocyte membranes. It was found that, during culture of the cells, the number of beta-receptors for catecholamine increases, while that of alpha-receptors decreases. The reverse changes in the numbers of receptors are seen in developing liver *in vivo*. The stimulations of cyclic AMP formation in hepatocytes by isoproterenol and glucagon are regulated by their respective receptor numbers (homologous desensitization), but treatment of hepatocytes with glucagon also caused desensitization to isoproterenol (heterologous desensitization). This is due to impairment of GTP-binding protein, which is necessary for post-receptor transduction of both hormonal signals. We also observed that hepatocyte membranes affect the actions of hormones on enzyme induction through cell-cell contact. The inductions of enzymes related to liver specific functions described above are high in cells cultured at high cell density, while those related to cell growth (such as glucose-6-phosphate dehydrogenase and DNA synthesis) are high at low cell density. These reciprocal regulations of enzymes are mediated by a membrane factor (cell surface modulator) through effects on gene expression. Therefore, enzyme activity is regulated not only by hormones *per se*, but also by cell density, which regulates hepatocyte growth. For studies on hormonal effects, it is necessary to culture cells for a long period in serum-free medium. However, hepatocytes do not survive for a long duration in this medium. We found that one of effective factor in serum for hepatocyte survival was a protease inhibitor and, subsequently, we found and characterized a membrane-bound trypsin-like protease, that causes damage of hepatocytes in serum-free medium. In this review we emphasize that enzyme amount in hepatocytes is regulated not only by hormones alone, but also by the conditions of cell membranes and the state of their growth cycle.

Introduction

In the mid 1950s Knox first observed the hormonal inductions of tyrosine aminotransferase (TAT) and tryptophan 2, 3-dioxygenase (TO) in liver *in vivo*. Since then, there have been numerous studies on the mechanisms of enzyme induction in liver. However, these studies have mainly been on liver *in vivo*, perfused liver or cultured hepatoma cells. These experimental systems have serious limitations, for instance that the results are influenced by the indirect effects of various endogenous factors, the duration of the experiments and limited hormonal responses of limited marker enzymes (27). These limitations were overcome in the early 1970s by the development of methods for the dispersion and primary culture of hepatocytes. Thus, it became possible to study hormonal regulation of liver enzymes *in vitro*. Today, many, if not all, workers agree that results obtained with primary cultures of hepatocytes reflect phenomena in liver *in vivo* (4, 16, 22, 24, 28). Among these studies on primary cultures of hepatocytes, however, some show only that these cells give clearer results than could be obtained *in vivo*. This review is limited to studies that were possible only with primary cultured hepatocytes. In particular, the importance of the plasma membranes of hepatocytes in cellular regulation is described by results showing the interactions of individual hepatocytes, and the effects of hormones and a membranous protease on them.

Induction and suppression of enzyme expression by various hormones

Among liver specific enzymes, TO and TAT are typical inducible enzymes; they are readily induced within a few hours *in vivo* by glucocorticoid. Their appearance in rat liver during development differs: neither of them is found in fetal rat liver, but after birth, TAT appears within a few hours and increases very rapidly, whereas TO does not appear till 2 weeks after birth and reaches the adult level in week 4. Thus, TO belongs to the 'late suckling cluster' of enzymes according to Greengard's classification of developmental patterns of liver enzymes (20). Therefore, these enzymes are very useful for studies on hormonal regulation of gene expression and the molecular mechanisms of cellular differentiation. *In vitro* studies on induction of these enzymes have been hampered by the absence of suitable systems: TO is not expressed in any established cultured cells and TAT is induced by glucocorticoid only in some cultured hepatoma cells. Furthermore, none of these cell lines responds to hormones other than glucocorticoid.

In 1980, we found that primary cultures of adult rat hepatocytes retain TO activity and that it is regulated by pancreatic hormones as well as glucocorticoid (43); glucagon and dexamethasone induced TO activity, whereas insulin suppressed this induction (Table 1). For its effect, glucagon could be replaced by dibutyryl cyclic AMP (bt$_2$cAMP). We also showed that catecholamine regulates this enzyme activity (51). Epinephrine suppressed the enzyme induction by glucagon and dexamethasone. This suppression was released by phenoxybenzamine, an α-adrenergic blocker and prazosin, an α_1-blocker, but not by yohimbine, an α_2-blocker, indicating that suppression of TO induction by catecholamine is through its α_1-adrenergic receptor. In general, regulation by sympathetic nerves has been thought to be very short-term, but our findings suggest that it may be long-term and involve transcription.

Hepatocytes in primary culture are also useful for studies of the developmental changes of TO (38). When cells from liver at various developmental stages were cultured with dexamethasone for 24 h, this steroid was found to cause precocious

Table 1. **Effects of epinephrine on inductions of TO, TAT and SDH by dexamethasone and glucagon.** Hepatocytes were cultured for 24 h and then the medium was replaced by fresh William's medium E containing 5% calf serum and the additions indicated. Antagonists were added before agonists. Enzyme activities were measured after culture for 24 h. Values are means from 3 dishes±sd (reference 51).

Additions	Concentration	Activity (mu/mg protein)		
	μM	TO	TAT	SDH
None		22.9± 3.69	9.03±0.67	3.02±0.79
Dexamethasone (D)	10	64.4± 5.11	17.7 ±0.86	3.75+0.88
D+glucagon (G)	0.1	132 ±10.7	92.2 ±6.87	21.0 ±1.32
D+G+insulin	0.1	41.7± 2.05	63.8 ±2.44	8.12±0.91
D+G+epinephrine (E)	10	53.3± 5.04	71.1 ±1.32	8.24±0.68
D+G+E+propranolol	20	54.3± 5.78	65.7 ±3.43	8.59
D+G+E+phenoxybenzamine	10	114 ±11.9	91.7 ±1.92	20.2

induction of TO to almost the adult level on day 9 after birth, when the activity is still undetectable *in vivo* (20) (Fig. 1). However, no response to glucagon or bt$_2$cAMP was observed at this stage, the responses to the latter hormone reaching the adult level about 2 weeks after birth when the TO level *in vivo* becomes just detectable. This was not due to a lack of response to glucagon on day 9 after birth, but to an immature state of gene expression of TO. This conclusion is supported by the facts that TAT is induced by glucagon at this stage and that the glucagon response and levels of cAMP and protein kinase in neonatal liver are similar to, or rather higher than, those in adult hepatocytes. When tryptophan was added to hepatocytes to stabilize TO protein, slight, but significant, increase of TO could be observed on day 5 after birth. This means that the TO gene is operative on day 5 and responds to glucocorticoid, but not to glucagon or cAMP. However, hepatocytes from rats on day 2 showed no induction of TO on addition of tryptophan, dexamethasone and glucagon, which are required for maximal TO induction in adult rat hepatocytes. This finding suggests that the TO gene of hepatocytes before day 5 is not influenced by these inducers. Therefore, the dormancy of the TO gene before day 2 is due to some unknown intrinsic mechanism, not to lack of a response to the above inducers; these inducers only stimulate transcription of the gene that is already operative. Hence, further study of the mechanism controlling expression of the TO gene during development could be helpful in clarifying the genetic mechanism of cellular differentiation. In a preliminary experiment, we found that when hepatocytes from rats of 9 days' old were cultured for 4 days, they acquired a response to glucagon to induce TO (38).

Other amino acid degrading enzymes in liver are under similar control to TO (Table 1). We studied the regulations of TAT (51), serine dehydratase SDH (52) and

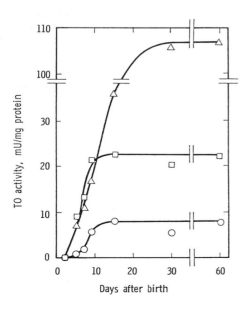

Fig. 1.

Developmental change in hormonal regulation of TO in primary cultures of rat hepatocytes. Hepatocytes were isolated on the indicated day after birth and cultured in hormone-free medium for 24 h, then the hormones were added with 2.5 mM tryptophan and the enzyme activity was assayed after 24 h. ○, no hormone; □, dexamethasone (0.1 μM); △, dexamethasone plus glucagon (0.1 μM). Values are means for duplicate experiments (reference 38).

L-lysine-2-oxo-glutarate reductase (67). It has long been puzzling that insulin, which suppresses gluconeogenesis, induces TAT in hepatoma cells and perfused liver. However, in hepatocytes in primary culture, we found that, in fact, in long-term (24 h) culture insulin suppresses the induction of TAT as well as other enzymes (42). In contrast, in short-term culture (a few hours), it induces TAT due to its stimulation of the syntheses of proteins with a short half-life in general.

TAT and TO were induced by either dexamethasone or glucagon alone, although their simultaneous addition had a synergistic effect. In contrast, both hormones were required for the induction of SDH (52) and L-lysine-2-oxo-glutarate reductase (67). This is a typical permissive effect of glucocorticoid, but its mechanism of action is unknown. We are now preparing cDNA containing the gene for SDH and this should be useful for elucidating the mechanism of the permissive effect of glucocorticoid at molecular and gene levels.

We have shown that changes in TO and SDH activity are due to changes in amounts of enzyme resulting from changes in rates of synthesis of the enzyme proteins (Table 2). These changes are also parallel with changes in the activities of mRNAs (50, 54). Recently, we prepared cDNA containing the TO gene and showed by the dot-blot hybridization technique that the changes of mRNA activity for TO by various hormones were parallel to those in the amount of mRNA (unpublished data). Previously, glucagon was thought to stimulate translation of mRNA, rather than transcription, but this study indicated that glucagon stimulates transcription of the TO gene and increases the amount of its mRNA. A similar conclusion was drawn from studies on phosphoenolpyruvate carboxykinase (PEPCK) in Reuber hepatoma cells (10), lactic dehydrogenase in C_6 glioma cells (29) and prolactin in pituitary GH_4 cells (37).

Table 2. Effects of various hormones on rates of enzyme synthesis, levels of translatable mRNA and amounts of mRNA of liver specific enzymes. Hepatocytes were cultured for one day and then treated with the indicated hormones as follows: cells were incubated with hormones for 7 h and then labelled with [^{3}H] leucine for 5 h to measure the rates of enzyme synthesis. They were incubated for 12 h with hormones and then their total RNA was extracted to measure mRNA activity (references 50, 54).

Additions	Rates of enzyme synthesis		Translatable mRNA	
	TO	SDH	TO	SDH
		%		
None	0.037		0.019	0.0023
Dexamethasone (D)	0.129	0.0044	0.304	0.0038
Glucagon (G)	0.049	0.0067	0.022	0.0035
D+G	0.24	0.025	0.75	0.0343
D+G+insulin	0.034	0.0115	0.123	0.0089
D+G+epinephrine		0.0097	0.308	0.0107

There is ample evidence that cAMP stimulates its dependent protein kinase, which phosphorylates various proteins including histones. But, details of the mechanism of transmission of the signal from cAMP to DNA and its effect on transcription are still unknown. It is possible that a soluble cytosolic factor is involved (35); its formation may be stimulated by cAMP and then it may be transferred to the nucleus. Such a factor has not been characterized, but its existence is suggested from the findings that added cytosol stimulated transcription of the heat-shock gene of isolated nuclei of *Drosophila* (14) and of β-casein of mammary cells (71).

The mechanism of the action of glucocorticoid at the gene level is clearer than that of glucagon. Results have shown that when glucocorticoid enters cells, it first binds to its receptor and is then transported into the nucleus where it binds to a specific site on DNA. This binding site of the glucocorticoid-receptor complex to DNA was determined by use of the mouse viral genome (MTV) of mammary tumor cells, which are sensitive to glucocorticoid (18, 64). Results indicated that the binding site of glucocorticoid was within the long-terminal repeat (LTR), which is located 100–150 bases up-stream from the initiation codon of the MTV gene, and that the binding site is within a sequence of 35 ± 6 base pairs. This finding was supported by experiments on transfection of the gene with different lengths of LTR (26). The base sequence of this binding site was determined to be AAGCTCTGA. Similar sequences were found in the genes for PEPCK (74), growth hormone (73), pro-opiomelanocortin (13) and TO (66), which are all regulated by glucocorticoid. However, it is still unknown how binding of the glucocorticoid-receptor complex to a specific site on the gene regulates transcription catalysed by RNA polymerase II.

In contrast to glucocorticoid and glucagon, which stimulate enzyme induction, insulin and catecholamine (α_1-action) suppress enzyme induction. Insulin suppresses PEPCK transcription (19), but the mechanism of its suppressive effect on the TO gene is still unknown. In fact, little is yet known at a molecular level about the mechanisms of action of insulin on cellular activities, such as post-receptor transfer of the signal, the possible involvement of a second messenger, the binding of this messenger, if it exists, to DNA, or the regulation of transcription by insulin.

Cell density-dependent regulation of hepatocyte growth and functions

In liver *in vivo*, hepatocytes are in tight contact with each other forming liver lobules. In these lobules, the cell density is about 3×10^5 cells/cm^2, which is twice that in cultures at high cell density. In this condition, hepatocytes do not grow being in the typical G$_o$ state of the cell cycle and show fully differentiated phenotypes. In regenerating liver, cell growth is stimulated and the characters of liver cells become immature. It was, therefore, very interesting to see how these changes during liver regeneration were regulated. As shown in Fig. 2 and Table 3, many characters of hepatocytes in culture are markedly regulated by cell density (47). In hepatocytes cultured at low cell density (2×10^4 cells/cm^2), the expressions and hormonal responses of differentiated liver specific enzymes, such as TO, TAT and SDH, are suppressed. Conversely, activities related to growth of the cells (44), such as the syntheses of DNA and glucose-6-phosphate dehydrogenase (G6PD) are markedly induced by insulin and EGF (75). It is interesting that the activities of G6PD and malic enzyme, both of which are lipogenic enzymes that have been thought to supply NADPH for fatty acid synthesis (48), are regulated reciprocally by cell density (47,

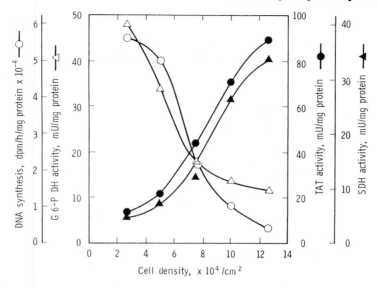

Fig. 2. Reciprocal modulation of growth and differentiated functions of hepatocytes by cell density. Experimental conditions were as for Table 3.

75). G6PD is induced by EGF and insulin at low cell density, whereas malic enzyme is suppressed by EGF and at low cell density. Therefore, G6PD seems to contribute to cell growth by supplying ribose-5-phosphate for nucleic acid synthesis and NADPH for cholesterogenesis, while the malic enzyme is involved only in fatty acid synthesis. Indeed, cholesterogenesis is high in cells at low density, presumably because it contributes to formation of membranes, whereas triglyceride synthesis is induced by insulin in cells at high density (75).

Table 3. Reciprocal effects of cell density on growth-related and hepatocyte-specific functions of primary cultured hepatocytes (reference 47). Hepatocytes were cultured at the indicated cell densities for 22 h and then various hormones were added. Various activities were assayed 24–45 h after hormone addition. Values are means for 3–5 experiments.

Function	Stimulators	Activity (% of maximum)		
		Cell density ($\times 10^4$ cells/cm^2)		
		2.5	*7.5*	*12.5*
DNA synthesis	Insulin (I) +EGF	100	36	5
Amino acid transport	I	100	67	42
Protein synthesis		100	84	52
Cholesterogenesis		100	75	37
G6PD induction	I+EGF	100	38	23
Triglyceride synthesis	I	33	88	100
Malic enzyme induction	I+T$_3$	34	50	100
TAT	Dexamethasone (D)	11	47	100
TO	D	13	55	100
SDH	D+glucagon	13	44	100

There are two possible explanations of this reciprocal regulation of hepatocyte activities by cell density. One is an autocrine mechanism, in which cellular activities are regulated by a factor secreted by the cells themselves. To test this possibility, we prepared conditioned medium from cultures at high cell density, and added it to cells at low cell density. However, it did not mimic the effect of high cell density. The second explanation is regulation by cell-cell contact, through a membrane signal. To test this possibility, we purified plasma membranes from mature rat liver and added them to cells at low cell density. As shown in Fig. 3, in the presence of the membranes, induction of TAT by dexamethasone increased dose-dependently and DNA synthesis was suppressed (47). Thus, addition of plasma membranes to cells at low density clearly mimicked the effect of high cell density. The size of hepatocytes in culture was also reduced at high cell density and dose-dependently by addition of plasma membranes.

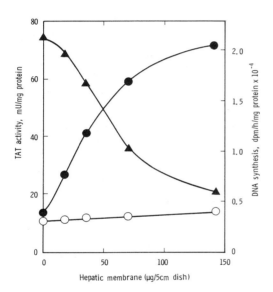

Fig. 3.
Stimulation of TAT induction and inhibition of DNA synthesis in sparse cultures of hepatocytes by addition of hepatic plasma membranes. Hepatocytes were cultured at a cell density (3×10^4 cells/cm^2) for 2 h and plasma membranes of rat liver were added. Hormones were added 22 h after membrane addition and TAT activity and DNA synthesis were measured 24 h after hormone addition (reference 47). ●, TAT without dexamethasone; ○, TAT with dexamethasone; ▲, DNA synthesis with insulin and EGF.

The above effects of plasma membranes were lost when the membranes were heated at 95°C for 5 min or treated with trypsin, indicating that their effect was due to a heat-labile protein. Next, we tried to extract the factor with various detergents. The factor could not be extracted with usual detergents, such as Triton X-100 and deoxycholate, but it was extracted with 4% octylglucoside containing 4M guanidine-HC1 (40). The molecular weight of the factor, determined by Sephacryl S-400 was about 67×10^4 and we tentatively named this factor 'cell surface modulator (CSM)'. Since CSM was found in the membranes of various tissues, such as liver, brain, kidney, red cells and even tumour cells, it is not tissue-specific. Thus, expression of tissue-specific phenotypes must be due to genetic control in the cells stimulated by this common factor. This conclusion was confirmed by immunochemical staining of TO and autoradiography of [³H]-thymidine incorporation into DNA in co-cultures of normal hepatocytes and Reuber hepatoma cells (41) (Fig. 4). Normal hepatocytes, when cultured alone at low density, do not express TO activity, but they did express this enzyme when co-cultured with Reuber hepatoma cells. Conversely, DNA synthesis is high in hepatocytes cultured alone at low cell density, but was low in cells at the same density co-cultured with Reuber hepatoma cells. Reuber hepatoma cells co-cultured had no TO or thymidine kinase and hence showed neither activity of TO nor of [³H]-thymidine incorporation.

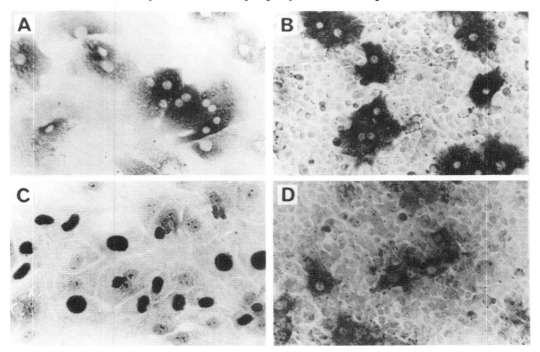

Fig. 4. Induction of TO and inhibition of DNA synthesis in sparse cultures of hepatocytes by co-culture with Reuber hepatoma cells (RY-121B). Hepatocytes at a cell density of 3×10^4 cells/cm^2 were plated and when they were attached sufficient RY-121B cells (1.5×10^5 cells/cm^2) were inoculated to cover almost all the spaces between hepatocytes in the dishes. Hormones were added to the culture 20 h after plating. Immunochemical staining of TO and radioautography of DNA synthesis were carried out 24 h after hormone addition. A, B, TO activity; C, D, DNA synthesis. A, C, hepatocytes alone; B, D, co-culture. In sparce culture of hepatocyte alone (A) TO was induced by dexamethasone, glucagon and tryptophan in hepatocytes contacted each other. Hepatocytes (C) were at similar cell density to those (A), but they appear to be at higher cell density owing to stimulation of cell spreading by insulin and EGF (reference 41).

From these studies we could explain the regulation of phenotypic expression by liver cells during liver regeneration and possibly during development, in which cell contact becomes loose, and during carcinogenesis in which cells become insensitive to CSM. In all these conditions, the effect of CSM is reduced, resulting in increased proliferation and decreased differentiation. As the cells proliferate, cell-cell contact becomes tighter resulting in decrease in cell growth and increase in expression of differentiated characters.

This is a new concept of cellular regulation, not only as individual cells, but also as tissue. It is a cytosocial or cytoarchitectural mechanism of cellular regulation. The mechanism involved is cell-cell interaction, not autocrine or endocrine regulation. This mechanism should be considered in understanding growth and gene expression of individual cells in homologous and heterologous cell groups.

Control of enzyme expression through change of hormone receptors

The first step in hormonal control of enzyme expression is the binding of the hormone to a cell receptor. Steroid hormones enter cells and bind to intracellular receptors, while peptide hormones and catecholamines bind to receptors on the cell surface. This binding provokes an intracellular messenger to transmit a signal to DNA to regulate enzyme expression. The only known messengers are cAMP and Ca^{2+} and inositol phospholipids. There are several types of catecholamine receptor: the β-receptor stimulates adenylate cyclase activity, while the α_2-receptor inhibits this activity. α_1-Receptor is related to Ca^{2+}-inositolphosphate turnover (65). β-Receptors can be classified as β_1- and β_2-receptors, both of which activate adenylate cyclase (31, 65). The glucagon receptor is also related to this system. The adenylate cyclase system consists of three components, receptor, guanine nucleotide regulatory proteins (G or N) and a catalytic protein (C). β-Adrenergic and glucagon receptors are connected with Ns (62, 63), and the α_2-receptor with Ni (30, 62) and they have stimulatory and inhibitory effects, respectively, on the C-protein. The Ns and Ni proteins are ADP-ribosylated by cholera and pertussis toxins (30, 62), respectively. Rat hepatocytes contain abundant Ni and Ns, but show no α_2-response (unpublished data). This is because they have very little α_2-receptor (65). Therefore, the role of Ni in hepatocytes is still unknown.

In mature rat liver, glycogenolysis is stimulated by glucagon and catecholamines. However, experiments on perfused liver (15) and isolated hepatocytes (9) showed that epinephrine does not increase cAMP in the liver, and thus that it stimulates glycogenolysis in rat liver through its α_1-receptor action (2, 9). Studies on slices of rat liver showed that the β-agonist, isoproterenol (Ip), markedly stimulates cAMP formation in neonatal rat liver and that the response decreases to almost zero during development (12). We confirmed this with isolated hepatocytes. Thus, the developmental change in the β-response occurs in parenchymal hepatocytes (45). Similarly, cAMP formation by glucagon is high in neonatal rat liver and decreased during development, but is still high in adult liver. The specific bindings of [^{125}I]-iodocyanopindolol ([^{125}I]-ICP), a β-antagonist, to liver plasma membranes of 7-day-old rats and adult rats had similar Kd values (about 140 pM), but there were 10 times more receptors in neonatal liver than in adult liver (Table 4). However, adult liver showed rather greater binding of [^{125}I]-iodoglucagon than neonatal liver, indicating that the over-all change of cAMP formation stimulated by glucagon during development cannot be explained only by change of the receptor number, and possibly involves changes in N- or C-protein as well.

On the contrary, control of glycogenolysis through the α_1-receptor is low in the liver of young rats (3, 36) and the binding of [^{3}H]-prazosin showed that α_1-receptor number increased during development (Table 4), but its Kd values did not change (about 200 pM). These results indicate that during the development of rats, the

Table 4. Developmental changes in receptor numbers of catecholamines and glucagon during development of rat liver. Purified plasma membranes of rat liver of different ages were used for binding assays of $[^{125}I]$-ICP and $[^{3}H]$-prazosin and isolated hepatocytes for that of $[^{125}I]$iodoglucagon (reference 45).

Days after birth	Number of binding sites		
	$[^{125}I]$-ICP (β-receptor)	$[^{3}H]$-Prazosin (α_1-receptor)	$[^{125}I]$-Iodo-glucagon (glucagon-receptor) sites $\times 10^{-3}$/cell
	(fmol/mg protein)		
7	185	483	9.1
17	110	373	—
60	20	1150	26.9

amount of α_1-receptor in the liver increases, while that of β-receptor decreases and control of glycogenolysis changes from β- to α_1-receptor mediated control.

This reciprocal change of α- and β-receptors, although it is opposite to that during development, was also observed in the liver of rats after adrenalectomy (8, 32), or with hypothyroidism (33, 59) or biliary obstruction (56). These changes have been thought to be due to conversion of α_1- to β-receptors, but recent studies show that the α_1- and β-receptors differ in molecular properties, indicating that they are not interconvertible. Moreover, the reciprocal changes observed in adrenalectomized rats were not due to changes in α_1-receptor number (17), but to change in the effect of GTP on the α_1-receptor. The amount of β-receptor increased under these conditions.

In hepatocytes in primary culture, changes in α_1- and β-receptors are the opposite

Table 5. Appearance of β-adrenergic responses during culture. Values are means of two experiments (reference 46). Activation of protein kinase is expressed as the ratio of activated form to the total activity.

Adult hepatocytes	Concentration µM	Glycogenolysis µmol/h/mg protein	cAMP-dependent protein kinase ratio
Freshly isolated			
None		0.39	0.20
Glucagon	0.1	0.99	0.64
Ip	10	0.40	0.22
7-h cultured			
None		0.47	0.23
Glucagon		1.11	0.63
Ip		1.02	0.64
7-h cultured with cycloheximide	10		
None		0.49	0.22
Glucagon		1.22	0.62
Ip		0.54	0.25

to those seen during development (45). During culture of adult rat hepatocytes, which show a very low β-adrenergic response *in vivo*, the responses increase rapidly (Table 5), (46, 55, 61). This acquisition of a β-response was inhibited by addition of cycloheximide or α-amanitin to the culture medium, suggesting that the syntheses of mRNA and protein are involved in the change. During culture of hepatocytes, their Kd value for $[^{125}I]$-ICP binding does not change, but the amount of binding sites increases 10 times (Fig. 5). Experiments on the effects of NaF, $G_{pp}(NH)_p$ and cholera toxin also showed that the components of the adenylate cyclase system, Ns- and C-proteins do not change much during culture. Therefore, increase in the β-response during culture is due solely to increase in the β-receptor number.

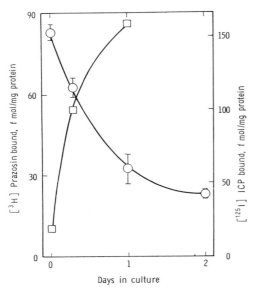

Days in culture

Fig. 5.
Decrease of α_1-adrenergic receptor sites and increase of β-adrenergic sites in adult rat hepatocytes during primary culture. At the indicated time plasma membranes were prepared and α_1- and β-receptors were measured by bindings of $[^3H]$-prazosin (○) and $[^{125}I]$-ICP (□), respectively (reference 45).

Conversely, the α_1-action decreases during culture of hepatocytes (45, 55). This is due to decrease in the α_1-receptor number, as shown by studies on $[^3H]$-prazosin binding. However, liver plasma membranes contain much more α_1-receptor than β-receptor and even after culture for 2 days, when the α_1-receptor has decreased and the β-receptor has increased, the cells still show considerable α_1-responses, such as stimulation of glycogenolysis (46, 55) and suppression of the induction of SDH and TO (51).

There is some indication that a high β-response and cell growth are related, because hepatocytes from young rats, regenerating liver (6), rats with biliary obstruction (56) and rats treated with carcinogens (5, 11) show a high β-response. However, the mechanism of this response is still unknown. An interesting possibility is that there is some factor regulating reciprocal change of α_1- and β-receptors in the serum during development. If this is so, the opposite changes of receptors of cells in culture from those *in vivo* could be due to lack of this regulator in the culture medium. However, the addition of various known hormones to hepatocytes in culture did not accelerate or suppress these changes of cells in culture, suggesting that if this regulatory factor exists *in vivo*, it is not one of the hormones examined

(45). Christoffersen also observed no effects of added hormones on acquisition of β-receptor during culture (61).

Desensitization of the adenylate cyclase system

When cells are treated continuously with a hormone for some time, their response to the hormone decreases. This is called desensitization or refractoriness. When hepatocytes in primary culture were incubated with glucagon or Ip, their rapid response to the two stimulators, such as increased glycogenolysis and cAMP accumulation, was the same, but their long-term responses to the two differed in extent, because transport of amino acids (57, 58) and induction of SDH (52) are stimulated by glucagon, but not by Ip. This difference was not because Ip has no long-term effect, since it increases PEPCK (7), TAT and TO (51). We found that when 1-methyl-3-isobutylxanthine, an inhibitor of phosphodiesterase, was added with Ip, then SDH was induced (51). This finding suggests that Ip cannot maintain a sufficient concentration of cAMP to induce SDH. This possibility was confirmed by the results in Fig. 6 showing that the maximum cAMP levels induced in 10–30 min by glucagon and Ip were very similar (52, 58), but that the level induced by Ip decreased rapidly returning to the basal level within 1 h, while the level induced by glucagon remained higher than the basal level for over 9 h.

The decrease in the cAMP level in these experiments, despite the continuous presence of Ip or glucagon, could be explained by desensitization of the hepatocytes to these agonists. Plas & Nunez first reported that increased glycogenolysis in fetal hepatocytes by glucagon was decreased during long-term culture due to desensitization of the hepatocytes to this hormone (60). Moreover, cAMP formation stimulated by either glucagon or Ip in adult hepatocytes varies inversely with the time of contact of the cells with these hormones (23, 53). The idea that desensitization to Ip is much faster than that to glucagon would explain the difference in the decay curves of the induced cAMP level (Fig. 6). This rapid desensitization to catecholamine seems reasonable in view of the very brief physiological effects of this hormone on biological activities, although catecholamine also has long-term effects as described earlier in this chapter.

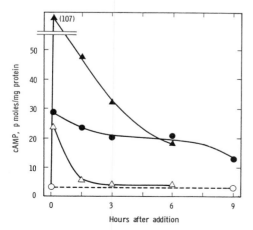

Fig. 6.
Changes of intracellular cAMP levels in cultured hepatocytes after addition of glucagon or Ip. Glucagon (0.5 μM, ●) or IP (10 μM, with (▲) or without (△) 1-methyl-3-isobutylxanthine 0.5 mM) were added 24 h after start of culture. ○, without hormone (reference 52).

Another difference between the desensitizations to Ip and glucagon is that Ip desensitizes only its own response (homologous desensitization), whereas glucagon desensitizes not only its own response, but also the response of Ip(heterologous desensitization) (23, 53). Homologous desensitization to catecholamine has been observed in various cells and is due to reduction in the β-receptor number (31). In cultures of hepatocytes during desensitization, the Kd value for binding of [^{125}I]-ICP did not change, but the number of receptors decreased markedly (53). Down-regulation of β-receptor in frog red cells, starts with internalization of the receptor without formation of coated pits (31). Since the internalized β-receptor still retains binding activity and its native molecular weight, it may be recycled to the membrane surface for use again. However, the mechanism of down-regulation in hepatocytes may be somewhat different from that in frog red cells.

Long-term pretreatment of hepatocytes with glucagon also resulted in decrease in their receptor number for [^{125}I]-iodoglucagon without any change in the Kd value (53). Therefore, down-regulation to these two agonists occurred at their respective receptors. Thus, the heterologous desensitization observed on long-term treatment of hepatocytes with glucagon should be due to changes in post-receptor events. The second messenger of glucagon and catecholamine is cAMP and hence the mechanism of its formation by these two hormones is common after they bind to their own receptors. From our studies on heterologous desensitization of hepatocytes to glucagon, we concluded that glucagon caused not only decrease of its receptor number, but also qualitative changes of Ns-protein (53). This conclusion was based on various findings. First, changes in the Kd value of the β-receptor induced by GTP were similar in membranes of hepatocytes with or without glucagon treatment, suggesting that coupling between the β-receptor and Ns-protein is normal. Second, cAMP formation and ADP ribosylation of Ns-protein stimulated by cholera toxin were the same in glucagon-treated and untreated cells. However, cAMP formation stimulated by glucagon, Ip, $G_{pp}(NH)_p$, NaF or forskolin was less in glucagon treated cells than in untreated cells (Table 6). All these results suggest that glucagon treatment, but not Ip treatment, impairs the ability of Ns-protein to couple with C-protein. But it is still unknown why and how Ns-protein is impaired. In hepatocytes, the amount of glucagon receptor is 10 times that of β-receptor and the rate of down-

Table 6. **Desensitization of adenylate cyclase by glucagon and isoproterenol treatments.** Hepatocytes were cultured with glucagon (0.5 μM) or Ip(10 μM) for 12 h and plasma membranes were prepared. Values are means ±S.D. for duplicate measurements in 2 experiments (reference 53).

Additions to membranes	Concentration	Adenylate cyclase		
	μM	Without pretreatment	With glucagon	With Ip
			pmol/min/mg protein	
None		8.1	3.2	7.7
GTP	10	9.3± 1.4	4.0± 0.5	7.4± 2.0
Glucagon+GTP	0.1	23.9± 2.8	7.5± 1.4	22.5± 2.3
Ip+GTP	10	19.1± 5.7	11.4± 3.9	9.3± 1.8
$G_{pp}(NH)_p$	10	27.8± 6.1	16.4± 3.5	24.6± 7.1
NaF	1×10^4	35.0± 1.4	27.5± 1.7	41.1± 1.1
Forskolin	100	100 ±10.6	79.8±10.1	102 ±11.1

regulation of this receptor is slower than that of the β-receptor. The relative insensitivity of glucagon desensitization compared with that of the β-response may be a second regulatory device to reduce the cAMP effect stimulated by both glucagon and catecholamine in hepatocytes. Recently, we also found that when hepatocytes were treated with bt$_2$cAMP for over 10 h, induction of SDH by bt$_2$cAMP and dexamethasone became very low (unpublished results). This suggests that there is also desensitization of the post-adenylate cyclase system although its mechanism is still unknown. Therefore, there are various regulatory mechanisms for transfer of cellular signals mediated by cAMP.

Protein catabolism and proteases in hepatocytes

It is known that protein breakdown in hepatocytes is catalysed by both lysosomal and non-lysosomal pathways (21, 49). The former plays the main role in degradation of proteins with long half-lives, such as structural and membranous proteins and those taken in by endocytosis, and increases during starvation or when the glucagon level increases. On the contrary, the non-lysosomal pathway is involved in breakdown of proteins with short half-lives, which are mostly related to cellular functions or are mistranslated and abnormal proteins. This pathway is also energy-dependent. Lysosomes contain an acidic protease (cathepsin D) and thiol proteases (cathepsins B, H and L). In primary cultures of hepatocytes, addition of leupeptin or pepstatin inhibits protein degradation, and the effects of the two are additive inhibiting almost 75% of total protein degradation under catabolic conditions (49, 68). Since leupeptin is a stronger inhibitor than pepstatin, thiol proteases are more important than the acidic protease and these two types of proteases degrade different proteins.

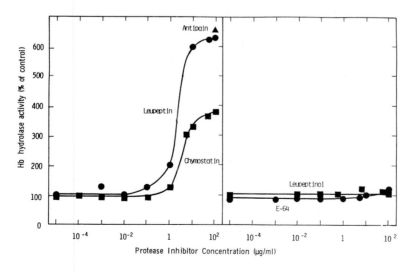

Fig. 7. **Dose-dependent effects of various protease inhibitors on the activity of hemoglobin hydrolase in hepatocytes.** After 2-day culture various inhibitors were added for 24 h (reference 68).

During studies with several protease inhibitors in primary cultures of hepatocytes, we observed induction of a new type of protease. Namely, it was found that, during culture of hepatocytes, the addition of leupeptin increased activity of an acidic, thiol protease that hydrolysed hemoglobin but was insensitive to pepstatin (68). Figure 7 shows that antipain and chymostatin caused similar inductions of this activity, but E-64, a specific inhibitor of thiol protease, did not cause induction. This means that inhibition of serine protease is involved in the enzyme induction. Increase in the enzyme activity seemed to involve protein synthesis and glycosylation, since induction was inhibited by addition of cycloheximide and tunicamycin (69). This enzyme was purified from the liver of rats that had been treated with leupeptin. During its purification, the enzyme was separated from cathepsin D on a pepstatin-Sepharose column and from cathepsins H and B on a phosphocellulose column, but remained associated with cathepsin L. The molecular weight (20 000) and substrate and inhibitor specificities of the two enzymes are very similar, but the leupeptin-induced protease is more stable than cathepsin L and it does not inactivate the enzyme substrates, aldolase and glucose-6-phosphate dehydrogenase, which are degraded by cathepsin L. Therefore, the induced protease differs from known cathepsins. This protease may be a precursor of cathepsin L. If the precursor has a very short half-life and is virtually non-existent in normal liver but accumulates on inhibition of its conversion to cathepsin L, then induction of this protease can be explained. However, the exact relation between these two proteases requires further study by immuno- and protein chemical techniques.

Protease activity in plasma membranes of hepatocytes and its relation to cell survival in culture

For studies on various functions of hepatocytes, it would be very useful to obtain a system in which the cells behave physiologically for a long time in serum-free culture. The additions of serum and various hormones have marked survival effects on hepatocytes. It should be mentioned that survival activity is activity for maintaining viable cells, but not for the promotion of growth. However, growth promoting activity may sometimes appear to be survival activity, because it results in a steady cell number due to a balance of cell growth and death.

Among various hormones, glucocorticoid and insulin show marked survival activity on cultured hepatocytes, but their mechanisms of action are still unknown. They may stimulate anabolism in hepatocytes including transport of amino acids and protein synthesis. Glucocorticoid stimulates secretion of fibronectin from hepatocytes, which is essential for cell attachment (34). Serum contains fibronectin and this is one reason why it is effective but cell attachment alone is not sufficient for hepatocytes survival (25). We found that serum contains a factor necessary for hepatocyte survival. We also found this factor at higher concentration in bovine pituitary extract. We purified this factor from the latter source to an homogeneous state (1). Further studies on its molecular weight (8000) and amino acid composition indicated that it is bovine pancreatic trypsin inhibitor (bPTI). This was confirmed by showing that the inhibitory activity of this factor on trypsin was parallel with its survival activity. This finding suggests that the survival activity found in serum is

Table 7. Correlation of hepatocyte survival activities of various protease inhibitors and their inhibitions of plasma membrane-bound protease (reference 39).

Inhibitor	Concentration	Survival activity	Concentration	Inhibition of protease
	($\mu g/ml$)	(%)	($\mu g/ml$)	(%)
bPTI	0.1	100	50	85
Soybean TI[a]	40	56	50	28
Egg white TI	40	24	50	8
Lima bean TI	40	16	50	32
Leupeptin	40	79	50	98
Chymostatin	50	0	50	19
Pepstatin	50	0	50	0
E-64	80	0	50	0
α_1-Antitrypsin	2000	80	100	95
α_2-Macroglobulin	2060	75		
α_2-Plasmin inhibitor	3.9	65	50	95
C_1-Inhibitor	280	29		
Antithrombin	179	6		
			(mM)	
Diisopropyl fluorophosphate			0.1	98
Phenylmethylsulfonylfluoride			10	95
5,5'-Dithiobis (2-nitrobenzoate)			1	0
N-Ethylmaleimide			1	
				0
EDTA			1	0

[a] Trypsin inhibitor.

due to trypsin inhibitor. Indeed, various serum protease inhibitors, such as α_2-plasmin inhibitor, α_1-antitrypsin, and α_2-macroglobulin showed survival activity (Table 7).

Thus, it seemed very interesting to study the mechanism of the effect of the protease inhibitor in causing survival of cultured hepatocytes. We found that protein degradation in hepatocytes was not affected by addition of bPTI and that α_2-plasmin inhibitor immobilized on Sepharose 4B also had survival activity (39). These results indicated that the survival factor acts on the cell surface, not in hepatocytes. In other words, there is a trypsin-like protease on the cell surface of hepatocytes that reduces hepatocyte survival.

Subsequently, we purified this surface protease from the plasma membranes of rat liver (70). The enzyme was solubilized with 4% octylglucoside or 0.2% Brij-35 and subjected to affinity chromatography on bPTI immobilized Sepharose. The purified enzyme, which appeared homogeneous on electrophoresis, hydrolysed various synthetic peptides that are substrates for trypsin and denatured albumin, but showed no activity of aminopeptidase, chymotrypsin or elastase. Table 7 shows the good parallel observed between the survival activities of various trypsin inhibitors on hepatocytes and their inhibitory activities on the purified protease. This protease was not inhibited by inhibitors of thiol-, metalo- or carboxylproteases or by chymostatin or elastatinal. But it was inhibited by various synthetic and natural trypsin inhibitors. The next question is whether this protease is involved in hepatocyte survival. When plasma membranes of hepatocytes were incubated, proteins with molecular weights of 200, 60 and 52 kD were found to be degraded very rapidly and this degradation was inhibited by the trypsin inhibitor described above. It is unknown, however, whether these proteins that disappeared are involved in the maintenance of hepatocytes in culture. Williams *et al.* (72) reported that hepatocytes in primary culture secrete a trypsin-like protease. This protease, however, is different from the membrane bound protease described above and it is not involved in hepatocyte survival.

From these results, we conclude that the reason for the short survival of hepatocytes in serum-free culture is that their plasma membranes undergo autodegradation. Trypsin-inhibitors in serum inhibit this degradation and thus prolong survival. Then, what is the natural role of this protease in the liver *in vivo*? It could have several roles, such as in membrane turnover, degradation of the intercellular matrix or splitting of peptides for protein secretion or endocytosis. It is noteworthy that this trypsin-like protease was found only in plasma membranes of normal hepatocytes, not in those of brain, red cells or hepatoma cells (70). These findings suggest that the protease may play a specific role in differentiated functions of normal hepatocytes.

REFERENCES

1 Asami O., Nakamura T., Mura T., Ichihara A.: Identification of trypsin inhibitor in bovine pituitary extracts as a survival factor for adult rat hepatocytes in primary culture. *J. Biochem.* 1984, **95**: 299–309.

2 Birnbaum M. J., Fain J. N.: Activation of protein kinase and glycogen phosphorylase in isolated rat liver cells by glucagon and catecholamines. *J. Biol. Chem.* 1977, **252**: 528–535.

3 Blair J. B., James M. E., Foster J. L.: Adrenergic control of glucose output and adenosine 3':5'-monophosphate levels in hepatocytes from juvenile and adult rats. *J. Biol. Chem.* 1979, **254**: 7579–7584.

4 Borek C., Williams G. M. (Eds): Differentiation and carcinogenesis in liver cell culture. *Ann. N.Y. Acad. Sci.* 1980, **349**: 1–415.

5 Boyed G., Martin T. J.: Changes in catecholamine- and glucagon-responsive adenylate cyclase activity in preneoplastic rat liver. *Molec. Pharmacol.* 1976, **12**: 195–202.

6 Brønstad G., Christoffersen T.: Increased effect of adrenaline on cyclic AMP formation and positive β-adrenergic modulation of DNA-synthesis in regenerating hepatocytes. *FEBS Lett.* 1980, **120**: 89–93.

7 Bulanyi G. S., Steele J. G., McGrath M. C., Yeoh G. C. T., Oliver I. T.: Hormonal regulation of phosphoenolpyruvate carboxykinase in cultured foetal hepatocytes from the rat. *Eur. J. Biochem.* 1979, **254**: 7579–7584.

8 Chan T. M., Blackmore P. F., Steiner K. E., Exton J. H.: Effects of adrenalectomy on hormone action on hepatic glucose metabolism. Reciprocal change in α- and β-adrenergic activation of hepatic glycogen phosphorylase and calcium mobilization in adrenalectomized rats. *J. Biol. Chem.* 1979, **254**: 2428–2433.

9 Cherrington A. D., Assimacopoulos F. D., Harper S. C., Corbin J. D., Park C. R., Exton J. H.: Studies on the β-adrenergic activation of hepatic glucose output. II. Investigation of the roles of adenosine 3':5'-monophosphate and adenosine 3':5'-monophosphate dependent protein kinase in the action of phenylephrine in isolated hepatocytes. *J. Biol. Chem.* 1976, **251**: 5209–5218.

10 Chrapkiewicz N. R., Beale E. G., Granner D. K.: Induction of the messenger ribonucleic acid coding for phosphoenolpyruvate carboxykinase in H4-II-E cells. *J. Biol. Chem.* 1982, **257**: 14428–14432.

11 Christoffersen T., Berg T.: Altered hormone control of cyclic AMP formation in isolated parenchymal liver cells from rats treated with 2-acetylaminofluorene. *Biochim. Biophys. Acta* 1975, **381**: 72–77.

12 Christoffersen T., Mørland J., Osnes J. B., Øye I.: Development of cyclic AMP metabolism in rat liver. A correlative study of tissue levels of cyclic AMP, and accumulation of cyclic AMP in slices, adenylate cyclase activity and cyclic nucleotide phosphodiesterase activity. *Biochim. Biophys. Acta* 1973, **313**: 338–349.

13 Cochet M., Chang A. C. Y., Cohen S.: Characterization of the structural gene and putative 5′-regulatory sequences for human pro-opiomelanocortin. *Nature* 1982, **297**: 335–339.

14 Craine B., Komberg T.: Transcription of the major *Drosophila* heatshock genes *in vitro*. *Biochemistry* 1981, **20**: 6584–6589.

15 Exton J. H., Robinson G. A., Sutherland E. W., Park C. R.: Studies on the role of adenosine 3′,5′-monophosphate in the hepatic actions of glucagon and catecholamines. *J. Biol. Chem.* 1971, **246**: 6166–6177.

16 Gerschenson L. E., Thompson E. B. (Eds): *Gene Expression and Carcinogenesis in Cultured Liver*: Academic Press, New York, 1975, pp 1–491.

17 Goodhardt M., Ferry N., Geynet P., Hanoune J.: Hepatic α_1-adrenergic receptors show agonist-specific regulation by guanine nucleotides. Loss of nucleotide effect after adrenalectomy. *J. Biol. Chem.* 1982, **257**: 11577–11583.

18 Govindan M. V., Spiess E., Majors J.: Purified glucocorticoid receptor hormone complex from rat liver cytosol binds specifically to cloned mouse mammary tumor virus long terminal repeats *in vitro*. *Proc. Natl. Acad. Sci.* 1982, **79**: 5157–5161.

19 Granner D., Andreone T., Sasaki K., Beale E.: Inhibition of transcription of the phosphoenol-pyruvate carboxykinase gene by insulin. *Nature* 1983, **305**: 549–551.

20 Greengard O.: Enzymatic differentiation in mammalian tissues. *Essays Biochem.* 1971, **7**: 159–205.

21 Grinde B., Seglen P. O.: Different effects of protease inhibitors and amines on the lysosomal and non-lysosomal pathways of protein degradation in isolated hepatocytes. *Biochim. Biophys. Acta* 1980, **632**: 73–86.

22 Guguen-Guillouzo C., Guillouzo A.: Modulation of functional activities in cultured rat hepatocytes. *Molec. Cell. Biochem.* 1983, **53/54**: 35–56.

23 Gurr J. A., Ruh T. A.: Desensitization of primary cultures of adult rat liver parenchymal cells to stimulation of adenosine 3′,5′-monophosphate production by glucagon and epinephrine. *Endocrinology* 1980, **107**: 1309–1319.

24 Harris R. A., Cornell N. (Eds): *Isolation, Characterization and Use of Hepatocytes*: Elsevier Biomedical Press, New York, 1983, pp 1–614.

25 Horiuti Y., Nakamura T., Ichihara A.: Role of serum in maintenance of functional hepatocytes in primary culture. *J. Biochem.* 1982, **92**: 1985–1994.

26 Hynes N., Van Ooyen A. J. J., Kennedy, N., Herrlich P., Ponta H., Groner B.: Subfragments of the large terminal repeat cause glucocorticoid responsive expression of mouse mammary tumor virus and of an adjacent gene. *Proc. Natl. Acad. Sci.* 1983, **80**: 3637–3641.

27 Ichihara A.: Relation of the characteristics of liver cells during culture, differentiation and carcinogenesis. *In: Control Mechanisms in Cancer*, W. E. Criss, T. Ono, J. R. Sabine (Eds): Raven Press, New York, 1976, pp 317–327.

28 Ichihara A., Nakamura T., Tanaka K.: Use of hepatocytes in primary culture for biochemical studies on liver functions. *Molec. Cell. Biochem.* 1982, **43**: 145–160.

29 Jungmann R. A., Kelley D. C., Miles M. F., Milkowski D. M.: Cyclic AMP regulation of lactate dehydrogenase. *J. Biol. Chem.* 1983, **258**: 5312–5318.

30 Katada T., Bokoch G. M., Smigel M. D., Ui M.: The inhibitory guanine nucleotide-binding regulatory component of adenylate cyclase. *J. Biol. Chem.* 1984, **259**: 3586–3595.

31 Lefkowitz R. J., Stadel J. M., Caron M. G.: Adenylate cyclase-coupled beta-adrenergic receptors. *Ann. Rev. Biochem.* 1983, **52**: 159–186.

32 Leray F., Chambaut A.-M. Perrenoud M.-L., Hanoune J.: Adenylate cyclase activity of rat liver plasma membranes. Hormonal stimulations and effect of adrenalectomy. *Eur. J. Biochem.* 1973, **38**: 185–192.

33 Malbon C. C.: Liver cell adenylate cyclase and β-adrenergic receptors. *J. Biol. Chem.* 1980, **255**: 8692–8699.

34 Marceau N., Goyette R., Deschenes J., Valet J.-P.: Morphological difference between epithelial and fibroblast cells in rat liver cultures, and the roles of cell surface fibronectin and cytoskeletal element organization in cell shape. *Ann. N.Y. Acad. Sci.* 1980, **349**: 138–152.

35 Meisner H., Lamers W. H., Hanson R. W.: Cyclic AMP and the synthesis of phosphoenolpyruvate carboxykinase (GTP) mRNA. *Trends Biochem. Sci.* 1983, **8**: 165–167.

36 Morgan N. G., Blackmore P. F., Exton J. H.: Age-related changes in the control of hepatic cyclic AMP levels by α_1- and β_2-adrenergic receptors in male rats. *J. Biol. Chem.* 1983, **258**: 5103–5109.

37 Murdoch G. H., Rosenfeld M. G., Evans R. M.: Eukaryotic transcriptional regulation and chromatin-associated protein phosphorylation by cyclic AMP. *Science* 1982, **218**: 1315–1317.

38 Nakamura T., Aoyama K., Tomomura A., Ichihara A.: Hormonal control of the development of tryptophan oxygenase in primary cultures of adult rat hepatocytes. *Biochim. Biophys. Acta* 1981, **678**: 91–97.

39 Nakamura T., Asami O., Tanaka K., Ichihara A.: Increased survival of rat hepatocytes in serum-free medium by inhibition of a trypsin-like protease associated with their plasma membranes. *Exp. Cell Res.* 1984, **155**: 81–91.

40 Nakamura T., Nakayama Y., Ichihara A.: Reciprocal modulation of growth and liver functions of mature rat hepatocytes in primary culture by an extract of hepatic plasma membranes. *J. Biol. Chem.* 1984, **259**: 8056–8058.

41 Nakamura T., Nakayama Y., Teramoto H., Nawa K., Ichihara A.: Loss of reciprocal modulations of growth and liver functions of hepatoma cells in culture by contact with cells and cell membranes. *Proc. Natl. Acad. Sci.* 1984, **81**: 6398–6402.

42 Nakamura T., Noda C., Ichihara A.: Two phase regulation of tyrosine aminotransferase activity by insulin in primary cultured hepatocytes of adult rats. *Biochem. Biophys. Res. Commun.* 1981, **99**: 775–780.

43 Nakamura T., Shinno H., Ichihara A.: Insulin and glucagon as a new regulator system for tryptophan oxygenase activity demonstrated in primary cultured rat hepatocytes. *J. Biol. Chem.* 1980, **255**: 7533–7535.

44 Nakamura T., Tomita Y., Ichihara A.: Density-dependent growth control of adult rat hepatocytes in primary culture. *J. Biochem.* 1983, **94**: 1029–1035.

45 Nakamura T., Tomomura A., Kato S., Noda C., Ichihara A.: Reciprocal expression of alpha$_1$- and beta-adrenergic receptors, but constant expression of glucagon receptor by rat hepatocytes during development and primary culture. *J. Biochem.* 1984, **96**: 127–136.

46 Nakamura T., Tomomura A., Noda C., Shimoji M., Ichihara A.: Acquisition of a beta-adrenergic response by adult rat hepatocytes during primary culture. *J. Biol. Chem.* 1983, **258**: 9283–9289.

47 Nakamura T., Yoshimoto K., Nakayama Y., Tomita Y., Ichihara A.: Reciprocal modulation of growth and differentiated functions of mature rat hepatocytes in primary culture by cell-cell contact and cell membranes. *Proc. Natl. Acad. Sci.* 1983, **80**: 7229–7233.

48 Nakamura T., Yoshimoto K., Aoyama K., Ichihara A.: Hormonal regulations of glucose-6-phosphate dehydrogenase and lipogenesis in primary cultures of rat hepatocytes. *J. Biochem.* 1982, **91**: 681–693.

49 Neff N. T., DeMartino G. N., Goldberg A. L..: The effect of protease inhibitors and decreased temperature on the degradation of different classes of proteins in cultured hepatocytes. *J. Cell. Physiol.* 1979, **101**: 439–458.

50 Niimi S., Nakamura T., Nawa K., Ichihara A.: Hormonal regulation of translatable mRNA of tryptophan 2,3-dioxygenase in primary cultures of adult rat hepatocytes. *J. Biochem.* 1983, **94**: 1697–1706.

51 Noda C., Nakamura T., Ichihara A.: Alpha-adrenergic control of enzymes of amino acid metabolism in primary cultures of adult rat hepatocytes. *J. Biol. Chem.* 1983, **258**: 1520–1525.

52 Noda C., Shinjyo F., Nakamura T., Ichihara A.: Requirement of prolonged presence of a high intracellular level of cyclic AMP for induction of serine dehydratase in primary cultured rat hepatocytes. *J. Biochem.* 1983, **93**: 1677–1684.

53 Noda C., Shinjyo F., Tomomura A., Kato S., Nakamura T., Ichihara A.: Mechanism of heterologous desensitization of the adenylate cyclase system by glucagon in primary cultures of adult rat hepatocytes. *J. Biol. Chem.* 1984, **259**: 7747–7754.

54 Noda C., Tomomura M., Nakamura T., Ichihara A.: Hormonal control of serine dehydratase mRNA in primary cultures of adult rat hepatocytes. *J. Biochem.* 1984, **95**: 37–45.

55 Okajima F., Ui M.: Conversion of adrenergic regulation of glycogen phosphorylase and synthase from an α to a β type during primary culture. *Arch. Biochem. Biophys.* 1982, **213**: 658–668.

56 Okajima F., Ui M.: Predominance of β-adrenergic over α-adrenergic receptor functions involved in

phosphorylase activation in liver cells of cholestatic rats. *Arch. Biochem. Biophys.* 1984, **230**: 640–651.

57 Pariza M. W., Butcher F. R., Becker J. E., Potter V. R.: 3':5'-Cyclic AMP: Independent induction of amino acid transport by epinephrine in primary cultures of adult rat liver cells. *Proc. Natl. Acad. Sci.* 1977, **74**: 234–237.

58 Pariza M. W., Butcher F. R., Kletzien R. F., Becker J. E., Potter V. R.: Induction and decay of glucagon-induced amino acid transport in primary cultures of adult rat liver cells. Paradoxical effects of cycloheximide and puromycin. *Proc. Natl. Acad. Sci.* 1976, **73**: 4511–4515.

59 Periksaitis H. G., Kan W. H., Kunos G.: Decreased α_1-adrenoceptor responsiveness and density in liver cells of thyroidectomized rats. *J. Biol. Chem.* 1982, **257**: 4321–4327.

60 Plas C., Nunez J.: Glycogenolytic response to glucagon of cultured fetal hepatocytes. Refractoriness following prior exposure to glucagon. *J. Biol. Chem.* 1975, **250**: 5304–5311.

61 Refsnes M., Sandnes D., Melien Ø., Sand T. E., Jacobsen S., Christoffersen T.: Mechanisms for the emergence of catecholamine-sensitive adenylate cyclase and β-adrenergic receptors in cultured hepatocytes. Dependence on protein and RNA synthesis and suppression by isoproterenol. *FEBS Lett.* 1983, **164**: 291–298.

62 Rodbell M.: The role of hormone receptors and GTP-regulatory proteins in membrane transduction. *Nature* 1980, **284**: 17–22.

63 Ross E. M., Gilman A. G.: Biochemical properties of hormone-sensitive adenylate cyclase. *Ann. Rev. Biochem.* 1980, **49**: 533–564.

64 Scheidereit C., Geisse S., Westphal H. M., Beato M.: The glucocorticoid receptor binds to defined nucleotide sequences near the promotor of mouse mammary tumor virus. *Nature* 1983, **304**: 749–752.

65 Schmelck P.-H., Hanoune J.: The hepatic adrenergic receptors. *Molec. Cell. Biochem.* 1980, **33**: 35–48.

66 Schmid W., Scherer G., Danesch U., Zentgraf H., Matthias P., Strange C. M., Rowekamp W., Schutz G.: Isolation and characterization of the rat tryptophan oxygenase gene. *EMBO J.* 1982, **1**: 1278–1293.

67 Shinno H., Noda C., Tanaka K., Ichihara A.: Induction of L-lysine-2-oxoglutarate reductase by glucocorticoid and glucagon: *in vivo* and *in vitro* studies. *Biochim. Biophys. Acta* 1980, **633**: 310–316.

68 Tanaka K., Ikegaki N., Ichihara A.: Effects of leupeptin and pepstatin on protein turnover in adult rat hepatocytes in primary culture. *Arch. Biochem. Biophys.* 1981, **208**: 296–304.

69 Tanaka K., Ikegaki N., Ichihara A.: Purification and characterization of hemoglobin-hydrolyzing, acidic, thiol-protease induced by leupeptin in rat liver. *J. Biol. Chem.* 1984, **259**: 5937–5944.

70 Tanaka K., Nakamura T., Ichihara A.: A unique kipsin-like protease associated with plasma membranes of rat liver – purification and characterization. *J. Biol. Chem.* 1986, **261**: (in press).

71 Teyssot B., Houdebine L.-M., Djiane J.: Prolactin induces release of a factor from membranes capable of stimulating β-casein gene transcription in isolated mammary cell nuclei. *Proc. Natl. Acad. Sci.* 1981, **78**: 6729–6733.

72 Williams G. M., Bermudez E., San R. H. C., Goldblatt P. J., Larpia M. F.: Rat hepatocytes in primary cultures IV. Maintenance in defined medium and the role of production of plasminogen activators and other proteases. *In Vitro* 1978, **4**: 824–337.

73 Woychik R. P., Camper S. A., Lyons R. H., Goodwin E. C., Rottman F. M.: Cloning and nucleotide sequencing of the bovine growth hormone gene. *Nucl. Acid Res.* 1982, **10**: 7197–7210.

74 Yoo-Warren H., Monahan J. E., Short J., Short H., Bruzeol A., Wynshaw-Boris A., Meisner H. M., Samols D., Hanson R. W.: Isolation and characterization of the gene coding for cytosolic phosphoenolpyruvate carboxykinase (GTP) from the rat. *Proc. Natl. Acad. Sci.* 1983, **80**: 3656–3660.

75 Yoshimoto K., Nakamura T., Ichihara A.: Reciprocal effects of epidermal growth factor on key lipogenic enzymes in primary cultures of adult rat hepatocytes: Induction of glucose-6-phosphate dehydrogenase and suppression of malic enzyme and lipogenesis. *J. Biol. Chem.* 1983, **258**: 12355–12360.

Research in *Isolated and cultured hepatocytes* A. Guillouzo & C. Guguen-Guillouzo eds, pp. 209–224
© 1986 John Libbey Eurotext Ltd./INSERM.

10

Synthesis of extracellular matrix components by cultured hepatocytes

Robert F. DIEGELMANN

Department of Surgery, Medical College of Virginia, Virginia Commonwealth University, Richmond, Virginia, USA

SUMMARY

Hepatocytes in culture maintain most of their specialized biochemical functions. However, with increasing time in culture they also begin to express some characteristics which are usually confined to the period of embryonic development. One additional parameter expressed is the production of a collagen-rich extracellular matrix. Recent studies in a number of laboratories have now confirmed and characterized the potential for the hepatocyte to produce multiple forms of collagen. Additional components such as fibronectin, laminin, and glycosoaminglycans are also synthesized. Part of the stimulus for this expression is probably due to the loss of extracellular material during the enzymatic dissociation of the liver to free the hepatocytes. The synthesis of collagen by the hepatocyte in culture is stimulated following *in vivo* regeneration and by carbon tetrachloride injury whereas it can be selectively inhibited *in vitro* by the presence of glucocorticoids. Expression of collagen by the hepatocyte in culture may be a manifestation of the cells' capacity to respond to injury *in vivo*. Based upon current cell culture studies, it is postulated that the hepatocyte may contribute significantly to the process of liver fibrosis.

Structure and function of the extracellular matrix

Enzymatic digestion of the hepatocellular matrix is necessary to isolate and place hepatocytes in culture. This is usually accomplished by perfusing the liver *in situ* with solutions of bacterial collagenases (Chapter 1). Bacterial collagenase is a mixture of collagenases and proteases which very effectively digests the supporting connective tissue matrix and allows for the release of hepatocytes. The hepatocyte must respond to this loss in extracellular matrix by repairing and replacing the damaged and lost structures. When the cells are placed directly on plastic surfaces, they require nutritional and hormone supplementation compared to hepatocytes placed on a variety of reconstituted extracellular matrices (57). An alternative method is to co-culture the hepatocytes with other cell types in an effort to allow a cooperation between the cells to regenerate a structural matrix (1, 6, 22). By far the most widely used technique is to place the hepatocytes on surfaces coated with collagen or fibronectin (Chapter 11). All of these techniques are attempts to provide the hepatocyte with a 'normal' extracellular matrix. Similar to the process of cellular differentiation during embryonic development (35), establishment of an extracellular matrix plays a critical role in the cellular interaction and reorganization of the hepatocyte in culture.

Collagen represents one of the most abundant constituents of the extracellular matrix. Fibrils of collagen are intimately associated with other glycoproteins and with proteoglycans to form a highly functional support structure. Although collagen is the most abundant protein in the animal kingdom and accounts for 30% of all mammalian proteins, it is composed of a most unusual molecular structure (for recent reviews see references 50 and 83). Three alpha chains, each approximately 1000 amino acids in length, are intercoiled to form a triple helical structure. There are five major types of genetically distinct collagens and perhaps as many as five additional forms of trace collagens. The most abundant form of collagen is Type I which is found in skin, bone, tendon, cornea, lung and liver. Type II collagen constitutes cartilagenous structures, whereas Type III collagen is found in fetal skin, uterus, placenta, aorta, liver and lung. These three types of collagen are referred to as interstitial collagens and function in a support capacity. Basement membrane, or Type IV collagen, forms unique structures in the lens capsule, placenta, glomerulus, aorta and a variety of tumours. Type IV collagen differs from interstitial forms of collagen since it is composed of characteristic triple helical collagenous structures containing segments of non-helical proteins. The fifth major collagen type has been described as cellular or cytoskeletal (19, 20) and can be found closely associated with the surface of smooth muscle cells as well as other cell types in a wide variety of tissues.

Collagen is synthesized on polysomes of the rough endoplasmic reticulum (8) and initially exists as a larger precursor molecule designated as a pre-pro alpha chain. As the molecules are processed through the vesicles of the endoplasmic reticulum, selected proline and lysine residues are hydroxylated by specific enzymes. Further processing of the procollagen alpha chains results in glycosylation of certain hydroxylysine moieties as initial alignment and helix formation begins. The next process is intracellular translocation of the procollagen molecules through the Golgi apparatus and packaging into vesicles in preparation for secretion. Microtubules then assist in the movement of the collagen-filled vesicles to the cell membrane (14) where they fuse with the membrane and the contents are extruded into the extracellular space. The amino terminal and carboxy terminal procollagen peptides are then cleaved by specific peptidases and the molecules are then capable of being crosslinked to form fibrils and eventually fibres.

Because of the many unique post-translational modifications made to the collagen molecule, the possibility of specific pharmacologic inhibition of collagen synthesis has been examined as a means of controlling fibrotic processes (5). The use of proline and lysine analogues to interfere with the normal collagen hydroxylation process has been suggested as a means to control collagen synthesis. However, this approach does not appear to be promising because these analogues are poorly incorporated into protein and they are not specific for collagen (5). Likewise, depletion of essential cofactors needed for collagen hydroxylation such as molecular oxygen, ascorbic acid and iron are not specific for collagen and can have toxic consequences. Microtubule-disruptive drugs such as colchicine and vinblastine have been suggested for use to block collagen secretion (14), but, once again, these drugs are not specific for collagen and appear to have only a transient effect on blocking secretion (10). One of the most promising approaches appears to be a selective interference with collagen crosslinking by such pharmacologic agents as beta aminopropionitrile (BAPN) and D-penicillamine (5). The rationale for this approach is based on the possibility that uncrosslinked collagen would have reduced structural stability and would have an increased rate of turnover. The possible use of these lathyrogenic agents to control fibrosis is being explored in a number of laboratories.

Another possible approach to block collagen accumulation is by the use of glucocorticoids (7). Indeed, a recent report from this laboratory has shown that glucocorticoids can specifically inhibit collagen synthesis by the hepatocyte (26). Unfortunately, steroids usually have many nonspecific secondary effects *in vivo*. At present, there is not a single specific agent available to inhibit collagen deposition. The future hope for controlling fibrotic processes will probably be found in the combined use of several anti-collagen therapies.

Collagen synthesis by the hepatocyte

The presence of significant amounts of collagen in the liver has been known for some time. Normally, this collagen functions as a support matrix and a filtration membrane in the sinusoid. However, following a variety of injuries, including chemical, metabolic and immunological insult, the collagen content is greatly increased. For example, normal human liver contains approximately 5.5 mg of collagen per gram of liver and this value is increased approximately six-fold in cirrhotic liver (62). In the past, it was always assumed that this remarkable increase in liver collagen was due to fibroblasts (46, 55), perisinusoidal cells (36, 39, 41, 54, 75) or cells derived from these cell types (2, 49, 64, 82). It has only been in recent years that we have come to appreciate the fact that the hepatocyte has the potential to produce collagen (12, 23, 27, 30, 34, 78). To what extent the hepatocyte actually contributes to the process of hepatic fibrosis is still being debated. However, it has been calculated that since hepatocytes constitute 70 to 80% of the cells in the liver, they could theoretically account for 80% of the hepatic collagen (31).

One of the first clues that the hepatocyte has the potential to produce collagen came from studies of an epithelial cell line derived from rat liver (67). Clones were obtained following long-term serial passage of liver-derived epithelial cells. Several of these subclones were then shown to have hydroxyproline associated with the cell layer. In addition, using electron microscopy, bundles of collagen fibrils could be demonstrated in the extracellular spaces of these cloned, liver-derived epithelial cells. Although these long-term cloned cells have been shown to produce albumin (32, 33), there still remains the question of altered gene expression *in vitro* (69) and just how accurately these derived cells from the liver and other chemically transformed cell lines (37, 73), actually represent *in vivo* behaviour of liver parenchymal cells.

To circumvent these problems, our laboratory has utilized a primary, isolated hepatocyte culture system, shown to have phenotypically stable characteristics of liver parenchymal cells (4). Hepatocytes can be isolated from either normal or regenerating rat liver by an *in situ* perfusion with a solution containing 0.03% bacterial collagenase. The hepatocytes are then separated from blood cells and other nonparenchymal cells of the liver by repeated centrifugation and resuspension in culture medium. The hepatocytes are then placed on 60 mm tissue culture plates coated with collagen. In our studies we have used purified bovine dermal collagen to coat the culture plates (Vitrogen, Collagen Corporation, Palo Alto, CA). The cells are plated at high density (3×10^6 hepatocytes per plate) and in the absence of serum to maintain a nonproliferating state. This culture technique allows the study of hepatocytes freshly removed from the liver where phenotypic stability is maintained (4). The culture medium is a modified Waymouth's MB752 formula where ornithine is substituted for arginine to preclude the possibility of fibroblast contamination (43). This medium also contains insulin (10^{-6}M) and fresh ascorbate (50 mg/l) which is changed every 24 hours. Under these conditions of cell isolation and culture, the hepatocytes form a monolayer by 4 hours and remain greater than 95% viable. Hepatocyte cultures have been maintained for up to 2 weeks under these conditions.

This well-defined, primary hepatocyte culture system was used to examine the potential of these cells to produce collagen. The first studies from our laboratory reported on biochemical and immunohistochemical evidence for the presence of prolyl hydroxylase in hepatocytes isolated from both normal and regenerating rat liver (23). It is of interest to note that the prolyl hydroxylase activity in hepatocytes isolated from regenerating liver was consistently about twice the specific activity of hepatocytes isolated from normal liver (23, 52). This observation suggested that the potential for collagen synthesis by the hepatocyte was linked to the *in vivo* proliferative state of the cell. The presence of insulin in the culture medium was found necessary for the maximal expression of prolyl hydroxylase activity by the hepatocyte (25).

It was of interest to note that the addition of peritoneal macrophages (2×10^5 macrophages per plate) at 24 hours (arrow) caused a prolonged potentiation of prolyl hydroxylase activity (Fig. 1). This finding suggests that inflammatory cells, or perhaps their products, may augment the hepatocytes' potential for the production of collagen. The influence of inflammation on formation of collagen in the liver is an important parameter to be considered especially in clinical situations such as in the hepatic fibrosis resulting from the granulomatous response to *Schistosoma* infection (16).

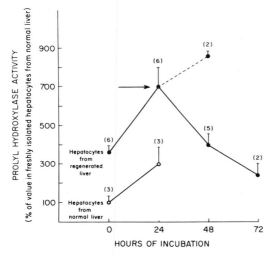

Fig. 1.
The effect of macrophages on hepatocyte prolyl hydroxylase activity. Freshly isolated hepatocytes were prepared 96 hours after partial hepatectomy (regenerated liver) or from normal animals, and were incubated in control medium. At 24 hours, 2×10^5 macrophages were added to hepatocytes from regenerated liver (2 plates) and incubation continued for an additional 24 hours. An equivalent amount of macrophages were cultured alone under these conditions and were found to be negative for prolyl hydroxylase activity. The results were expressed as the per cent of the average value in freshly isolated hepatocytes derived from normal liver. Brackets indicate the sem with the number of experiments given in parentheses. Control data were previously reported (23).

Further evidence for collagen synthesis by the hepatocyte was obtained when cultures were incubated with radioactive proline and radioactive hydroxyproline was produced (23). However, greater than 90% of the radioactive hydroxyproline produced during the first 48 hours in culture was found to be dialysable and soluble in 5% trichloroacetic acid (23). This observation was then explained in part by the fact that freshly isolated hepatocytes retain some of the bacterial collagenase used in the liver perfusion to liberate the cells (24). Therefore, investigators using freshly isolated hepatocytes, especially those studying collagen metabolism, should be cautious of possible collagenase and other protease retention by these cells and associated problems due to the presence of these enzymes.

After 3 days in cell culture, with 3 exchanges of medium, the residual bacterial collagenase contamination is no longer a problem (24), and one can readily detect hydroxyproline in the large molecular weight protein fraction. If purified collagen is added to cultures following a 24-hour exposure to radioactive proline, newly synthesized hepatocyte collagen can be trapped and co-purified with a non-radioactive collagen standard (27). When this technique was applied to 72-h hepatocyte cultures, all of the purified radioactive collagen subsequently chromatographed on an agarose molecular seive column was of high molecular weight, and was eluted in the gamma, or triple helical region (27). By the ninth day, purified radioactive collagen in the alpha and beta regions could also be detected (27). Therefore, these initial studies suggested that the hepatocyte in culture has the potential to produce multiple types of collagen and this phenotypic expression changes with increasing time of incubation.

We have now refined the technique needed to measure collagen synthesis by hepatocytes in culture (26). For each determination 5, 60 mm culture plates (approximately 1.5×10^7 cells), are incubated for 24 hours in the standard culture medium plus 10 μCi of ^{3}H-proline substituted for the nonradioactive proline. The medium and cell layer are scraped into a centrifuge tube on ice and the plates are rinsed once with cold deionized water which is added to the original harvest. We have now found that it is important to next immerse the samples into a boiling water bath for 5 minutes to destroy endogenous proteases contained in hepatocytes. The samples are then chilled to 4°C and nonincorporated ^{3}H-proline is removed from the radioactive protein by four repeated washings with 5% trichloroacetic and centrifugations ($1000 \times$ g, 4°C). After removal of the last trichloroacetic acid wash, the protein pellet is resuspended in a small volume of 0.2 M NaOH and distributed into three fractions. One aliquot is digested with purified bacterial collagenase under optimal conditions and a second fraction serves as an enzyme blank (53). The third fraction can be used for DNA analysis to quantitate collagen synthesis per cellular DNA (58). After incubation for 90 minutes at 37°C, the non-collagenous proteins are reprecipitated by addition of an equal volume of 10% trichloroacetic acid — 0.5% tannic acid in the cold. Radioactivity in both fractions is determined by liquid scintillation counting and the enzyme blank supernatant is subtracted. A calculation is used to correct for the enriched amino acid content of collagen compared to non-collagen protein (15) and results are expressed on a relative basis as the percentage collagen synthesis per amount of total non-collagen protein synthesized. This technique avoids some of the technical problems associated with other assays such as degree of collagen hydroxylation, uptake of isotope and the size of the endogenous proline pool within the cell (53).

Using this assay, we have been able to characterize the dynamics of collagen expression by hepatocytes from regenerating liver compared to normal liver and as a function of time in culture (Fig. 2). During the first several days, hepatocytes derived from normal liver produce about 0.01% of their total protein as collagen. By the ninth day, this level increases to about 1% of their total protein. In contrast, hepatocytes from regenerating liver synthesize approximately 2 to 3 times more collagen throughout this period of culture (26). These observations suggest that the *in vivo* metabolic state of the hepatocyte influences the potential for collagen synthesis in cell culture. Since these cells are not proliferating *in vitro*, it is unlikely that there is an enrichment of collagen-producing hepatocytes. Studies using cDNA probe analysis are now in progress to address the questions of how collagen

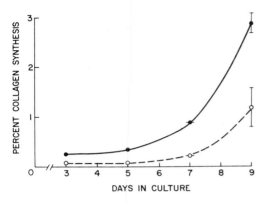

Fig. 2.
Time course of collagen synthesis in hepatocyte cultures. Freshly isolated hepatocytes were prepared by collagenase perfusion of normal rat liver (○ – – – – – ○) or of regenerated liver 4 days after partial hepatectomy (● ——— ●) and were incubated for the indicated times. On culture days 2, 4, 6 and 8, replicate dishes of monolayer cultures, derived from a single liver, were incubated for 24 hours in medium containing [³H]-proline. At the indicated times, cells plus medium from these labelled cultures were harvested, proteins were precipitated, and the radioactivity in collagen and non-collagen protein was measured. The results were calculated as synthesis of collagen relative to synthesis of non-collagen protein expressed as a percentage. Data from experiments in cultures derived from the liver from 4 normal rats or from 19 regenerating livers are shown with brackets indicating S.E.M. The other time points reflect the average of two experiments. Reprinted with permission (26).

expression by the hepatocyte is regulated at the molecular genetic level.

Some of the initial studies had suggested that there were multiple forms of collagen being expressed by the hepatocyte in culture and that the phenotypic expression was changing with the duration of culture (27). Indeed, this proved to be the explanation once the collagen was purified and identified by slab gel electrophoresis and specific immunohistochemical reacting (12). During the first two days in culture, hepatocytes produced only Type IV basement membrane collagen and by the eighth day, collagen Types I, III and IV were also detected (12). It is important to reiterate that under those conditions of culture, the hepatocytes are not proliferating.

It is also important to point out that simultaneous staining of the fixed hepatocytes with specific antibodies to albumin and fibrinogen proved that all of the hepatocytes retained these characteristic liver functions while producing the multiple types of collagen (12). With the use of *in situ* cDNA hybridization techniques, Saber *et al.* (66) have also shown that freshly isolated mouse hepatocytes contain both albumin and pro-alpha$_2$ (I) mRNA. Additional laboratories have been investigating collagen metabolism by hepatocytes in primary culture and have reported also the production of the collagen Types I, III, IV (30, 42, 68) and perhaps Type V (79).

Not only does the hepatocyte have the capacity to synthesize collagen, but this highly multipotential cell can very effectively degrade collagen. The mammalian form of collagenase has been demonstrated in culture medium removed from hepatocytes (45, 48) and we have reported on the rapid degradation of newly synthesized collagen by the hepatocyte (9). Beyond the period of bacterial collagenase contamination (72 hours of culture), approximately 40% of the total collagen synthesized is found as trichloroacetic acid soluble material (9). Since the hepatocyte probably only produces trace amounts of collagen under normal conditions *in vivo*, when it is stimulated to synthesize collagen following injury or altered environment such as cell culture, it may produce much of the collagen as 'defective' collagen. Therefore, this rapid degradation of newly synthesized collagen may be an expression of a 'quality control' mechanism (3) to ensure that the collagen destined for the extracellular matrix is properly assembled and functional collagen. Irrespective of the explanation for this process, it is certainly a very important aspect to be considered with regards to hepatic fibrosis and more research needs to be devoted to the process of collagen resorption by the liver.

Now that the potential for collagen synthesis by the hepatocyte has been confirmed by a variety of studies, factors which may modulate this potentiated phenotypic expression are being examined. Glucocorticoids represent one of the first groups of compounds to be examined. The rationale for these studies is based on the fact that collagen synthesis by fibroblasts can be inhibited by glucocorticoids (7) and because methylprednisolone is used clinically to treat hepatic fibrosis.

When hepatocyte cultures were incubated for up to 8 days with glucocorticoids, there was a significant inhibition of collagen synthesis (26). For example, treatment of hepatocyte cultures with dexamethasone at concentrations of 10^{-8}M and above resulted in greater than 80% inhibition of collagen synthesis (Fig. 3). The dose needed for a 50% inhibition of maximal collagen synthesis was 5×10^{-9} M; a concentration considered to be in the 'physiological' range. There were two striking differences between these observations and the studies of glucocorticoid inhibition of fibroblast collagen synthesis. First, the effective dose range needed to block hepatocyte collagen synthesis is much less than that needed to inhibit collagen synthesis by fibroblasts. Secondly, there was a selective inhibition of hepatocyte collagen synthesis by the glucocorticoids and non-collagen protein synthesis was not diminished. The inhibition of collagen deposition was due to decreased synthesis and not increased degradation. The same observations were made when hepatocytes were exposed to various concentrations of methylprednisolone, triamcinolone, prednisone, and hydrocortisone whereas progesterone, testosterone and estradiol were noneffective (26).

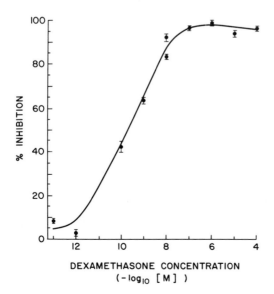

Fig. 3.
Dose-response of dexamethasone on inhibition of collagen synthesis in hepatocyte cultures. After the first 24 hours of incubation in serum-free medium, cultures prepared from regenerated liver were divided into groups receiving one of the indicated concentrations of dexamethasone. Incubation was carried out for 9 days, including a terminal 24-hour period with radio labelled [^{3}H]-proline added to the medium. The cells plus medium were harvested and radioactivity in collagen was determined. The results for dexamethasone-treated cultures are presented as per cent inhibition compared with control cultures incubated in standard glucocorticoid-free medium for the full 9-day period. Reprinted with permission (26).

These studies suggest that perhaps *in vivo* there is some 'steroid-like' factor(s) which normally suppress collagen synthesis by the hepatocyte. When hepatocytes are removed from the *in vivo* environment and placed in culture, repression by this 'factor' is lost and the cells begin to express their potential for collagen formation. Studies are now in progress using *in vitro* protein synthesis systems and collagen specific cDNA probes to analyse the alteration in the expression of collagen synthesis at the molecular genetic level by the hepatocyte following steroid treatment.

In addition to understanding the mechanisms involved in the down-regulation of hepatocyte collagen synthesis, it is also important to elucidate the processes responsible for enhanced collagen production. It has been observed that there is a significant increase in prolyl hydroxylase activity and isotope incorporation into collagen following acute exposure to CCl_4 (18). Mice were given a single oral dose of CCl_4 and 3 days later, liver explant cultures were established and analysed. After 11 days in culture there was a 10-fold increase in collagen production by explants obtained from the damaged liver compared to controls (18). However, the cell types responsible for the increased collagen synthesis were not identified.

To eliminate these problems, pure cultures of hepatocytes were isolated from livers of rats treated for 3 weeks with CCl_4 and their potential to synthesize collagen was determined (11). These initial studies indicated that there is an enhanced capacity for collagen production by hepatocytes obtained from *in vivo* injured liver (see Table 1). On each day examined, there was increased collagen produced per culture and a decrease in noncollagen protein synthesis. This finding suggests that following the *in vivo* injury due to CCl_4 administration, the hepatocyte responds by producing scar tissue at the expense of its normal protein production. If the hepatocytes isolated from the CCl_4-injured liver were incubated in culture for six days with dexamethasone (10^{-9} M), there was a 74% selective inhibition of collagen synthesis. These observations in cell culture suggest that indeed there may be some benefit in the clinical use of glucocorticoids to treat hepatic fibrosis.

Table 1. Influence of *in vivo* CCl_4 treatment for three weeks on synthesis of collagen and non-collagen protein by hepatocytes in culture

In Vivo treatment	Period of culture (days)	Collagen	Non-collagen	Relative collagen synthesis (%)
		$CPM \times 10^{-3}$/culture		
Control	4	8.2	610.8	0.25
CCl_4	4	13.9	537.1	0.48
Control	6	23.3	483.1	0.88
CCl_4	6	28.5	263.6	2.0
Control	8	37.6	213.5	3.1
CCl_4	8	45.0	169.8	4.7

Rats were injected every third day with 0.3 ml (ip) of a 30% solution of CCl_4 in mineral oil or with mineral oil alone (control) for three weeks. Hepatocytes were isolated by the standard *in situ* perfusion with 0.03% bacterial collagenase and placed in culture. On the indicated days, the cultures were exposed to ^{3}H-proline for 24 hours and the amount of radio activity incorporated into collagen and noncollagen protein was determined (53). Relative collagen synthesis was calculated after correcting for the enriched amino acid content of collagen compared to non-collagen protein (15).

Since collagen secretion is facilitated by movement of secretory vesicles along microtubules (14), it has been suggested that disruption of microtubules with colchicine might provide an effective method to inhibit fibrosis (63). Although several animal and human studies have been directed at the possible use of colchicine for the treatment of cirrhosis (40, 61, 63, 77) the potential efficacy of this drug remains unclear. We have recently examined the effect of colchicine on blocking collagen secretion by the hepatocyte in culture and have found only limited disruption of collagen secretion (10). When hepatocytes were treated for 2 hours with 100 μM colchicine, there was greater than 77% blockage of collagen secretion. However, as the incubation time increased, the degree of inhibition was reduced and by 24 hours was no longer significant. Therefore, after long exposure to colchicine, the hepatocytes, and also fibroblasts, appear to become resistant to the action of the drug. There still remains the possibility that colchicine can prevent fibrosis by enhancing collagen breakdown (29) and by reducing inflammation (44). These potential mechanisms of colchicine need to be more fully explored with regards to hepatic fibrosis.

A variety of other anti-collagen drugs such as proline analogues, beta-amino-propionitrile, alpha-alpha-dipyridyl and penicillamine have been suggested for possible use in the treatment of hepatic fibrosis (5, 47, 56, 59), but they remain to be thoroughly examined using hepatocyte cell culture systems. An extract of berries of Japanese ampelopsis has been tested using liver cells in culture and was found to prevent the formation of collagen fibres (38). This extract has been used by various Japanese populations to treat liver disease, but the actual effectiveness and chemical composition have not been documented.

Non-collagenous components of the extracellular matrix produced by hepatocytes in culture

In addition to collagen, the extracellular matrix can contain other glycoproteins such as fibronectin, laminin, as well as elastin, glycosaminoglycans and proteoglycans. Of these non-collagenous components, hepatocytes or cells derived from the liver have been shown to produce fibronectin, laminin, and glycosaminoglycans (for a recent review see reference 62). The first of these, cellular fibronectin, is a glycoprotein of approximately 400 000 molecular weight and is found on the surface of many cells and forms an integral component of the extracellular matrix in most tissues (65). Fibronectin can form complexes with collagen, actin, fibrin and glycosaminoglycans as it binds these various components to specific sites on the surface of the cell. In this manner, fibronectin provides a key role in the interaction of the cell with the extracellular matrix. A liver-derived epithelial line, ARL-6 cells, has been reported to produce fibronectin as well as collagen Types I, III and IV (17). In more recent work, primary cultures of rat hepatocytes have been shown to synthesize significant amounts of plasma fibronectin, a more soluble form of the attachment protein (75). These authors speculate that the hepatocyte may be one of the major contributors to the circulating pool of fibronectin.

Laminin is another important component found in the extracellular matrix and produced by hepatocyte-like cells in culture (17). Laminin is also a large molecular weight glycoprotein (approximately 800 000 daltons) thought to provide integrity to basement membrane-like structures. Frequently, laminin co-distributes with Type IV collagen and may facilitate the attachment of epithelial cells to basement collagen (80).

The remaining constituents of the extracellular matrix reported to be produced by hepatocytes in culture are glycosaminoglycans. These materials not only provide an important influence on the normal physio-chemical characteristics of the extra-cellular matrix, but they also provide key functions during tissue repair and embryonic development. The most abundant glycosaminoglycan produced by liver-derived cells in culture appears to be heparan sulfate (74). Chondroitin sulfate, dermatan sulfate and hyaluronic acid have also been observed in cultures of these cells and the relative quantities of these glycosaminoglycans varies with cell proliferation, transformation (51), levels of cyclic AMP (74), treatment with (+)-catechin (72) and from *in vivo* thioacetamide liver injury (21).

Speculation as to the possible contribution by the hepatocyte to liver fibrosis

Normally, when the liver is subjected to injury, the repair is facilitated by the elegant process of regeneration. Following regeneration, the stromal and parenchymal components of the liver are replaced in their normal architectural relationships and normal hepatic function is restored. However, sometimes normal regeneration does not occur and collagenous scar tissue accumulates in excess of parenchyma and normal liver function is disrupted. There is no question that fibroblasts and 'fibroblast-like' cells from the liver can synthesize collagen. The more important question remains as to how the process of hepatic fibrosis is initiated and what cells participate.

In recent years as our methods for detecting, identifying, and quantifying collagen have become highly sensitive, it has become apparent that many cell types in the body have the capacity to produce collagen (13). This potential for expression of collagen synthesis can be greatly influenced by the state of differentiation as well as the extracellular environment. As discussed in the preceding sections of this paper, when hepatocytes are enzymatically stripped from their normal *in vivo* environment and placed in cell culture, they express multiple forms of collagen. We view the cell culture environment as one which places the cell in a 'traumatized' state. Under these conditions the cell begins to respond by first producing its normal basement membrane (Type IV) collagen and then eventually the scar forms of collagen (Types I and III). Perhaps this is a recapitulation of the hepatocyte's repair response which can occur *in vivo*. This hypothesis is strengthened by our recent observation that increased amounts of Type IV collagen is the initial form deposited by hepatocytes following injury induced by bile duct ligation (12). An initial increase in the deposition of Type IV collagen also has been reported in studies of human liver fibrosis (19, 28). Since fibroblasts do not normally produce Type IV collagen, it is unlikely that they are the source of the initial collagen deposition. The initial deposit of Type IV collagen is then followed by the accumulation of collagen Types I and III (19, 60, 71). The hepatocyte becomes walled-off as the sinusoid forms a complete basement membrane (55), further causing parenchymal damage with eventual necrosis. By this time, significant quantities of collagen Types I and III could be deposited by the traumatized hepatocytes. Finally, fibroblasts and other collagen producing cells are attracted to the sites of inflammation resulting in the formation of permanent scar tissue. This concept may explain why hepatic fibrosis is sometimes reversible (hepatocyte involvement) whereas in advanced stages it is not (fibroblasts).

Hopefully, in the coming years, as our technologies become more advanced we will be able to address some of these questions. By reconstituting the various cellular components of the liver using *in vitro* culture techniques, we can analyse how they normally interact resulting in normal matrix formation. Once this is understood, then inflammatory cells and their products as well as various pharmacologic agents and heptotoxins can be studied. Analyses are now extending to the molecular genetic level with the hope of understanding, and perhaps controlling the mechanisms involved in the process of hepatic fibrosis.

ACKNOWLEDGEMENTS

I wish to express my sincere thanks to Dr Philip S. Guzelian who initially stimulated my interest in liver fibrosis and who continues to provide companionship and a strong scientific base for our shared studies. The thoughtful comments of Dr William J. Lindblad and manuscript preparation by Fay Akers and Rae Carole Spivey are all greatly appreciated. This work supported by NIH Grant AM 18976.

REFERENCES

1　Baffet G., Clement B., Glaise D., Guillouzo A., Guguen-Guillouzo C.: Hydrocortisone modulates the production of extracellular material and albumin in long-term co-cultures of adult rat hepatocytes with other liver epithelial cells. *Biochem. Biophys. Res. Commun.* 1982, **109**: 507–512.

2　Bhathal P. S.: Presence of modified fibroblasts in cirrhotic livers in man. *Pathology* 1972, **4**: 139–144.

3　Bienkowski R. S., Coman M. J., McDonald J. A., Crystal R. G.: Degradation of newly synthesized collagen. *J. Biol. Chem.* 1978, **253**: 4356–4363.

4　Bissell D. M., Guzelian P. S.: Phenotypic stability of adult rat hepatocytes in primary monolayer culture. *Ann. N.Y. Acad. Sci.* 1980, **349**: 85–98.

5　Chvapil M.: Experimental modifications of collagen synthesis and degradation and their therapeutic applications. *In: Collagen in Health and Disease*, J. B. Weiss, M. I. V. Jayson (Eds): Churchill Livingstone, Edinburgh, 1982, pp 206–217.

6　Clement B., Guguen-Guillouzo C., Campion J. P., Glaise D., Bourel, M., Guillouzo A.: Long-term co-culture of adult human hepatocytes with rat liver epithelial cells: Modulation of albumin secretion and accumulation of extracellular material. *Hepatology* 1984, **4**: 373–380.

7　Cutroneo K. R., Rokowski R., Counts D. F.: Glucocorticoids and collagen synthesis: Comparison of *in vivo* and cell culture studies. *Coll. Relat. Res.* 1981, **1**: 557–568.

8　Diegelmann R. F., Bernstein L., Peterkofsky B.: Cell-free collagen synthesis on membrane-bound polysomes of chick embryo connective tissue and the localization of prolyl hydroxylase on the polysome-membrane complex. *J. Biol. Chem.* 1973, **248**: 6514–6521.

9　Diegelmann R. F., Cohen I. K., Guzelian P. S.: Rapid degradation of newly synthesized collagen by primary cultures of adult rat hepatocytes. *Biochem. Biophys. Res. Commun.* 1980, **97**: 819–826.

10　Diegelmann R. F., Guzelian P. S.: Colchicine is only a transient blocker of collagen secretion by rat hepatocytes in cultures. *Gastroenterology* 1983, **84**: 1137.

11　Diegelmann R. F., Guzelian P. S.: Influence of carbon tetrachloride injury to rat liver on synthesis of collagen by the hepatocyte in primary monolayer culture. *Fed. Proc.* 1984, **43**: 384.

12 Diegelmann R. F., Guzelian P. S., Gay R., Gay S.: Identification of the collagen phenotype synthesized by primary cultures of adult rat hepatocytes. *Science* 1983, **219**: 1343–1345.

13 Diegelmann R. F., Lindblad, W. J.: Cellular sources of fibrotic collagen. *Fund. Appl. Toxicol.* 1985, **5**: 219–227.

14 Diegelmann R. F., Peterkofsky B.: Inhibition of collagen secretion from bone and cultured fibroblasts by microtubular disruptive drugs. *Proc. Natl. Acad. Sci.* 1972, **69**: 892–896.

15 Diegelmann R. F., Peterkofsky B.: Collagen biosynthesis during connective tissue development in chick embryo. *Dev. Biol.* 1972, **28**: 443–453.

16 Dunn M. A., Kamel R., Kamel I. A., Biempica L., El Kholy A., Hait P. K., Rojkind M., Warren K. S., Mahound A. A. F.: Liver collagen synthesis in *Schistosomiasis mansoni*. *Gastroenterology* 1979, **76**: 978–982.

17 Foidart J. M., Berman J. J., Paglia L., Rennard S., Abe S., Perantoni M. S., Martin G. R.: Synthesis of fibronectin, laminin, and several collagens by a liver-derived epithelial line. *Lab. Invest.* 1980, **42**: 525–532.

18 Galligani L., Lonati-Galligani M., Fuller G. C.: Collagen synthesis in explant cultures of normal and CCl$_4$-treated mouse liver. *Toxicol. Appl. Pharmacol.* 1979, **48**: 131–137.

19 Gay S.: Collagen in liver fibrosis. *Ital. J. Gastroenterol.* 1980, **12**: 30–32.

20 Gay S., Rhodes R. K., Gay R. E., Miller E. J.: Collagen molecules comprised of alpha 1 (V)-chains (B-chains): An apparent localization in the exocytoskeleton. *Coll. Relat. Res.* 1981, **1**: 53–58.

21 Gressner A. M., Grouls P.: Stimulated synthesis of glycosaminoglycans in suspension cultures of hepatocytes from subacutely injured livers. *Digestion* 1982, **23**: 259–264.

22 Guguen-Guillouzo C., Guillouzo A.: Modulation of functional activities in cultured rat hepatocytes. *Molec. Cell. Biochem.* 1983, **53/54**: 35–56.

23 Guzelian P. S., Diegelmann R. F.: Localization of collagen prolyl hydroxylase to the hepatocyte: Studies in primary monolayer cultures of parenchymal cells from adult rat liver. *Exp. Cell. Res.* 1979, **123**: 269–279.

24 Guzelian P. S., Diegelmann R. F.: Retention of clostridial collagenase by primary cultures of parenchymal cells prepared from adult rat liver. *Life Sci.* 1979, **24**: 513–518.

25 Guzelian P. S., Diegelmann R. F., Lamb R. G., Fallon H. J.: Effects of hormones on changes and cytochrome P-450, prolyl hydroxylase, and glycerol phosphate acyltransferase in primary monolayer cultures of parenchymal cells from adult rat liver. *Yale J. Biol. Med.* 1979, **52**: 5–12.

26 Guzelian P. S., Lindblad W. J., Diegelmann R. F.: Glucocorticoids suppress formation of collagen by the hepatocyte: studies in primary monolayer cultures of parenchymal cells prepared from adult rat liver. *Gastroenterology* 1984, **86**: 897–904.

27 Guzelian P. S., Qureshi G. D., Diegelmann R. F.: Collagen synthesis by the hepatocyte. *Coll. Relat. Res.* 1981, **1**: 83–93.

28 Hahn E., Wick G., Pencev D., Timpl R.: Distribution of basement membrane proteins in normal and fibrotic human liver: Collagen type IV, laminin, and fibronectin. *Gut* 1980, **21**: 63–71.

29 Harris E. D., Krane S. M.: Effects of colchicine on collagenase in cultures of rheumatoid synovium. *Arthritis Rheum.* 1971, **14**: 669–684.

30 Hata R., Nagai Y.: Differentiation of hepatocytes into type I collagen producing cells during primary culture in the presence of alphidicolin (inhibitor of DNA polymerase α). *Biochem. Int.* 1980, **1**: 567–573.

31 Hata R., Ninomiya Y.: Hepatocytes (hepatic parenchymal cells) produce a major part of liver collagen *in vivo*. *Biochem. Int.* 1984, **8**: 181–186.

32 Hata R., Ninomiya Y., Nagai Y., Sakakibara K., Tsukada, Y.: Active synthesis of collagen by albumin-producing liver parenchymal cell clones in cultures. *Proc. Japan Acad.* 1978, **54**: 391–396.

33 Hata R., Ninomiya Y., Nagai Y., Tsukada Y.: Biosynthesis of interstitial types of collagen by albumin-producing rat liver parenchymal cell (hepatocyte) clones in culture. *Biochemistry* 1980, **19**: 169´176

34 Hatahara T., Seyer J. M.: Procollagen production by rat hepatocytes in primary culture. *Biochim. Biophys. Acta* 1982, **716**: 431–438.

35 Hay E. D.: Collagen and embryonic development. *In: Cell Biology of Extracellular Matrix*, E. D. Hay (Ed.): Plenum Press, New York, 1981, pp 379–409.

36 Jezequel A. M., Koch M. M., Orlandi F.: Hepatic fibrosis. Role of perisinusoidal cells? *Ital. J. Gastroenterol.* 1980, **12**: 37–40.

37 Karasaki S., Raymond J.: Formation of intercellular collagen matrix by cultured liver epithelial cells and loss of its ability in hepatocarcinogenesis *in vitro*. *Differentiation* 1981, **19**: 21–30.

38 Katasuta H., Takaoka T.: An attempt in tissue culture at preventing and treating the collagen fiber formation of liver cells. *Japan J. Exp. Med.* 1980, **50**: 275–282.

39 Kent G., Gay S., Inouye T., Bahu R., Minich O. T., Popper H.: Vitamin A-containing lipocytes and formation of type III collagen in liver injury. *Proc. Natl. Acad. Sci.* 1976, **73**: 719–722.

40 Kershenobich D., Uribe M., Suarez G., Mata J. M., Pérez-Tamayo R., Rojkind M.: Treatment of cirrhosis with colchicine: A double-blind randomized trial. *Gastroenterology* 1979, **77**: 532–536.

41 Kobayashi Y., Fujiyama S.: Pathological study of gold impregnation of fat-storing cells in human liver. *Acta Pathol. Jpn.* 1981, **31**: 65–74.

42 Konomi H., Hata R., Sano J., Sunada H., Nagai Y.: Evidence for the production of type I collagen by adult rat hepatocytes in primary culture: immunohistochemical observations. *Biomed. Res.* 1982, **3**: 341–344.

43 Leffert H. L., Paul D.: Studies on primary cultures of differential fetal liver cells. *J. Cell Biol.* 1972, **52**: 559–568.

44 Malawista S. E.: Colchicine: a common mechanism for its anti-inflammatory and anti-mitotic effects. *Arthritis Rheum.* 1968, **11**: 191–197.

45 Maruyama K., Okazaki I., Kobayashi T., Suzuki H., Kashiwazaki K., Tsuchiya M.: Collagenase production by rabbit liver cells in monolayer culture. *J. Lab. Clin. Med.* 1983, **102**: 543–550.

46 McGee J. O. D., Patrick R.: The role of perisinusoidal cells in hepatic fibrogenesis. *Lab. Invest.* 1972, **26**: 429–440.

47 Mezey E., Potter J. J., Iber F. L., Maddrey W. C.: Hepatic collagen proline hydroxylase activity in alcoholic hepatitis: effect of d-penicillamine. *J. Lab. Clin. Med.* 1979, **93**: 92–100.

48 Nagai Y., Hori H., Hata R., Konomi H., Sunada H.: Collagenase production by adult rat hepatocytes in primary culture. *Biomed. Res.* 1982, **3**: 345–349.

49 Nakano M., Worner T. M., Lieber C. S.: Perivenular fibrosis in alcoholic liver injury: ultrastructure and histologic progression. *Gastroenterology* 1982, **83**: 777–785.

50 Nimni M. E.: Collagen: Structure, function, and metabolism in normal and fibrotic tissues. *Arthritis Rheum.* 1983, **13**: 1–86.

51 Ninomiya Y., Hata R., Nagai Y.: Glycosaminoglycan synthesis by liver parenchymal cell clones in culture and its change with transformation. *Biochim. Biophys. Acta* 1980, **629**: 349–358.

52 Patrick R. S., Martin J., Thompson W. D.: The collagen prolyl hydroxylase activity of hepatocytes and mesenchymal cells isolated from normal and regenerating rat liver. *Diag. Histopathol.* 1981, **4**: 95–98.

53 Peterkofsky B., Diegelmann R. F.: Use of a mixture of proteinase-free collagenases for the specific assay of radioactive collagen in the presence of other proteins. *Biochemistry* 1971, **10**: 988–994.

54 Popper H., Lieber C. S.: Histogenesis of alcoholic fibrosis and cirrhosis in the baboon. *Am. J. Pathol.* 1980, **98**:6695–716.

55 Popper H., Udenfriend S.: Hepatic fibrosis: correlation of biochemical and morphologic investigations. *Am. J. Med.* 1970, **49**: 707–721.

56 Pott G., Rauterberg J., Voss B., Gerlach U.: Connective tissue components of the normal and fibrotic human liver. *Klin. Wochenschr.* 1982, **60**: 1–7.

57 Reid L., Jefferson D. M.: Culturing hepatocytes and other differentiated cells. *Hepatology* 1984, **4**: 548–559.

58 Richards G. M.: Modifications of the diphenylamine reaction giving increased sensitivity and simplicity in the estimation of DNA. *Anal. Biochem* 1974, **57**: 369–376.

59 Rojkind M.: Inhibition of liver fibrosis by L-azetidine-2-carboxylic acid in rats treated with carbon tetrachloride. *J. Clin. Invest.* 1973, **52**: 2451–2456.

60 Rojkind M., Giambrone M. A., Biempica L.: Collagen types in normal and cirrhotic liver. *Gastroenterology* 1979, **76**: 710–719.

61 Rojkind M., Kershenobich D.: Effect of colchicine on collagen, albumin and transferrin synthesis by cirrhotic rat liver slices. *Biochim. Biophys. Acta* 1975, **378**: 415–423.

62 Rojkind M., Ponce-Noyola P.: The extracellular matrix of the liver. *Coll. Relat. Res.* 1982, **2**: 151–175.

63 Rojkind M., Uribe M., Kershenobich D.: Colchicine and the treatment of liver cirrhosis. *Lancet* 1973, **1**: 38–39.

64 Rudolph R., McClure W. J., Woodward M.: Contractile fibroblasts in chronic alcoholic cirrhosis. *Gastroenterology* 1979, **76**: 704–709.

65 Ruoslahti E., Engvall E., Hayman E. G.: Fibronectin: current concepts of its structure and functions. *Coll. Rel. Res.* 1981, **1**: 95–128.

66 Saber M. A., Zern M. A., Shafritz D. A.: Use of *in situ* hybridization to identify collagen and albumin mRNAs in isolated mouse hepatocytes. *Proc. Natl. Acad. Sci.* 1983, **80**: 4017–4020.

67 Sakakibara K., Saito M., Umeda M., Enaka K.: Native collagen formation by liver parenchymal cells in culture. *Nature* 1976, **262**: 316–318.

68 Sakakibara K., Suzuki T., Tsukada Y., Nagai Y.: Distribution of type I collagen and basement membrane proteins in the cultures of cloned epithelial liver cells. *Cell. Struct. Funct.* 1982, **7**: 213–228.

69 Sakakibara K., Takaoka T., Katsuta H., Umeda M., Tsukada Y.: Collagen fiber formation as a common property of epithelial liver cell lines in culture. *Exper. Cell Res.* 1978, **111**: 63–71.

70 Sakakibara K., Umeda M., Satto S., Nagase S.: Production of collagen and acidic glycosaminoglycans by an epithelial liver cell clone in culture. *Exper. Cell Res.* 1977, **111**: 159–165.

71 Seyer J. M., Hutcheson E. T., Kang A. H.: Collagen polymorphism in normal and cirrhotic human liver. *J. Clin. Invest.* 1977, **59**: 241–248.

72 Sinn W., Sudhakaran P. R., Von Figura K.: Stimulation of heparan sulfate synthesis in cultured rat hepatocytes by (+)-catechin. *Biochem. J.* 1981, **200**: 51–57.

73 Smith, B. D., Niles R.: Characterization of collagen synthesized by normal and chemically transformed rat liver epithelial cell lines. *Biochemistry* 1980, **19**: 1820–1825.

74 Sudhakaran P. R., Sinn W., Von Figura K.: Regulation of heparan sulphate metabolism by adenosine 3′:5′-cyclic monophosphate in hepatocytes in culture. *Biochem. J.* 1980, **1922**: 395–402.

75 Tankum J. W., Hynes R. O.: Plasma fibronectin is synthesized and secreted by hepatocytes. *J. Biol. Chem.* 1983, **258**: 4641–4647.

76 Tanaka M., Fukunaga M., Watanabe K., Kaneko Y., Takahashi T., Ishikawa E.: Fat-storing cells (Ito's cell) of human liver. *Acta Pathol. Jpn.* 1981, **31**: 55–63.

77 Tanner M. S., Jackson D., Mowat A. P.: Hepatic collagen synthesis in a rat model of cirrhosis, and its modification by colchicine. *J. Pathol.* 1981, **135**: 179–187.

78 Tseng S. C. G., Leep P. C., Ells P. F., Bissell D. M., Smuckler E. A., Stern R.: Collagen production by rat hepatocytes and sinusoidal cells in primary monolayer culture. *Hepatology* 1982, **2**: 13–18.

79 Tseng S. C. G., Smuckler E. A., Stern R.: Types of collagen synthesized by normal rat liver hepatocytes in primary culture. *Hepatology* 1983, **3**: 955–963.

80 Vlodavsky I., Gospodarowicz D.: Respective involvement of laminin and fibronectin in the adhesion of human carcinoma and sarcoma cells. *Nature* 1980, **289**: 304–306.

81 Voss B., Allam S., Rauterberg J., Ullrich K., Gieselmann V., Von Figura K.: Primary cultures of rat hepatocytes synthesize fibronectin. *Biochem. Biophys. Res. Commun.* 1979, **90**: 1348–1354.

82 Voss B., Rauterberg J., Pott G., Brehmer U., Allam S., Lehmann R., Von Bassetwitz D. B.: Nonparenchymal cells cultivated from explants of fibrotic liver resemble endothelial and smooth muscle cells from blood vessel walls. *Hepatology* 1982, **2**: 19–28.

83 Weiss J. B., Ayad S.: An introduction to collagen. *In: Collagen in Health and Disease*, J. B. Weiss, M. I. V. Jayson (Eds): Churchill Livingstone, Edinburgh, 1982, pp 1–17.

Research in *Isolated and cultured hepatocytes* A. Guillouzo & C. Guguen-Guillouzo eds., pp. 225–258
© 1986 John Libbey Eurotext Ltd./INSERM.

11

Matrix and hormonal regulation of differentiation in liver cultures

Lola M. REID, Masaki NARITA, Michiyasu FUJITA,
Zenobia MURRAY, Clifford LIVERPOOL and
Lawrence ROSENBERG

Department of Molecular Pharmacology, Albert Einstein College of Medicine, 1300 Morris Park Avenue, Bronx, New York 10461 (LMR, MN*, MF, ZM, CL) and Orthopedic and Connective Tissue Research Laboratories, Montefiore Hospital and Medical Center, 111 East 210 Street, Bronx, New York 10467, USA (LR)

* Current address: Department of Pediatric Stomatology, School of Dentistry, Hokkaido University, Sapporo, Hokkaido 060, Japan.

SUMMARY

The potential for studying differentiated liver cells under defined conditions in culture has been greatly enhanced by recent innovations in cell culture. The innovations under development are designed to mimic critical cell-cell interactions that are thought to effect differentiation *in vivo*. These cell-cell interactions are mimicked by the use of serum-free, hormonally defined media and substrata of extracellular matrix, each carefully designed for a specific cell type. In the case of liver, there are now several hormonally defined media (HDM) described for both normal and neoplastic hepatocytes. The use of HDM in combination with tissue culture plastic has resulted in culture conditions that permit the cells to survive for approximately one week, that strongly select for the parenchymal cells, and that achieve high levels of cytoplasmic mRNAs encoding liver-specific functions. However, the maintenance of normal liver-specific mRNA levels under these conditions has been shown due to increased mRNA stability and not due to sustained liver-specific transcriptional signals. The use of matrix substrata in combination with the hormonally defined media has resulted in liver cultures that can last for weeks to months (depending on the type of matrix substrata), that select for parenchymal cells, that determine whether or not the hepatocytes can grow (influenced by the type of collagens) and that maintain stably for weeks high cytoplasmic concentrations of liver-specific mRNAs and lowered levels of common gene mRNAs. It is unknown at this time if the maintenance of differentiated functions under these conditions is via transcriptional or post-transcriptional regulation. These findings indicate both the rapid development of new culture technologies for liver cells and other differentiated cell types. They also indicate important new perspectives on the regulation of differentiation. One of the most important is that whereas in the past and from investigations *in vivo*, it was thought that differentiation is primarily regulated at the transcriptional level, recent evidence, especially evidence derived from cells cultured using the new technologies, indicates that post-transcriptional regulation of differentiation is much more important than hitherto realized. Thus, hormonal or matrix induced changes in the output of a specific differentiated product may reflect changes in any of a number of regulatory sites including: transcription (rate of sythesis of messenger RNA), splicing, messenger RNA half life, efficiency of translation, post-translational modifications, rate of secretion or incorporation into an appropriate cellular compartment. As sophistication in cell culture technology grows with the development of more defined media and defined matrix substrata, the ability to manipulate the differentiation of the liver cells at one or more of these regulatory levels should be achieved. Such achievements are the hopes for the many investigators working to define culture technology and to ascertain the critical hormonal and matrix regulatory factors in liver cell differentiation.

Introduction

Hepatocytes are typical of differentiated cells expressing a variety of tissue-specific functions which are altered qualitatively and quantitatively in various physiological circumstances. However, until recently these processes could not be studied *in vitro*, since procedures used in preparing liver cells for culture have invariably led to their dedifferentiation and death within a matter of 1–2 weeks (7, 8, 39). Consequently, investigators wishing to study some differentiated function(s) in liver have resigned themselves to studying the liver *in vivo* or studying liver slices or small chunks of tissues *in vitro*, conditions under which tissue-specific functions are maintained.

Recent breakthroughs in cell culture technology (which are reviewed in references 4, 5, 55, 59, 117, 162, 163) are providing methods by which to establish individual cell types, including hepatocytes, in culture with retention of their differentiated phenotype. The breakthroughs include the elimination of serum (now shown to be toxic and/or inhibitory to hepatocytes and various epithelial cells) (4, 5, 35, 44, 72, 117), the development of better basal media and serum-free, hormonally defined media designed for each cell type (4, 5, 139) and the use of substrata of tissue-specific extracellular matrix or matrix components (35, 66, 67, 89, 90, 120–123, 162, 204, 205, 215–217).

In this review, we will not discuss in any detail hormonal or matrix regulation of growth of liver cells in culture, since a review on regeneration studies is presented elsewhere in this volume (see Chapter 2 by McGowan). We will restrict our attention to studies on the new cell culture technologies developed for liver cells and on the findings on hormonal and matrix regulation of gene expression in liver cells under these new cell culture conditions.

Classical cell culture conditions

As a background for the discussion of the new culture conditions, it is necessary to acknowledge the classical cell culture conditions that are the mainstay in most laboratories today. The usual methods of preparing cells for culture start with the disruption of the tissue and dispersal into single cell suspensions. The cells are then plated onto a tissue culture plastic (TCP) substratum and provided with a medium. The medium is composed of a basal medium with a specific mixture of salts, amino acids, trace elements, carbohydrates etc and which is supplemented from 5–25% with a biological fluid, usually serum (see Fig. 1). Although some investigators utilize the autologous serum to the cell types to be cultured, it is more common that the serum derives from animals that are routinely slaughtered for commercial usage such as cows, horses, sheep or pigs.

As shown diagramatically in Fig. 2, when the tissues are disrupted and first plated into culture, the cultures are referred to as 'primary cultures'. Under classical cell culture conditions, such primary culture last typically for 1–2 weeks. If one is successful at isolating a specific cell type by cloning the cells (deriving an entire cell

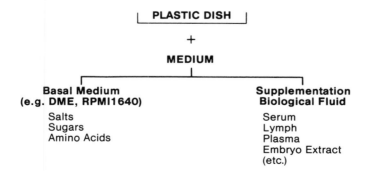

CLASSICAL CELL CULTURE

Fig. 1. Classical cell culture conditions. Under classical cell culture conditions, tissues or stock cultures are dissociated into single cell suspensions and seeded onto tissue culture plastic dishes and in medium. The medium contains a specific mixture of salts, sugars, amino acids, trace elements etc and is supplemented with one or more biological fluids. The most common biological fluid used is serum usually derived from animals such as cows, horses, sheep or other animals that are routinely slaughtered for commercial purposes.

culture from one cell) and by passaging the cells from dish to dish, the cultures are referred to as a 'cell strain'. By definition, cell strains have a limited life span, usually 50–60 passages. If a permanent, cloned cell population is established, the cultures are referred to as a 'cell line'. Cell lines can occur, but do so infrequently, as a result of spontaneous 'transformation' of a cell strain. However, the frequency of conversion of a cell strain to a cell line is greatly augmented by exposing the cells to some oncogenic event: treatment with radiation, chemicals or viruses. Thus, a standard approach to the establishment of a specific cell type in culture is to establish a cell strain and then intentionally transform it. This approach entails significant risks: usually the differentiative potential of the cells can be partially or completely lost (7, 39). An alternative has been to resort to minimally deviant neoplastic cells carried as transplantable tumour lines in syngeneic or immunosuppressed hosts. Such tumour lines can be adapted more readily to culture than can normal cells. Using this approach many partially differentiated cell cultures have been established (39).

Hepatocytes under standard, classical cell culture conditions spread to a squamous-like shape, appear increasingly translucent and agranular, and rapidly lose their granular endoplasmic reticulum. Rapid morphological deterioration is accompanied by decreased biochemical functions resulting in a loss, within 3–5 days, of all tissue-specific functions and, within one to two weeks, of viable cells (7, 39).

FORMS OF CELL CULTURE

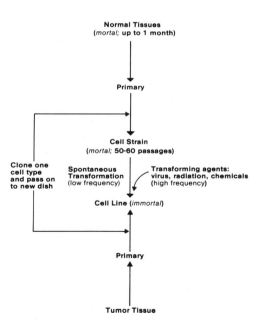

Fig. 2.
The forms of cell culture. Three forms of cell culture exist: primary cultures, cell strains and cell lines. When normal or neoplastic tissue is dissociated and put into culture, it is referred to as a primary culture. In primary cultures, there are usually multiple cell types present. The cultures survive under classical cell culture conditions for 1–2 weeks or, if plated onto collagenous substrata, for approximately 1 month. If the investigator(s) succeed(s) at cloning a specific cell type (deriving an entire population from one cell) from the primary cultures of normal cells and succeed(s) at passaging the cells from dish to dish, the cloned cell population is referred to as a 'cell strain'. Preparing cell strains has been routinely successful for most types of normal fibroblasts but rarely so for epithelial cell types. Most cell strains survive for approximately 50–60 passages and then undergo 'senescence', in which they gradually slow their growth rate, then stop mitosis and then die. If a cell strain continues proliferating idefinitely and becomes a permanent cell population, it is referred to as a 'cell line'. Although the rate of spontaneous transformation from cell strains to cell lines is quite low, that rate can be dramatically increased by using various transforming agents such as tranforming viruses, radiation or chemical carcinogens. Experimental transformation of cell strains is a standard approach for establishing certain cell types in culture. Cloned cell populations from tumours are easier to establish in culture than normal cells and usually automatically become permanent cell populations. All cell lines, whether from spontaneously or experimentally transformed cell strains or from cloned tumour cell populations, have properties that deviate from normal and show a loss in differentiated functions.

The morphological and biochemical findings have been extended in recent years by analyses using recombinant DNA technologies and examining specific gene expression. Within a few hours of dissociation, the transcription of most tissue-specific mRNAs in liver was significantly reduced, and by 24 hours was less than 1% of normal. By contrast, the transcription of mRNAs for common genes such as actin and tubulin increased many fold within a few hours but returned to normal by 24 hours (19, 72). Over the life span of these primary cultures, usually 1–2 weeks, the tissue-specific mRNA transcriptional signals remained low or not detectable, whereas the common gene mRNA transcription remained at levels comparable to *in vivo*. Furthermore, those tissue-specific mRNAs already transcribed at the time of dissociation of the liver, degraded at an exponential rate such that by 5 days of culture, the cytoplasmic mRNA levels for even the most abundant tissue-specific mRNA species were no longer detectable, resulting in dedifferentiation of the cultures (71–73).

There is substantial evidence that these classical culture conditions have been inadequate for maintaining normal cells primarily because the technologies involve the destruction of critical cell-cell relationships that *in vivo* sustain the viability and differentiative function of the tissues (4–6, 21, 55, 131, 163). Malignant tumours, known to contain one (or at most two or three) cell types proliferating in an unregulated fashion, would, therefore, be cells that are qualitatively or quantitatively autonomous to the cellular interactions. That autonomy gives them a selective advantage *in vitro*, and makes them more easily adaptable to cell culture conditions.

The corollary is that development of culture conditions for normal cells requires maintenance of or simulation of critical cell-cell relationships (21, 54, 55, 122, 163). For example, in contrast to the findings with the dissociated liver cells, Clayton & Darnell (20) showed that if liver is put into culture in the form of tissue slices or small chunks of tissue, the transcription of tissue-specific functions is sustained for as long as the slices or chunks are intact, usually up to 2 days. In classical cell culture technologies an especially important cell-cell interaction, the epithelial-mesenchymal relationship, has been simulated, in part, by the use of feeder layers of cells or co-cultures, techniques found valuable for primary cultures of many types of differentiated epithelial cells (21, 54, 55, 122, 163; and discussed in considerable detail for liver cultures elsewhere in this volume). Now numerous research efforts are focused on analysing and defining the factors mediating such relationships to develop cell culture technologies permitting maintenance of many cell types under completely defined conditions (5, 6, 117). As shown in Figs 3 & 4, the factors found relevant to the maintenance of differentiated cells are:

Soluble factors — hormones, growth factors, specific nutrients and trace elements and derived from autocrine, paracrine and endocrine cell-cell interactions. Although there are some hormonal requirements needed by all cell types (eg transferrin and insulin-like growth factors), the composition of factors is cell-type specific. The requirements for a given cell type can be defined empirically by methods developed by Sato and associates (4, 5) and by Ham & McKeehan (59). These factors are presented in the form of serum-free, 'hormonally defined' media (HDM). The requirements change somewhat depending on whether the cells are to grow or to be fully differentiated. There appear to be some factors that are required both for growth and differentiation, and some that act only as

**COMPONENTS NEEDED FOR MAINTENANCE OF
DIFFERENTIATED CELLS**

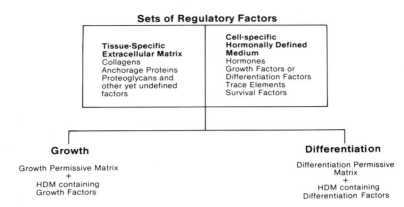

Fig. 3.   Components needed for maintenance of differentiated cells. Numerous studies in recent
years have determined that adult differentiated cells can be maintained in culture with
retention of many of their tissue-specific functions. Two groups of factors have been found
essential for such cultures: soluble factors that include hormones and growth factors
stemming from autocrine, paracrine, and endocrine cellular interactions and insoluble ones
found in the extracellular matrix and usually presented as a substratum for the cells. The
identity of the soluble factors required by a specific cell type can be deduced empirically by
determining the requirements for a minimally deviant neoplastic cell to grow clonally in a
serum-free medium. The resulting serum-free, hormonally defined medium (HDM) for the
tumour cells is the starting point for deducing the factors required for a HDM for the normal
cells. The realization underlying this approach, is that tumour cells are hormonally regulated
by a subset of the factors regulating their normal counterparts, or that neoplastic
transformation results in cells that are qualitatively and/or quantitatively autonomous to
specific growth factors. For attachment, long-term survival, normal cell shapes and sustained
expression of tissue-specific functions, cells need extracellular matrix substrata containing
specific collagens, anchorage proteins, proteoglycans and other factors. Some of the factors,
eg the proteoglycans, are tissue-specific. *In vivo* the chemistry of the extracellular matrix
changes when cells shift from a quiescent to regenerating state. Thus, chemically distinct
matrix substrata are needed for optimal growth and differentiation of cells.

mitogens or only as differentiation factors.

Insoluble factors — extracellular matrix components are usually presented as a
substratum for the cells. In some instances, when a purified matrix component is
soluble, it is presented in the medium. The matrices used today are either isolated,
purified matrix components (87, 88, 215–217) or crude extracts of tissues or cell
layers enriched in extracellular matrix (reviewed in reference 162).

Hormonally defined media for liver

In recent years, one of the revolutionary changes in cell culture has been the
introduction of serum-free, hormonally defined media (HDM). The history and
technologies for HDM have been extensively reviewed recently by Barnes & Sato (4)
and by Mather (117). In general, the development of an HDM begins by defining the
hormonal and growth factor requirements for a minimally deviant neoplastic cell

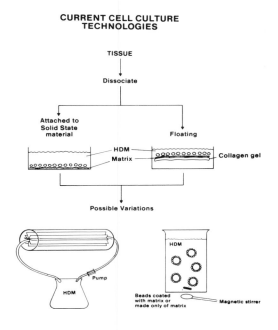

CURRENT CELL CULTURE TECHNOLOGIES

Fig. 4.
Current cell culture technologies. The current approaches to establishing cells into culture are to dissociate the tissues and attach the cells to an appropriate matrix substratum and in an appropriate serum-free, hormonally defined medium (HDM). The matrix substratum and the HDM must be the appropriate ones for a specific cell type and must be the appropriate composition to effect either growth and/or differentiation of the cells. These conditions can be presented in many ways. Several examples are shown. The matrix can be smeared onto any culture dish and the cells seeded on the immobile matrix substratum and into an HDM. To permit optimal cell shape changes that might bring about some aspects of differentiation, the matrix can be coated onto collagen gels. After the cells are attached to the matrix on the gels, the gels are detached from the dishes and allowed to float in the HDM. Cells can also be attached to matrix-coated beads or beads made of matrix, and the beads-matrix-cells kept suspended in an HDM by a magnetic stirrer. The matrix can be used to coat the vanes in a mass mammalian cell culture apparatus, and the HDM pumped through the apparatus.

line. Since a cell line is already adapted to culture, it can readily be used in clonal growth assays to define growth requirements under serum-free conditions. The HDM for the tumour cells usually contains a subset of the requirements and is, therefore, a starting point in defining the requirements for the normal cellular counterparts to the tumour cells (17, 35, 40).

This approach has been used to develop an HDM for hepatocytes. Since the mid-70s, an increasing number of studies have utilized serum-free media to which one or more hormonal or growth factors were tested for their influence on growth or on some differentiative function (35, 48, 71–73, 91, 104, 110–112, 128, 150, 178–180, 187, 211). In serum-free medium or in serum-free medium to which only one or two hormones or growth factors are added, hepatocyte cultures survive for 4–5 days, approximately half the life span of the cells in SSM. However, the differentiated functions in the cells in serum-free medium were at higher levels and were more stable than ever seen in cultures in SSM (55, 102, 211).

An HDM that permitted more long-term cultures was developed by Gatmaitan *et al.* (40), who systematically screened over 70 factors to deduce an HDM for hepatoma cells. They found that the HDM's composition was dependent upon the type of substratum used for the cells (see Table 1). Thus, on collagenous substrata as opposed to tissue culture plastic, the cells required fewer factors for clonal growth. The same medium was found effective with hepatoma cell lines derived from mice, rats, and humans. Utilizing the HDM developed by Gatmaitan *et al.* (40) as a starting point, Enat *et al.* (35) developed an HDM for primary cultures of normal rat liver cells. This HDM was found to select for parenchymal cells even when the cells were on tissue culture plastic (35, 72) resulting in cultures that were mostly hepatocytes

Table 1. Constituents of 'hormonally defined media' for normal and neoplastic rat hepatocytes.

Factor	Hepatocytes on tissue culture plastic	Hepatomas on tissue culture plastic	Hepatomas on Type I collagen
Epidermal growth factor	50 ng/ml	Not required	Not required
Insulin	10 μg/ml	100 μg/ml	1–5 μg/ml
Glucagon	10 μg/ml	10 μg/ml	5 μg/ml
Hydrocortisone	not required	1×10^{-8}M	not required
Transferrin	not required	10 μg/ml	not required
* Linoleic acid	5 μg/ml	10 μg/ml	5 μg/ml
Triiodothyronine	not required	1×10^{-9}M	not required
Prolactin	20 mU/ml	2 mU/ml	2 mU/ml
Growth hormone	10 μU/ml	10 μU/ml	10 μU/ml
Trace elements			
Zinc	1×10^{-10}M	1×10^{-10}M	1×10^{-10}M
Copper	1×10^{-7}M	1×10^{-7}M	1×10^{-7}M
Selenium	3×10^{-10}M	3×10^{-10}M	3×10^{-10}M

These culture conditions permit clonal growth of many hepatoma cell lines (human, rat and mouse cell lines have been tried). However, normal hepatocytes will grow at high densities ($>10^5$ cells/60 mm dishes) but not at clonal seeding densities (10^2–10^3 cells/60 mm dishes) when maintained in the above hormonally defined medium. Furthermore, unless protease inhibitors and/or specific matrix substrata are used, the cells must be seeded in a mixture of 5–10% serum plus the hormones for a few hours (4–6 hours) and then transferred into the serum-free hormonally defined medium.
* Linoleic acid must be present in combination with fatty acid-free bovine serum albumin (Pentax, Inc.) at a 1:1 molar ratio. If added alone, it is quite toxic to the cells.
Pituitary hormones can be purchased from commercial sources or alternatively obtained through the NIH hormone distribution service.
Details of the development of these defined media are available in references 35, 40, 71–73, 117.

within a few days. However, the life span of the primary cultures was found to be only 1 week, at which time the cells peeled off the plates in sheets. However, achievement of culture life spans in excess of 3 weeks was achieved by using collagenous or matrix substrata in combination with the HDM (see next section).

Serum-free media and/or HDM improved the differentiation of the liver cultures when they were assayed at the protein levels for liver-specific functions (35, 48, 71–73, 91, 104, 110–112, 187). Furthermore, in contrast to the cultures in SSM in which liver-specific transcriptional signals were undetectable, the cultures in HDM had liver-specific transcriptional signals that were detectable, albeit low (3–12% of normal) (19, 20, 71–73). Of considerable interest, the cytoplasmic mRNA concentrations for liver-specific mRNAs were expressed at almost *in vivo* levels during the life span of these cultures on tissue culture plastic (72) (Fig. 5). The discrepancy between the low transcriptional activity and yet normal cytoplasmic levels of specific mRNA species was found due to mRNA stabilization in the serum-free, hormonally defined medium (72). Although the dogma in molecular biology has been that differentiation is mostly transcriptionally regulated (24, 31), there has been increasing evidence from *in vivo* studies on other tissues or organisms for post-transcriptional mechanisms playing important roles in the expression of tissue-specific functions (14, 18). It is now evident that post-transcriptional regulation occurs also in hepatocytes and is the primary form of regulation in primary cultures on tissue culture plastic (19, 20, 71, 72).

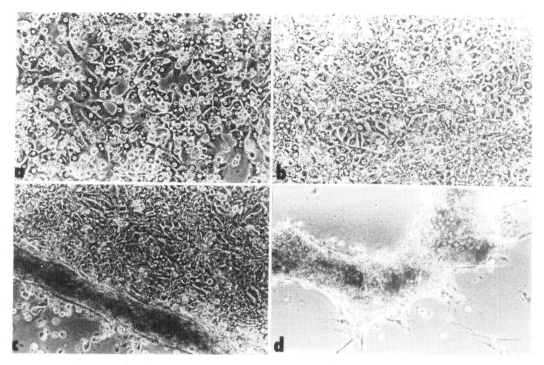

Fig. 5. Primary cultures of normal hepatocytes on tissue culture plastic and in serum-free, hormonally defined medium. Adult, hepatocyte-specific functions deteriorate rapidly in cultures in serum supplemented media (reviewed in references 162 & 163). Furthermore, serum supplementation selects for non-parenchymal cells. If cells are cultured in a serum-free, hormonally defined medium designed for hepatocytes, selection occurs for the parenchymal cells and the adult, tissue-specific functions are maintained for as long as the cultures last. If the cells are plated onto tissue culture plastic, the culture life span is approximately one week. In these phase photomicrographs, cultures are shown at 24 hours (*a*), 5 days (*b*), 7 days (*c*) and 9 days (*d*) after plating. Although most of the cells in cultures are hepatocytes, and although measures of cytoplasmic levels of tissue-specific mRNA remain at normal levels through day 7 of culture, the cells do not remain attached to the dishes. After approximately 7 days in culture, the cell layer rolls up like a sheet and detaches from the dish (see *c*). Thereafter, only a few clumps of contracted cells remain on the dishes (*d*).

The expression of common genes, represented by actin and tubulin, was quite distinct from that of the tissue-specific genes (19, 20, 72). *In vivo* in quiescent liver, the common genes show strong transcriptional signals but extremely low cytoplasmic levels of mRNA, implicating some mechanism of down regulation in expression. When the liver was dissociated into single cell suspensions, the transcriptional signals for common genes increased many fold within a few hours but returned to normal by 24 hours (19, 20). Thereafter, in primary liver cultures, rates of transcription for these genes remained at levels comparable to that seen in quiescent liver *in vivo*. However, measures of cytoplasmic mRNA levels by Northern blots for the common genes were at high levels under all medium conditions tested: with and without serum, and in all the combinations of hormones (19, 20, 71, 72). Thus, similar to the tissue-specific genes, there were changes observed in the cytoplasmic mRNA levels that did not correlate with a comparable change in the transcriptional signals for those genes. This implies that the expression of common genes in cultured liver cells was also regulated by a post-transcriptional, presumably mRNA stabilization, phenomena. However, the mRNAs for the common genes were stabilized in serum supplemented medium (SSM), in serum-free media and in HDM.

Of the hormones tested by various groups, dexamethasone has proved to be one of the most beneficial in maintaining primary liver cultures and in stabilizing differentiated functions (48, 55, 57, 73, 110–112, 127, 187, 211). Addition of dexamethasone to serum-free media or to SSM resulted in cultures that attached better, that lasted longer, and that showed an increase in tissue-specific functions such as albumin secretion (48, 55, 57, 73, 110–112, 127, 211). Marceau *et al.* (110–112) showed that dexamethasone induced the formation of a fibronectin-rich

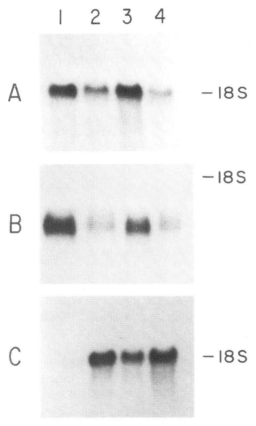

Fig. 6.
Influence of media on gene expression in primary liver cultures. Normal rat liver cells are plated onto tissue culture plastic and into RPMI 1640 supplemented with 10% fetal bovine serum plus the hormones and growth factors given for normal hepatocytes (SSM/HDM) in the Table. After 24 hours, some of the cultures were switched into RPMI 1640 supplemented with 10% fetal bovine serum (SSM); some were switched into a serum-free, hormonally defined medium containing only the components given in the Table for normal hepatocytes (HDM); and some were maintained in the mixture of the serum plus hormonally supplemented medium (HDM/SSM). After 5 days in culture, the cytoplasmic RNA was purified and assayed by Northern blot analysis using cDNA probes. The details of the methods and the experiment are as described by Jefferson *et al.* (72). The blots indicate that the concentrations of cytoplasmic mRNA for liver-specific functions are greatly reduced in cells cultured in SSM but are maintained at levels approximating those *in vivo* in cells in HDM. The loss of the tissue-specific mRNAs in cells in SSM is not due to the absence of specific hormones, since cells cultured in HDM/SSM also lose their tissue-specific mRNAs albeit at a slightly slower rate. Rather, serum supplementation is itself inhibitory to liver-specific gene expression. As explained in more detail in the text, the sustained cytoplasmic mRNA levels for tissue-specific functions in cultures in HDM are due to mRNA stabilization, not due to sustained tissue-specific transcription. Lane 1 = RNA was prepared from freshly isolated liver tissue (*in vivo*); Lane 2 = RNA was prepared from liver cultures maintained in HDM/SSM; Lane 3 = RNA was prepared from liver cultures maintained in HDM; Lane 4 = RNA was prepared from liver cultures maintained in SSM; Panel A = Hybridized with a cDNA probe to rat albumin; Panel B = Hybridized with a cDNA probe to α_1-antitrypsin; Panel C = Hybridized with a cDNA probe to actin.

extracellular matrix, a finding interesting in light of the findings by Diegelmann & Guzelian, and subsequently by Jefferson *et al.* (73), that dexamethasone suppressed the synthesis of Type I collagen in primary liver cultures (32, 57). These results suggest that dexamethasone may trigger the liver cells to replace one type of extracellular matrix for another. Recently, it was reported that addition of dexamethasone to HDM for primary liver cultures resulted in a significant effect on the transcriptional signals and on the cytoplasmic mRNA levels encoding matrix proteins (eg fibronectin and collagen) but not on any tissue-specific mRNA species such as albumin or ligandin (73). Different findings were reported for cultures in SSM. Dexamethasone altered the transcriptional signals and the mRNA levels for the matrix genes in a pattern similar to that observed in HDM. It also showed no effect on the transcriptional signal for any tissue-specific mRNA species in liver cultures in SSM. However, in the cultures in SSM, dexamethasone significantly augmented cytoplasmic tissue-specific mRNA levels over that found in cultures in SSM but without dexamethasone (73). Thus, at a transcriptional level, dexamethasone was shown to have an effect only on matrix genes, regardless of the medium conditions; and in terms of cytoplasmic mRNA levels, dexamethasone altered expression for matrix genes in a fashion correlated with its effect on the transcription of those genes; but it showed an effect on cytoplasmic levels of tissue-specific mRNAs (eg albumin) only in cultures in SSM. Therefore, the effect of dexamethasone in liver cultures in SSM must be indirect and somehow blocking the deleterious influence of serum on mRNA stability. Whether this protective effect against serum is due to dexamethasone's influence on the synthesis of specific matrix factors is unknown at this time.

In later studies, it was found that even in serum-free medium with no hormonal additives, liver-specific mRNAs achieved some measure of stability such that cytoplasmic levels were at least at 25–50% of levels seen *in vivo* (71). With the addition of the hormones and growth factors found active on liver cultures, the cytoplasmic concentrations of tissue-specific mRNAs increased to normal levels even though the transcriptional signals for these same mRNAs remained at levels similar to that in serum-free medium with no hormonal additives. Varying combinations of the hormones and growth factors preferentially stabilized specific mRNA species (71). For example, ligandin mRNAs were optimally stabilized in an HDM containing insulin, growth hormone, prolactin, epidermal growth factor, linoleic acid/BSA and trace elements. By contrast, albumin mRNAs were best stabilized in an HDM with the same factors plus glucagon and the most critical hormone in the HDM for stabilization of albumin was epidermal growth factor.

In all the investigations to date on liver cultures on tissue culture plastic and in any serum-free HDM, the differentiation of the cells has been primarily post-transcriptionally regulated, presumably by mRNA half life (19, 20, 71–73). These findings are in sharp distinction to the results on liver *in vivo* or in which the liver tissue structure remains intact, conditions under which differentiation of liver is well documented to be under transcriptional control (20, 24, 31). Empirically, some aspect(s) of tissue structure, destroyed when cells are dispersed into single cell suspensions, is essential for maintenance of tissue-specific transcription (20). Possible candidates include extracellular matrix components.

Extracellular matrix for liver cultures

General comments

Interest in the extracellular matrix has increased dramatically in recent years due to increasing awareness of its relevance in the regulation of growth and differentiation. Several recent reviews and books, especially those of Bornstein & Sage (12), Miller (124, 126), Yamada (215, 216), Hay (62), Kleinman *et al.* (87–89), Reid & Jefferson (162–163), Bernfield (6), Barnes (5) and Trelsted (199) provide excellent coverage of the past and present studies on extracellular matrix. Studies on the relevance of matrix in biological processes have utilized two approaches: 1) studies of one, two or a few purified components (5, 53, 78, 87, 88, 97, 98, 195, 201, 215–217); and, 2) use of crude extracts enriched for matrix (162, 204, 205). Crude extracts of cell layers or of whole tissues are made with protocols designed to select for the insoluble components in extracellular matrix. The crude extracts are then utilized as cell culture substrata for either clonal cell lines and/or primary cultures of tissues (35, 109, 133, 168, 204, 205).

Both approaches have been essential. Much of the matrix is inherently insoluble due to extensive crosslinking of its components. Therefore, many of its components are difficult to isolate intact (for example, Type IV collagen; 5, 88, 95, 96, 166, 197) and often require extraction methods which destroy parts of the molecules. Most of the matrix components studied to date (eg Type I collagen, fibronectin) are those which are amenable to solubilization by standard methods of chemical isolation and purification. There are presumed to be matrix components which have not been isolated and purified because of the inherent insolubility of matrix.

In addition to the technical problems, the influence of the matrix on cells is the net result of a complex mixture of molecules not just one or two. The tendency of scientists to analyse one component by itself, albeit an essential approach, cannot exclude the need for studies which acknowledge that the matrix is a mixture of components operating in synchrony.

The chemistry of extracellular matrix

Although the chemistry of extracellular matrix has been studied for many years (3, 12, 37, 45, 62, 87, 95, 114, 124, 126, 216, 217), the studies have focused mostly on only a few of the components of extracellular matrix, particularly those that were soluble in standard extraction solutions. With increasing sophistication in methods for purifying matrix components (95, 124, 126) and especially with methods for cloning matrix genes (eg 10, 92, 113) there has been an expansion in the number of matrix components under investigation as well as an increase in the number of matrix components identified. Thus, the chemistry of extracellular matrix is still incompletely understood. Even so, there is now widespread appreciation of the fact that there are multiple forms of extracellular matrix in every tissue, and each matrix type may play a distinct biological role(s). Although no type of matrix has been studied sufficiently to know all of its components, all matrices consist of collagen scaffoldings (12, 95, 96, 124, 126) to which the cells are bound by multiple types of anchorage proteins (3, 15, 87, 89, 214, 217). Various forms of glycosaminoglycans (GAGs) and proteoglycans (PGs) are present in association with the anchorage

EXTRACELLULAR MATRIX

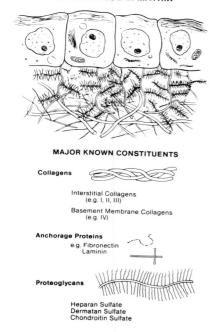

MAJOR KNOWN CONSTITUENTS

Collagens

Interstitial Collagens
(e.g. I, II, III)

Basement Membrane Collagens
(e.g. IV)

Anchorage Proteins
e.g. Fibronectin
Laminin

Proteoglycans

Heparan Sulfate
Dermatan Sulfate
Chondroitin Sulfate

Fig. 7.
Components of the extracellular matrix. All metazoan cells synthesize and are associated with extracellular matrices. The cells are attached by multiple anchorage proteins to a collagen scaffolding. Various proteoglycans are found in association with the anchorage proteins. Both anchorage proteins and proteoglycans are bound to the cell surface via receptors, or, in the case of some proteoglycans, intercalated into the cell membrane via a core protein.

Representative Families of Extracellular Matrix

Collagen Type	Subunits	Molecular Composition	Major Locations	Associated Anchorage Proteins	Major Proteoglycans
Type I	α1 (I) and α2 (I)	[α1 (I)]₂ α2 (I)	Tendon, Skin, Bone	Fibronectin	Dermatan sulfate Chondroitin sulfate
Type II	α1 (II)	[α1 (II)]₃	Cartilage	Chondronectin	Chondroitin sulfate
Type III	α1 (III)	[α1 (III)]₃	Skin, Placenta Blood vessels	Fibronectin	Heparan sulfate
Type IV	α1 (IV) and α2 (IV)	[α1 (IV)] ₃ [α2 (IV)] ₃	Basement membranes	Laminin	Heparan sulfate
Type V	α1 (V), α2 (V), and α3 (V)	[α1(V)]₂α2(V)	Pericellular and matrix	Laminin	Heparan sulfate

Fig. 8. Families of extracellular matrix. Multiple families of extracellular matrices have been described. The different families are identified in terms of the type of collagen forming the scaffolding. As described in more detail in the text, the different collagen types have distinct amino acid compositions and appear to serve somewhat distinct biological functions. Each collagen type is found in association with a particular anchorage protein (plus other anchorage proteins that vary with the cell type) and several proteoglycans, although the proteoglycan named is usually the one in abundance.

proteins (63, 64, 99, 100) and/or operating as transmembrane molecules connecting the cells' cytoskeleton to the extracellular matrix (6, 90, 140, 144–146, 213). These known components are shown in schematic forms in Fig. 7. The different types of matrix are defined in terms of the type of collagen used as the scaffolding. Each collagen type has, in turn, specific anchorage proteins and proteoglycans which are typically associated with it. For example, a 'Type I' matrix consists of Type I collagen, fibronectin (plus other anchorage proteins), and chondroitin sulfate or dermatan sulfate proteoglycans. By contrast, a 'Type IV' matrix consists of Type IV collagen, laminin (plus other anchorage proteins) and heparan sulfate proteoglycans. In Fig. 8 the most well known matrix families in mammalian tissues are listed.

Every cell that is bound into a tissue structure, secretes and is associated with one or more types of matrix, and all contain a collagen (12, 124, 126), multiple anchorage proteins (215) and multiple proteoglycans (63, 124, 126). When the cell undergoes a change in its physiological status (eg from quiescence to growth), it secretes either an altogether distinct matrix or alters one or more components in the matrix (15, 116, 169, 209). The story is less clear for free floating cells such as haemopoietic cells, although increasingly certain matrix components are being found to be produced by these cells and to play a critical role in their functioning.

The extracellular matrix of the liver

General considerations. Chemical analysis of liver as well as immunochemistry and localization studies on matrix components (discussed in more detail in the next sections on individual matrix components) have indicated that the liver contains multiple matrix types (mostly types I, III, IV & V) which are susceptible to change during regeneration or during pathological conditions (2, 23, 41, 51, 116, 118, 119, 134, 169, 176, 181, 206). Localization studies of liver matrix components at light microscopic and ultrastructural levels have been done using antibodies to matrix components and immunoperoxidase or fluorescent staining (23, 52, 58, 61, 176, 206). They have found that there are several matrix types (types I, III & IV) in between the layer of hepatocytes and endothelial cells forming the sinusoids. In the quiescent liver, the hepatocyte contributes a Type III matrix; the endothelial cells contribute a Type IV matrix; and fibroblasts contribute a Type I matrix. Over most of the hepatocyte-sinusoidal surface, the matrix is a mixture of Type III and Type IV matrices. However, in regions of architectural stress, Type I matrix is present. In the regenerating liver, the chemistry of the matrix changes: the hepatocytes convert to synthesizing a Type IV matrix. Thus, the hepatocyte-sinuscidal area becomes an intact basal lamina produced both by the hepatocytes and by the endothelial cells. Under pathological conditions in which the liver endures chronic insults and becomes cirrhotic, the matrix chemistry again changes: now the hepatocytes as well as certain non-parenchymal cellular components synthesize a Type I matrix. These results are particularly useful for interpreting some of the findings of studies in cell culture.

Anchorage proteins in liver. Anchorage protein is a generic term for molecules that attach cells to collagens (or to a substratum) (3, 13, 129, 215, 216). There are only two anchorage proteins that have been identified and well characterized in liver: fibronectin and laminin (15, 38, 74, 177, 181, 194, 216). Several other putative anchorage proteins have been identified but very little is known about them (138, 141, 155, 171). These include hepatonectin (155) and liver cell adhesion molecules (141). All of these factors are known to facilitate attachment of hepatocytes to dishes.

Fibronectin is a glycoprotein that exists in at least two different forms, differing in solubility and molecular weight (3, 92, 216). One form is known as plasma fibronectin, is synthesized by the liver, and is a major protein in blood plasma (300 μg/ml). A related form, known as cellular fibronectin, is found on the surface of many different cell types. Fibronectin is composed of polypeptide sub-units linked by disulfide bonds. There is a cell binding domain of fibronectin responsible for cell surface interactions (217). Proteolytic fragments containing only this region are capable of mediating cell attachment and spreading on plastic substrata. Recent data indicate that the minimum signal necessary for the binding of cells to fibronectin resides in the tetrapeptide, arginine-glycine-asparagine-serine, and that this amino acid sequence is found in at least five other proteins (154). Other distinctions in either chemistry or biology between plasma and cellular fibronectin have been extensively reviewed by Yamada (3, 129, 215, 216) and will not be presented here.

Plasma fibronectin is synthesized and secreted by hepatocytes of rats and hamsters in primary culture (38, 74, 194). Fibronectin has been implicated in adhesive and ligand binding functions for hepatocytes (38, 74, 171, 177, 194). Purified plasma fibronectin, used as a precoated film on plastic can replace the serum dependence for cell attachment in primary liver cultures and in hepatomas (74). Fibronectin affects cell morphology; cells spread more on fibronectin-coated dishes than on tissue culture plastic. If plated on to dishes coated with fibronectin, hepatocytes remain attached to culture dishes longer, whether in SSM, in serum-free media or in HDM. Although fibronectin has been shown to have significant influence on the differentiation of other cell types (extensively reviewed by Yamada: 216, 217), its demonstrated influence on primary cultures of hepatocytes has been as an attachment factor (38, 171, 194). Thus far, there has been no evidence that fibronectin will significantly alter gene expression, either in terms of transcription or in terms of cytoplasmic mRNA levels, in primary liver cultures (Reid, unpublished results).

Laminin is a glycoprotein found in basal lamina and responsible for anchoring most epithelial cells and endothelial cells to Type IV collagen (15, 38, 195, 198, 215). Laminin was first purified by Timpl *et al.* (198) from transplantable tumour tissue. Chemical characterization of basement membranes in normal tissues has been difficult because the constituents are highly cross-linked and therefore not soluble without pepsin digestion, which destroys some of the matrix components. Moreover, purification from normal tissues usually results in a small amount of material available for examination (45, 81, 82, 124, 126). A technical breakthrough occurred with the discovery of tumours such as the EHS sarcoma and parietal endoderm cell lines which constitutively produce large amounts of basement membrane proteins that are not as cross-linked or as insoluble as in normal tissues (11, 101, 198). The tumours are used as a reliable source of large quantities of basement membrane proteins that can readily be purified (198).

The structure of laminin is composed of 3 α chains, each 200 kdaltons and 1 β of 400 kdaltons, and contains about 14–20% carbohydrates (215). The chains are covalently linked by disulfide bonds to form a molecule which is approximately 1 000 000 daltons. Laminin has a distinctive cruciform shape with at least 3 identical short arms and 1 long arm as well as at least 7 globular domains. For an extensive discussion of its chemistry and structure, see the reviews by Timpl (198) and Yamada (215).

Functionally, laminin serves as an anchorage protein for almost all epithelial cells. It can also mediate the attachment of fibroblasts and other mesenchymal cells to plastic or glass substrata, although it is less effective than fibronectin. Hepatocytes attach to either laminin or fibronectin by functionally independent receptors (15), but show preference for one or the other depending on whether the cells are in a quiescent or regenerating condition (15, 116, 181). Furthermore, in the adult quiescent liver, fibronectin is the preferred anchorage protein, whereas in fetal and regenerating liver, laminin is preferred (15). This indicates that adhesion properties of liver cells are dependent on specific physiological states (15). Further supporting this realization are the findings that the attachment of regenerating or fetal liver cells to dishes can be inhibited by the presence of anti-laminin but not by the presence of anti-fibronectin. Conversely, attachment of adult, quiescent liver cells to dishes is inhibited by antibodies to fibronectin and not by anti-laminin. With fetal cells, laminin has been found effective in promoting not only their attachment to dishes but also in prolonging their growth and their ability to produce and secrete albumin and alphafetoprotein (66). There was a higher degree of DNA synthesis and cell proliferation exhibited during the culture of fetal liver cells on laminin-coated dishes as opposed to fibronectin-coated dishes (66). Preliminary studies on the effects of laminin on liver cell gene expression indicate that, like fibronectin, its effects are minimal.

Collagens. More than 10 types of collagens, each with a somewhat distinct amino acid composition, have been reported (12, 95, 124, 126). However, only 5 have been chemically or biologically characterized to any degree, of which four (types I, III, IV & V) have been found or well characterized in the liver (32, 41, 51, 52, 56, 57, 77, 113, 116, 118, 186, 206). The component polypeptide chains are products of separate genes (10, 17, 126). Their distributions and molecular chain compositions are shown in Fig. 8. The collagens are characterized by an amino acid composition containing 33% glycine and 20% proline and hydroxyproline. The basic structure of the α-chain has been shown to contain sequences of repeating Gly-X-Y triplets. The repetitive triplet structure of the chain contributes to the triple helix formation via hydroxyproline residues (12, 37, 42, 95, 124).

There are two basic structural types: fibrillar collagens (eg types I–III) and basement membrane collagens (Type IV) having a nonfibrillar, chicken-wire-like structure (12, 37, 42, 81, 82, 108, 124, 166, 197). The amino acid composition of Type IV collagen shows a higher degree of hydroxylation of the proline and lysine residues, a low content of alanine and arginine, and a high amount of large hydrophobic amino acids. Timpl and co-workers proposed a model of macromolecular structure of Type IV collagen by using a rotary shadowing technique (197). The existance of a 7S cross-linked 'domain' structure of the Type IV collagen molecules was revealed in human placenta (45, 95) bovine lung and murine EHS tumours (95, 96, 197).

Biosynthesis and maturation of collagen. The biosynthesis and maturation of collagens have been described in some detail elsewhere and will be mentioned only briefly in this review (1, 12, 29, 33, 36, 43, 103, 114, 149, 159, 160, 174, 183). The newly synthesized collagen polypeptide chain, referred to as pre-pro-collagen, has an additional hydrophobic amino-terminal signal or leader sequence. Similar to other proteins characterized in the 'Signal Hypothesis' (9), the signal sequence for pre-pro-collagen binds to the rough endoplasmic reticulum and leads the nascent polypeptide chain into the membrane. However, the amino acid sequence of pre-pro-collagen may be significantly longer than that of most other proteins (29, 36). The pre-pro-collagen sequence is cleaved by endopeptidase (36, 114). Hydroxylation and glycosylation reactions are initiated while the pro-peptide chains are being assembled on the ribosomes and continues after the synthesis of complete pro-collagen chains. These reactions terminate when the chains assume a helical formation (1, 12, 36 43, 84).

To form Type I pro-collagen, two pro-α1(I) chains and one pro-α2(II) chain associate, form disulfide bonds at the carboxy terminal end and coil into a triple helical protein (43). The conversion of pro-collagen to collagen requires at least two enzymes: one to remove the amino terminal pro-peptide and the other the carboxy terminal pro-peptide (12, 36, 43, 47, 84, 124, 126). The collagen molecules formed by removal of the pro-peptides assemble spontaneously in the specific membrane to form collagen fibrils (36) and then cross-linked by a series of covalent bonds of certain lysyl and hydroxlysyl residues formed by the enzyme lysyl oxidase (84, 114, 183).

Native collagens are resistant to most proteases (105, 106, 114, 153). The initial step in their breakdown is carried out by a specific collagenase for which there is a collagen type specificity (105, 106). Types IV & V collagens are resistant to cleavage by vertebrate collagenase and appear to require the newly described type-specific collagenase (106). Although trypsin is not found in normal sites of collagen degradation, it is able to degrade types III, IV & V collagens (105, 106, 125).

Localization of collagens in liver. Repeated digestion of normal human liver with pepsin has solubilized types I & III as well as Type V collagen and results in approximately equal amounts of Types I & III (58, 169). From immunocytochemical studies it has been shown that Type I and Type III collagens are present in the matrix around the portal vein and other large blood vessels (23, 51, 52, 176, 206). However, in some studies antibodies failed to detect Type I collagen within the liver lobules or detected it in the periportal areas but not in the sinusoids (51, 52). Other studies, however, clearly showed a reaction of antibodies to Type I collagen along the sinusoidal walls (116). These differences could be related to different specificity of the antibodies used. Types IV & V collagen have been found localized in the basement membranes of portal tract blood vessels, lymphatics, nerves, bile ducts and central vein (58, 116, 176, 206). They are also present between the endothelial lining of the sinusoids and hepatocytes, ie in the space of Disse (116, 176, 206).

In liver cirrhosis (whether due to hepatitis, alcohol, schistosomiasis etc), the collagen content of the liver increases from four- to seven-fold (41, 58, 169). Immunofluorescence studies showed quantitative changes of collagen types in cirrhosis (41). It has been shown that whereas cirrhotic liver produces relatively larger quantities of Type I collagen, regenerating liver synthesizes relatively greater amount of Types IV & V collagen (15, 58, 116, 176, 206).

Collagen synthesis by liver cells. Four cell types exist in the sinusoidal site: hepatocytes, Kupffer cells, endothelial cells and fat-storing cells. Studies have shown that hepatocytes *in vivo* produce Type III, the Kupffer cells produce Type I and the endothelial cells and fat-storing cells produce Type IV collagen (30, 32, 116, 172). Outside the sinusoidal area, the fibroblasts synthesize Types I & III collagen (51, 52, 116). It has been demonstrated that most cell types in culture, including hepatocytes and hepatomas, produce some type of collagen (30, 32, 38, 56, 57, 172, 174, 186). Experiments have suggested that during the first few days in culture, adult rat hepatocytes produce collagen types IV or V. At later stages, the hepatocytes produce Type I collagen (32, 38, 61). Recently, these findings were also corroborated by *in situ* hybridization methods using cDNA probes to detect pro- collagen mRNA levels encoding Type I collagen (172). Plating epithelial cells into culture onto Type I collagen stabilizes the types IV and V collagen synthesized and slows their degradation (6, 25–27). Whether the same occurs to hepatocytes plated onto Type I collagen is unknown.

Collagen as a substratum for liver cell cultures. Hepatocytes, like most epithelial cells, attach better and maintain differentiated properties for longer periods of time when maintained on collagenous substra (5, 34, 40, 53, 66, 67, 70, 87, 88, 120, 121, 123, 185, 191, 208, 217). In most studies, an acid extract of rat tail tendon has been prepared in a variety of forms due to its ease of isolation and preparation. Such an extract consist mostly of Type I collagen with variable amounts of impurities. Several variations in the collagen gel technique have proven useful for hepatocyte cultures: 1) collagen-coated substra (40, 66, 67, 70); 2) floating collagen gels (121, 123); and, 3) nylon meshes coated with collagen (185). The life span of primary hepatocytes cultures can be extended for 2 or 3 weeks on Type I collagen-coated plates. If the collagenous substra are detached and permitted to float, the hepatocytes remain viable and functional for 4–5 weeks (121, 123). Analogous phenomena have been described with other epithelial cell types (34). Another technique is the use of a nylon mesh support system for the collagen gel (185). The advantage of this technique is that it requires very small amounts of collagen material, and the cells can be easily removed intact after a short period of treatment with collagenases.

The augmented differentiative state of liver cells plated onto Type I collagenous substra is associated with more three-dimensional shapes which are permitted by the flexible collagenous substratum (121, 123) and with other matrix components synthesized by the hepatocytes and temporarily stabilized by the Type I collagen gels (25–27). Morphologically, the cells are distinctly different when plated onto collagen gels in contrast to plastic. On collagen gels, the cells assume polygonal shapes which become cuboidal over time. Histology and ultrastructure indicate formation of cellular junctions, and development of polarity, and well-developed endoplasmic reticulum and Golgi bodies. Some functions, such as cytochrome P450 and glucocorticoid-inducible tyrosine aminotransferase, survive for 10–14 days (121, 123, 185). Some functions (eg albumin) are expressed throughout the life span of the culture (121, 123, 185). However, as the cultures age, there is gradual fetalization in which adult- specific functions, such as albumin synthesis, are replaced by fetal-specific ones, such as AFP synthesis (185). Thus, albumin levels, which peak in a

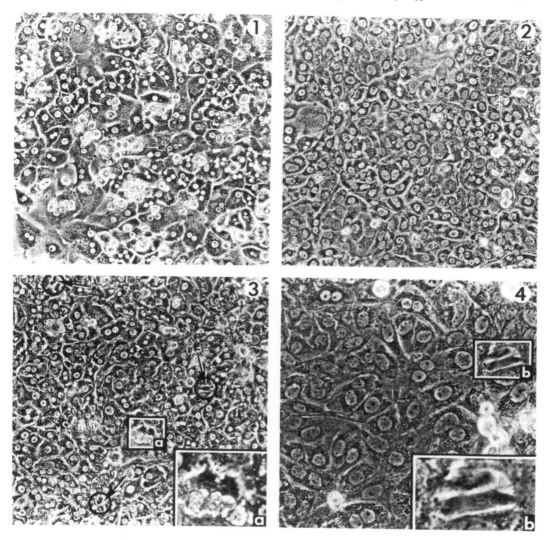

Fig. 9. **Primary cultures of normal rat hepatocytes on purified Type IV collagen and in serum-free hormonally defined medium.** Primary liver cultures can be sustained for approximately one month if plated onto substrata of purified collagens (types I or IV). However, if liver cells are plated onto purified Type I collagen, the liver cultures show little growth, whereas on purified Type IV collagen, they show extensive growth until confluence is achieved. The cultures shown have been seeded on to purified Type IV collagen and given serum-free, hormonally defined medium (as described in Table 1). Mitotic figures are evident throughout the cultures. Panel 1, 24h after plating; panel 2, 5 days after plating; panel 3, 2 weeks after plating; panel 4, 3 weeks after plating.

few days and remain on a plateau for about two weeks, gradually decrease over the next 2–4 weeks; in a parallel fashion, AFP is not expressed for 2–3 weeks, and then increases, peaking by the end of the life of the culture. By 4–6 weeks, the cultures, although viable, express few or very low levels of their tissue-specific functions and express high levels of embryonic proteins.

In recent years, there have been some efforts to culture cells on different types of collagens that are more typical of the *in vivo* substrata of specific cell types. For example, epithelia have been found to attach preferentially to Type IV collagen (65, 66, 70, 87, 88, 132, 208). Rubin *et al.* (171) showed that the hepatocyte attached equally well to all collagen types I–V. However, Narita *et al.* (138) have shown that different collagen types elicit qualitatively and quantitatively different physiological responses in primary liver cultures. The liver cultures attached slowly to purified Type I collagen, requiring up to 36 hours to fully spread and requiring either addition of fibronectin or culturing the cells in a SSM for 4–6 hours. Little to no growth of the cultures occurred when they were plated onto purified Type I collagen. In the first 1–2 weeks of culture on Type I collagen, the liver cells expressed normal levels of tissue-specific functions but then gradually lost the adult-specific functions and increasingly expressed fetal proteins such as AFP. By contrast, liver cultures plated onto purified Type IV collagen attached and spread within 4 hours even in a serum-free medium. The cultures showed sustained growth until the cells were confluent. During the growth phase, the cells expressed intermediate levels of adult-specific functions which increased to normal levels once the cells became confluent. At least over a 4-week period, these cultures never underwent fetalization; thus, they continued to express only their adult-specific functions (Figs 9 and 10).

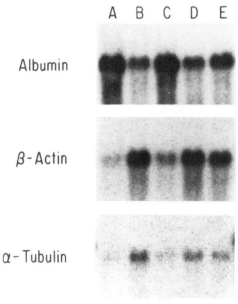

Fig. 10.
Gene expression in primary liver cultures on various matrix substrata and in serum-free hormonally defined medium. If primary liver cultures are plated onto collagens or crude extracts enriched in extracellular matrix (eg biomatrices) and in serum-free, hormonally defined medium, the cells will sustain their liver-specific functions at levels approximating those *in vivo* for 2–3 weeks. When the cells are plated onto purified Type IV collagen or on biomatrices prepared from EHS tumours (the tumour cells constitutively secrete basement membrane proteins), the cells grow rapidly for the first week in culture. During this time, the liver-specific mRNAs are intermediate in levels to those *in vivo* and to those when the cells become confluent. Throughout the life span of the cultures, the cells express only adult tissue-specific functions. By contrast, on Type I collagen, there is little growth of the hepatocytes, and the liver-specific mRNAs remain at levels approximating those *in vivo* for about 2 weeks. Thereafter, the hepatocytes begin to fetalize and to express fetal proteins such as AFP. In this figure Northern blots from primary liver cultures plated onto various collagens or biomatrices and in HDM and maintained for 5 days are shown. For each blot, 10 μg RNA was used and hybridized to the indicated cDNA probe. (A) Control rat liver; (B) Primary liver cultures plated onto purified Type IV collagen and in serum-free, hormonally defined medium (Table); (C) Primary liver cultures plated onto purified Type IV collagen mixed with heparan sulfate; (D) Primary liver cultures plated onto biomatrix substrata prepared from the EHS tumour and in hormonally defined medium; (E) Primary liver cultures plated onto purified Type I collagen prepared from skin, and in hormonally defined medium.

Proteoglycans. Proteoglycans (PGs) are macromolecules which consist of variable numbers of glycosaminoglycan chains covalently bound to a protein core (reviewed in reference 170*b*). Glycosaminoglycans (GAGs) are sugar polymers usually composed of alternating glucuronic acid and sulfated hexosamine residues, which carry closely spaced negatively charged groups. Several different classes of proteoglycans have now been described, which are present in the extracellular matrix of connective tissues such as cartilage and blood vessel wall; in the basement membranes associated with epithelial cells; and in the plasma membranes of cells. These classes of protoglycans are now being characterized and differentiated from one another, in terms of the kinds of GAGs which are bound to the protein core of the proteoglycan, the primary structure (amino acid sequence) of the protein core, and the peptide maps and the immunologic identity of the protein core.

Cationic dyes (ruthenium red, Alcian blue, acridine orange and safranin O) are useful stains for histochemically localizing proteoglycans in tissues. Histochemical

STRUCTURES OF THE GLYCOSAMINOGLYCANS
AND THEIR LINKAGE REGIONS TO PROTEIN

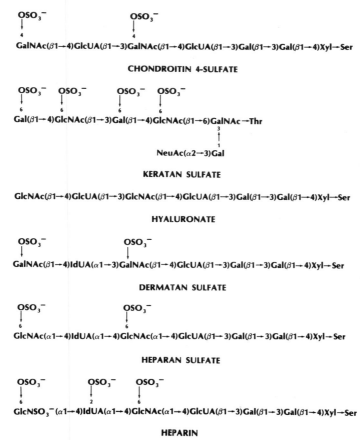

Fig. 11. Classes of proteoglycans.

observations have shown that proteoglycans exist as extended 'bottle brush' structures within the extracellular matrices of various tissues.

The structures of the GAGs and their linkage regions to the protein core of the proteoglycan are shown in Fig. 11. The GAGs are made up of two different sugar residues which alternate regularly in the sugar polymer chain. Thus, the GAG chains are composed of repeating disaccharide units. One class of proteoglycans, which is present in the plasma membranes of cells such as hepatocytes, is heparan sulfate proteoglycan. It is about 80 000 in molecular weight and contains 4 heparan sulfate chains bound to a core protein which is intercalated and anchored within the plasma membrane and/or bound to cell surface receptors (heparin-releasable) (67, 75, 93, 94, 170). It has been isolated and characterized from many types of cells including hepatomas (79, 80, 135), glial cells, muscle cells and fibroblasts (46, 140, 148), bovine aortic endothelial cell (147), teratocarcinoma cells (76, 157, 200), EHS tumour (60, 142) and mouse mammary epithelial cells (25–28, 90, 161). The heparan sulfate PG present in plasma membranes of quiescent hepatocytes (and in other cell types) forms complexes with fibronectin, and these complexes mediate cell attachment to an appropriate form of interstitial collagen (63, 64, 70, 89, 213). In an analogous fashion, epithelial cells (or presumably hepatocytes during regeneration) are connected to Type IV collagen by fibrils containing laminin associated with heparan sulfate PG (100, 101). Heparin and/or heparan sulfate apparently induce conversion of soluble fibronectin (and similarly laminin) to fibrils which have more affinity for collagen molecule. Hyaluronic acid, dermatan sulfate, and chondroitin sulfate suppress this effect (69).

Another class of heparan sulfate proteoglycans is present in renal glomerular basement membrane, where it contributes to the selective permeability of the basement membranes involved in glomerular filtration (75). While the ultra-structural localization, functional role and structure of this heparan sulfate PG have been studied most extensively in renal glomerular basement membrane, similar heparan sulfate PGs appear to be present in the basement membranes of other organs and tissues (25–27, 58, 60).

Synthesis, secretion and deposition. Liver tissue or liver-derived cells have been demonstrated to synthesize GAGs *in vivo* and *in vitro* (2, 50, 58, 80, 85, 86, 135, 139, 143–145, 158, 167, 207). Primary cultures synthesized heparan sulfate PG predominantly, and less amounts of chondroitin sulfate, dermatan sulfate, and hyaluronic acid (144, 145, 158, 192). Most of heparan sulfate PGs were associated with the cell layer (145). Rat liver parenchymal cells mainly synthesized heparan sulfate and distributed them predominantly into the cell layer (139). After synthesis, most GAGs move rapidly to cell-surface, then they are released immediately to the medium or accumulate at the membrane to be shed more slowly at a later time or to be degraded (200).

Heparan sulfate PGs were isolated from rat liver microsomal fractions. Their molecular weights were 75–80 000. The molecule consists of a core protein of molecular weight of approximately 17 000–40 000 and polysaccharide chains of an average molecular weight of 14 000 (145). These data agree with the interpretation that heparan sulfate PGs from plasma membrane of rat hepatocyte cultures consists of 3–4 heparan sulfate chains bound to a core protein (135, 145). Smaller amounts of other GAGs (chondroitin sulfate, dermatan sulfate and hyaluronic acid) were also

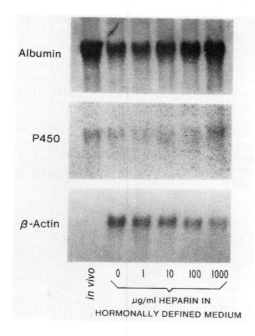

Albumin

P450

β-Actin

in vivo   0   1   10   100   1000

μg/ml HEPARIN IN
HORMONALLY DEFINED MEDIUM

Fig. 12.
Influence of heparin on gene expression in primary liver cultures in serum-free hormonally defined medium. The addition of purified glycosaminoglycans or proteoglycans to the culture medium (or used as a substratum) can result in a significant augmentation of liver-specific functions. Some of the glycosaminoglycans tested, such as heparin, also caused suppression of the mRNAs of common genes such as actin and tubulin. The Northern blots shown are from primary liver cultures maintained for 5 days in hormonally defined medium supplemented with the indicated concentrations of heparin (derived from porcine intestinal mucosa). For each blot, 10 μg of cytoplasmic RNA was used.

synthesized, but more than 90% of chondroitin sulfate was secreted into medium. During the 8 day culture of rat liver parenchymal cells, the synthesis of chondroitin sulfate, dermatan sulfate and hyaluronic acid increased markedly coincidently with the increase of Type I collagen production (139).

An epithelial cell line cloned from rat liver (passage level was 100) synthesized two kinds of GAGs, hyaluronic acid and dermatan sulfate. The GAGs were detected within the same cell layers, and the amount of synthesis rapidly increased concurrently with an accumulation of Type I collagen (173). Apparently, different patterns of GAGs (PGs) synthesis are affected by the length of time cells are in culture.

Factors influential to the synthesis of proteoglycans. 1) *Influences of other matrix components.* Collagen gel substrata remarkably reduced the degradation of GAGs synthesized by epithelial cells and caused those GAGs synthesized to remain in the substratum of the cells rather than being secreted into the medium (25–27, 107). The GAGs and PGs synthesized by cells are bound into the pericellular matrix by a fibrillar network of fibronectin via strong non-covalent linkages (64). Collagens have been shown also to alter the types of GAGs synthesized by cells. In various mesenchymal cells cultured on TCP, heparan sulfate was the major sulfated GAG released in trypsin extracts of the cells, whereas dermatan sulfate was a minor component. When cells were cultured on Type I collagen gels, the synthesis of dermatan sulfate increased more than 3-fold making it the principal sulfated GAG released by trypsinization (40*b*). 2) *Pharmacological and hormonal influences on proteogylcan synthesis.* Factors that increase or decrease the synthesis or deposition of GAGs and/or PGs in the extracellular matrix cause significant changes in the differentiation of the cells. Treatment of primary cultures of rat hepatocytes with

1 mM cycloheximide has been shown to decrease ^{35}S-incorporation to heparan sulfate to 5% of normal levels and to result in reduced cell spreading (192). By contrast, monensin, a drug which disrupts the Golgi apparatus and which inhibits hyaluronic acid synthesis, did not inhibit cell spreading. Tunicamycin, known as an inhibitor of N-glycosylation of proteins, also has marked inhibitory effects (up to 75%) on proteoglycan synthesis, and results in alterations in cell shape and an increase in surface microvilli and blebs (156). Dibutyryl cyclic-AMP has been demonstrated to decrease significantly the synthesis of heparan sulfate PGs in rat hepatocyte cultures (192).

Factors such as β-xyloside, whch inhibit the synthesis and/or deposition of GAGs and PGs into the matrix, also inhibits the differentiation of those tissues *in vivo* and in organ culture (13, 193, 196).

Retinoic acids are known to induce significant qualitative and quantitative changes in the PGs and GAGs synthesized by cells, changes that are associated with the differentiation of various epithelial cell types including embryonic stem cells such as teratocarcinomas (76, 157, 184) and adult cells such as haemopoietic cells or chondrocytes (151, 182, 188).

Influence of proteoglycans on the biology of liver cultures. Evidence for biological functions of the proteoglycans has been obtained in many different cell types including the differentiation of muscle cells (70, 97); the outgrowth of retinal neurites (98); cell polarity and cell attachment in normal and neoplastic hepatocytes and various other cell types (99, 170, 189, 201); and, cell growth (137, 143). In recent studies on gene expression in primary rat liver cultures in an HDM, Fujita, Reid & Rosenberg (39a) have found that heparin and liver-specific heparan sulfate (but not chondroitin sulfate or dermatan sulfate) can greatly augment the cytoplasmic mRNA concentrations for albumin, ligandin, cytochrome P450 and a number of other liver-specific functions (above that observed in an HDM), while simultaneously suppressing the expression of actin and tubulin (see Fig. 12). The proteoglycans are the first factors known which simultaneously increased tissue-specific functions and decreased common gene functions in liver cultures. These differentiative effects were due both to transcriptional and post-transcriptional regulation of the mRNA levels (39a).

Implications for biological roles of proteoglycans have also derived from studies on tumours. Transformed cells usually do not assemble a normal extracellular matrix (3, 28, 134, 167, 170, 202, 203, 212, 216). On tissue culture plastic, transformed mammary epithelial cells and their normal, parental counterparts have identical rates of GAGs synthesis and secretion into the medium. On collagen substrata, the parental cells incorporated the GAGs into a basal lamina, whereas transformed cells continued to secrete the GAGs into the medium. This impairment, thought to be due to production of matrix-degrading enzymes, may prevent the neoplastic cells from forming an appropriate matrix, and therefore allow local invasion (28, 167). The ability of tumour cells to be invasive and metastatic has been shown to be strictly correlated with production of enzymes such as Type IV collagenase and/or endoheparinase that degrade components of the extracellular matrix (105, 106, 138b, 204, 205).

Cultured normal rat kidney cells displayed a fibrillar network of heparan sulfate PG identified immunochemically at the cell surface, whereas virally transformed cell lacked such a surface network of the PG (63). By contrast, the distribution of chondroitin sulfate PG showed a similar punctate pattern on the surface of both normal and transformed cell types. Heparan sulfate PGs in the matrix of normal cells were found to co-distribute with fibronectin or laminin, while chondroitin sulfate did not. Treated with sodium butyrate, transformed cells successfully formed complexes of fibronectin or laminin and heparan sulfate PG at their cell surface and changed their morphology to a pattern resembling that of normal cells. These results suggest a relationship between morphology and formation of the anchorage protein-heparan sulfate PG complex (63).

Many types of tumor cells including hepatomas and virally transformed cells have been shown to produce undersulfated heparan sulfate PG (28, 107, 137, 167, 189, 202, 212). Robinson *et al.* (189) demonstrated that hepatoma cells synthesize aberrant forms of heparan sulfate PGs that are undersulfated and had lowered affinity for fibronectin. Sulfation decreased by 20–40% particularly in $GlcNH_2$ residues bearing 6–O–sulfate groups (18, 189, 212). Uneven distribution of sulfate groups in oligosaccharide chains were also observed (212). The reduced negative charge of the PGs due to undersulfation was shown to affect not only the formation of complexes with collagen, anchorage proteins, and other matrix components but also the permeability of matrix around the cells.

Thus, even with the limited studies to date, it is apparent that various classes of proteoglycans, especially heparin and heparan sulfate, are present in liver, and that they potentially are among the biologically active matrix components regulating growth and differentiation of liver cells and that aberrations in proteoglycan chemistry or synthesis are commonly associated with neoplastic transformation. The future studies on proteoglycan biology are likely to be among the most important for new understandings of the regulation of differentiation in liver as well as other tissues.

ACKNOWLEDGEMENTS

Dr Martinez-Hernandez (Hahnemann University, Philadelphia) and Dr T. Miller (University of Alabama, Birmingham) generously discussed data and shared information from unpublished results. Thanks are owed to Dr Douglas Jefferson for providing constructive criticisms and for contributing one of the figures (Fig. 6). We thank Dorothy Occhino for her technical assistance and Rosina Passela for her secretarial assistance. This research was supported by a grant from the American Cancer Society (BC-439D) and by NIH grants (P30CA1330, CA30117, AM17702–12, and CA33164). Lola Reid receives salary support through a career development award (NIH CA00783).

REFERENCES

1 Adams E., Frank L.: Metabolism of proline and hydroxyproline. *Ann. Rev. Biochem.* 1980, **49**: 1005.

2 Akasaki M., Kawasaki, T., Yamashina, I.: The isolation and characterization of glycopeptides and mucopolysaccharides from plasma membranes of normal and regenerating livers of rats. *FEBS Letts* 1975, **59**: 100–104.

3 Akiyama S. K., Yamada K. M.: Fibronectin in disease. A Review. *Monogr. Pathol.* 1983, **24**: 55–96.

4 Barnes D., Sato G.: Serum-free culture: a unifying approach. *Cell* 1980, **22**: 649–655.

5 Barnes D., Sato, G.: *Methods for Serum-free Culture of Cells. Cell Culture Methods for Molecular and Cellular Biology*, Vols 1–4: Alan R. Liss, Inc, New York, 1984.

6 Bernfield M., Banerjee S. D., Koda J. E., Rapraeger A. C.: Remodeling of the basement membrane: morphogenesis and maturation. *In: Basement Membranes and Cell Movement*: Ciba Foundation Symposium no. 108, 1984, pp 1–17.

7 Bissell D. M., Guzelian P.: Phenotypic stability of adult rat hepatocytes in primary monolayer culture. *Ann. N.Y. Acad. Sci.*, 1981, **349**: 86–98.

8 Bissell M. J.: The differentiated state of normal and malignant cells or how to define a 'normal' cell in culture. *Int. Rev. Cytol.* 1981, **70**: 27–100.

9 Blobel G.: Synthesis and segregation of secretory proteins: The signal hypothesis. *Int. Cell Biol.* 1977, 318.

10 Boedtker H., Fuller F., Tate, U.: The structure of collagen genes. *Int. Rev. Connective Tiss. Res.* 1983, **10**: 1–63.

11 Bonaldo, D. F. M., Cassaro-Strunz, C. M., Machado-Santelli, G. M.: Sulfated glycosaminoglycan and collagen patterns in parietal yolk sac carcinoma (PYSC). *Cell Different.* 1982, **11**: 99–106.

12 Bornstein P., Sage H.: Structurally distinct collagen types. *Ann. Rev. Biochem.* 1980, **49**: 957–1003.

13 Brennan M. J., Oldberg A., Hayman E. G., Ruoslahti E.: Effect of a proteoglycan produced by rat tumor cells on their adhesion to fibronectin-collagen substrata. *Cancer Res.* 1983, **43**: 4302–4307.

14 Brock M. L., Shapiro D. J.: Estrogen stabilizes vitelogenin mRNA against cytoplasmic degradation. *Cell* 1983, **34**: 207–213.

15 Carlsson R., Engvall E., Freeman A., Ruoshlahti E.: Laminin and fibronectin in cell adhesion: Enhanced adhesion of cells from regenerating liver to laminin. *Proc. Natl. Acad. Sci.* 1981, **78**: 2403–2406.

16 Cherington P. V., Smith B. L., Pardee A. B.: Loss of epidermal growth factor requirement and malignant transformation. *Proc. Natl. Acad. Sci.* 1980, **76**: 3937–3941.

17 Cheah K. S. E., Grant M. E.: Procollagen genes and messenger RNAs. *In: Collagen in Health and Disease*, eds, J. B. Weiss and M. I. V. Jayson, Churchill Livingstone, Edinburgh, 1982, pp 73–100.

18 Chung S., Landfear S. M., Blumber D. D., Cohen N. S., Lodish, H. F.: Synthesis and stability of developmentally regulated Dictyostelium mRNA are affected by cell-cell contact and cAMP. *Cell* 1981, **24**: 785–797.

19 Clayton D. F., Darnell J. E.: Changes in liver-specific compared to common gene transcription during primary culture of mouse hepatocytes. *Molec. Cell. Biol.* 1983, **3**: 1552–1561.

20 Clayton D. F., Harrelson A. L., Darnell J. E.: Dependence of liver-specific transcription on tissue organization. (Submitted.)

21 Clement B., Guguen-Guillouzo C., Campion J. P., Glaise D., Bourel M., Guillouzo A.: Long-term co-cultures of adult human hepatocytes with rat liver epithelial cells: Modulation of albumin secretion and accumulation of extracellular material. *Hepatology* 1984, **4**: 373–380.

22 Daniel J. C., Kosher R. A., Hamos J. E., Lash J. W.: Influence of external postassium on the synthesis and deposition of matrix components by chondrocytes *in vitro. J. Cell Biol.* 1974, **63**: 843–854.

23 Dardenne A. J., Burns J., Sykes B. C., Kirkpatrick P.: Comparative distribution of fibronectin and type III collagen in normal human tissues. *J. Pathol.* 1983, **141**: 55–69.

24 Darnell J. E.: Variety in the level of gene control in eukaryotic cells. *Nature* 1982, **297**, 365–371.

25 David G., Bernfield M.: Collagen reduces glycosaminoglycan degradation by cultured mammary epithelial cells: Possible mechanism for basal lamina formation. *Proc. Natl. Acad. Sci.* 1979, **76**: 786–790.

26 David G. Bernfield M.: Type I collagen reduces the degradation of basal lamina proteoglycans by mammary epithelial cells. *J. Cell Biol.* 1981, **91**: 281–286.

27 David G. Bernfield M.: Defective basal lamina formation by transformed mammary epithelial cells: A reduced effect of collagen on basal lamina (heparan sulfate-rich) proteoglycan degradation. *J. Cell Physiol.* 1982, **110**: 56–62.

28 David G., Van Den Berghe H.: Transformed mouse mammary epithelial cells synthesize undersulfated basement membrane proteoglycan. *J. Biol. Chem.* 1983, **258**: 7338–7344.

29 Davidson J. M., McEneary S. G.: Intermediates in the limited proteolytic conversion of procollagen to collagen. *Biochem.* 1975, **14**: 5188.

30 de Leeuw A. M., McCarthy S. P., Geerts A., Knook D. L.: Purified rat liver fat-storing cells in culture divide and contain collagen. *Hepatology* 1984, **4**: 392–403.
31 Derman E., Krauter K., Walling L., Weinberger C., Ray M., Darnell J. E., Jr.: Transcriptional control in the production of liver-specific mRNAs. *Cell* 1981, **23**: 731–739.
32 Diegelmann R. F., Guzelian P. S., Gay R., Gay S.: Collagen formation by the hepatocyte in primary monolayer culture and *in vivo*. *Science* 1983, **219**: 1343–1345.
33 Duksin P., Bornstein P.: Impaired conversion of procollagen to collagen by fibroblasts and bone treated with tunicamycin, an inhibitor of protein glycosylation. *J. Biol. Chem.* 1977, **252**: 955–962.
34 Emmerman J. T., Pitelka D. R.: Maintenance and induction of morphological differentiation in dissociated mammary epithelium on floating collagen membranes. *In Vitro* 1977, **13**: 346–348.
35 Enat R., Jefferson D. M., Ruiz-Opazo N., Gatmaitan Z., Leinwand L. A., Reid L. M.: Hepatocyte proliferation *in vitro*: Its dependence on the use of serum-free hormonally defined medium and substrata of extracellular matrix. *Proc. Natl. Acad. Sci.* 1984, **81**: 1411–1415.
36 Fessler J. H., Fessler L. I.: Biosynthesis of procollagen. *Ann. Rev. Biochem.* 1978, **47**: 129–142.
37 Fietzek P. P., Kuhn K.: The primary structure of collagen. *In: International Review of Connective Tissue Research*, D. A. Hall, D. S. Jackson (Eds), 1976, **7**: 1–60.
38 Foidart J. M., Berman J. J., Paglia L., Rennard S., Abe S., Perantoni A., Martin G. R.: Synthesis of fibronectin, laminin, and several collagens by a liver-derived epithelial line. *Lab. Invest.* 1980, **42**: 525–532.
39 Freshney R. I.: *Culture of Animal Cells. A Manual of Basic Technique*: Alan R. Liss, Inc, New York.
39a Fujita M., Spray D., Choi H., Saez J., Rosenberg L., Reid L.: Glycosaminoglycans and proteoglycans, extracellular matrix components that are inducers of gap junctions and of tissue-specific gene expression in liver. *In: Proceedings of the Conference on Liver Cells in Culture*. (In press).
40 Gatmaitan Z., Jefferson D., Ruiz-Opazo N., Leinwand L., Reid L.: Regulation of growth and differentiation of a rat hepatoma cell line by the synergistic interactions of hormones and collagenous substrata. *J. Cell. Biol.* 1983, **97**: 1179–1190.
40b Gallagher J. T., Gasiunas N., Schor S. L.: Synthesis of glycosaminoglycans by human skin on collagen gels. *Biochem. J.* 1980, **190**: 243–254.
41 Gay S., Fietzek P. P., Remberger K., Eder M., Kuhn K.: Liver cirrhosis: Immunofluorescence and biochemical studies demonstrate two types of collagen. *Klin. Wochenschr.* 1975, **53**: 205–208.
42 Gay S., Miller E. J.: What is collagen? What is Not?: *Ultrastruct. Pathol.* 1983, **4**: 365–377.
43 Gelman R. A., Poppka D. C., Piez K. A.: Collagen fibril formation *in vitro*: The role of the non-helical terminal regions. *J. Biol. Chem.* 1979, **254**: 11741–11745.
44 Georgoff I., Secott T., Isom H. C.: Effect of simian virus 40 infection on albumin production by hepatocytes cultured in chemically defined medium and plated on collagen and non-collagen attachment surfaces. *J. Biol. Chem.* 1984, **259**: 9595–9602.
45 Glanville R. W., Rauter A., Fiezek P. P.: Isolation and characterization of a native placental basement membrane collagen and its component α-chains. *Eur. J. Biochem.* 1979, **95**: 383–389.
46 Glimelius B., Busch C., Hook M.: Binding of heparin on the surface of cultured human endothelial cells. *Thrombosis Res.* 1978, **12**: 773–782.
47 Goldberg B., Taubman M. B., Radin A.: Procollagen peptidase: Its mode of action on the native substrata. *Cell* 1975, **4**: 45–50.
48 Gomez-Lechon M. J., Garcia M. D., Castell J. V.: Effect of glucocorticoids on the expression of γ-glutamyltransferase and tyrosine aminotransferase in serum-free-cultured hepatocytes. *Hoppe-Seyler's Z. Physiol. Chem. Bd.* 1983, **364**: 501–508.
49 Green H.: The keratinocyte as differentiated cell type: a review. *Harvey Lect.* 1979, **74**: 101–139.
50 Gressner A. M., Pazen H., Greiling H.: The biosynthesis of glycosaminoglycans in normal rat liver and in response to experimental hepatic injury. *Hoppe-Seyler's Z. Physiol. Chem. Bd.* 1977, **358**: 825–833.
51 Grimaud J. A., Borojevic R.: Intercellular formation of collagen in human liver. *Cell. Molec. Biol.* 1980, **26**: 555–562.
52 Grimaud J. A., Druguet M., Peyrol S., Chevalier O., Herbage G., El Badrawy N.: Collagen immunotyping in human liver, light and electronmicroscopic study. *J. Histochem. Cyto. Chem.* 1980, **28**: 1145–1156.

53 Grinnel F.: Cell-collagen interactions: overview. *Methods Enzymol.* 1982, **82**: 499–508.
54 Guguen-Guillouzo C., Clement B., Baffet G., Beaumont C. Morel-Chany E., Glaise D., Guillouzo A.: Maintenance and reversibility of active albumin secretion by adult rat hepatocytes co-cultured with another liver epithelial cell type. *Exp. Cell. Res.* 1983, **143**: 47–54.
55 Guguen-Guillouzo C., Guillouzo A.: Modulation of functional activities in cultured rat hepatocytes. *Molec. Cell Biochem.* 1983, **53/54**: 35–56.
56 Guzelian P. S., Diegelmann R. F.: Localization of collagen prolyl hydroxylase to the hepatoctye. *Exp. Cell Res.* 1979, **123**: 269–279.
57 Guzelian P. S., Lindblad W. J., Diegelmann R. F.: Glucocorticoids suppress formation of collagen by the hepatocyte: Studies in primary monolayer cultures of parenchymal cells prepared from adult rat liver. *Gastroenterology* 1984, **86**: 897–904.
58 Hahn E., Wick G., Pencer D., Timpl R.: Distribution of basement membrane proteins in normal and fibrotic human liver: collagen Type IV, laminin and fibronectin. *Gut.* 1980, **21**: 63–71.
59 Ham R., McKeehan W.: Media and growth requirements. *Meth. Enzymol.* 1979, **58**: 44–93.
60 Hassell J. R., Robey P. G., Barrach H., Wilczek J., Rennard S. I., Martin G. R.: Isolation of a heparan sulfate-containing proteoglycan from basement membrane. *Proc. Natl. Acad. Sci.* 1980, **77**: 4494–4498.
61 Hata R., Ninomiya Y., Nagai Y., Tsukada Y.: Biosynthesis of interstitial types of collagen by albumin-producing rat liver parenchymal cell (hepatocyte) clones in culture. *Biochem.* 1980, **19**: 169–176.
62 Hay E. D.: Cell and extracellular matrix: their organization and mutual dependence. *In: Spatial Organization of Eukaryotic Cells*, J. R. McIntosh, (Ed.): Alan R. Liss Inc., New York, 1983, pp 509–548.
63 Hayman E. G., Oldberg A., Martin G. R., Ruoslahti E.: Codistribution of heparan sulfate proteoglycan, laminin, and fibronectin in the extracellular matrix of normal rat kidney cells and their coordinate absence in transformed cells. *J. Cell Biol.* 1982, **94**: 28–35.
64 Hedman K., Johansson S., Vartio T., Kjellen L., Vaheri A., Hook M.: Structure of the pericellular matrix: Association of heparan and chondroitin sulfates with fibronectin-procollagen fibres. *Cell* 1982, **28**: 663–671.
65 Herberg J., Codina J., Rich K. A., Rojas F., Iyengar R.: The hepatic glucagon receptor. *J. Biol. Chem.* 1984, **259**: 9285–9294.
66 Hirata K., Usui T., Koshiba H., Maruyama Y., Oikawa I., Freeman A. E., Shiramatsu K., Hayasaka H.: Effects of basement membrane matrix on the culture of fetal mouse hepatocytes. *Gann* 1983, **74**: 687–692.
67 Hirata K., Yoshida Y., Shiramatsu K., Freeman A. E., Hayasaka H.: Effects of laminin, fibronectin and Type IV collagen on liver cell cultures. *Exp. Cell Biol.* 1983, **51**: 121–129.
68 Hirsiger H., Giger U., Meyer U. A.: Stimulation of DNA synthesis and mitotic activity of chick embryo hepatocytes in primary culture. *In Vitro* 1984, **20**: 172–181.
69 Hormann H., Jelinic V.: Regulation by heparin and hyaluronic acid of the fibronectin-dependent association of collagen, type III, with macrophages. *Hoppe-Seyler's Z. Physiol. Chem. Bd.* 1981, **362**: 87–94.
70 Huw A. J., Hazel L.: The effect of different collagen types used as substrata on myogenesis in tissue culture. *Coll Biol. Int. Rep.* 1980, **4**: 841–850.
71 Jefferson D. M., Liverpool C., Reid L.: Hormonal modulation of steady state levels of specific mRNAs in primary cultures of adult rat hepatocytes. *J. Cell. Biol.* 1984, **99**: 201a.
72 Jefferson D. M., Clayton D. F., Darnell J. E., Reid L. M.: Post-transcriptional modulation of gene expression in cultured rat hepatocytes. *Molec. Cell. Biol.* 1984, **4**: 1929–1934.
73 Jefferson D. M., Reid L. M., Giambrone M., Shafritz D. A., Zern M. A.: Effects of dexamethasone on albumin and collagen gene expression in primary cultures of adult rat hepatocytes. *Hepatology* 1985, **5**: 14–20.
74 Johansson S., Hook M.: Substrate adhesion of rat hepatocytes: On the mechanism of attachment to fibronectin. *J. Cell. Biol.* 1984, **98**: 810–817.
75 Kanwar Y. S., Farquhar M. G.: Presence of heparan sulfate in the glomerular basement membrane. *Proc. Natl. Acad. Sci.* 1979, **76**: 1303–1307.
76 Kapoor R., Prehm P.: Changes in proteoglycan composition of F9 teratocarcinoma cells upon differentiation. *Eur. J. Biochem.* 1983, **137**: 589–595.

77 Karasaki S., Raymond J.: Formation of intercellular collagen matrix by cultured liver epithelial cells and loss of its ability in hepatocarcinogenesis *in vitro. Differentia.* 1981, **19**: 21–30.

78 Karasek M. A., Charlton M. E.: Growth of post-embryonic skin epithelial cells on collagen gels. *J. Invest. Dermatol.* 1971, **51**: 247–252.

79 Kawakami H., Terayama H.: Cell surface proteoglycans as a negative modulator in concanavalin A-mediated agglutination of hepatoma cells. *Biochim. Biophys. Acta.* 1980, **599**: 301–314.

80 Kawakami H., Terayama H.: Liver plasma membranes and proteoglycan prepared from them inhibit the growth of hepatoma cells *in vitro. Biochim. Biophys. Acta* 1981, **646**: 161–168.

81 Kefalides N. A.: Isolation of collagen from basement membrane containing three identical α chains. *Biochem. Biophys. Res. Comm.* 1971, **45**: 226–234.

82 Kefalides N. A., Alper R., Clark C. C.: Biochemistry and metabolism of basement membrane. *Int. Rev. Cytol.* 1979, **61**: 167–228.

83 Kent G., Gay S., Inouye T., Bahn R., Minick O. T. , Popper H.: Vitamin A containing lipocyte and formation of Type III collagen in liver injury. *Proc. Natl. Acad. Sci.* 1976, **73**: 3719–3722.

84 Kivirikko K. I., Myllyla R.: Post-translational modifications. *In: Collagen in Health and Disease*: eds. J. B. Weiss & M. I. V. Jayson, Churchill Livingstone, Edinburgh, 1982, pp 101–120.

85 Kjellen L., Oldberg A., Hook M.: Cell-surface heparan sulfate: Mechanisms of proteoglycan-cell association. *J. Biol. Chem.* 1980, **255**: 10407–10413.

86 Kjellen L., Pettersson I., Hook M.: Cell-surface heparan sulfate: An intercalated membrane proteoglycan. *Proc. Natl. Acad. Sci.* 1981, **78**: 5371–5375.

87 Kleinman H. K., Klebe R. J., Martin G. R.: Role of collagenous matrices in the adhesion and growth of cells. *J. Cell Biol.* 1981, **88**: 473–485.

88 Kleinman H. K., Rohrbach D. H., Terranova V. P., Varner A. T., Hewitt G. R., Grotendorst G. R., Wilkes C. M., Martin G. R., Seppa H., Schiffman E.: Collagenous matrices as determination of cell function. *In: Immunochemistry of the Extracellular Matrix*, H. Furthmayr (Ed.): CRC Press, 1982, pp 151–174.

89 Kleinman H. K., Wilkes C. M., Martin G. R.: Interaction of fibronectin with collagen fibrils. *Biochem.* 1981, **20**: 2325–2330.

90 Koda J. E., Bernfield M. R.: Heparan sulfate proteoglycans from mouse mammary epithelial cells: basal extracellular proteoglycan binds specifically to native type I collagen fibrils. *J. Biol. Chem.* 1984, **259**: 1–23.

91 Koch K. S., Shapiro P., Skelly H., Leffert H. L.: Rat hepatocyte proliferation is stimulated by insulin-like peptides in defined medium. *Biochem. Biophys. Res. Comm.* 1982, **109**: 1054–1063.

92 Kornblihtt A. R., Vibe-Pederson K., Baralle F. E.: Human fibronectin: Molecular cloning evidence for two mRNA species differing by an internal segment coding for a structural domain. *EMBO J.* 1984, **3**: 221–226.

93 Kraemer P. M.: Heparan sulfates of cultured cells. I. Membrane-associated and cell-sap species in Chinese hamster cells. *Biochemistry* 1971, **10**: 1437–1445.

94 Kraemer P. M.: Heparan sulfates of cultured cells. II. Acid-soluble and acid-precipitable species of different cell lines. *Biochemistry* 1971, **10**: 1445–1451.

95 Kuhn K.: Chemical properties of collagen. *In: Immunochemistry of the Extracellular Matrix*, H. Furthmayr (Ed.): Vol. I, CRC Press, 1981, pp 1–29.

96 Kuhn K., Wiedemann H., Timpl R., Risteli J., Dieringer H., Voss T., Glanville R. W.: Macromolecular structure of basement membrane collagens: Identification of 7S collagen as a crosslinking domain of Type IV collagen. *FEBS Lett.* 1981, **125**: 123–129.

97 Kujawa M. J., Tepperman K.: Culturing chick muscle cells on glycosaminoglycan substrates: Attachment and differentiation. *Dev. Biol.* 1983, **99**: 277–286.

98 Lander A. D., Fujii D. K., Gospodarowicz D., Reichardt L. F.: Characterization of a factor that promotes neurite outgrowth: Evidence linking activity to a heparan sulfate proteoglycan. *J. Cell Biol.* 1982, **94**: 574–585.

99 Laterra J., Silbert J. E., Culp L. A.: Cell surface heparan sulfate mediates some adhesive responses to glycosaminoglycan-binding matrices, including fibronectin. *J. Cell. Biol.* 1983, **96**: 112–123.

100 Leivo I.: Basement membrane-like matrix of teratocarcinoma-derived endodermal cells: Presence of laminin and heparan sulfate in the matrix at points of attachment to cells. *J. Histochem. Cytochem.* 1983, **31**: 35–45.

101 Leivo I., Alitalo K., Risteli L., Vaheri A., Timpl R., Wartiovaara J.: Basal lamina glycoproteins

laminin and type IV collagen are assembled into a fine-fibered matrix in cultures of a teratocarcinoma-derived endodermal cell line. *Exp. Cell Res.* 1982, **137**: 15–23.

102 Lerouz-Nicollet I., Noel M., Baribault H., Goyette R., Marceau N.: Selective increase in cytokeratin synthesis in cultured rat hepatocytes in response to hormonal stimulation. *Biochem. Biophys. Res. Comm.* 1983, **114**: 556–563.

103 Leung M. K. F., Fessler L. I., Greenberg D. B.: Separate amino and carboxy procollagen peptides in chick embryo tendon. *J. Biol. Chem.* 1979, **254**: 224–232.

104 Lin Q., Blaisdell J., O'Keefe E., Earp H. S.: Insulin inhibits the glucocorticoid-mediated increase in hepatocyte EGF binding, *J. Cell. Physiol.* 1984, **119**: 267–272.

105 Lindblad W. J., Fuller G. C.: An improved assay of mammalian collagenase activity, and its use to determine hepatic extracellular matrix susceptibility to degradation. *Clin. Chem.* 1982, **28**: 2134–2138.

106 Liotta L. A., Abe S., Robey P. G., Martin G. R.: Preferential digestion of basement membrane collagen by an enzyme derived from a metastatic murine tumor. *Proc. Natl. Acad. Sci.* 1979, **76**: 2268–2272.

107 Luikart S. D., Maniglia C. A., Sartorelli A. C.: Influence of collagen substrata on glycosaminoglycan production by B16 melanoma cells. *Proc. Natl. Acad. Sci.* 1983, **80**: 3738–3742.

108 Madri J. A., Foellmer H. G., Furthmayr H.: Ultrastructural morphology and domain structure of a unique collagenous component of basement membranes. *Biochem.* 1983, **22**: 2797–2804.

109 Mai S., Chung A. E.: Cell attachment and spreading on extracellular matrix-coated beads. *Exp. Cell. Res.* 1984, **152**: 500–509.

110 Marceau N., Goyette R., Valet J. P., Deschenes J.: The effect of dexamethasone on formation of a fibronectin extracellular matrix by rat hepatocytes *in vitro. Exp. Cell. Res.* 1980, **125**: 497–502.

111 Marceau N., Goyette R., Guidoin R., Antakly T.: Hormonally-induced formation of extracellular biomatrix in cultured normal and neoplastic liver cells: Effect of dexamethasone. *Scan. Electron. Microsc.* 1982, Pt. 2, 815–823.

112 Marceau N., Goyette R., Pelletier G., Antakly T.: Hormonally-induced changes in the cytoskeleton organization of adult and newborn rat hepatocytes cultured on fibronectin precoated substratum: Effect of dexamethasone and insulin. *Cell. Molec. Biol.* 1983, **29**: 421–435.

113 Marsillo E., Sobel M. E., Smith B. D.: Absence of procollagen α2 (I) mRNA in chemically transformed rat liver epithelial cells. *J. Biol. Chem.* 1984, **259**: 1401–1404.

114 Martin G. R., Byers P. H., Piez K. A.: Procollagen. *Adv. Enzymol.* 1975, **42**: 167–191.

115 Martin G. R., Kleinman H. K.: Extracellular matrix proteins give new life to cell culture. *Hepatology* 1981, **1**: 264–266.

116 Martinez-Hernandez A.: The hepatic extracellular matrix. I: Electron immunohistochemical studies in normal rat liver. *Lab. Inv.* 1984, **51**: 57–74.

117 Mather J. (Ed.) *Mammalian Cell Culture*: Plenum Press, Inc, New York, 1984.

118 McGee J. O. D., Patrick R. S.: The role of perisinusoidal cells in hepatic fibrogenesis. *Lab. Inv.* 1972, **26**: 429–440.

119 McGee J. O. D.: Liver. *In: Collagen Health and Disease,* J. B. Weis, M. I. V. Jayson (Eds): Churchill Livingstone, New York, 1982, pp 414–423.

120 Michalopoulos G., Cianciulli H. D., Novotry A. R., Kligerman A. D., Strom S. C., Jirtle R. L.: Liver regeneration on studies with rat hepatocytes in primary culture. *Cancer Res.* 1982, **42**: 4673–4682.

121 Michalopoulos G., Pitot H. C.: Primary culture of parenchymal liver cells on collagen membranes. *Exp. Cell Res.* 1975, **94**: 70–78.

122 Michalopoulos G., Russell F., Biles C.: Primary cultures of hepatocytes on human fibroblasts. *In Vitro* 1979, **15**: 796–806.

123 Michalopoulos G., Sattler G. L., Pitot H. C.: Maintenance of microsomal cytochrome B-5 and P-450 in primary cultures of parenchymal liver cells on collagen membranes. *Life Sci.* 1976, **18**: 1139–1144.

124 Miller E. J.: Biochemical characteristics and biological significance of the genetically-distinct collagens. *Molec. Cell. Biochem.*, 1976, **13**: 165–192.

125 Miller E. J., Finch E. J. Jr, Chung E., Butler W. T.: Specific cleavage of the native type III collagen molecule with trypsin. *Arch. Biochem. Biophys.* 1976, **173**: 631–637.

126 Miller E. J., Gay S.: Collagen: an overview. *Meth. Enzymol.* 1982, **82**: 3–32.

127 Miyanaga O., Evans C., Cottam G. L.: The effect of dexamethasone on pyruvate kinase activity in primary cultures of hepatocytes. *Biochim. Biophys. Acta* 1983, **758**: 42–48.

128 Morin O., Fehlmann M., Freychet P.: Binding and action of insulin and glucagon in monolayer cultures and fresh suspensions of rat hepatocytes. *In: Molecular and Cellular Endocrinology*: Elsevier/North-Holland Scientific Publishers, Ltd., 1982, **25**: 339–352.

129 Mosher D. F.: Physiology of fibronectin. *Rev. Ann. Rev. Med.* 1984, **35**: 561–575.

130 Morriss-Kay G. M., Crutch B.: Culture of rat embryos with β-D-Xyloside: Evidence of a role for proteoglycans in neurulation. *J. Anat.* 1982, **134**: 491–506.

131 Motta P. M.: The three-dimensional microanatomy of the liver. *Arch. Histol. Jpn.* 1984, **47**: 1–30.

132 Murray J. C., Stingl G., Kleinman H. K., Martin G. R., Katz S. I.: Epidermal cells adhere preferentially to Type IV (basement membrane) collagen. *J. Cell Biol.* 1979, **80**: 197–202.

133 Muschel R., Khoury G., Reid L.: Regulation of insulin mRNA adenylation: its dependence on hormones and matric substrata. *Mol. Cell. Biol.* (In press.)

134 Muto M., Yoshimura M., Okayama M., Kaji A.: Cellular transformation and differentiation. Effect of Rous sarcoma virus transformation on sulfated proteoglycan synthesis by chicken chondrocytes. *Proc. Natl. Acad. Sci.* 1977, **74**: 4173–4177.

135 Mutoh S., Funakoshi I., Nobuo U., Yamashina I.: Structural characterization of proteoheparan sulfate isolated from plasma membranes of an ascites hepatomas, AH66. *Arch. Biochem. Biophy.* 1980, **202**: 137–143.

136 Mutoh S., Funakoshi I., Yamashina I.: Isolation and characterization of proteoheparan sulfate from plasma membranes of an ascites hepatoma, AH66. *J. Biochem.* 1978, **84**: 483–489.

137 Nakamura T., Nakayama Y., Ichihara A.: Reciprocal modulation of growth and liver functions of mature rat hepatocytes in primary culture by an extract of hepatic plasma membranes. *J. Biol. Chem.* 1984, **259**: 8056–8058.

138 Narita M., Jefferson D. M., Miller E. J., Clayton D. F., Rosenberg L.: Hormonal and matrix regulation of differentiation in primary liver cultures. *In: Growth and Differentiation of Cells in Defined Environments*: Springer Verlag, New York. (In press.)

138b Nicolson G. L.: Cell surface molecules and tumor metastasis: Regulation of metastastic phenotypic diversity. *Exp. Cell. Res.* 1984, **150**: 3–22.

139 Ninomiya Y., Hata R., Nagai Y.: Active synthesis of glycosaminoglycans by liver parenchymal cells in primary culture. *Biochim. Biophys. Acta* 1981, **675**: 248–255.

140 Norling B., Glimelius B., Wasteson A.: Heparan sulfate proteoglycan of cultured cells. Demonstration of a lipid- and a matrix-associated form. *Biochem. Biophys. Res. Comm.* 1981, **103**: 1265–1272.

141 Ocklind C., Odin P., Obrink B.: Two different cell adhesion molecules-cell-CAM 105 and a calcium-dependent protein-occur on the surface of rat hepatocytes. *Exp. Cell Res.* 1984, **151**: 29–45.

142 Oegeme T. R. Jr, Hascall V. C., Dziewiatkowski D. D.: Isolation and characterization of proteoglycans from the swarm rat chondrosarcoma. *J. Biol. Chem.* 1975, **250**: 6151–6159.

143 Ohnishi T., Ohshima E., Ohtsuka M.: Effect of liver cell coat acid mucopolysaccharide on the appearance of density-dependent inhibition in hepatoma cell growth. *Exp. Cell Res.* 1975, **93**: 136–142.

144 Oldberg A., Hook M.: Structure and metabolism of rat liver heparan sulphate. *J. Cell. Biol.* 1977, **164**: 75–81.

145 Oldberg A., Kjellen L., Hook M.: Cell-surface heparan sulfate: Isolation and characterization of a proteoglycan from rat liver membranes. *J. Biol. Chem.* 1979, **254**: 8505–8510.

146 Oldberg A., Ruoslahti E.: Interactions between chondroitin sulfate proteoglycans, fibronectin, and collagen. *J. Biol. Chem.* 1982, **257**: 4859–4863.

147 Oohira A., Wight T. N., Bornstein P.: Sulfated proteoclycans synthesized by vascular endothelial cells in cultures. *J. Biol. Chem.* 1983, **258**: 2014–2021.

148 Pacifici M., Molinaro M.: Developmental changes in glycosaminoglycans during skeletal muscle cell differentiation in culture. *Exp. Cell Res.* 1980, **126**: 143–152.

149 Palmiter R. D., Davidson J. M., Gagnon J., Rowe D. W., Bornstein P.: NH$_2$-terminae sequence of the chick pro α$_1$ (I) chain synthesized in the reticulocyte lysate system. *J. Biol. Chem.* 1979, **254**: 1433.

150 Patsch W., Franz S., Schonfeld G.: Role of insulin in lipoprotein secretion by cultured rat

heptocytes. *J. Clin. Invest.* 1983, **7**: 1161–1174.

151 Pennypacker J. P., Lewis C. A., Hassell J. R.: Altered proteoglycan metabolism in mouse limb mesenchyme cell cultures treated with vitamin A. *Arch. Biochem. Biophys.* 1978, **186**: 351–358.

152 Pessac B., Defendi V.: Cell aggregation: Role of acid mucopolysaccharides. *Science* 1971, **175**: 898–900.

153 Piez K. A.: Crosslinks of collagen and elastin. *Ann. Rev. Biochem.* 1968, **37**: 547–570.

154 Plant P. W., Deeley R. G., Grieninger G.: Selective block of albumin gene expression in chick embryo hepatocytes cultured without hormones and its partial reversal by insulin. *J. Biol. Chem.* 1983, **258**: 15355–15360.

155 Ponce P., Cordero J., Rojkind M.: A noncollagenous matrix component for attachment of rat hepatocytes in culture. *Hepatology* 1981, **1**: 204–210.

156 Pratt R. M., Yamada K. M., Olden K., Ohanian S. H., Hascall V. C.: Tunicamycin-induced alterations in the synthesis of sulfated proteoglycans and cell surface morphology in the chick embryo fibroblast. *Exp. Cell Res.* 1979, **118**: 245–252.

157 Prehm P.: Induction of hyaluronic acid synthesis in teratocarcinoma stem cells by retinoic acid. *FEBS Lett.* 1980, **111**: 295–298.

158 Prinz R., Klein U., Sudhakaran P. R., Sinn W., Ullrich K. von Figura K.: Metabolism of sulfated glycosaminoglycans in rat hepatocytes. Synthesis of heparan sulfate and distribution into cellular and extracellular pools. *Biochim. Biophys. Acta* 1980, **630**: 402–413.

159 Prockop D. J., Kivirikko J. J., Tuderman L., Guzman N. A.: The biosynthesis of collagen and its disorder. *N. Eng. J. Med.* 1979, **301**: 13–23.

160 Ramachandran G. N., Reddi A. M. (Eds): *Biochemistry of Collagen*: 1976, Plenum, New York, pp 536.

161 Rapraeger A. C., Bernfield M.: Heparan sulfate proteoglycans from mouse mammary epithelial cells. A putative membrane proteoglycan associates quantitatively with lipid vesicles. *J. Biol. Chem.* 1983, **258**: 3632–3636.

162 Reid L. M., Jefferson D. M.: Cell culture studies using extracts of extracellular matrix to study growth and differentiation in mammalian cells. *In: Mammalian Cell Culture*, J. P. Mather (Ed.), 1984, pp 239–280.

163 Reid L. M., Jefferson D. M.: Culturing hepatocytes and other differentiated cells. *Hepatology* 1984, **4**: 548–559.

164 Remberger K., Gay S., Fietzek P. P.: Immunohistochemische untersuchungen zur kollagen charakterisierung in lebercirrhosen. *Virchows Arch. Pathol. Anat. Histol.* 1975, **367**: 231–367.

165 Rich A. M., Pearlstein E., Weissmann G., Hoffstein S. T.: Cartilage proteoglycans inhibit fibronectin-mediated adhesion. *Nature* 1981, **293**: 224–226.

166 Risteli J., Bachinger H. P., Engel J., Furthmayr H., Timpl R.: 7–S collagen: Characterization of an unusual basement membrane structure. *Eur. J. Biochem.* 1980, **108**: 239–250.

167 Robinson J., Viti M., Hook M.: Structure and properties of an undersulfated heparan sulfate proteoglycan synthesized by a rat hepatoma cell line. *J. Cell Biol.* 1984, **98**: 946–953.

168 Rojkind M., Gatmaitan Z., Mackensen S., Giambrone M.-A., Ponce P., Reid L. M.: Connective tissue biomatrix: Its isolation and utilization for long-term cultures of normal rat hepatocytes. *J. Cell Biol.* 1980, **87**: 255–263.

169 Rojkind M., Ponce-Noyola P.: The extracellular matrix of the liver. A Review. *Coll. Relat. Res.* 1982, **2**: 151–175.

170 Rollins B. J., Culp L. A.: Glycosaminoglycans in the substrate adhesion sites of normal and virus-transformed murine cells. *Biochem.* 1979, **18**: 141–148.

170b Rosenberg L., Varma R. An overview of proteoglycans in physiology and pathology. *In: Glycosaminoglycans and Proteoglycans in Physiological and Pathological Processes of Body Systems*, R. Varma, (Ed): Karger, Basel, Switzerland, 1982, pp 1–15.

171 Rubin J., Hook M., Obrink B., Timpl R.: Substrate adhesion of rat hepatocytes: Mechanism of attachment to collagen substrate. *Cell* 1981, **24**: 463–470.

172 Saber M. A., Zern M. A., Shafritz D. A.: Use of *in situ* hybridization to identify collagen and albumin mRNA in isolated mouse hepatocytes. *Proc. Natl. Acad. Sci.* 1983, **80**: 4017–4020.

173 Sakakibara K., Umeda M., Saito S., Nagase, S.: Production of collagen and acidic glycosamino-glycans by an epithelial liver cell clone in culture. *Exp. Cell Res.* 1977, **110**: 159–165.

174 Sakakibara K., Takaoka T., Katsuta H., Umeda M., Tsukada Y.: Collagen fibre formation as a

common property of epithelial liver cell lines in culture. *Exp. Cell Res.* 1978, **111**: 63–71.

175 Salomon D. S., Liotta L. A., Kidwell W. R.: Differential response to growth factor by rat mammary epithelium plates on different collagen substrata in serum-free medium. *Proc. Natl. Acad. Sci.* 1981, **78**: 382–386.

176 Sano J., Sato S., Ishizaki M., Yajima G., Konomi H., Fujiwara S., Najai Y.: Types I, III and IV (basement membrane) collagens in the bovine liver parenchyma: Electron microscopic localization by the peroxidase-labelled antibody method. *Biomed. Res.* 1981, **2**: 546–551.

177 Schwartz C. E., Ruoslahti E.: Concurrent modulation of cell surface fibronectin and adhesion to fibronectin in hepatoma cells. *Exp. Cell. Res.* 1983, **143**: 456–461.

178 Schwarze P. E., Solheim A. E., Seglen P. O.: Amino acid and energy requirements for rat hepatocytes in primary culture. *In Vitro* 1982, **18**: 43–54.

179 Schudt C.: Hormonal regulation of glucokinase in primary cultures of rat hepatocytes. *Eur. J. Biochem.* 1979, **98**: 77–82.

180 Seglen P. O.: Hepatocyte suspensions and cultures as tools in experimental carcinogenesis. A Review. *J. Toxicol. Environ. Health.* 1979, 5: 551–560.

181 Sell S., Ruoslahti E.: Expression of fibronectin and laminin in the rat liver after partial hepatectomy, during carcinogenesis, and in transplantable hepatocellular carcinomas. *J. Natl. Can. Inst.* 1982, **69**: 1005–1014.

182 Shapiro S. S., Poon J. P.: Effect of retinoic acid on chondrocyte glycosaminoglycan biosythesis. *Arch. Biochem. Biophys.* 1976, **174**: 74–81.

183 Siegel R. C.: Lysyl oxidase. *Int. Rev. Conn. Tiss. Res.* 1979, **8**: 73–118.

184 Sinn W., Sudhakaran P. R., Von Figura K.: Stimulation of heparan sulphate synthesis in cultured rat hepatocytes by (+)-catechin. *Biochem. J.* 1981, **200**: 51–57.

185 Sirica A. E., Richards W., Tsukada Y., Sattler C. A., Pitot H. C.: Fetal phenotypic expression by adult rat hepatocytes on collagen gel/nylon meshes. *Proc. Natl. Acad. Sci.* 1979, **76**: 283–287.

186 Smith B. D., Niles R.: Characterization of collagen synthesized by normal and chemically transformed rat liver epithelial cell lines. *Biochem.* 1980, **19**: 1820–1825.

187 Spagnoli D., Dobrosielski-Vergona K., Widnell C. C.: Effects of hormones on the activity of glucose-6-phosphatase in primary cultures of rat hepatocytes. *Arch. Biochem. Biophys.* 1983, **226**: 182–189.

188 Spooner E., Gallagher J. T., Kirzsa F., Dexter T. M.: Regulation of haemopoiesis in long-term bone marrow cultures. IV. Glycosaminoglycan synthesis and the stimulation of haemopoiesis by β-D-Xylosides. *J. Cell Biol.* 1983, **96**: 510–514.

189 Stamatoglou S. C., Keller J. M.: Correlation between cell substrate attachment *in vitro* and cell surface heparan sulfate affinity for fibronectin and collagen. *J. Cell Biol.* 1983, **96**: 1820–1823.

190 Straus D. S.: Growth-stimulatory actions of insulin *in vitro* and *in vivo*. *Endocrine Rev.* 5: 356–369.

191 Strom S. C., Michalopoulos G.: Collagen as a substrata for cell growth and differentiation. *Meth. Enzymol.* 1982, **82**: 544–555.

192 Sudhakaran P. R., Sinn W., Von Figura K.: Regulation of heparan sulphate metabolism by adenosine 3′:5′-cyclic monophosphate in hepatocytes in culture. *Biochem. J.* 1980, **192**: 395–402.

193 Sudhakaran P. R., Sinn W., Von Figura K.: Initiation of altered heparan sulphate by β-D-xyloside in rat hepatocytes. *Hoppe-Seyler's Z. Physiol. Chem. Bd.* 1981, **362**: 39–46.

194 Tamkun J. W., Hynes R. O.: Plasma fibronectin is synthesized and secreted by hepatocytes. *J. Biol. Chem.* 1983, **258**: 4641–4647.

195 Terranova V. P., Rohrbach D. H., Martin G. R.: Role of laminin in the attachment of PAM 212 (epithelial) cells to basement membrane collagen. *Cell.* 1980, **22**: 719–726.

196 Thompson H. A., Spooner B. S.: Proteoglycan and glycosaminoglycan synthesis in embryonic mouse salivary glands: Effects of β-D-Xyloside, an inhibitor of branching morphogenesis. *J. Cell Biol.* 1983, **96**: 1443–1450.

197 Timpl R., Wiedemann H., Van Delden V., Furthmayr H., Kuhn K.: A network model for the organization of type IV collagen molecules in basement membranes. *Eur. J. Biocehm.* 1981, **120**: 203–211.

198 Timpl R., Rohde H., Risteli L., Ott U., Robey P., Martin G.: Laminin. *Meth. Enzymol.* 1982, **82**: 831–838.

199 Trelsted R. L. (Ed.): *The Role of Extracellular Matrix in Development*: Alan R. Liss, Inc, New York, 1984.

200 Tyree B., Ledbetter S., Hassell J. R.: Basement membrane proteoglycans processing. *J. Cell Biol.* 1983, **97**: A230.

201 Underhill C., Dorfman A.: The role of hyaluronic acid in intercellular adhesion of cultured mouse cells. *Exp. Cell. Res.* 1978, **117**: 155–164.

202 Underhill C. B., Keller J. M.: A transformation-dependent difference in the heparan sulfate associated with the cell surface. *Biochem. Biophys. Res. Comm.* 1975, **63**: 448–454.

203 Vaheri A., Mosher D. F.: High molecular weight, cell surface-associated glycoprotein (fibronectin) lost in malignant transformation. *Biochim. Biophys. Acta.* 1978, **516**: 1–25.

204 Vlodavsky I., Lui G. M., Gospodarowicz D.: Morphological appearance, growth behaviour and migratory activity of human tumor cells maintained on extracellular matrix versus plastic. *Cell* 1980, **19**: 607–616.

205 Vlodavsky I., Ariav Y., Atzmon R., Fuks Z.: Tumor cell attachment to the vascular endothelium and subsequent degradation of the subendothelial extracellular matrix. *Exp. Cell Res.* 1981, **140**: 149–159.

206 Voss B., Ranterberg J., Allam S., Pott G.: Distribution of collagen type I and type III and of two collagenous components of basement membrane in the human liver. *Pathol. Res. Pract.* 1980, **170**: 50–60.

207 Weber W., Kehrer T., Gressner A. M., Stuhlsatz H. W., Greiling H.: Changes in the catalytic activities of proteoglycan-degrading lysosomal enzymes in parenchymal and non-parenchymal liver cells and in serum during the development of experimental liver fibrosis. *J. Clin. Chem. Clin. Biochem.* 1983, **21**: 287–293.

208 Wicha M. S., Liotta L. A., Garbisa S., Kidwell W. R.: Basement membrane collagen requirements for attachment and growth of mammary epithelium. *Exp. Cell. Res.* 1979, **124**: 181–190.

209 Wick G., Brunner H., Penner E., Timpl R.: The diagnostic application of specific anti procollagen sera: II. Analysis of liver biopsies. *Int. Arch. Allergy Appl. Immunol.* 1978, **56**: 316–324.

210 Williams G. M., Bermudez E., San R. H. C., Goldblatt P. J., Laspia M. F.: Rat hepatocyte primary cultures: IV. Maintenance in defined medium and the role of production of plasminogen activator and other proteases. *In Vitro.* 1978, **14**: 824–837.

211 Wilson E. J., McMurray W. C.: Effects of hormones on the maintenance and mitochondrial functions of rat hepatocytes cultured in serum-free medium. *Can. J. Biochem. Cell Biol.* 1983, **61**: 636–643.

212 Winterbourne D. J., Mora P. T.: Cells selected for high tumorigenicity or transformed by simian virus 40 synthesize heparan sulfate with reduced degree of sulfation. *J. Biol. Chem.* 1981, **256**: 4310–4320.

213 Woods A., Hook M., Kjellen L., Smith C. G., Rees D. A.: Relationship of heparan sulfate proteoglycans to the cytoskeleton and extracellular matrix of cultured fibroblasts. *J. Cell. Biol.*

214 Yamada M., Okigaki T.: Promotion of epithelial cell adhesion on collagen by proteins from rat embryo fibroblasts. *Cell Biol. Int. Rep.* 1983, **7**: 1115–1121.

215 Yamada K.: Cell surface interactions with extracellular materials. *Ann. Rev. Biochem.* 1983, **52**: 761–799.

216 Yamada K.: Fibronectin and Interactions at the Cell Surface. *Prog. Clin. Biol. Res.* 1984, **151**: 1–15.

217 Yang J., Nandi S.: Growth of cultured cells using collagen as substrate. *Int. Rev. Cytol.* 1983, **81**: 249–286.

218 Yoshimoto K., Nakamura T., Ichihara A.: Reciprocal effects of epidermal growth factor on key lipogenic enzymes in primary cultures of adult hepatocytes. *J. Biol. Chem.* 1983, **258**: 12355–12360.

Research in *Isolated and cultured hepatocytes* A. Guillouzo & C. Guguen-Guillouzo eds., pp. 259–284.
© 1986 John Libbery Eurotext Ltd./INSERM.

12

Role of homotypic and heterotypic cell interactions in expression of specific functions by cultured hepatocytes

Christiane GUGUEN-GUILLOUZO

Unité de Recherches Hépatologiques, INSERM U49, Hôpital Pontchaillou, 35033 Rennes Cédex, FRANCE

SUMMARY

Intercellular adhesions are fundamental in embryonic induction by mediation of the early expression of two CAMs: N-CAM (neuronal CAM) and L-CAM (liver CAM). These molecules are integral membrane proteins. They must play a direct role during early events of development in the control of morphogenetic movements, cellular adhesion and motility. Cell-cell interactions also play a critical role in later stages of tissue organogenesis. Liver results from necessary cellular interactions between the endoderm, which differentiates into parenchymal cords, and the mesoderm, which gives rise to the endothelial cells lining the blood sinusoids. L-CAM appears as a major cell adhesion molecule on embryonic liver cells. In addition cell-cell interactions remain essential for maintaining and modulating the hepatocyte functional capacities in adult life. Adult hepatocytes are able to communicate between each of them and to express cell density dependence. Gap junctions are the morphological specialization in plasma membranes that enable contacting cells to communicate. The synthesis rates of albumin and total cellular proteins as well as the total RNA are increased in cells at low density. However, this increased functional activity corresponds only to a transient stimulation which may suggest principally stabilization of mRNAs for a few days. Functional changes and cell death occur early. Therefore, these homotypic hepatocyte-hepatocyte interactions would be useful for quantitatively determining the level of specific expression whereas another type of cell-cell interactions involving cell contacts between hepatocytes and biliary cells may fundamentally influence the specific liver expression. Using a co-culture system it is observed that this type of heterotypic binding with hepatocytes improves cell viability and controls the maintenance or the disappearance of specific gene expression, at least in part, at the transcriptional level for several weeks.

Introduction

Intercellular adhesion is of fundamental importance in embryonic induction, in growth and differentiation, in the maintenance and regeneration of tissues as well as in certain pathological conditions. But, the underlying molecular mechanisms involved in these processes remain obscure and complex.

It would be difficult to consider that the form and pattern of tissues could arise solely from any one molecular mechanism. Indeed, we have to account for three major events in the course of development before reaching adult life: the early embryonic events with their coordinated series of morphogenetic movements; the secondary events of histogenesis; and, the perinatal changes. Moreover, the molecular basis of tissue differentiation must take into consideration at least four primary processes: cell adhesion, migration, growth and differentiation.

Cell adhesion has been the most extensively studied in embryonic induction (18). One strategy has been to search for molecules mediating cell adhesion and to study their structure and the way they work in relation to key morphogenetic events during early development. Two conflicting hypotheses have arisen concerning the nature of specific cell surface proteins that mediate primary events. The strict chemo-affinity hypothesis suggests that specificity results from the presence of a number of different surface marker molecules (88). This would require the expression of many different gene products in various sites of a single tissue. In contrast, modulation theory asserts that tissues will have only a few cell-cell adhesion molecules (CAMs) with potential modulation mechanisms of their binding activities by epigenetic means (17). In its rigorous form, this last theory requires that different binding regimes can occur for the same kind of cell adhesion molecule, in different regimes of a tissue.

A few years ago, Edelman and several other groups began their search for cell adhesion molecules (CAMs) with the assumption that they must be protein-like molecules displayed on the cell surface and that they are likely to be present in small numbers (17). To date, they have accumulated data which favour the modulation theory rather than the strict chemo-affinity theory of cell-cell recognition. Indeed, so far it can be assumed that two CAMs account for more than two-thirds of the early embryonic surface: N-CAM (neuronal CAM) (91) and L-CAM (liver CAM) (29). One or two other molecules may be necessary to complete the map but in any case it is likely that the number required for embryogenesis will not be very large (19). It is notable that each CAM persists into adult life only in tissues derived from the germ layer in which it was originally expressed. One interpretation of these observations suggests how structures, even though they originate in different layers, can meet to give rise to organs and complex tissues: what they have in common is a CAM.

Intercellular adhesion can, therefore, be considered of fundamental importance in embryonic induction by mediation of the early expression of two CAMs. These CAMs must play a direct role in the control of morphogenetic movements, cellular adhesion and motility. They must, however, be generally independent of the other kinds of molecular systems involved in cellular interactions which are cell substrate adhesion mediated by SAMs (substrate adhesion molecules), and cell contacts via intercellular (gap) junctions and those involved in defined interactions of cells with extracellular matrix (46). CAM expression must be also independent of cell differentiation because a given CAM appears in regions which will later form different cell types of quite different organs.

In the later stages, additional heterotypic interactions appear to require other CAMs with new specificities needed to generate certain patterns. Histogenesis of mouse brain, the best studied organ, affords an example of this increasing complexity with late development. In this system, besides N-CAM, a new molecule N_gCAM has already been found on neuron surface in order to develop heterotypic interactions with glial cells (50). Furthermore, modulation mechanisms by chemical modifications of these proteins or by changes of their local distribution have been described to play a specific control in this tissue maturation.

Thus, in view of the need for specificity and the diverse structural requirements made upon cells in different tissues, a variety of different mechanisms can be hypothesized.

Compared with brain, liver organogenesis and maturation are much less understood. The interest in the study of intercellular adhesion in liver cells has arisen from the ability of the liver to express numerous functions but also to retain the peculiar capacity *in vivo* to regenerate normally to form a well organized tissue. Moreover, when isolated and plated in tissue culture, hepatocytes reconstitute cell trabeculae and also show adhesive affinity for a wide variety of surfaces including plastic, fibronectin, collagen and heterologous cells.

Most of the liver specific functions including production of export proteins and several groups of enzymes are located in the hepatocytes. But these cells represent only about 65 per cent of the total cell population. Thus, cultures of pure hepatocyte populations have been studied in order to better define their own functional regulation. Indeed, these pure hepatocyte cultures eliminated complexities involved in heterogeneous populations and permitted studies of cell to cell adhesion and cell-matrix interactions. However, a number of studies over the last 10 years have shown that although cultured hepatocytes reconstituted trabeculae and transiently reformed bile canaliculi, they were unable to retain a stable differentiated state (15, 34, 38, 87). After a few days of culture they had invariably lost most of the differentiated functions despite efforts of cell biologists to rigorously define culture environment (medium and support). One conclusion that can be drawn from this universal phenomenon is that very few, if any, tissue-specific functions are 'constitutive'. Moreover, the decrease in function that occurs in this primary culture model could be regarded as an asset rather than a liability; it suggests that a complex tissue such as liver, which has diverse functions and an intricate structure, does require a much more complex micro-environment for the maintenance of its differentiated state. It is, therefore, reasonable to question whether heterotypic cell interactions are necessarily required for the regulation processes of hepatic differentiation in later stages of development and in adult life as well as during early embryogenesis.

This review, after considering the role of cell adhesion in early embryonic liver formation, will describe different mechanisms of interactions between mature hepatocytes or between hepatocytes and other hepatic cells and will focus attention on their role on differentiation *in vitro*.

Liver organogenesis results from cellular interactions between the endoderm and the mesoderm

At the primitive streak stage, the prospective hepatic area is localized in the anterior half of the blastoderm so that the liver endodermal and mesenchymal potencies are at first located in the same embryonic area (58). Later, after the gastrulation process, liver endodermal and mesodermal areas evolve differently. The presumptive hepatic endoderm migrates ventrally and becomes restricted anteriorily to a small surface while the liver mesodermal component extends posteriorly in the septum transversum. During the closure of the foregut, liver endodermal buds develop and proliferate. They give rise to epithelial cords which invade the mesenchyme of the septum transversum and the lateral mesenchymal areas, and differentiate into parenchymal cells. Mesenchyme gives rise to the endothelial cells lining the blood sinusoids. Necessary invasion of hepatic mesenchymal areas by endoderm for the differentiation of hepatocytes to occur has been well established (52). Mouse hepatic endoderm has been cultivated alone or in association with chick mesenchyme by placing the two tissues in contact with each other for two days at 38°C. The explants were then grafted into the somatopleure of 3-day chick embryos. When cultivated alone, the mouse hepatic endoderm failed to differentiate and rapidly became necrotic, whereas when associated with mesenchyme it differentiated into parenchymal cells. The results were the same regardless of substrate or culture medium. It is interesting to note that the presumptive hepatic endoderm appeared committed to differentiate into hepatocytes at a very early stage, while the action of the mesodermal component remained non-specific since mesenchyme of another species and even of another tissue could replace the hepatic mesoderm. In addition, this morphogenetic interaction required close apposition of the interacting cells.

This progressive regrouping of cells which occurs throughout liver organogenesis might be mediated by specific CAMs which differ from the molecules involved in gap junctions and substrate adhesion (18). Liver CAM (L-CAM) is a cell surface glycoprotein, one of the two primitive CAMs found in early embryonic epochs (20). It is a major cell adhesion molecule on embryonic liver cells, originally isolated from embryonic liver tissue by Gallin *et al.* (29). L-CAM, like N-CAM appears to be an integral membrane protein but differs from it markedly in structure with a molecular weight of 124 000 daltons whereas N-CAM is 160 000 daltons and without the polysialic acid found in N-CAM (16, 29, 51). They also differ markedly in their mechanisms of binding. Unlike N-CAM, L-CAM mediates cell adhesion only when calcium ions are present (29). In addition, they have different immunological properties. The distribution of L-CAM and N-CAM during organogenesis also suggests that these molecules are associated with different histogenetic adhesion processes. During pregastrulation and gastrulation, L-CAM remains present on ectoderm but is not detected on mesodermal and definitive endodermal cells. During neurulation and organogenesis, L-CAM disappears from the neural ectoderm in which N-CAM increases markedly. It appears and remains on all endodermally derived structures including liver (15). However, it remains possible that detailed analysis will reveal some evolutionary similarities for these two CAMs (29).

The role of the L-CAM molecule has not yet been strictly defined by functional and biochemical experiments. Nonetheless, the sequence of enhanced staining and disappearance is strikingly correlated with both primary and secondary inductions during early development. Hyafil *et al.* (54) have described uvomorulin, a molecule involved in the adhesion and compaction of the early embryo that is released from embryonal carcinoma cells by trypsin in the presence of calcium. Yoshida & Takeichi (100) have also described a molecule on teratocarcinoma cells that appears as a species of Mw 140 000. There is a possibility that all of these molecules are closely related or identical molecules that could be comparable to L-CAM. These similarities raise the possibility that L-CAM carries out major functions during early events of development including cell adhesion and movement, as well as cell-cell recognition, but the causal signals for the differential expression of this CAM are not known.

The fundamental shaping event of liver organogenesis, the endodermal to mesenchymal transition, might be accounted for by the prevalent modulation of L-CAM and also by the coordinate rise and fall of a substrate molecule (SAM), as in the case of migration of neural crest cells studied by Rovasio *et al.* (81). These authors describe fibronectin forming a carpet on which the cells move. To date, such interaction of L-CAM with SAM or an extracellular matrix component has not been described in liver organogenesis. No chemical modulation event has been observed for L-CAM, but L-CAM modulation could be possible by changes in cell surface prevalence.

Thus, heterotypic cell interactions play a critical role on parenchymal differentiation of endoderm during embryogenesis. Cell-cell interactions will remain essential for maintaining and modulating the functional capacities of hepatocytes in later stages of development as well as in adult life.

Hepatocytes isolated from animals at different developmental stages can reaggregate spontaneously *in vitro* and communicate

Hepatocytes isolated from animals of later stages of development or of adult life may be maintained alive in suspension in nutritive medium for only 6 h. However, in order to survive longer they must attach to a substratum. This observation suggests that interactions of cells with the substratum do occur. Moreover, hepatocytes reaggregate spontaneously and reconstitute cell trabeculae as observed *in vivo*, suggesting a specific adhesive behaviour.

Hepatocyte adhesive affinity is specific

Assay conditions have been devised whereby isolated hepatocytes can express adhesive specificity. Adhesive affinity can be defined as the preference cells show for adhering to homologous rather than to heterologous cell types. If isolated cells given a choice of surfaces, show adhesive specificity by binding to homologous rather than to heterologous cells we assume that they retain cell surface components involved in specific adhesion and reflect the events that occur *in vivo*. Initial studies on cell adhesion were performed with embryonic tissue culture cells (93, 95) and later with young adult animals (71). Kuhlenschmidt *et al.* (57) have performed studies on the intercellular adhesion of rat and chicken hepatocytes. They showed marked adhesive specificity (71). However, the possibility that specificity was observed because the hepatocytes were obtained from divergent species might be raised due to possible mediation of histocompatibility antigens or other similar determinants located on cell surfaces. As shown by Albanese *et al.*, mixtures of hepatocytes and myocytes isolated from a single animal also show dramatic adhesive specificity and therefore rule out the previous hypothesis (1).

In an assay for molecules involved in this liver specific cell aggregation, isolated hepatocytes obtained from 8- to 14-day chicken embryos were seeded onto culture dishes (9). They reaggregated rapidly. This aggregation was experimentally inhibited by FAb' fragments of antibodies prepared against the cells. Moreover, an aqueous extract of liver cell membrane appeared to contain antigens that neutralized the adhesion-blocking properties of the FAb' fragments. The molecule involved in this aggregation of embryonic liver cells was named L-CAM, then purified and characterized. This approach was also used to detect surface components involved in adult rat hepatocyte adhesion (72). Staining for L-CAM has been found in early embryonic epochs and also recently demonstrated in adult liver. It appeared on all surfaces of parenchymal cells with an apparently brighter staining on surfaces between adjacent hepatocytes. There was no apparent staining of blood cells or of cells lining blood vessels and sinusoids (92).

Determination of the exact nature of mechanisms of binding and modulation of binding affinities for L-CAM remain to be elucidated. It is already known that N-CAM undergoes local surface modulation leading to a decrease in sialic acid residues (16, 18) whereas, so far, no chemical modulation event has been observed for L-CAM. Nevertheless, L-CAM shows modulation by change in cell surface prevalence in adult tissues as well as during critical epochs for development. Determination of its relation to formation and maintenance of hepatic structures and functions require more experiments.

Some other proteins and carbohydrates have also been implicated in various cellular interactions (28). They might be involved in hepatocyte adhesive affinity. Both are possibly capable of encoding large degrees of specificity into their structure by variations in the sequence of their constituent residues. In fact, as recalled by Shur (85), variations in structure of surface proteins might be responsible for a variety of cell surface receptor specificities, such as histocompatibility antigens (69) and cell surface carbohydrates might be also instrumental in cell migration, tissue interactions, immune recognition – to mention only a few examples. It can be assumed that these macromolecules, which are thought to mediate cellular interactions, probably function by binding to specific cell surface receptors, analogous to the way hormones elicit specific responses by binding to their appropriate target cell receptors.

So, an orientation appropriate for a quantitative receptor involved in cellular interactions could be plasma membrane molecules capable of recognizing complex carbohydrate residues. A variety of proteins have been identified which can bind complex carbohydrates with high specificity (28). These include the enzymes responsible for their synthesis (glycosyltransferases), the enzymes responsible for their degradation (glycosidases) and proteins with no known enzymatic action but which, nevertheless, interact specifically with carbohydrates (lectins and certain antibodies). Thus, glycosyltransferases synthesize all the known complex carbohydrates, including glycoproteins, glycolipids and glycosaminoglycans, and most of glycosyltransferases are membrane-bound.

Lectins have been suggested to function during cellular interactions by serving as receptors for extracellular complex carbohydrates (5). However, some of these lectins appear to be predominantly intracellular proteins and thus, their role in cellular adhesion awaits clarification. In a series of elegant studies, Pricer & Ashwell showed that liver membranes from mammalian species contain a receptor (eg a binding protein) which is specific for galactose-terminated glycoproteins (75) and which requires Ca^{2+} for activity. Electron microscopy studies have determined that this binding protein is located primarily on the serosal face of the hepatocytes (94).

Isolated hepatocytes, therefore, contain active hepatic carbohydrate-binding proteins, as they do in the intact liver and extensive studies have recently been reported on their kinetic properties and their sugar specificity (56, 98). But, in an attempt to refine the conditions under which the specificity of hepatocyte adhesion was observed, Kulhlenschmidt *et al.* (57) have examined the effects of different sera and divalent cations. Dependent upon certain experimental conditions, they observed that hepatocytes could adhere in a random manner suggesting adhesive nonspecificity. The authors concluded that this nonspecificity was mediated by the hepatic glycoprotein binding proteins. Since they showed that antibodies directed against the purified chicken hepatic agalactoglycoprotein binding protein did not induce a detectable effect on the rate of intercellular adhesion of hepatocytes, they ruled out the possibility that the hepatic carbohydrate binding proteins may be normally involved in adhesive specificity of hepatocytes.

However, this does not preclude a role for these proteins in preferentially selecting other appropriate cells; it is possible that they may be involved in the selection of non-parenchymal cells. An example is found in the nervous system where adhesive specificity is displayed towards heterologous as well as homologous cell types.

Cells *in vitro* as *in vivo* are remarkably specific with respect to their adhesive affinity not only for homologous cells but also for a wide variety of surfaces including fibronectin and collagens (45). For example, the effects of fibronectin on cell morphology, motility and adhesion are likely to be due to the interactions of the 'cellular surface binding' domain of the fibronectin molecule with its specific cell receptor. Fibronectin (2), laminin (2, 77), two examples of adhesive factors, collagens (82) and agglutinines, such as lectins (75) have been demonstrated to be involved in hepatocyte morphology, viability or adhesion. However, it is difficult to imagine that these molecules, while having clear effects on cell social behavior, account for the degree of specificity that characterizes hepatocyte specific recognition and, more generally, for the various cellular interactions that occur throughout development and tissue organogenesis.

When aggregated, hepatocytes are able to communicate undergoing changes in their growth and functional activities as a function of cell density.

Contacting hepatocytes are able to communicate for regulating their functions

Many investigations in a variety of systems have suggested a central role for cell to cell contacts in development as well as in the regulation of cell growth of proliferative cell lines. More recently, specific protein synthesis was also concluded to be cell density dependent, such as prolactin synthesis and secretion from pituitary cells (8) or collagen production from cultured fibroblasts (3).

Assay conditions have been devised where isolated hepatocytes maintained in pure population can also exhibit cell density dependence. When cultured at lower cell density, stimulation of hepatocyte DNA synthesis by insulin and epidermal growth factor was greatly increased (67). However, it is important to note that even if more than 50% of cells, instead of 5%, were labelled by [^{3}H]-thymidine exposure at lower density, only very few cells were able to enter into mitosis. It may, therefore, be hypothesized that most of the cells remained blocked in the G_2 phase.

Ichihara and his coworkers have reported that only growth related functions including DNA synthesis and glucose-6-phosphate dehydrogenase are stimulated at low cell density, whereas hepatocyte specific characters like tyrosine amino-transferase, succinate dehydrogenase or malic enzymes are stimulated at higher cell density (68, 101). For these authors, this reciprocal regulation is due to cell contacts through a membrane signal. By preparing plasma membranes from mature rat liver and adding them to cells at low density they mimicked the effect of high cell density and they defined this factor as a protein-like 'cell surface modulator'.

However, when measuring albumin secretion, a non-growth related function, and the rate of synthesis of total cellular proteins from hepatocytes seeded either at low or high density, we found that both of them were increased in cells at low density (Figs 1 & 2) (26). This functional stimulation would, therefore, be not only concerning the growth-related functions as suggested by Ichihara, but also the other specific and common proteins. Recent data have allowed us to confirm this hypothesis (Table 1): 1) the amounts of total RNAs from cells at low density were higher; and, 2) the patterns of the translational products of mRNAs prepared from hepatocytes cultured at low and high cell densities were identical suggesting that most, if not all, the

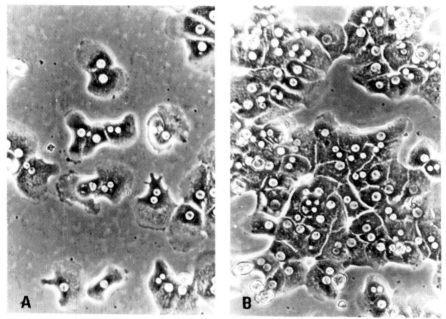

Fig. 1. Phase-contrast micrograph of adult rat hepatocytes seeded at low and high density and observed after one day of culture. 2.5×10^6 cells were seeded in 25 cm^2 (*a*) and 75 cm^2 (*b*) dishes respectively. Magnification $\times 190$.

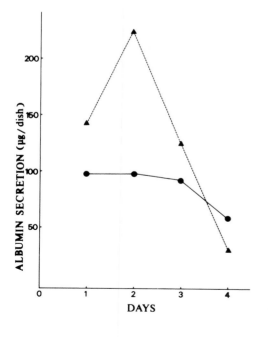

Fig. 2.
Daily quantitation of albumin secretion by hepatocytes seeded at low (▲ . . . ▲) and high density (● – ●). Medium was changed daily and albumin was measured by immunonephelometry using a specific antibody. The values are expressed in μg/dish/24 h. Higher amounts of albumin were secreted in low density cultures.

Table 1. Cell density dependence of two non-growth related functions and of the synthesis rate of total cellular proteins and RNAs in cultured hepatocytes.

	Cell density		
	High density (2.5×10^6 cells/25 cm² dish)	Low density (2.5×10^6 cells/75 cm² dish)	Ratio $\dfrac{Low}{High}$ density
Albumin secretion (μg/24h/dish)	70±6	139±8	2
Level of tyrosine aminotransferase induction	3.6	7.6	2.1
³H-Leucine incorporation (cpm/mg of protein)			
Intracellular proteins	111 500	171 000	1.5
Secreted proteins	171 000	398 000	2.3
Total RNA (μg/50×10⁶ cells)	360	624	1.7
³H-Uridine incorporation (cpm/μg DNA)	87	101	1.2

hepatocyte mRNA sequences undergo the same relative changes when cell density is modified. It is interesting to note that hepatocytes seeded at low density, although having a higher functional activity, show a decreased cell survival when compared with that of cells maintained at high density. Therefore, it may be suggested that the increased functional activity observed at low density would be the consequence of a post-transcriptional regulation involving principally stabilization of mRNAs for a few days.

Gap junctions represent regions of morphological specialization in cell plasma membranes that enable contacting cells to communicate with each other by the relatively nonselective passage of small molecules (7). Recent investigations in a variety of systems have suggested a central role for gap junctional communication in development as well as in the regulation of cell growth (31, 62, 99). Isolated gap junctions were first characterized in livers from mouse and rat (23, 47). It is now widely accepted that the major liver gap junction protein corresponds to a polypeptide with an apparent molecular weight of about 27 000 on SDS-poly-acrylamide gels (70). By immunochemical criteria, a protein similar to the liver gap junction protein was identified as common to many cell types and organisms (49). However, while the gap junction polypeptides may be the same in all tissues, it appears that the regulation of gap junctional communication is not uniform. This communication may be affected in different tissues by many different stimuli including pH (90), calcium concentration (80) and transjunctional potential (89). Indeed, the cells which have gap junctions are ionically coupled and gaps are reported to be low-resistance junctions (53). This heterogeneity might be conferred by specific regulatory proteins which would act as gates for the gap junction channels. There is, as yet, no firm evidence for the existence of such specific cytoplasmic proteins. However, a potential candidate would be the Ca^{++} sensitive protein, calmodulin which has been shown to bind to liver gap junction polypeptides *in vitro* (48).

Contacting hepatocytes are unable to maintain their functional specificity

Despite limited alterations of morphological characteristics and the absence of mitotic activity (15, 35, 96), adult hepatocytes have a limited survival and lose the major part of their functional capacities within 1 week in culture. Although the changes reach a wide spectrum of functions, the more specific ones are preferentially modified. In various metabolic pathways, an early decrease of several specific enzyme activities occurs.

In the soluble cytosolic fraction, the activity of non-specific enzymes such as lactate dehydrogenase or glucose-6-phosphate dehydrogenase (40) was slightly reduced while that of specific enzymes dramatically declined within the first 2 days. This was true for pyruvate kinase, aldolase, tyrosine aminotransferase and glucokinase (11, 40, 73, 87), as well as for some enzymes of the urea cycle such as arginase (61). Some of these enzymes possess several molecular protein forms which have been characterized as genetically determined and may therefore be considered as isozymes. Although exerting the same catalytic function, they are easily distinguishable by electric charges and kinetic constants. Predominant isozymic forms are present exclusively in adult hepatocytes, eg L for pyruvate kinase, B for aldolase and L for phosphofructokinase — and, therefore, may be considered as specific markers. During culture, these specific adult isozymic forms gradually disappear whereas the minor forms, normally synthesized by fetal hepatocytes as well as adult non-parenchymal cells, appear to be the only ones detectable after 7 days (24, 34, 40). The loss of adult isozymes in cultured adult hepatocytes suggests that cell adaptation to standard cell culture conditions results in repression of the synthesis of certain specific proteins and in a shift towards a more fetal-like state. Furthermore, these changes are accelerated and amplified under certain culture conditions, especially those which favour cell attachment and spreading (38, 39).

The induction in cultured hepatocytes of certain enzymes such as tyrosine aminotransferase, alanine aminotransferase and phosphoenolpyruvate carboxy-kinase by hormones, in particular glucocorticoids, has been well documented (11, 40, 44, 61, 84). Several authors have reported decreased basal tyrosine amino-transferase levels within the first 3 days of culture. Enzyme inducibility in the presence of 5×10^{-6} to 10^{-5} M dexamethasone initially increased 4 to 5-fold and only 2-fold on day 6 (11, 40, 44). Five enzymes or groups of enzymes are involved in the conversion of CO_2 and ammonia to urea. The activity of these different enzymes (both mitochondrial and cytoplasmic) has been found to be well maintained for 24 to 72 hours and at a lower level up to 96 hours in cells incubated in serum-free medium without hormone supplementation (61). Later on, enzyme activities rapidly declined. Drug metabolizing enzymes also disappear in a sequential manner in cultured adult hepatocytes. Cytochrome P-450-dependent enzymes and conjugating enzymes which are absent or low in the fetal liver are rapidly lost whereas reduction reactions, which are active drug metabolic pathways found in the fetal liver, are maintained for longer. Therefore, like isozymic changes, these modifications could be interpreted as an adult to fetal transition under culture conditions.

Most plasma proteins with the exception of immunoglobulins are produced by the hepatocytes. Several of them have been found in hepatocyte cultures, including albumin, transferrin, α_1-acid glycoprotein and α_2u-globulin (86). All hepatocytes participate in albumin production and the amounts secreted are related to the degree of cell ploidy (41, 59). However, the rate of albumin secretion by adult rat hepatocytes rapidly declines after a few days of culture (38, 41, 64, 86). These different observations indicate that the biosynthetic machinery of hepatocytes is rapidly altered during culture. The phenotypic changes appear to correspond to an ordered adaptation to an *in vitro* environment and to be related to selective degradation, release or synthesis of certain proteins (21, 24, 40, 86). This leads the cells toward a dedifferentiated state, close to that of fetal cells. Therefore, it is likely that regulation of gene expression is involved in this cell dedifferentiation process.

As might have been predicted, knowing the liver specific protein synthesis changes described above, the concentration of the great majority of liver-specific mRNAs declined with time in culture (13, 27). In addition a dramatic early decrease within 24 h in liver-specific gene transcription was indicated by measuring nascent RNAs from isolated nuclei, while transcription of common genes such as actin did not decline. Thus, a prompt differential transcriptional effect seems to underline the gradual loss of tissue specificity of the primary cultures. It may be noted that drastic changes of chromatin structure, especially of non-histone chromatin proteins, parallels this decline in the rate of transcription (40).

Various exogenous factors have been found to improve cell survival and/or to regulate a number of functions in cultured hepatocytes. Among them are hormones, growth factors, vitamins and co-factors (4, 22). Recently, Reid and her co-workers have compared the transcriptional rates of several mRNA sequences in primary cultures of hepatocytes maintained in a serum supplemented medium or a serum-free hormonally defined medium (55). They demonstrated that, even in conditions in which specific functional activities are better maintained, the transcription level of specific genes remained very low, and they concluded that there was a post-transcriptional regulation involving principally stabilization of mRNAs.

All the present observations show that whatever the cell density and the composition of the medium used, cell viability and *in vitro* functional stability of hepatocyte monolayers do not exceed a few days and that neither interactions between each other nor the presence of various soluble factors are sufficient for maintaining liver specific gene transcription in postnatal and mature hepatocytes. Therefore, it can be questioned whether heterotypic cell interactions are playing a critical role in the regulation processes of hepatic differentiation in later stages of development and in adult life.

Possible *in vitro* control of hepatocyte differentiation by mimicking tissue heterotypic interactions

Hepatocyte and mesenchymal cell interactions can improve longevity of culture

During early hepatic morphogenesis it has been shown that interactions between the endoderm and the mesoderm are required for hepatocyte proliferation and differentiation. Since contacts exist between the two tissues, factors other than soluble ones should be involved. These findings led several authors to hypothesize that the difficulties of maintaining functionally stable hepatocytes *in vitro* were at least partly due to the separation of parenchymal cells from other hepatic cells and their pericellular matrix and therefore to the loss of critical cell-cell relationships, particularly interactions between parenchymal and mesenchymal cells (10, 76).

In the last 5 years, a number of authors have taken into account the possible role of mesenchymal factors in cultured hepatocytes. As proposed by Reid *et al.* (76), the interactions between parenchymal and mesenchymal cells could occur by means of soluble signals or an insoluble collagenous material forming the basement membrane. The soluble signals if present, should be found in conditioned culture medium of the relevant cells. Although some reports have indicated that conditioned medium can be critical for growth and differentiation of target cells, nobody has thus far demonstrated that hepatocytes can maintain their functional activities in the presence of a conditioned medium.

Numerous studies have dealt with the influence of insoluble mesenchymal factors on cultured hepatocytes. Various components of the extracellular connective tissue matrix have been used as substrates (74, 86). Rat hepatocytes have been plated on collagen (11, 66) or fibronectin-coated plastic (63), floating collagen membranes and collagen-coated meshes (86). These cells adhere to both native and denatured collagen, without the aid of fibronectin (83). We have used another complex matrix for cultivating adult hepatocytes which was the extracellular material secreted by bovine corneal endothelial cells (32, 39). These organic substrates promote cell attachment, spreading and survival. However, cell survival rate does not exceed two weeks and phenotypic changes leading to partial loss of differentiated functions occurs within a few days of culture. Therefore, Rojkind *et al.* (79) postulated that, as occurs *in vivo*, hepatocytes required a specific complex matrix *in vitro* and they prepared a 'basement membrane' extract of rat liver containing both glycoproteins and collagenous material.

These data together have shown that normal levels of specific liver functions were not maintained for a very long period when hepatocytes were cultured on organic substrates. Thus, the question arises as to whether the matrices used are adequate since their preparation involves the action of denaturing agents. It cannot be ruled out also that complex cells such as hepatocytes will require a much more complex microenvironment than that obtained with an organic substrate for the maintenance of the differentiated state. Therefore, assays for culturing hepatocytes with other cell types were performed.

Michalopoulos *et al.* (65) have compared the maintenance of some hepatic functions in hepatocytes cultured on collagen membranes and on confluent diploid human fibroblasts. The avidity with which hepatocytes attach on fibroblasts was very high. Moreover, the basal levels of cytochrome P-450 were not measurable after day 3 in hepatocytes cultured on collagen-coated plates, whereas measurable levels were maintained in the hepatocytes cultured on fibroblasts. However, a drastic decrease was regularly observed.

Symbiotic cultures of adult rat hepatocytes and sinus-lining cells, isolated separately by specific enzymatic procedures, were also performed by Wanson *et al.* (97). They included endothelial and Kupffer cells. The survival period of the cultured hepatocytes was increased from 3 to 8 days. For longer periods of culture, the cells underwent partial dedifferentiation and became more flattened. No cell membrane junctions, such as tight or gap junctions, or desmosomes occurred between the adjacent membranes of endothelial cells and hepatocytes. Since the major role of sinusoidal cells is to form an efficient barrier between parenchymal cells and the blood, it is not surprising that their presence *in vitro* does not dramatically affect hepatocyte behaviour. Cell contacts *in vivo* do not exist between hepatocytes and fibroblasts. Furthermore, Type I collagen which is actively synthesized by fibroblastic cells is absent or rare in the Disse space (78).

Only one cell type has direct contact with hepatocytes *in vivo*. These are the epithelial cells, which form the transitional canals of Hering through which bile is transported from bile canaliculi to ductules and ducts. It has been assumed that rat liver epithelial cell lines are derived from this cell type (33). The presence of some hepatic functions in these lines particularly after their transformation (12, 30) could be explained by their close embryonic relationship with hepatocytes.

Taking into account these data, we hypothesized that when mixed with liver epithelial cell lines, hepatocytes would be able to recreate *in vitro* an adequate pericellular environment and maintain a stable phenotype. Our recent results are in agreement with this hypothesis.

Hepatocyte and liver epithelial cell interactions are essential for the maintenance of the long-term functional integrity of adult hepatocytes

When co-cultured with an untransformed epithelial cell line derived from 10-day old rat liver, adult rat hepatocytes survived for more than 2 months (Fig. 3) and secreted high albumin levels throughout the culture period (36) (Fig. 4). Albumin production was shown to be restricted to parenchymal cells. Other proteins including acute-phase proteins were also actively synthesized (43). Tyrosine aminotransferase specific activity remained high and normally inducible by corticosteroids. Cytochrome P-450 levels and the L form of pyruvate kinase which rapidly declined in pure hepatocyte cultures, were analysed during the first 10 days of co-culture and

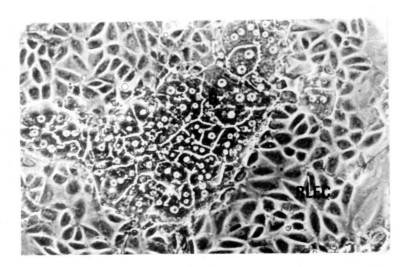

Fig. 3. Phase-contrast micrograph of adult rat hepatocytes co-cultured for 3 weeks with rat liver epithelial cells (RLEC). Magnification ×190.

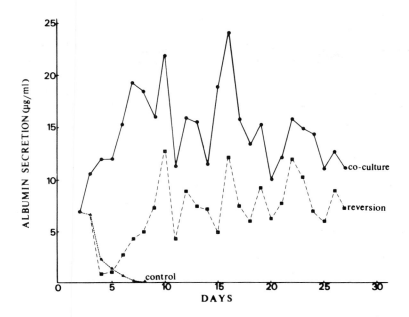

Fig. 4. Secretion of albumin by adult rat hepatocytes cultured alone (▲ . . . ▲) or in association with RLEC (● – ●). Epithelial cells were added either as early as 3 h after hepatocyte seeding or 3 days later for reversion studies (■ . . . ■). The medium was changed daily and used for assays. The values are expressed in µg/ml of medium/24 h.

were also found to be well maintained (6, 42). Long-term maintenance of taucholate uptake was also maintained in co-culture (25). Hepatocytes from various species including man and isolated from either adults or fetuses may interact with rat liver cells and retain high functional capacities for a prolonged period (14, 37, 60).

Interestingly, the qualitative and quantitative maintenance of specific functions in co-cultured hepatocytes appeared to be related to the active production of an extracellular material (36). This material, revealed by reticulin staining, was primarily located between the two cell populations, and later covered the hepatocyte cords and infiltrated epithelial cell areas (Figs 5 & 6). The maintenance of specific liver functions and the production of an extracellular material did not occur in the absence of cell-cell contacts between the two cell populations and conditioned medium or cell extracts from epithelial cells were ineffective. Moreover, the loss or decrease of specific functions which occurred rapidly in pure hepatocyte cultures could be reverted after epithelial cell addition. The increase of specific functions following late addition of epithelial cells was always preceded by establishment of cell-cell contacts and correlated with the production of extracellular material. These findings indicate that the loss of liver functions in cultured hepatocytes is a reversible phenomenon due to modifications of control mechanisms and not to irreversible alterations of cellular structures. Therefore, the expression or the non-expression of a specific function *in vitro* appears to be modulated by a major subset of regulator

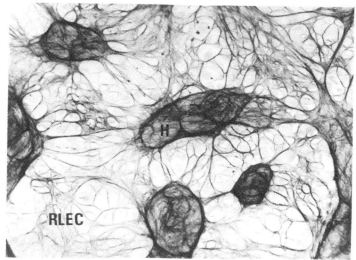

Fig. 5. Reticulin staining of a 7 day rat hepatocyte co-culture. Reticulin fibres are much more abundant on hepatocytes (H) than on rat liver epithelial cells (RLEC). Magnification ×110.

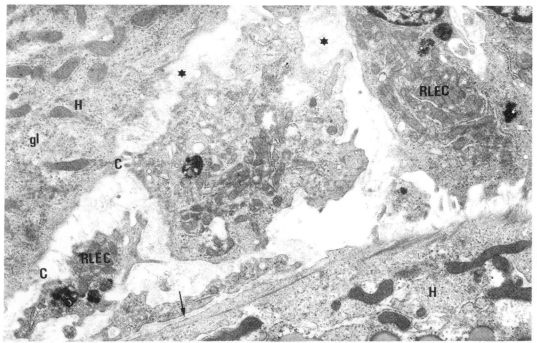

Fig. 6. Electron microscopic appearance of hepatocytes co-cultured with rat liver epithelial cells. Hepatocytes (H) were isolated from an adult human liver by collagenase perfusion and co-cultured with rat liver epithelial cells (RLEC) for 18 days. Hepatocytes still contain glycogen particles (gl) and show discontinuous intimate contacts with rat cells (C). Extracellular material is visible between the two cell types. It appears as either amorphous or fibrillar material (★) or in places as a continuous layer resembling a basement membrane (arrow). Magnification ×12 000.

molecules effected through specific cellular interactions.

We have tried to identify the mechanism of the changes in the amounts of a number of proteins including albumin. Their abundance appears to be determined by their rate of synthesis and, in turn, by the relative concentration of specific mRNA sequences (27). Various specific mRNAs (albumin, aldolase B, pyruvate kinase L etc.) dramatically decline in hepatocytes maintained as pure population as early as day 2 and disappear after 5 days, whereas in co-culture they gradually increase until day 8 and large amounts of various specific mRNAs are still present by day 12 (Figs 7 & 8). Therefore, the principal, if not the only, factor in determining the rate of protein synthesis during co-culture appears to be the mRNA level. The increased amounts of liver specific mRNAs following late addition of RLEC during reversion could also support such a conclusion.

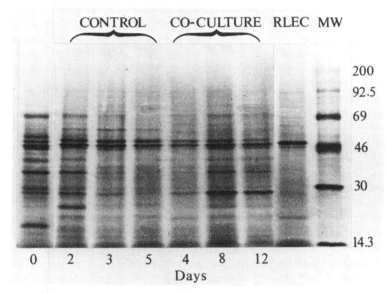

Fig. 7. Translation *in vitro* of cultured hepatocyte RNAs. Hepatocytes were maintained either in pure (control) or mixed (co-culture) cultures. Translation was carried out in reticulocyte lysates using 5 μg of total RNA and 55 μCi of [^{35}S]-methionine. The products were separated electrophoretically and autoradiographed. For comparison, translation products from freshly isolated hepatocytes (O) and rat liver epithelial cells (RLEC) are included. (MW) standard proteins.

In order to determine whether the increased levels of liver specific mRNAs in co-cultured cells resulted from a stabilization of these mRNAs or whether a change of the transcriptional activity takes place we carried out *in vitro* transcription assays in nuclei isolated from control and co-cultured cells (27). Nuclei were isolated and the previously initiated RNA chains were allowed to elongate in the presence of [α^{32}P]UTP. Elongated transcripts were then isolated and hybridized to 'Gene Screen Plus' filters containing DNA from various liver specific genes (Fig. 8). We found: 1) a rate of transcription in co-cultures twice that of pure cultured hepatocytes, on day 4; 2) no significant change in this level of transcriptional activity for at least 2 weeks; and 3) a variation in transcripts from one gene to another when compared to freshly

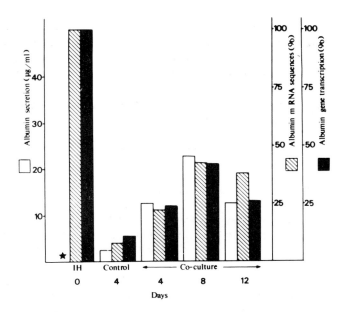

Fig. 8. Graphic representation of albumin secretion (□) and the corresponding mRNA concent-
ration (▨) and transcription level (■) in hepatocyte cultures as a function of time. (IH)
freshly isolated hepatocytes; (control) hepatocytes in conventional culture conditions; (co-
culture) hepatocytes in co-culture conditions. For determination of albumin mRNA concentration, equal amounts of total RNAs from the different sources were used; for transcription
rate analysis equal amounts of labelled RNAs, transcribed *in vitro* in the 'run-on' transcription
system, were hybridized with an excess of specific cDNA. Data are percentage of the freshly
isolated hepatocyte values.

isolated hepatocytes. In co-cultured cells, the transcription of the transferrin gene
continued at a high rate corresponding to 60 to 80% of the initial value, whereas the
transcription of the more specific genes such as albumin was retained at a rate of 20 to
40%. Moreover, it was shown that mRNAs, especially those corresponding to
specific functions could revert to high levels by addition of liver epithelial cells to 3-
day-old hepatocyte cultures. This strongly suggests that a transcriptional event is
also involved in these 'reverted' cultures. By contrast, as previously mentioned,
Jefferson *et al.* (55) demonstrated that even in a hormonally defined medium in
which specific functional activities are better maintained, the transcription level of
specific genes remained very low. In addition, they found that switching cells from
basal to hormonally defined culture medium at 72 h resulted in only stabilization of
the remaining mRNAs.

It may, therefore, be assumed that at least part of the mechanism involved in
long-term functional stability in co-culture is of transcriptional origin and that this
increased transcription is sufficient to enable the cells to survive for several weeks
and to express differentiated functions. This efficient liver specific transcription
could be dependent upon a factor provided by the rat liver epithelial cells since close
contacts were required for stimulation of liver functions, suggesting a key role for
plasma membranes. Cell-to-cell contacts have already been reported as necessary for
liver differentiation during embryogenesis. The co-culture system provides evidence

that heterotypic interactions also play a key role in the maintenance of liver specificity in mature cells. However, the nature of the signal remains unknown. It may be hypothesized that it involves, as a first step, specific cell adhesion via a molecule similar to the L-CAM that induces, as a secondary event, a specific signal which will act on gene transcription either via secretion of a soluble factor and/or extracellular matrix components or via a change of a plasma membrane property under the control of corticosteroids.

A signal from heterotypic cell interactions can be propagated to the whole hepatocyte population

In co-culture, hepatocytes form colonies of cells surrounded by liver epithelial cells so that only a few hepatocytes have close contacts with the other cell type. However, all the hepatocytes from one colony have a prolonged cell survival and the same level of albumin synthesis as shown by immunolocalization experiments. This observation demonstrates that the signal due to co-culture is propagated from one hepatocyte to another.

In addition, the protein synthesis rate of hepatocytes remains cell density-dependent in co-culture since albumin secretion is two-fold higher in co-culture when hepatocytes are seeded at low compared to high density (26). This increase appears strikingly maintained during time in co-culture (Fig. 9). Thus, hepatocytes maintained in co-culture as well as in pure populations can communicate with each other within the same colony to modulate their protein synthesis.

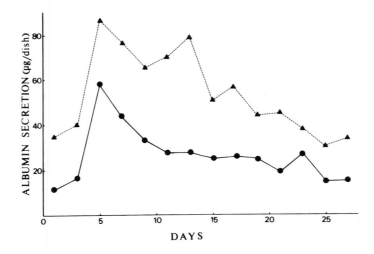

Fig. 9. Daily quantitation of albumin secretion as a function of culture time, by human adult hepatocytes seeded at low (▲ . . . ▲) and high (● – ●) cell density in co-culture. 2×10^6 cells were seeded in 25 cm^2 (● – ●) or 75 cm^2 (▲ . . . ▲) dishes. The medium was changed every day and collected for assay. Albumin is expressed in µg/dish/24 h.

It may be postulated that a post-transcriptional regulation involving principally stabilization of mRNAs may be responsible for these functional changes in co-cultured hepatocytes as well as in pure hepatocyte populations in relation to cell density.

It is interesting to note that hepatocyte DNA synthesis is completely arrested in co-culture whatever the hepatocyte number seeded per plate while labelled thymidine incorporation is highly increased in pure populations of hepatocytes at low cell density.

Conclusions

The results described in this review demonstrate that very few, if any, tissue specific functions are able to be irreversibly expressed in differentiated adult cells. Hepatocytes as well as other cells, such as neurons or pancreatic β cells, must be continuously stimulated by various exogeneous factors to retain their differentiated state. It is now quite obvious that besides the soluble factors like hormones or growth factors that modulate the hepatocyte functional level, cell-cell interactions may play a critical role.

At least two types of cell-cell interactions, described in this review are concerned: (1) the heterotypic cell interactions between hepatocytes and biliary cells; and, (2) the homotypic hepatocyte-hepatocyte interactions. They influence the specific liver functions at two different levels. One is fundamental since it controls the maintenance or the disappearance of the specific gene expression, at least in part at the transcriptional level. As illustrated with the co-culture system the heterotypic binding between hepatocytes and biliary cells plays this key role. The second level of regulation is for quantitatively determining the level of expression, and stabilization of mRNAs seems principally involved. Homotypic hepatocyte-hepatocyte interactions may act at this level.

Soluble factors, especially hormones, would also be essential for modulating both levels of regulation by acting either on heterotypic cell-cell interactions or on hepatocytes themselves.

Thus, cell-cell interactions which have been described as essential during early embryogenesis and late development for allowing liver organogenesis and parenchymal cell differentiation remain also critical during adult life for allowing the maintenance of the hepatic tissular specificity. However, in view of the needs that are different in embryonic and adult tissues, CAMs with different specificities are probably involved and a variety of different modulation mechanisms can be hypothesized.

ACKNOWLEDGMENTS

I wish to express my sincere appreciation to my collaborators who have contributed to personal data. I thank Professor J. Kruh and Dr A. Strain for their thoughtful criticism of the review and Mrs A. Vannier for typing the manuscript. Personal research was supported by the Institut National de la Santé et de la Recherche Médicale.

REFERENCES

1 Albanese J., Kuhlenschmidt M. S., Schmell E., Slife C. W., Roseman S.: Studies on the intercellular adhesion of rat and chicken hepatocytes. *J. Biol. Chem.* 1982, 257: 3165–3170.

2 Alitalo K., Kurkinen M., Vaheri A., Krieg T., Timpl R.: Extracellular matrix components synthesized by human amniotic epithelial cells in culture. *Cell* 1980, **19**: 1053–1062.

3 Aumailley M., Krieg T., Razaka G., Muller P. K., Bricaud H.: Influence of cell density on collagen biosynthesis in fibroblast cultures. *Biochem. J.* 1982, **202**: 505–510.

4 Barnes D., Sato G.: Serum-free culture: a unifying approach. *Cell* 1980, **22**: 649–655.

5 Barondes S. H.: Lectins: their multiple endogenous cellular functions. *Ann. Rev. Biochem.* 1981, **50**: 207–231.

6 Begue J. M., Guguen-Guillouzo C., Pasdeloup N., Guillouzo A.: Prolonged maintenance of active cytochrome P-450 in adult rat hepatocytes co-cultured with another liver cell type. *Hepatology* 1984, **4**: 839–842.

7 Bennett, M. V. L., Goodenough D. A.: Gap junctions, electronic coupling and intercellular communication. *Neurol. Res. Prog. Bull.* 1978, **16**: 473–486.

8 Bentley A. M., Wallis M.: Cell density dependence of the rate of prolactin secretion from perifused rat anterior pituitary cells. *J. Endocr.* 1983, **97**: 221–228.

9 Bertolotti R., Rutishauser U., Edelman G. M.: A cell surface molecule involved in aggregation of embryonic liver cells. *Proc. Natl. Acad. Sci.* 1980, **77**: 4831–4835.

10 Bissell D. M., Guzelian P. S.: Phenotypic stability of adult rat hepatocytes in primary monolayer culture. *Ann. N.Y. Acad. Sci.* 1980, **349**: 85–98.

11 Bonney R. J., Becker J. E., Walker P. R., Potter V. R.: Primary monolayer cultures of adult rat liver parenchymal cells suitable for study of the regulation of enzyme synthesis. *In Vitro* 1974, **9**: 399–413.

12 Borek C.: Neoplastic transformation *in vitro* of a clone of adult liver epithelial cells into differentiated hepatoma-like cells under conditions of nutritional stress. *Proc. Natl. Acad. Sci.* 1972, **69**: 956–959.

13 Clayton D. F., Darnell J. E.: Changes in liver-specific compared to common gene transcription during primary culture of mouse hepatocytes. *Molec. Cell Biol.* 1983, **3**: 1552–1561.

14 Clement B., Guguen-Guillouzo C., Campion J. P., Glaise D., Bourel M., Guillouzo A.: Long-term co-cultures of adult human hepatocytes with rat liver epithelial cells: modulation of albumin secretion and accumulation of extracellular material. *Hepatology* 1984, **4**: 373–380.

15 Chapman G. S., Jones A. L., Meyer U. A., Bissell D. M.: Parenchymal cells from adult rat liver in non proliferating monolayer culture. II. Ultrastructural studies. *J. Cell. Biol.* 1973, **59**: 735–745.

16 Cunningham B. A., Hoffman S., Rutishauser U., Hemperly J. J., Edelman G. M.: Molecular topography of N-CAM: surface orientation and the location of sialic acid-rich and binding regions. *Proc. Natl. Acad. Sci.* 1983, **80**: 3116–3120.

17 Edelman G. M.: Surface modulation in cell recognition and cell growth. Some new hypotheses on phenotypic alteration and transmembranous control of cell surface receptors. *Science* 1976, **192**: 218–226.

18 Edelman G. M.: Cell adhesion molecules. *Science* 1983, **219**: 450–457.

19 Edelman G. M.: Cell adhesion molecules: a molecular basis for animal form. *Sci. Am.* 1984, **251**: 80–91.

20 Edelman G. M., Gallin W. J., Delouvee A., Cunningham B. A., Thiery J. P.: Early epochal maps of two different cell adhesion molecules. *Proc. Natl. Acad. Sci.* 1983, **80**: 4384–4388.

21 Edwards A. M.: Regulation of γ-glutamyltranspeptidase in rat hepatocyte monolayer cultures. *Cancer Res.* 1982, **42**: 1107–1115.

22 Enat R., Jefferson D. M., Ruiz-Opazo N., Gatmaitan Z., Leinwand L. A., Reid L. M.: Hepatocyte proliferation *in vitro*: its dependance on the use of serum-free, hormonally defined medium and substrata of extracellular matrix. *Proc. Natl. Acad. Sci.* 1984, **81**: 1411–1415.

23 Evans W. H., Gurd J. W.: Preparation and properties of nexuses and lipid-enriched vesicles from mouse liver plasma membranes. *Biochem. J.* 1972, **128**: 691–700.

24 Feliu J. E., Coloma J., Gomez-Lechon M. J., Garcia M. D., Baguena J.: Effect of dexamethasone on the isozyme pattern of adult rat liver parenchymal cells in primary cultures. *Molec. Cell. Biochem.* 1982, **45**: 73–81.

25 Foliot A., Glaise D., Erlinger S., Guguen-Guillouzo C.: Long-term maintenance of taurocholate uptake by adult rat hepatocytes co-cultured with a liver epithelial cell line. *Hepatology* 1985, **5**: 215–219.

26 Fraslin J. M., Kneip B., Saunier A., Guguen-Guillouzo C.: Cell density dependence of functional activities in non-proliferating hepatocytes maintained in primary culture. (Submitted).)

27 Fraslin J. M., Kneip B., Vaulont S., Glaise D., Munnich A., Guguen-Guillouzo C.: Dependence of hepatocyte specific gene expression on cell-cell interactions in primary culture. *Embo J.* 1985, 4: 2487–2491.

28 Frazier W., Glaser L.: Surface components and cell recognition. *Ann. Rev. Biochem.* 1979, **48**: 491–523.

29 Gallin W. J., Edelman G. M., Gunningham B. A.: Characterization of L-CAM, a major cell adhesion molecule from embryonic liver cells. *Proc. Natl. Acad. Sci.* 1983, **80**: 1038–1042.

30 Gerschenson L. E., Anderson M., Molson J., Okigaki T.: Tyrosine transaminase induction by dexamethasone in a new rat liver cell line. *Science* 1970, **170**: 859–861.

31 Ginzberg R. D., Gilula N. B.: Modulation of cell junctions during differentiation of the chicken otocyst sensory epithelium. *Dev. Biol.* 1979, **68**: 110–129.

32 Gospodarowicz D., Moran J., Braun D., Birdwell C. A.: Clonal growth of bovine endothelial cells in tissue culture: fibroblast growth factor as a survival agent. *Proc. Natl. Acad. Sci.* 1976, **73**: 4120–4124.

33 Grisham J. W.: Cell types in long-term propagable cultures of rat liver. *Ann. N.Y. Acad. Sci.* 1980, **349**: 128–137.

34 Guguen C., Gregori C., Schapira F.: Modification of pyruvate kinase isozymes in prolonged primary cultures of adult rat hepatocytes. *Biochimie* 1975, **57**: 1065–1071.

35 Guguen C., Guillouzo A., Boisnard M., Le Cam A., Bourel M.: Etude ultrastructurale de monocouches d'hépatocytes de rat adulte cultivés en présence d'hémisuccinate d'hydrocortisone. *Biol. Gastroenterol.* 1975, **8**: 223–231.

36 Guguen-Guillouzo C., Clement B., Baffet G., Beaumont C., Morel-Chany E., Glaise D., Guillouzo A.: Maintenance and reversibility of active albumin secretion by adult rat hepatocytes co-cultured with another liver epithelial cell type. *Exp. Cell Res.* 1983, **143**: 47–54.

37 Guguen-Guillouzo C., Clement B., Lescoat G., Glaise D., Guillouzo A.: Modulation of human fetal hepatocyte survival and differentiation by interactions with a rat liver epithelial cell line. *Dev. Biol.* 1984, **105**: 211–220.

38 Guguen-Guillouzo C., Guillouzo A.: Modulation of functional activities in cultured rat hepatocytes. *Molec. Cell Biochem.* 1983, **53/54**: 35–56.

39 Guguen-Guillouzo C., Seignoux D., Courtois Y., Brissot P., Marceau N., Glaise D., Guillouzo A.: Amplified phenotypic changes in adult rat and baboon hepatocytes cultured on a complex biomatrix. *Biol. Cell* 1982, **46**: 11–20.

40 Guguen-Guillouzo C., Tichonicky L., Szajnert M. F., Schapira F., Kruh J.: Changes of some chromatin and cytoplasmic enzymes in primary cultures of adult rat hepatocytes. *Biol. Cell* 1978, **31**: 225–234.

41 Guillouzo A., Beaumont C., Le Rumeur E., Rissel M., Latinier M. F., Guguen-Guillouzo C., Bourel M.: New findings on immunolocalization of albumin in rat hepatocytes. *Biol. Cell* 1982, **43**: 163–172.

42 Guillouzo A., Beaune P., Gascoin M. N., Begue J. M., Campion J. P., Guengerich F. P., Guguen-Guillouzo C.: Maintenance of cytochrome P-450 in cultured adult human hepatocytes. *Biochem. Pharmacol.* 1985, **34**: 2991–2995.

43 Guillouzo A., Delers F., Clement B., Bernard N., Engler R.: Long term production of acute-phase proteins by adult rat hepatocytes co-cultured with another liver cell type in serum-free medium. *Biochem. Biophys. Res. Commun.* 1984, **120**: 311–317.

44 Gurr J. A., Potter V. R.: Independent induction of tyrosine aminotransferase activity by dexamethasone and glucagon in isolated rat liver parenchymal cells in suspension and in monolayer culture in serum-free medium. *Exp. Cell Res.* 1980, **126**: 237–248.

45 Hay E. D.: Extracellular matrix. *J. Cell Biol.* 1981, **91**: 205–223.

46 Hay E.: Collagen and embryonic development. *In: Cell Biology of Extracellular Matrix*, E. Hay (Ed.): Plenum Publishing Corporation, New York, 1981, pp 379–409.

47 Hertzberg E. L., Gilula N. B.: Isolation and characterization of gap junctions from rat liver. *J. Biol. Chem.* 1979, **254**: 2138–2147.

48 Hertzberg E. L., Gilula N. B.: Liver gap junctions and lens fibre junctions: comparative analysis and cadmodulin interaction. *Cold Spring Harbor Symp. Quant. Biol.* 1981, **46**: 639–645.

49 Hertzberg E. L., Skibbens R. V.: A protein homologous to the 27 000 dalton liver gap junction protein is present in a wide variety of species and tissues. *Cell* 1984, **39**: 61–69.

50 Hoffman S., Edelman G. M.: Kinetics of homophilic binding by embryonic and adult forms of the neural cell adhesion molecule. *Proc. Natl. Acad. Sci.* 1983, **80**: 5762–5766.

51 Hoffman S., Sorkin B. C., White P. C., Brackenbury R., Mailhammer R., Rutishauser U., Cunningham B. A., Edelman G. M.: Chemical characterization of a neural cell adhesion molecule purified from embryonic brain membranes. *J. Biol. Chem.* 1982, **257**: 7720–7729.

52 Houssaint E.: Differentiation of the mouse hepatic primordium. I. An analysis of tissue interactions in hepatocyte differentiation. *Cell Diff.* 1980, **9**: 269–279.

53 Hulser D. F., Webb D. J.: Relation between ionic coupling and morphology of established cells in culture. *Exp. Cell Res.* 1973, **80**: 210–222.

54 Hyafil F., Morello O., Babinet C., Jacob F.: A cell surface glycoprotein involved in the compaction of embryonal carcinoma cells and cleavage stage embryos. *Cell* 1980, **21**: 927–934.

55 Jefferson D. M., Clayton D. F., Darnell J. E., Reid L. M.: Post-transcriptional modulation of gene expression by media conditions in cultured rat hepatocytes. *Molec. Cell. Biol.* 1984, **4**: 1929–1934.

56 Kawaguchi K., Kuhlenschmidt M., Roseman S., Lee Y. C.: Differential uptake of D-galactosyl- and D-glycosyl-neoglycoproteins by isolated rat hepatocytes. *J. Biol. Chem.* 1981, **256**: 2230–2234.

57 Kuhlenschmidt M. S., Schmell E., Slife C. W., Kuhlenschmidt T. B., Sieber F., Lee Y. C., Roseman S.: Studies on the intercellular adhesion of rat and chicken hepatocytes. Conditions affecting cell-cell specificity. *J. Biol. Chem.* 1982, **257**: 3157–3164.

58 Le Douarin N. M.: An experimental analysis of liver development. *Med. Biol.* 1975, **53**: 427–455.

59 Le Rumeur E., Guguen-Guillouzo C., Beaumont C., Saunier A., Guillouzo A.: Albumin secretion and protein synthesis by cultured diploid and tetraploid rat hepatocytes separated by elutriation. *Exp. Cell Res.* 1983, **147**: 247–254.

60 Lescoat G., Theze N., Clement B., Guillouzo A., Guguen-Guillouzo C.: Control of albumin and α-fetoprotein secretion by fetal and neonatal rat hepatocytes maintained in co-culture. *Cell Diff.* 1985, **16**: 259–268.

61 Lin R. C., Snodgrass P. J.: Primary culture of normal adult rat liver cells which maintain stable urea cycle enzymes. *Biochem. Biophys. Res. Commun.* 1975, **64**: 725–734.

62 Loewenstein W. R.: Junctional intercellular communication and the control of growth. *Biochim. Biophys. Acta* 1979, **560**: 1–65.

63 Marceau N., Noel M., Deschenes J.: Growth and functional activities of neonatal and adult rat hepatocytes cultured on fibronectin-coated substratum in serum-free medium. *In Vitro* 1982, **18**: 1–11.

64 May C., Popowski A., Mosselmans R., Wanson J. C.: Albumin synthesis in hepatocytes and preneoplastic nodules isolated from diethylnitrosamine-treated livers. *Biol. Cell* 1979, **35**: 66a.

65 Michalopoulos G., Russel F., Biles C.: Primary cultures of hepatocytes on human fibroblasts. *In Vitro* 1979, **15**: 796–806.

66 Michalopoulos G., Pitot H. C.: Primary culture of parenchymal cells on collagen membranes: morphological and biochemical observations. *Exp. Cell Res.* 1975, **94**: 70–78.

67 Nakamura T., Tomita Y., Ichihara A.: Density-dependent growth control of adult rat hepatocytes in primary culture. *J. Biochem.* 1983, **94**: 1029–1035.

68 Nakamura T., Yoshimoto K., Nakayama Y., Tomita Y., Ichihara A.: Reciprocal modulation of growth and differentiated functions of mature rat hepatocytes in primary culture. *J. Biochem.* 1983, **94**: 1029–1035.

69 Nathenson S. G., Uehara H., Ewenstein B. M., Kindt J. J., Coligan J. E.: Primary structural analysis of the transplantation antigens of the murine H-2 major histocompability complex. *Ann. Rev. Biochem.* 1981, **50**: 1025–1052.

70 Nicholson B. J., Takemoto L. J., Hunkapiller M. W., Hood L. E., Revel J. P.: Differences between liver gap junction protein and lens MIP 26 from rat: Implications for tissue specificity of gap junctions. *Cell* 1983, **32**: 967–978.

71 Obrink B., Kuhlenchmidt M. S., Roseman S.: Adhesive specificity of juvenile rat and chicken liver cells and membranes. *Proc. Natl. Acad. Sci.* 1977, **74**: 1077–1081.

72 Obrink B., Ocklind C.: Cell surface component(s) involved in rat hepatocyte intercellular

adhesion. *Biochem. Biophys. Res. Comm.* 1978, **85**: 837–843.

73 Pariza M. W., Yager J. D. Jr., Goldfarb S., Gurr J. A., Yanachi S., Grossmann S. H., Becker J. E., Barber T. A., Potter V. R.: Biochemical, autoradiographic and electron microscopic studies of adult rat liver parenchymal cells in primary cultures. *In: Gene Expression and Carcinogenesis in Cultured Liver*, L. E. Gershenson, E. B. Thompson (Eds): Academic Press, New York, 1975, pp 137–167.

74 Ponce P., Cordero J., Rojkind M.: A noncollagenous matrix component for attachment of rat hepatocytes in culture. *Hepatology* 1981, **1**: 204–210.

75 Pricer W. E. Jr, Ashwell G.: The binding of desialylated glycoproteins by plasma membranes of rat liver. *J. Biol. Chem.* 1971, **246**: 4825–4833.

76 Reid L., Morrow B., Jubinsky P., Schwartz E., Gatmaitan Z.: Regulation of growth and differentiation of epithelial cells by hormones, growth factors, and substrates of extracellular matrix. *Ann. N.Y. Acad. Sci.* 1981, **372**: 354–370.

77 Rhode H., Wick G., Timpl R.: Immunochemical characterization of the basement membrane glycoprotein, laminin. *Eur. J. Biochem.* 1979, **102**: 195–201.

78 Rojkind M.: The extracellular matrix. *In: The liver: Biology and Pathobiology*, I. Arias, H. Popper, D. Schachter, D. A. Schafritz (Eds): Raven Press, New York, 1982, pp 537–548.

79 Rojkind M., Mackensen S., Giambrone M. A., Ponce P., Reid L.: Connective tissue biomatrix: its isolation and utilization for long-term cultures of normal rat hepatocytes. *J. Cell. Biol.* 1980, **87**: 255–283.

80 Rose B., Rick R.: Intracellular pH, intracellular free Ca and junctional cell-cell coupling. *J. Membrane Biol.* 1978, **44**: 377–415.

81 Rovasio R. A., Delouvee A., Yamada K. M., Timpl R., Thiery J. P.: Neural crest cell migration: requirements for exogenous fibronectin and high cell density. *J. Cell Biol.* 1983, **96**: 462–473.

82 Rubin K., Hook M.: Substrate adhesion of rat hepatocytes: Mechanism of attachment to collagen substrates. *Cell* 1981, **24**: 463–470.

83 Rubin K., Johansson S., Pettersson I., Ocklind C., Obrink B., Hook M.: Attachment of rat hepatocytes to collagen and fibronectin: a study using antibodies directed against cell surface components. *Biochem. Biophys. Res. Commun.* 1979, **91**: 86–94.

84 Savage C. R., Bonney R. J.: Extended expression of differentiated functions in primary cultures of adult liver parenchymal cells maintained on nitrocellulose filters. I. Induction of phosphoenol-pyruvate carboxylase and tyrosine aminotransferase. *Exp. Cell Res.* 1978, **114**: 307–315.

85 Shur B. D.: The receptor function of galactosyltransferase during cellular interactions. *Molec. Cell Biochem.* 1984, **61**: 143–158.

86 Sirica A. E., Richards W., Tsukada C., Sattler C., Pitot H. C.: Fetal phenotypic expression by adult rat hepatocytes on collagen gel/nylon meshes. *Proc. Natl. Acad. Sci.* 1979, **76**: 283–287.

87 Spence J. T., Haars L., Edwards A., Bosch A., Pitot H. C.: Regulation of gene expression in primary cultures of adult rat hepatocytes on collagen gels. *Ann. N.Y. Acad. Sci.* 349: 99–110.

88 Sperry R. W.: Chemoaffinity in the orderly growth of nerve fibre patterns and connections. *Proc. Natl. Acad. Sci.* 1963, **50**: 703–710.

89 Spray D. C., Harris A. L., Bennett M. V. L.: Voltage dependence of junctional conductance in early amphibian embryos. *Science* 1979, **204**: 432–434.

90 Spray D. C., Stern J. H., Harris A. L., Bennett M. V. L.: Gap junctional conductance: comparison of sensitivities to H^+ and Ca^{2+} ions. *Proc. Natl. Acad. Sci.* 1982, **79**: 441–445.

91 Thiery J. P., Brackenbury R., Rutishauser U., Edelman G. M.: Adhesion among neural cells of the chick embryo. II Purification and characterization of a cell adhesion molecule from neural retina. *J. Biol. Chem.* 1977, **252**: 6841–6845.

92 Thiery J. P., Delouvee A., Gallin W. J., Cunningham B. A., Edelman G. M.: Ontogenetic expression of cell adhesion molecules: L-CAM is found in epithelia derived from the three primary germ layers. *Dev. Biol.* 1984, **102**: 61–78.

93 Umbreit J., Roseman S.: A requirement for reversible binding between aggregating embryonic cells before stable adhesion. *J. Biol. Chem.* 1975, **250**: 9360–9368.

94 Wall D. A., Wilson G., Hubbard A. L.: The galactose-specific recognition system of mammalian liver: the route of ligand internalization in rat hepatocytes. *Cell* 1980, **21**: 79–93.

95 Walther B. T., Ohman R., Roseman S.: A quantitative assay for intercellular adhesion. *Proc. Natl. Acad. Sci.* 1973, **70**: 1569–1573.

96 Wanson J. C., Drochmans P., Mosselmans R., Ronveaux M. F.: Adult rat hepatocytes in primary monolayer culture. Ultrastructural characteristics of intercellular contacts and cell membrane differentiations. *J. Cell. Biol.* 1977, **74**: 838–877.

97 Wanson J. C., Mosselmans R., Brouwer A., Knook D. L.: Interaction of adult rat hepatocytes and sinusoidal cells in co-culture. *Biol. Cell.* 1979, **56**: 7–16.

98 Weigel P. H.: Characterization of the asialoglycoprotein receptor on isolated rat hepatocytes. *J. Biol. Chem.* 1980, **255**: 6111–6120.

99 Weir M. P., Lo C. W.: Gap-junctional communication compartments in the Drosophila wing imaginal disk. *Dev . Biol.* 1984, **102**: 130–146.

100 Yoshida C., Takeichi M.: Teratocarcinoma cell adhesion: Identification of a cell surface protein involved in calcium-dependant cell aggregation. *Cell* 1982, **28**: 217–224.

101 Yoshimoto K., Nakamura T., Ichihara A.: Reciprocal effects of epidermal growth factor on key lipogenic enzymes in primary cultures of adult rat hepatocytes. Induction of glucose-6-phosphate dehydrogenase and suppression of malic enzyme and lipogenesis. *J. Biol. Chem.* 1983, **258**: 12356–12360.

Research in *Isolated and cultured hepatocytes* A. Guillouzo & C. Guguen-Guillouzo eds., pp. 285–312.
© 1986 John Libbey Eurotext Ltd./INSERM

13

Drug metabolism in cultured fetal hepatocytes

Pierre KREMERS

Laboratoire de Chimie Médicale, Institut de Pathologie, Bâtiment B 23, Université de Liège, B–4000 Sart Tilman par Liège 1, BELGIUM

SUMMARY

One of the purposes of drug metabolism studies is to analyse the metabolic fate of a given compound, as well as to look at the influence of endo- and exogenous factors on its metabolism. Cells in culture constitute an attractive *in vitro* model for these toxicological and pharmacological studies. This chapter is mainly concerned with the use of fetal rat liver cells for the study of drug metabolizing enzymes and their regulation. An important methodological section is devoted to the culture conditions and to the development of sensitive methods for the measurement of the enzymatic activities in small biological samples. The present review illustrates how fetal hepatocytes have been used to elucidate several problems linked to the regulation of drug metabolizing enzymes: the mechanisms of induction of cytochrome P-450 by polycyclic hydrocarbons, the expression of various mono-oxygenase activities as a function of the culture conditions, the imprinting of new cytochrome P-450 species in culture by dexamethasone and the maturation of the fetal hepatocytes allowing for long term culture.

Drug metabolism: the need for a good experimental model

Generalities

Like most other xenobiotics, such as hydrocarbons, pesticides or food additives, drugs are often so hydrophobic that they would accumulate in the body in toxic amounts if they were not metabolized into more polar compounds.

Living organisms have developed a complex enzymatic system which is responsible for the metabolism of exogenous compounds: this system is composed of the drug metabolizing enzymes, which are classified into two categories based on their action on xenobiotics. Phase I enzymes, the cytochrome P-450 dependent mono-oxygenases, introduce a functional group, usually a hydroxyl group, into the molecules. This functional group is then conjugated to a hydrophilic function by Phase II enzymes, to transform the products into water-soluble metabolites (23).

The mono-oxygenases constitute an enzyme system located in the endoplasmic reticulum which contains a haemoprotein, cytochrome P-450, which exists in many forms characterized by their substrate specificity, electrophoretic, chromatographic and immunological properties. One of the most striking properties of the microsomal mono-oxygenase system is its lack of specificity which enables it to attack practically any lipophilic compounds. The mono-oxygenases are inducible by environmental chemicals such as polycyclic hydrocarbons, drugs such as phenobarbital, and steroids such as pregnenolone-16α-carbonitrile. These enzymes are also regulated by various endogenous factors such as hormones, age, sex and nutritional conditions (60). All the endogenous, pharmacological and pathological parameters qualitatively and quantitatively modify the expression of the mono-oxygenase activity (15, 23).

Phase II enzymes are responsible for conjugation reactions. They add hydrophilic groups such as glucuronic acid, sulfate or glutathione to the foreign compound or to its first phase metabolites. Quantitatively speaking, glucuronidation is the most important conjugation reaction. This reaction takes place via an heterogenous group of enzymes located in the endoplasmic reticulum. The other conjugation reactions occur in the cytosol and require activated forms of the added group for the reaction to take place: S-adenosylmethionine and acetyl-CoA, for example.

The role of hepatocytes in culture in pharmacological and toxicological studies

The liver plays an important role in handling foreign chemicals, since it is the first organ to receive the chemicals absorbed in the organism. The liver is also the most active mammalian tissue with respect to xenobiotic metabolism (44), and it contains a large variety of enzymes which are able to transform xenobiotics.

Isolated hepatocytes have become more attractive as a model for the study of drug toxicity. They could also be an excellent approach to problems linked to metabolic interactions between various drugs, or drugs and endogenous compounds, or even between drugs and other chemicals found in the environment. Hepatocytes may be used in various ways for toxicological studies. They can also serve for the solution of general cytotoxicity problems such as the study of a toxic effect at a real molecular level; or to decipher the molecular events linked to the toxicity of a compound: what enzymes, organelles, or other structures are involved, and what are the biochemical modifications induced by the chemical?

Hepatocytes may be used to measure quantitatively the effect of xenobiotics on several biological and biochemical parameters such as carbohydrate metabolism, protein synthesis and membrane integrity. One of their most interesting applications is the study of xenobiotic metabolizing capacity. Without a doubt, they represent a particularly interesting model for the analysis of the metabolic fate of a given compound, and the effect of numerous exogenous and endogenous factors on metabolism (71).

The purpose of experimental toxicology and pharmacology is to provide scientific evidence for the assessment of the toxic potential of a substance and its metabolites, and to furnish valuable information about the various factors concerning its safe use by man.

Procedures for estimating safety levels are largely based on animal experiments. For various reasons, particularly due to the number of parameters involved, animal testing procedures present a number of shortcomings. Consequently, *in vitro* systems have become increasingly attractive alternatives. Various *in vitro* models have been studied: liver perfusion (65), hepatocytes in suspension (1, 45), primary cells in culture (68), cell lines (68), fetal hepatocytes in culture and isolated enzymes (35). Each method has specific advantages and limitations.

Two models involving fetal hepatocytes have been extensively used: chicken liver cells and fetal rat hepatocytes. Chicken liver cells offer certain advantages. The material is readily accessible, the embryonic development is relatively easy to control and the embryos can be treated prior to the isolation of the hepatocytes (3). Cytochrome P–450 levels are well maintained in these cultures (3). Problems arise with the extrapolation of the results to the mammalian and human situations. Furthermore, most of the observations and results collected via drug metabolism studies have been obtained from rat liver. Hence, models derived from other animal species should be developed. Nevertheless, chicken liver cells can be an excellent model for the study of regulation problems and can provide clearcut answers to particular questions.

Nebert *et al.* have used primary fetal rat liver hepatocytes for the study of drug metabolizing enzymes (47). These cells divide in culture, are inducible by polycyclic hydrocarbons and phenobarbital, but unfortunately, only express cytochrome

P_1-450 linked activities. However, within the past few years, our laboratory has developed a culture medium in which these cells can express other P-450 linked activities, namely those which are induced by phenobarbital in the adult liver. This model, ie primary fetal liver cells in culture, is the main topic of this chapter.

Drug metabolizing enzymes in primary culture and drug metabolism studies have been limited for many years by the sensitivity of the assay methods used to detect and measure the drug metabolites formed. However, present analytical methods can detect very low amounts of drugs in complex biological fluids (11).

The first use of fetal liver cells for the study of mono-oxygenase induction was reported by Nebert & Gelboin (47). Nebert *et al.* (50) demonstrated that the AHH activity in these fetal cells could be induced by a wide variety of compounds. Numerous experiments conducted on hepatocyte monolayers have led to a documented study of the mechanism behind enzyme induction. Most of these experiments would not have been possible on intact animals. Hepatocyte monolayers can be treated for specific periods of time with precise concentrations of various products: hormones, inducers, inhibitors etc. Large doses of inducers or inhibitors may be used in tissue cultures, whereas they could be toxic when used *in vivo* on other tissues.

Methodological aspects

Preparation of cell cultures

Livers of 18- to 20-day-old rat fetuses are used to prepare the primary cultures. Pregnant rats are treated intraperitoneally with 15 mg oxytetracycline, 24 h before removal of the fetuses. The fetal livers are rinsed, minced and washed in a Ca-Mg-free Dulbecco solution enriched with glucose (1 g/l) under aseptic conditions, and finally suspended in the same solution which is supplemented with trypsin (0.2%).

The suspension is first maintained at 0°C for 2 h and then incubated for 15 min at 37°C. After trypsin decantation, the tissue fragments are resuspended in the culture medium and dissociated by gentle shaking in the presence of glass microspheres (1 mm diameter).

The culture medium is made of Eagle's minimum essential medium with Hanks salts, supplemented with sodium bicarbonate (12 μM), penicillin (100 U/ml), streptomycin (100 μg/ml) and newborn calf serum (10%). After sedimentation, the medium containing the isolated cells is removed and the same procedure is repeated until complete dissociation of the liver fragments. The cells are then washed twice in the culture medium, resuspended at a final concentration of 4–6$\times 10^5$ cells/ml of complete medium and distributed in appropriate tissue culture dishes (2.5 ml cell suspension in a 60-mm diameter dish). The cultures are grown at 37°C in an atmosphere of humidified air with CO_2 (5%). Cell debris and red cells are washed out 24 h later and the firmly attached hepatocytes are cultured in a medium enriched with dexamethasone. This treatment preferentially slows down the growth of the fibroblasts which do not represent more than 10% of the entire cell population, even after 8 days of continuous culture. The media are routinely replaced at 48 h intervals (25, 75).

Cell homogenization

The cells are scraped off the dishes, washed twice in a Dulbecco solution and kept as a dry pellet at −20°C. For preparation of the homogenate, the cells are suspended in a Tris (0.05 M, pH 7.6), sucrose (0.25 M), EDTA (0.001 M) buffer and sonicated for 20 seconds (setting 8; MSE, type L 667). The whole homogenate is used for the determination of enzymatic activities.

Enzymatic activities

Ethoxycoumarin deethylase. In rat liver, ethoxycoumarin deethylase is supported by various cytochrome P-450s. It is mainly induced by methylcholanthrene, but also by phenobarbital and ethanol (73).

Ethoxycoumarin deethylase is measured by a spectrofluorimetric assay. Various methods have been proposed. The method described by Weber & Ullrich is based on a direct recording of the fluorescence of hydroxycoumarin which appears during incubation in the sample cuvette (72). This method produces direct kinetic measurements. Two other methods have been proposed, but both require an extraction step (2, 26). To measure low activities, the method of Poland seems to be the most practical (26).

We have developed a method based on GC-MS (12). This method is very specific and sensitive but requires the use of GC-MS equipment which is not always available in every biochemical laboratory.

Ethoxyresorufin deethylase. Ethoxyresorufin is a specific substrate of the methyl-cholanthrene-induced cytochrome P-450 (8). This deethylase is not induced by phenobarbital, ethanol or steroids, and remains at very low levels of activity in control microsomes. Its activity increases by a factor of 100 after induction by polycyclic hydrocarbons (73). This activity can be monitored by direct measurement of the increase in fluorescence in the fluorimetric cuvette in which the reaction takes place (9).

Burke *et al.* have developed an assay for the direct measurement of this activity in cells in culture (8). Ethoxyresorufin deethylase is a very sensitive assay, but it requires a certain amount of care in the preparation and handling of the substrates and product solutions in order to avoid rapid degradation and loss of fluorescence.

Aryl hydrocarbon hydroxylase. Aryl hydrocarbon hydroxylase is the most widely measured enzyme in cells in culture. This is for two principal reasons, primarily because polycyclic hydrocarbons are metabolized into mutagenic products and a very sensitive assay has been available for several years. Two different assays are used for the measurement of this enzyme. 1) A radiometric assay (74) based on the tritium exchange from a general labelled benzopyrene; this method accounts for the various hydroxylations which occur on the various carbon atoms of the benzopyrene ring. 2) The oldest assay is based on the fluorescence of the main metabolite, 3-hydroxy-benzopyrene (47). This assay accounts for the contribution of cytochrome P_1-450, the cytochrome induced by methylcholanthrene. However, the validity of the assay as a means for measuring cytochrome P_1-450 specifically has been subject to debate

(58). Indeed, this assay reflects the production of 3-hydroxy- and 9-hydroxy-derivatives, and 3-hydroxybenzopyrene is further metabolized with a loss of fluorescence. Several authors have drawn attention to the limitations of this assay (14, 30).

Aldrin epoxidase. Aldrin is transformed by liver microsomes into a stable epoxide, dieldrin. After extraction with hexane and gas chromatography, this compound can be easily measured by electron capture according to the method of Wolff *et al.* (77). A significant improvement in the reproducibility and exactitude of the assay has been achieved by the use of 1-1-1-trichloro-2, 2bis-(p-chlorophenyl)ethane (DDT) as an internal standard (76). This rapid and sensitive assay requires high quality solvents and reagents (free from chlorinated compounds). Aldrin epoxidase activity is specifically supported by the phenobarbital and/or cyanopregnenolone inducible cytochrome P-450.

Steroid hydroxylase. Liver microsomes hydroxylate steroids on various positions: 16α, 6β, 7α, 2α etc. Due to their particular structures, steroids are useful for the study of the stereospecificity of the cytochrome P-450 responsible for their metabolism. A similar molecule (for example, testosterone) can be hydroxylated on various positions, probably by different cytochrome P-450s (64), and different steroid molecules can be hydroxylated on a same position (for example, progesterone and testosterone on 16α). Moreover, steroid hormones are natural, endogenous substrates. Their liver metabolism directly influences their blood levels and consequently their hormonal activity on target tissues.

Steroid hydroxylations have been demonstrated in fetal hepatocytes in culture (38), in which they reflect the activity of different cytochrome P-450s.

The measurement of steroid hydroxylase activity requires the separation of the various metabolites formed after incubation in order to quantify each of them. This is the major difficulty with this assay, since all these metabolites have very similar physico-chemical properties and are consequently not easily separated by chromatography. High performance-liquid chromatography or gas liquid chromatography on capillary columns is commonly used for this purpose. We use a mass fragmentographic method (13, 38) that provides obvious advantages: high specificity and sensitivity. Providing that the necessary reference compounds are available, this method can accurately measure any metabolite of a steroid hormone.

Epoxide hydrolase. Epoxide hydrolase is often measured in cells in culture as a representative of Phase II enzymes, mainly in association with studies on the activation or deactivation of some compounds such as aromatic hydrocarbons. Epoxide hydrolase transforms the epoxide produced by the mono-oxygenase (Phase I enzyme) into metabolically inactive diols. Unfortunately, some of them, particularly benzopyrene 7,8-diol, can be recycled via the mono-oxygenase process to form the highly mutagenic 7,8-dihydroxy-9,10-epoxybenzopyrene. Epoxide hydrolase is measured by a radiometric assay developed by Schmassman *et al.* (61).

Cytochrome P-450. 1) *Spectrophotometric method.* Cytochrome P-450 may be determined spectrophotometrically on the basis of its CO-induced difference spectrum, giving rise to the well known peak at 450 nm (16, 49). This will provide a measurement of the overall cytochrome P-450 concentration, providing that the protein remains intact and contains a functional heme. The spectral observation relies on the interaction of reduced heme with carbon monoxide and does not discriminate between various isozymes, if it is not by the very small spectral modifications, ie a blue shift to 448 nm of the spectral band in the induced microsomes. The spectrophotometrical determinations of cytochrome P-450 are obtained from hepatocytes cultured for periods varying from 1 to 7 days. Due to the low level of cytochrome in cells in culture, it is recommended to use microcuvettes and to be very careful during CO bubbling and dithionite addition.

2) *Immunological methods*. Several recent immunological methods are available for measuring individual isozymes recognized by their apoprotein moeity. Depending on the titre and specificity of the antibody, these methods are very sensitive measurements of simple isozymes (54). The recent appearance of monoclonal antibodies directed against P-450 isozymes and other drug metabolizing enzymes will increase the possibilities for investigating cytochrome P-450 multiplicity and for measuring individual isozymes.

Several ELISA and RIA methods have been proposed for measuring drug metabolizing enzymes (54, 63, 67). Moreover, inhibition of enzymatic activities by antibodies have enabled us to correlate enzymatic activities with various isozymes with greater precision (36, 70).

Another convenient and powerful technique for separating and quantifying the individual cytochrome P-450 isozymes relies on SDS-PAGE (41) followed by Western blots (17, 27, 40). We have successfully applied this method to the analysis of the composition of cytochrome P-450 in cultured fetal hepatocytes (40).

3) *HPLC*. A third method for analysing cytochrome P-450 content is to separate the different cytochrome P-450 isozymes by high pressure liquid chromatography. Some publications (5, 37) indicate that this technique is very promising. This method has been applied in our laboratory to the separation of microsomal cytochrome P-450 from rat liver and hepatocytes in culture (7). This method is rapid, reproducible and enables us to differentiate the various cytochrome P-450 isozymes with relatively high accuracy on relatively small samples (less than 1 mg microsomal protein).

Drug metabolizing enzymes in cells in culture

Drug metabolizing enzymes are studied in cell cultures for various reasons. 1) Evaluation of the metabolic capacities of the cells. 2) Comparison of the metabolism of a compound between cells in culture and animals *in vivo*, and/or liver enzymes *in vitro*. 3) Study of the biochemical properties of the drug metabolizing enzymes; effect of different inducers and varying culture conditions. 4) Regulation studies on the expression of these enzymes.

Cells in culture offer many advantages in the approach to regulation studies, primarily in that the cellular environment can be controlled very carefully.

Most published drug metabolism studies on isolated hepatocytes are performed on adult liver cells maintained in culture for a short period of time which never exceeds a few days (3, 28, 29, 69). The main difficulties with these cells is their loss of enzymatic activity and their dedifferentiation during culture. This type of cell is the main topic of the next chapter.

Drug metabolizing enzymes in cultured chick embryo hepatocytes

An interesting model for the study of cytochrome P-450 and drug metabolizing enzymes was developed by Meyer and colleagues (3, 4, 20, 21, 22, 33). They used chick embryo hepatocytes as starting material. These cells were cultivated and analysed with respect to their cytochrome P-450 content and drug metabolizing activities. Different species of cytochrome P-450 could be induced in these embryo hepatocytes and, moreover, the responses to the inducers resembled that of adult mammalian livers (3, 44) (Table 1).

Table 1. Phenobarbitone-mediated changes in cytochrome P-450 concentration, 7-ethoxy-coumarin deethylase and 5-aminolevulinate synthitase activity in chick embryos *in ovo* and in cultured chick embryo hepatocytes

	In ovo		*In hepatocyte culture*	
	Control	*Phenobarbitone-treated*	*Control*	*Phenobarbitone-treated*
Cytochrome P-450 concentration (pmol cytochrome P-450/mg protein)	195 ± 13 (9)	465 ± 37 (10)*	112 ± 5 (9)	213 ± 8 (13)*
(% of control)		237 ± 9 (10)		196 ± 3 (12) .
7-Ethoxycoumarin deethylase activity (pmol hydroxycoumarin/mg protein/min)	774 ± 77 (8)	1782 ± 191 (9)*	328 ± 12 (6)	725 ± 33 (4)*
(% of control)		205 ± 9 (9)		224 ± 4 (4)
5-Aminolevulinate synthitase activity (ALA) (pmol ALA/mg protein/30 min)	153 ± 11 (6)	1327 ± 157 (8)*	293 ± 25 (8)	661 ± 56 (9)*
(% of control)		817 ± 92 (8)		229 ± 8 (9)

In ovo chick embryos were treated with 5 mg of phenobarbitone dissolved in 0.1 ml of water 16 h before killing on day 17. The controls were injected with solvent. In hepatocyte culture, hepatocytes from 15-day-old chick embryos were cultured for 44 h in William's E medium. Monolayers were exposed to 0.4 mM phenobarbitone for the last 16 h of culture. Hepatic cytochrome P-450 concentration and 7-ethoxycoumarin deethylase activity were measured in microsomes and 5-aminolevulinate synthitase activity was determined in homogenates. Results are means ± sem. The numbers of experiments are indicated in parentheses.
*$P < 0.001$, compared with control values (Student's *t*-test). From reference 20.

The authors characterized two *de novo* synthesized haemoproteins after induction by phenobarbital or methylcholanthrene. These proteins have spectral, electrophoretic and enzymatic properties which are very similar to those of the corresponding proteins from rat liver microsomes (3, 4).

The turnover of cytochrome P-450 proteins in these cultures and the mechanisms of induction have been investigated (3, 4). Basal and induced P-450 have a half-life of about 10 hours (4). These results also indicate that apocytochrome P-450 synthesis can be increased by induction, independently of heme synthesis. An inhibition of heme biosynthesis does not decrease the synthesis of the apoprotein.

In chicken embryo hepatocytes, metyrapone and nicotinamide induce and stabilize the cytochrome P-450 (22) as in primary adult liver cells (52). This induction of cytochrome P-450 by metyrapone is accompanied by an increase in 5-

Table 2. Effect of metyrapone on two mono-oxygenase activities in cultured chick embryo hepatocytes.

Metyrapone (mM)	Time of presence (h)	Inducing compound (28–44 h)	7-Ethoxycoumarin deethylase activity		Aryl hydrocarbon hydroxylase activity	
			pmoles OH-coumarin/ mg protein/min	pmoles OH-coumarin/ pmole P-450/min	pmoles OH-benzopyrene/ mg protein/min	pmoles OH-benzopyrene/ pmole P-450/min
		—	332± 31 (6)	3.05	163± 31 (5)	1.45
0.25	24–44	—	447± 27 (3)†	1.78	130± 17 (3)	0.52
0.5	24–44	—	558± 58 (4)*	1.69	150± 25 (3)	0.45
0.25	0–44	—	551± 72 (4)†	2.21	188± 38 (3)	0.76
0.5	0–44	—	594± 74 (4)*	1.93	202± 43 (3)	0.66
		Phenobarbital (0.4 mM)	709± 47 (4)*	3.19	213± 55 (4)	0.96
0.25	0–44	(0.4 mM)	654± 87 (3)*	1.92	194± 58 (3)	0.57
0.5	0–44	(0.4 mM)	809± 30 (3)*	1.73	194± 30 (3)	0.42
		β-Naphthoflavone (11 μM)	1304±118 (4)*	3.75	962±149 (4)*	2.76
0.25	0–44	(11 μM)	1220±108 (3)*	2.65	700± 98 (3)*	1.52
0.5	0–44	(11 μM)	1285±147 (3)*	2.39	917±106 (3)*	1.70

Cytochrome P-450, 7-ethoxycoumarin deethylase and aryl hydrocarbon hydroxylase activities were determined in microsomes. Results are expressed as the mean±se with the numbers of experiments in parentheses.
*$P \leq 0.01$ and †$P \leq 0.05$, compared to the untreated control (Student's t-test). From reference 22.

aminolevulinate synthetase (21). The newly synthesized heme is required for providing a prosthetic group to the newly synthesized apocytochrome P-450. The induced P-450 shares some common properties with the phenobarbital induced P-450 (similar molecular weight, electrophoretic mobility, differential spectrum) but shows some differences, namely its catalytic properties (affinity for ethoxycoumarin and benzopyrene). This is particularly well illustrated by Fig. 1 and Table 2.

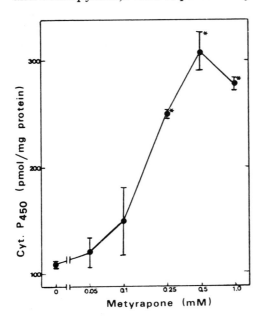

Fig. 1.
Effect of metyrapone on microsomal cytochrome P-450 in cultured chick embryo hepatocytes. Hepatocytes from 15-day old chick embryos were cultured for 44 h in William's E medium containing 1.5 μM triiodothyronine. Monolayers were exposed to various concentrations of metyrapone during the entire culture period. Each point represents the mean$\pm$se of 3–9 experiments.
*$P \leq 0.001$, compared to the untreated control (Student's t-test). From reference 22.

Schneider *et al.* (62) showed that chick embryo liver cells were also able to metabolize steroid hormones and namely estradiol that was hydroxylated on positions 2 and 16. These hydroxylation reactions were inducible by phenobarbital and methylcholanthrene. The 16α hydroxylation was the most sensitive to phenobarbital and did not change in the presence of aromatic hydrocarbons. The two hydroxylation, much more active, was induced by methylcholanthrene. This example further illustrates that several P-450s may be expressed and induced in these cultures. A similar illustration is provided by the observation of Sinclair *et al.* (66) who showed that ethanol was also able to induce benzphetamine demethylase in cultured chick embryo hepatocytes.

Drug metabolizing enzymes in fetal hepatocytes

Fetal hepatocytes can proliferate in culture. A suspension of cells is seeded at a cell density of 4 to 8×10^6 cells/ml, the hepatocytes attach to the plastic culture dish and start to divide. Divisions and proliferations are observed until the cells are confluent and form a monocellular layer. The active growth period occurs between 24 and 96 h after plating. After 5 to 6 days, the cells leave their artificial support and die (50).

The mono-oxygenase activity, the most widely studied in these cells, is benzopyrene hydroxylase or AHH. This enzyme has been selected as a model reaction for cytochrome P-450 catalysed reaction. The specific activity of this enzymes is quite high, and it may be easily induced by a wide variety of compounds.

AHH induction. AHH activity is optimally induced between the second and fourth days of culture, when the cells are in the proliferation and growing phases. The enzymatic activity is multiplied by a factor of 2 within 3 h of contact with the inducer (48).

AHH is induced by a wide variety of products: β-naphthoflavone, 2-naphtho-flavone, methylcholanthrene, benzanthracene, 2,5-diphenyloxazole, metyrapone, SKF 525-A, phenobarbital, transtilbene oxide, piperonyl butoxide, biogenic amines and cigarette smoke condensate (18, 19, 25, 50). These compounds may, never-theless, be separated into two distinct groups. The first contains all the aromatic hydrocarbons and products such as β-naphthoflavone; it is usually represented by methylcholanthrene or benzanthracene. The second group is usually represented by phenobarbital. For each inducer, an optimal concentration can be defined. If two products from the same category are mixed, both at their optimal concentrations, no additional induction is observed. But when the mixed compounds originate from both groups, an additive effect is observed (Fig. 2) (18).

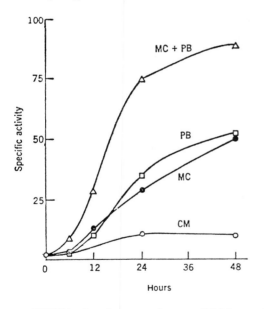

Fig. 2.
Aryl hydrocarbon hydroxylase induction in hepatocytes grown in 0.75 μM MC, 2 mM PB, or both inducers together. The activity of the hydroxylase system in cells grown in control medium only is shown by curve CM. From reference 18.

AHH induction requires an RNA synthesis followed by a translation into a newly synthesized protein by the ribosomal protein synthesis machinery. This was already demonstrated in 1971 by Nebert & Gielen who showed that actinomycin D prevented a rise in hydroxylation activity (48).

The effect of actinomycin D on protein synthesis and the synthesis of AHH is illustrated by Fig. 3. Actinomycin D rapidly inhibits RNA synthesis, but a delay of at least 6 h is necessary to affect the protein synthesis. The phenobarbital induced enzymatic activity is affected by lower doses of actinomycin D than the benzanthracene induced enzyme, indicating that both inducers act in different ways.

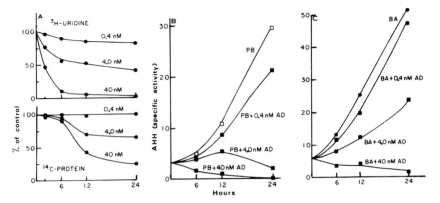

Fig. 3. **Effect of low doses of actinomycin D (AD) on total RNA and protein synthesis and on the induction of aryl hydrocarbon hydroxylase activity initially in fetal rat hepatocyte cultures by PB or BA.** The experiment was begun after the primary cultures had grown for 36 h. The incorporation of ^{3}H-uridine and ^{14}C-protein hydrolysate added together in the same dish for 30-min periods, in the presence of varying concentrations of actinomycin D, is compared to that found in cells grown in control medium alone (A). The specific activity of duplicate samples varied by less than 15%. The effects of various levels of actinomycin D on the stimulation of hydroxylase activity by 2.0 mM PB (B), or 13 μM BA (C), are shown. The inhibitor was added simultaneously with the inducer to the cell culture dishes. The ordinate is expressed as specific activity, units per mg of cellular protein. The specific activity of duplicate samples varied less than 10%. From reference 48.

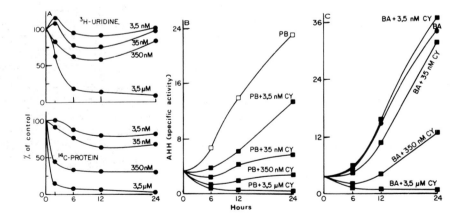

Fig. 4. **Effect of low doses of cycloheximide (CY) on total RNA and protein synthesis during initial induction of aryl hydrocarbon hydroxylase activity initially in fetal rat liver cells by PB or BA.** Cycloheximide was added to the cultures at the same time as the inducer. The levels of gross RNA and protein synthesis (A), and the kinetics of hydroxylase induction by either 2.0 mM PB (B), or 13 μM BA (C), were determined in the same manner as that described in Fig. 3. The experiment was begun 36 h after the plating of the primary fetal hepatocyte cultures. From reference 48.

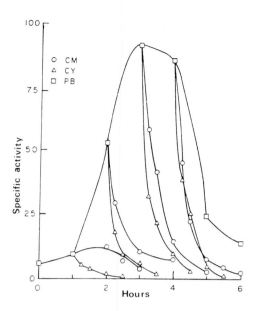

Fig. 5.
Degradation of the PB-induced aryl hydrocarbon hydroxylase activity in the presence of control medium alone (CM), or 3.5 μM cycloheximide (CY). Exposures of the hepatocytes to 2.0 mM PB was begun 6 h after the fetal liver cells had been plated and was continued for as long as 6 days. The half-lives were determined by the method of least squares from the data of 6 similar experiments. From reference 48.

Cycloheximide inhibits protein synthesis rapidly (Fig. 4). At low doses, it already inhibits phenobarbital induction, but rather higher concentrations are required to prevent benzanthracene induction. These experiments have been interpreted as a strong indicator that the induction process relies on a mRNA synthesis. The differences in sensitivity to the inhibitors observed between the two types of inducers, benzanthracene and phenobarbital, may rely on the fact that the role of ribosomal RNA is of greater importance for phenobarbital induction (48). Since phenobarbital induces the proliferation of many cellular proteins, a greater amount of mRNA may be necessary in order to stimulate AHH activity by phenobarbital up to a level similar to that obtained with benzanthracene. Replacement of the culture medium by a fresh one or the addition of cycloheximide to the medium at various intervals during phenobarbital induction results in a decay of AHH activity. This decay allows for the measurement of the half-life of the induced enzyme (Fig. 5). A half-life of 8.5±2.5 hours and 10.5±3.6 hours, respectively, was found in hepatocytes grown in fresh medium and in medium supplemented with cycloheximide (3.5 μM) (48). This experiment also showed that the decay of the enzymatic activity was independent of the level of hydroxylase activity attained during induction.

Benzopyrene metabolism. Fetal hepatocytes in culture not only show an AHH activity, but they can really metabolize benzopyrene into various compounds that are excreted from the cell into the culture medium as sulfates and glucuronide conjugates (Fig. 6).

The pattern of metabolites is influenced by the substrate concentration (Table 3). At low doses of benzopyrene (0.8 μM), the relative amount of polar metabolites is twice as high as that of primary phenols, and twice as low when compared to those

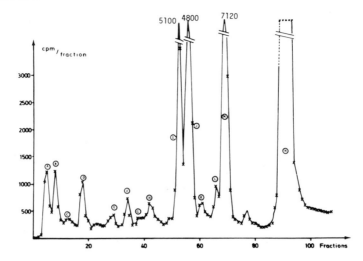

Fig. 6. Pattern of metabolites excreted by the cells. Cells were treated with benzanthracene (25 μM) for 48 h. The medium was then replaced by a new medium containing [^{3}H]BP (80 μM; 65 000 dpm/nmol) and the cell cultures were further incubated for 60 min. The metabolites were then analysed by HPLC. Some of the radioactive peaks have the same retention time as reference BP derivatives: A, B, C, polar metabolites; D, BP-9, 10-dihydrodiol; E, non-enzymatic metabolites, F, BP-4, 5-dihydrodiol; G, BP-7, 8-dihydrodiol; H, unknown; I, BP-1, 6-quinone; J, BP-3, 6-quinone; L, 9-hydroxy-BP, M, 3-hydroxy-BP; N, BP. From reference 75.

Table 3. Profile of the BP metabolites obtained after treatment of the fetal hepatocyte culture with the indicated amount of BP.

BP concentration (μM)	Class of metabolites	BP metabolites					
		% of total metabolites			nmol/plate		
		Control medium	PB	BA	Control medium	PB	BA
	Polar derivatives	7.1	7.7	7.9	0.07	0.82	1.02
	Dihydrodiols	19.3	18.1	18.6	0.21	1.92	2.40
80	Quinones	54.9	49.6	47.5	0.58	5.26	6.13
	Phenols	18.6	24.6	26.0	0.20	2.61	3.35
	Total	100	100	100	1.06	10.6	12.9
	Polar derivatives	—	16.4	15.5	—	0.102	0.110
	Dihydrodiols	—	16.2	20.4	—	0.100	0.145
8	Quinones	—	52.8	48.2	—	0.327	0.342
	Phenols	—	14.6	15.9	—	0.091	0.112
	Total	—	100	100	—	0.62	0.71

[^{3}H]BP was incubated for 60 min with fetal hepatocytes pretreated with BA (25 μM) or PB (2 mM) or not (control medium). The metabolites were extracted and analyzed by HPLC. The results are presented per class of metabolites grouped as follows: Polar derivatives: peak A+B+C; dihydrodiols: peak D+F+G: quinones: peak I+J; phenols: peak L+M (see Fig. 6). The results correspond to the mean values obtained from two experiments. From reference 75.

produced by cells treated with high doses of benzopyrene (80 μM). The AHH activity drastically modifies the overall rate of benzopyrene metabolism but does not affect the qualitative pattern of the excreted metabolites (75). The fetal hepatocytes are characterized by an active 6-hydroxylation since the major products excreted are benzopyrene-1-6-quinone and 3-6-quinone (75).

Drug metabolizing enzymes in human fetal hepatocytes in culture

Pelkonen *et al.* have extensively studied the cytochrome P-450 concentrations, benzopyrene metabolism and AHH activity in human liver samples as well as in human fetal cells in culture (55, 56, 57). Human fetal hepatic AHH is not inhibited by 7,8-benzoflavone and thus exhibits properties specific to the phenobarbital induced enzyme. This contrasts with the placental enzyme which is strongly inhibited by 7, 8-benzoflavone and exhibits properties that are typical of the polycyclic hydrocarbon-induced enzyme. The benzopyrene hydroxylase activity in human fetal cells in culture is induced by exposure for 24 h to benzanthracene and methylcholanthracene (55). In human cells, it has also been observed that benzopyrene is metabolized into known polar metabolites such as dihydrodiols, phenols and quinones (57). Compared to *in vitro* incubation of human liver microsomes, cultured hepatocytes produce a higher proportion of secondary metabolites. *In vivo*, most of the radioactivity associated with the incubated benzopyrene is excreted as soluble metabolites into the culture medium (57).

Other enzymatic activities in fetal hepatocytes in culture

Mono-oxygenase activities other than AHH have been described in fetal rat liver cells. In our laboratory, we routinely measure ethoxycoumarin deethylase, aldrin epoxidase, and several steroid hydroxylase activities (38).

Lambiotte (42) has described the hydroxylation of biliary acids by fetal rat liver cells in the presence of glucocorticoids (10, 43).

Husson *et al.* (34) have shown that in fetal hepatocytes urea cycle enzymes such as argininosuccinate synthetase and argininosuccinase are modulated by the hormonal composition of the culture medium.

Regulation of mono-oxygenase activities in cultured fetal liver cells

Tissue culture offers many advantages for studying regulation problems, because cells may be maintained in a perfectly controlled environment so that various parameters may be modified individually and their contribution to the enzymatic activity verified.

Serum

The different cell culture media contain either fetal or newborn calf serum. It is well known that the growth and functions of the cell may be modified by the serum. From one batch of serum to another, it is possible to obtain different results.

Serum is necessary during the first hours of culture to allow the cells to adhere to their plastic support. The serum contains growth factors, hormones, vitamins and various unidentified essential compounds. Serum can be heat-inactivated and dialysed without losing its stimulating effect on the cells, indicating that the essential factors are relatively small and are heat-stable molecules. The presence of serum is a prerequisite for AHH induction by phenobarbital; on the other hand, methyl-cholanthrene can induce the enzymatic activity by 30%–50% of its maximum potential in the absence of serum (19) (Table 4).

Table 4. Aryl hydrocarbon hydroxylase activity as a function of serum concentration.

Inducer	Fetal calf serum			
	0%	1%	3%	10%
None	4*	7	7	10
Phenobarbital	11	38	75	263
Benzanthracene	191	200	170	203

*picomoles.min^{-1}.mg protein^{-1}

Several unsuccessful attempts have been made to replace the serum by a completely synthetic medium of specifically known composition. Most likely, several factors are involved in cell growth and maturation, and the involvement of these factors in the sequence of events is not well understood.

Ligands

Various cytochrome P-450 ligands have been added to the culture medium, mainly to adult hepatocytes in culture, to try to prevent the loss of cytochrome P-450. The most widely used products are pyridine derivatives (51), nicotinamide (52) and ascorbic acid (6). These compounds have no direct effect on protein synthesis, but rather protect pre-existing cytochrome P-450 from the normal degradation process (53). However, these studies have only been concerned with the measurement of the total cytochrome P-450 content based on the integrity of the heme moeity. Variations between different isozymes may have been overlooked.

In fact, none of these treatments can completely sustain the original functions of the hepatocytes. They are always partial, or even typical, solutions to the difficult problem of cellular development and cell differentiation in culture. It would be more advantageous to define with precision a 'working model' in order to understand in depth their possibilities and limitations. This is the aim of various laboratories, and important progress in this field can be expected in the very near future.

Nicotinamide and mono-oxygenase activity in fetal hepatocytes

Paine *et al.* have shown that nicotinamide can prevent the rapid loss of cytochrome P-450 in adult liver cells in culture (52). We have investigated whether this compound can modify the cytochrome P-450 content and the expression of the mono-oxygenase activity in fetal cells in culture. Cells were treated with increasing concentrations of nicotinamide and their AHH activity measured 96 hours after treatment. The nature of the cytochrome P-450 supporting AHH activity was determined by the sensitivity of the enzymatic activity to the *in vitro* effect of metyrapone and α-naphthoflavone (24). Figure 7 illustrates that nicotinamide selectively induces the cytochrome P-448 dependent AHH activity, ie that which is already present in control cells (not treated with dexamethasone) and which is inhibited by α-naphthoflavone *in vitro*. When the effect of nicotinamide is studied as a function of the duration of the treatment, nicotinamide seems to act primarily by stabilizing rather than by inducing the cytochrome P-448. When the fetal cytochrome P-448 is no longer synthesized (24 to 48 h after the onset of dexamethasone treatment), the effect of nicotinamide is rapidly reversed.

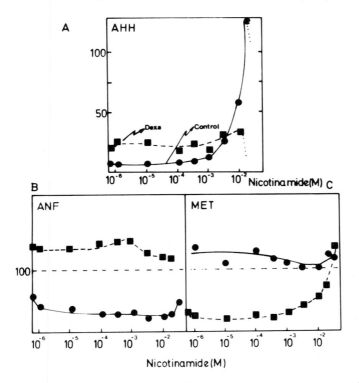

Fig. 7. Effect of nicotinamide on the AHH activity of primary fetal rat liver cells in culture. The AHH activity (pmol/min/mg protein) (panel A) and its *in vitro* sensitivity to 5.10^{-4}M α-naphthoflavone (% of control) (panel B) and 5.10^{-4}M metyrapone (% of control) (panel C) were measured in cells which had been cultured for 96 hours in the presence of various concentrations of nicotinamide. The experiment was performed on control (● - - - ●) and dexamethasone treated (■ - - - ■) cells.

The selective effect of nicotinamide is further illustrated by its lack of action on aldrin epoxidase, an enzymatic activity which is specifically supported by adult-like forms of cytochrome P-450.

The role of dexamethasone in the regulation of fetal hepatocyte drug metabolizing enzymes

Our approach to the problems linked to the regulation and expression of cytochrome P-450 in culture is based on the comparison with the *in vivo* situation during the perinatal period of life. This period is mainly characterized by the onset, imprinting and maturation of various important processes. The perinatal period is critical to the quantitative and qualitative development of the microsomal mono-oxygenases.

These activities increase rapidly either just prior to birth or during the first days of extrauterine life. This phenomenon is regulated by various physiological stimuli controlled by hypophysic hormones and is modulated by glucocorticoids (39). The important question which arises is whether or not it is possible to reproduce *in vitro* in culture dishes, or at least partially, the sequence of biological events observed *in vivo* during the perinatal period.

When AHH is measured in cells harvested at various times after seeding (Fig. 8*A*), the activity first rises and then falls with the age of the culture (39). The presence of dexamethasone in the culture medium prevents this loss of activity. In one-day-old cells, AHH activity is inhibited by α-naphthoflavone and is insensitive to metyrapone. The presence of dexamethasone in the culture medium has a decisive effect on this feature (Fig. 8*B*). Enzymatic activity of cells cultivated in the presence of dexamethasone is no longer inhibited by β-naphthoflavone but is inhibited by metyrapone, indicating that AHH is supported by a cytochrome P-450 isozyme similar to that found in adult rat liver after induction by phenobarbital. In the absence of dexamethasone, primary fetal hepatocytes continue to express a cytochrome P_1-450.

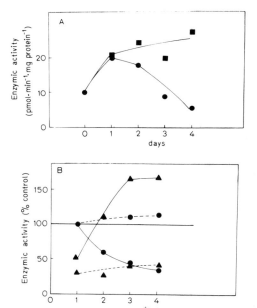

Fig. 8.
Aryl hydrocarbon hydroxylase activity in cultured fetal hepatocytes (A), and the effect of α-naphthoflavone and metyrapone (B). Dexamethasone (5 μM) was (■) or was not (●) added to the culture medium on day 0, 24 hours after the culture had started. (A) Enzymatic activity is expressed in pmol.min^{-1} mg protein^{-1} and was determined on a whole cell homogenate. (B) The enzymatic activity is expressed as a percentage of the corresponding control activity measured in the absence of inhibitors. Inhibitor concentrations for the inhibition *in vitro* were 50 μM for α-naphthoflavone (▲), and 0.5 mM for metyrapone (●). Aryl hydrocarbon hydroxylase inhibition was measured on an homogenate of cells cultivated in the presence (—) or absence (- - -) of 5 μM dexamethasone. From reference 38.

This observation has been further confirmed in several ways. 1) Aldrin epoxidase activity is only detected in cells treated with dexamethasone. This enzymatic activity is known to be dependent on adult forms of cytochrome P-450 and namely, the isozymes induced by phenobarbital and/or by pregnenolone-16β-carbonitrile. 2) The absorption peak for the cytochrome P-450-CO complex is spectrally located at 450 nm for microsomes from cells cultivated in the presence of dexamethasone and at 447-448 nm for cells induced with benzanthracene or with a mixture of benzanthracene and phenobarbital. 3) In the presence of dexamethasone, even at low concentrations (10^{-8}M), the cells can hydroxylate testosterone on the 2, 6, 7 and 16α positions. 16α-Hydroxylation is turned on at very low concentrations of dexamethasone and its activity does not vary with the dexamethasone concentration. On the other hand, 6β-hydroxylase activity increases with the amount of dexamethasone present in the culture medium (65). 4) The SDS PAGE analysis of the microsomal proteins obtained from these cell shows that the protein composition in the 40 000 to 60 000 molecular weight region varies significantly as a function of the cell treatment (Fig. 9). 5) This is further confirmed by an immunological study.

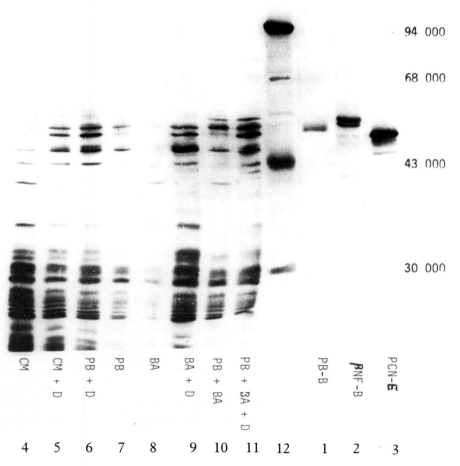

Fig. 9. SDS PAGE analysis of microsomes prepared from fetal hepatocytes in culture. Gels were 0.75 mm thick and acrylamide concentrations were 7.5%. The gels were revealed by staining with silver nitrate. Molecular weight standards are in lane 12. Lanes 1, 2 and 3 contained purified cytochrome P-450 fractions: PBB, βNFB, and PCNE, respectively. Lanes 4 to 11 correspond to the different microsomal proteins from hepatocytes cultured in a control medium (CM, 4), in a medium supplemented with dexamethasone (CM+D, 5), in the presence of phenobarbital (PB, 7), benzanthracene (BA, 8), phenobarbital and dexamethasone (PB/D, 6), benzanthracene and dexamethasone (BA+D, 9), benzanthracene and phenobarbital (PB+BA, 10) benzanthracene plus phenobarbital plus dexamethasone (PB+BA+D, 11).

Proteins are electroblotted from the acrylamide gel onto a nitrocellulose sheet that is incubated with appropriate antibodies. Three different cytochrome P-450 isozymes are recognized: P-450 PB-B (the main form induced by phenobarbital in adult rat liver) P-450 PCN-E (the form induced by pregnenolone-16α-carbonitrile); and P-450 βNF-B (the form induced by polycyclic hydrocarbons). This latter form is only detected in cells treated with both phenobarbital and benzanthracene or with phenobarbital alone, but always in the absence of dexamethasone (40).

The P-450 PB-B is detected in cells treated by both dexamethasone and phenobarbital. The P-450 PCN-E (Fig. 10) is observed in all cells treated with the glucocorticoid.

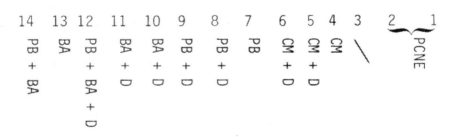

Fig. 10. Immunoelectrophoresis of the microsomal preparations from the different hepatocytes with anti-PCNE as an antibody. The antibody used was raised in rabbits against the purified rat liver PCNE cytochrome P-450. Lanes 1 and 2 correspond to 5 and 10 pmoles of PCNE Cytochrome P-450, respectively. Other lanes are as for Fig. 9.

All of these experiments clearly demonstrate that dexamethasone can provoke a physiological mechanism which can trigger the expression of cytochrome P-450 supported mono-oxygenase activities normally absent from the fetal cells and only present in adult hepatocytes.

The effect of dexamethasone varies as a function of its concentration in the culture medium. At low concentrations ($10^{-9}M$), dexamethasone allows for the induction of aldrin epoxidase by phenobarbital (Fig. 11) and produces a qualitative change in the expression of cytochrome P-450; the various enzymatic activities (AHH and ethoxycoumarin deethylase) become inhibited *in vitro* by metyrapone and are no longer sensitive to α-naphthoflavone (38). At higher concentrations ($5.10^{-6}M$), dexamethasone can induce the enzymatic activities by itself in cultured fetal hepatocytes.

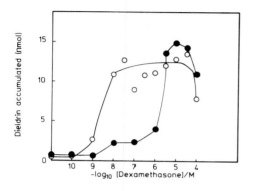

Fig. 11
Enhancement of aldrin metabolism as a function of the concentration of dexamethasone in the culture medium. Cells were cultivated in a control medium (closed symbols) or in the presence of 2 mM phenobarbital (open symbols). From reference 39.

Effect of other glucocorticoids

The specificity of dexamethasone action was studied by comparison with several other hormonal steroids, androgens, estrogens and competitor steroids were added to the culture medium to determine whether they modified the expression of cytochrome P-450 in the fetal cells in culture (Tables 5 & 6). Dexamethasone ($10^{-6}M$) in the culture medium leads to a significant increase in aldrin epoxidase and tyrosine aminotransferase activity, and to a shift from the α-naphthoflavone sensitive AHH activity to a metyrapone sensitive activity. Tyrosine aminotransferase is measured as an indicator of the involvement of the glucocorticoid receptor.

Table 5: Effect of hormonal treatments on various enzymatic activities of primary fetal rat hepatocytes in culture.

Treatment	Aldrin epoxidase	AHH (ANF; MET)	TAT
None	1.6	5.6 (33; 115)	1.6
Dexa $10^{-6}M$	11.6	3.3 (170; 69)	42
DMP $10^{-5}M$	13.0	11.1 (130; 45)	20.8
DMP + Dexa	34.6	15.9 (175; 31)	38.5
Prog $10^{-5}M$	0.5	5.8 (40; 109)	1.3
Prog + Dexa	22.5	8.0 (238; 48)	27.7

The activity of aldrin epoxidase (pmol/min/mg protein), AHH (pmol/min/mg protein) and TAT (milliunits/min/mg protein) has been measured in primary fetal rat hepatocytes which had been cultured for 96 hours in the presence of the indicated hormones: Dexa (dexamethasone), DMP (6α, 16α-dimethylprogesterone), Prog (progesterone). The sensitivity *in vitro* of AHH to α-naphthoflavone ($5.10^{-4}M$) and metyrapone (5.10^{-4} M) is indicated as a percentage of the control (numbers in parentheses).

Table 6. Effect of hormonal treatments on various enzymatic activities of primary fetal rat hepatocytes in culture.

Treatment (M)	Aldrin epoxidase	AHH (ANF; MET)	TAT
None	1.6	5.6 (33; 115)	1.6
Dexa 10^{-6}	11.1	3.3 (170; 69)	42
DMP 10^{-6}	11.4	5.9 (174; 75)	12.5
10^{-5}	13.0	11.1 (130; 45)	20.8
Prog 10^{-6}	0.6	3.7 (39; 111)	1.9
10^{-5}	0.5	5.8 (40; 109)	1.3
Doc 10^{-5}	1.9	7.2 (65; 107)	3.9
10^{-4}	46.9	13.2 (208; 58)	7.7
RU$_{2999}$ 10^{-5}	1.5	9.5 (40; 122)	7.5
10^{-4}	23.4	21.1 (135; 98)	8.6
DHT 10^{-5}	1.5	10.3 (42; 109)	1.9
10^{-4}	30.2	36.8 (78; 109)	9.8
Testo 10^{-4}	34.7	26.4 (98; 93)	11.7
DHEA 10^{-5}	1.5	8.0 (43; 117)	1.7
10^{-4}	39.9	20.3 (141; 88)	4.8
Estradiol 10^{-6}	0.2	4.9 (41; 109)	1.4
10^{-5}	0.3	5.6 (38; 113)	1.6
10^{-4}	—	27.9 (31; 85)	1.3

See footnote to Table 5. Abbreviations: AHH (aryl hydrocarbon hydroxylase), ANF (α-naphtho-flavone), MET (metyrapone), TAT (tyrosine aminotransferase), Dexa (dexamethasone), Prog (progesterone), DMP (6α, 16α-dimethylprogesterone), DOC (11-dexyocorticosterone), RU$_{2999}$ (a synthetic progestagen), DHT (5α-dihydro-testosterone), DHEA (dehydroepiandrosterone).

Progesterone alone, an antagonist, does not induce aldrin epoxidase nor tyrosine aminotransferase. Dimethylprogesterone alone, a suboptimal inducer, suboptimally induces the tyrosine aminotransferase activity, but induces aldrin epoxidase to the same extent as dexamethasone (Tables 5 & 6). Estradiol has no effect on aldrin epoxidase and tyrosine aminotransferase (Table 6).

Imprinting

Cells are cultured in the presence of 10^{-5}M dexamethasone for 48 h and then cultured for an additional 48 h in a fresh medium without dexamethasone, but with or without phenobarbital (Fig. 12). The basal level of aldrin epoxidase rises with the concentration of dexamethasone and decreases abruptly after the removal of the corticoid. The induction of aldrin epoxidase is nearly absent when low concentrations of dexamethasone are used for the pretreatment and progressively increases when higher concentrations are added to the culture medium. Conversely, the AHH activity is induced to a greater extent by phenobarbital when the cells are pretreated with low concentrations of dexamethasone, but at this time, phenobarbital induces an α-naphthoflavone sensitive AHH activity. The induction of AHH disappears progressively when the cells are pretreated with higher concentrations of dexamethasone but the induced enzyme is then sensitive to metyrapone. This experiment clearly indicates that dexamethasone can turn on a mechanism triggering the expression of a new cytochrome P-450 isozyme, even if the glucocorticoid is no longer present in the culture medium.

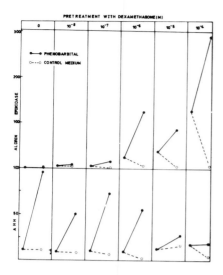

Fig. 12.
Induction of aldrin epoxidase and aryl hydrocarbon hydroxylase activity by phenobarbital as a function of the concentration of dexamethasone used for the pretreatment of the fetal hepatocytes. The enzymatic activities ($pmol.min^{-1}.mg$ protein^{-1}) were measured in primary fetal hepatocytes which had been pretreated for 2 days with the indicated concentrations of dexamethasone, and cultured for 2 more days without dexamethasone in a control medium (O - - - O), or in the presence of phenobarbital, 2.10^{-3} M (● - - - ●).

Long-term culture of fetal hepatocytes

In a culture medium supplemented with dexamethasone (10^{-8}M or 10^{-6}M), fetal liver cells may be maintained in culture for several weeks. They continue to metabolize aldrin at an appreciable rate (Table 7) indicating that the glucocorticoid may trigger a physiological mechanism involved in long-term cell maturation processes. This effect can also be obtained when cells are cultivated in a so-called 'conditioned' medium, ie a culture medium collected from dishes in which cells have grown in the presence of 10^{-8}M dexamethasone for at least 48 h. This medium does not contain sufficient amounts of dexamethasone to produce this maturation effect, but seems to contain some other factors which are produced in the medium under the influence of the corticoid, and that can turn on the physiological maturation mechanism. A possible factor might result from the organization of the extracellular matrix. The cultures are prepared from whole livers and hence contain different cell types originating from this tissue. This represents an ideal situation for the initiation of cell-cell and cell-biomatrix interactions which are important for long-term survival of the cells, and corticoids may be important for these cell-cell communications and interactions. However, additional experiments are required to unravel the mechanisms by which corticoids produce a maturation of the fetal hepatocytes.

Culture on biomatrix and cell-cell interactions

A recent development in tissue culture is in the use of biomatrix or cell-cell interactions in order to maintain the physiological functions of the hepatocytes in for long periods of time. Various supports have been studied. From these studies it appears that interactions of cells with their surrounding surfaces regulate many fundamental biological processes such as growth, differentiation, and metabolic function, but no clear-cut information is available at the present (59). Only some working hypotheses and preliminary information have been published in this new

Table 7. **Aldrin epoxidase activity in primary fetal hepatocytes in culture. Enzymatic activity is expressed in pmoles of aldrin epoxidase per culture dish and per h.**

Dexa	Days						
	8	13	17	22	27	34	48
—	13.7*	55					
	19.4	51					
	19	51					
10^{-8}M	129.5	352	706	1040	957	295	727
	110.2	289					
10^{-6}M	406	682	1173	1037	1154	566	661
	406	727					

*pmoles of dieldrin. hour^{-1}. dish^{-1}.

but rapidly developing field. Various supports have been tested for cell attachment and growth. This varies from different cell types, fibroblasts or epithelial cells, to pigskin substrate (31) and various purified proteins or glycoproteins such as different types of collagen, fibronectin and laminin, all of which are major components of the basement membranes (32). Laminin seems to be necessary for cellular growth and functional maintenance of fetal mouse hepatocytes (32). Fetal mouse hepatocytes cultured on pigskin epidermal substrate grow for 7 weeks and after 2 weeks are even able to produce albumin instead of alphafetoprotein, indicating that a maturation process has been turned on (31).

More recently, Nakamura *et al.* have shown that cell growth as well as many metabolic functions of the hepatocytes are regulated by cell density (46), suggesting that the reciprocal regulation of cell growth and hepatocyte functions are mediated by some surface components via cell-cell contact.

In this area, numerous studies are in progress and it may be that important information and explanations will be obtained in the very near future.

ACKNOWLEDGMENTS

The author is grateful to Ms Janice Lynn Delaval for her expert and considerable help in preparing this manuscript.

REFERENCES

1 Aarbakke J., Bessessen A., Morland J.: Metabolism of ^{14}C-antipyrine in suspensions of isolated rat liver cells. *Acta Pharmacol.* 1977, **41**: 225–234.
2 Aitio A.: A simple and sensitive assay of 7-ethoxycoumarin deethylation. *Anal. Biochem.* 1978, **85**: 488–492.
3 Althaus F. R., Sinclair J. F., Sinclair P., Meyer U. A.: Drug-mediated induction of cytochrome(s) P-450 and drug metabolism in cultured hepatocytes maintained in chemically defined medium. *J. Biol. Chem.* 1979, **254**: 2148–2153.
4 Althaus F. R., Meyer U. A.: Effects of phenobarbital, beta-naphthoflavone, dexamethasone and formamidoxime on the turnover of inducible microsomal proteins in cultured hepatocytes. *J. Biol. Chem* 1981, **256**: 3079–3094.
5 Bansal S. K., Love J., Gurtoo H. L.: High pressure liquid chromatographic separation of multiple forms of cytochrome P-450. *Biochem. Biophys. Res. Commun.* 1983, **117**: 268–274.
6 Bissell D. M., Guzelian P.S.: Ascorbic deficiency and cytochrome P-450 in adult rat hepatocytes in

primary monolayer culture. *Arch. Biochem. Biophys.* 1979, **192**: 569–576.

7 Bollinne A., Kremers P., Gielen J. E.: Induction of cytochrome P-450 isozymes in cultured fetal hepatocytes: analysis by HPLC. Abstract, Third International Symposium on Microsomes and Drug Metabolism. Brighton, UK, 5–10 August 1984.

8 Burke M. D., Hallman H.: Microfluorimetric analysis of cytochrome P-448 associated ethoxyresorufin O-deethylase activities of individual isolated rat hepatocytes. *Biochem. Pharmacol.* 1978, **27**: 1539–1544.

9 Burke M. D., Prough R. A., Mayer R. T.: Characteristics of a microsomal cytochrome P-448 mediated reaction: ethoxyresorufin O-deethylase. *Drug Metab. Disp.* 1976, 5: 1–8.

10 Croizot B., Granelli-Piperno A., Lambiotte M., Gros F.: Conversions isozymiques de l'aldolase en culture primaire de foie foetal. *Biochimie* 1972, **54**: 375–380.

11 De Graeve J., Gielen J. E., Heusghem C.: The selection of an appropriate methodology for drug determination in biological samples: A conceptual approach. *In*: *Mises au point de biochimie pharmacologique, II*, G. Siest, C. Heusghem (Eds): Masson, Paris, 1979, pp 1–50.

12 De Graeve J., Kremers P., Frankinet C., Gielen J. E.: A new highly sensitive assay for ethoxycoumarin deethylase in cultured hepatocytes. *Analyt. Biochem.* 1980, **104**: 419–424.

13 De Graeve J., Kremers P., Gielen J. E.: Measurement of progesterone and pregnenolone-16α-hydroxylase activities by a tritium exchange method. *Eur. J. Biochem.* 1977, **74**: 561–566.

14. DePierre J. W., Ernster L.: The metabolism of polycyclic hydrocarbons and its relationship to cancer. *Biochem. Biophys. Acta* 1977, **473**: 149–186.

15 Estabrook R. W., Lindenlaub E.: *The Induction of Drug Metabolism*: F. K. Schattauerverlag, Stuttgart, 1978.

16 Estabrook R. W., Werringloer J.: The measurement of different spectra: application to the cytochromes of microsomes. *In*: *Methods in Enzymology*, Vol. 52, S. P. Colowick, S. N. O. Kaplan (Eds): Academic Press, New York, 1978, pp 212–220.

17 Gershoni J. M., Palade G. E.: Protein blotting: principles and application. A review. *Anal. Biochem.* 1983, **131**: 1–15.

18 Gielen J. E., Nebert D. W.: Microsomal hydroxylase induction in liver cell culture by phenobarbital, polycyclic hydrocarbon and pp'-DDT. *Science* 1971, **172**: 167–169.

19 Gielen J. E., Nebert D. W.: Aryl hydrocarbon hydroxylase induction in mammalian liver cell culture. III. Effect of various sera, hormones, biogenic amines and other endogenous compounds on the enzyme activity. *J. Biol. Chem.* 1972, **247**: 7591–7602.

20 Giger U., Meyer U. A.: Role of heme in the induction of cytochrome P-450 by phenobarbitone. *Biochem. J.* 1981, **198**: 321–329.

21 Giger U., Meyer U. A.: Induction of delta-aminolevulinate synthase and cytochrome P-450 hemoproteins in hepatocyte culture. Effect of glucose and hormones. *J. Biol. Chem.* 1981, **256**: 1182–1190.

22 Giger U., Meyer U. A.: The substituted pyridines metyrapone and nicotinamide are inducers of 5-aminolevulinate synthase and cytochrome P-450 in hepatocyte culture. *Biochem. Pharmacol.* 1983, **31**: 1735–1741.

23 Gillette J. R.: Effects of induction of cytochrome P-450 enzymes on the concentration of foreign compounds and their metabolites and on the toxicological effects of these compounds. *Drug Metab. Rev.* 1979, **10**: 59–87.

24 Goujon F. M., Nebert D. W., Gielen J. E.: Genetic expression of aryl hydrocarbon hydroxylase induction. IV. Interaction of various compounds with different forms of cytochrome P-450 and the effect of benzo (a) pyrene metabolism *in vitro*. *Molec. Pharmacol.* 1972, **8**: 667–680.

25 Goujon F., Van Cantfort J., Gielen J. E.: Comparison of aryl hydrocarbon hydroxylase and epoxide hydrolase induction in primary fetal rat liver cells. *Chem.-Biol. Interactions*, 1980, **31**: 19–33.

26 Greenlee W. F., Poland A.: An improved assay of 7-ethoxycoumarin O-deethylase activity: Induction of hepatic enzyme activity in C57B1/6J and DBA/2J mice by phenobarbital, 3-methylcholanthrene, and 2, 3, 7, 8-tetrachlorodibenzo-p-dioxin. *J. Pharmacol. Exp. Therap.* 1978, **205**: 596–605.

27 Guengerich F. P., Dannan G. A., Wright S. T., Martin M. V., Kaminsky L. S.: Purification and characterization of liver microsomal cytochrome P-450: elecrophoretic, spectral, catalytic and immunochemical properties and inducibility of eight isozymes isolated from rats treated with

phenobarbital and β-naphthoflavone. *Biochemistry* 1982, **21**: 6019–6030.

28 Guguen-Guillouzo C., Guillouzo A.: Modulation of functional activities in cultured rat hepatocytes. *Molec. Cell. Biochem.* 1983, **53/54**: 35–56.

29 Guillouzo A. (ed): Drug metabolism by cultured adult hepatocytes. *In: Isolated and cultured hepatocytes*, London: John Libbey, 1986.

30 Hansen A. R., Fouts U. R.: Some problems in Michaelis-Menten kinetic analysis of benzpyrene hydroxylase in hepatic microsomes from polycyclic hydrocarbon-pretreated animals. *Chem.-Biol. Interactions* 1972, **5**: 167–182.

31 Hirata K., Shiramatsu K., Usui T., Yoshida Y., Freeman A. E., Hayasaka H.: Modulation of fetal mouse liver cells cultured on a pigskin substrate. *Tohoku J. Ep. Med.* 1983, **140**: 15–28.

32 Hirata K., Usui T., Koshiba H., Maruyama Y., Oikawa I., Freeman A. E., Shiramatsu K., Hayasaka H.: Effects of basement membrane matrix on the culture of fetal mouse hepatocytes. *Gann* 1983, **74**: 687–692.

33 Hirsiger H., Giger U., Meyer U. A.: Stimulation of DNA synthesis and mitotic activity of chick embryo hepatocytes in primary culture. *In Vitro* 1984, **20**: 172–182.

34 Husson A., Bouazza M., Buquet C., Vaillant R.: Hormonal regulation of two urea-cycle enzymes in cultured foetal hepatocytes. *Biochem. J.* 1983, **216**: 281–285.

35 Johnson E. F., Schwab G. E.: Constitutive forms of rabbit liver microsomal cytochrome P-450: Enzymatic diversity, polymorphism and allosteric regulation. *Xenobiotica* 1984, **14**: 3–18.

36 Kaminsky L. S., Dannan G. A., Guengerich F. P.: Composition of the cytochrome P-450 isozymes from hepatic microsomes, of C57Bl/6 and DBA/2 mice assessed by warfarin metabolism, immunoinhibition, and immunoelectrophoresis with anti-rat cytochrome P-450. *Eur. J. Biochem.* 1984, **141**: 141–148.

37 Kotacke A. N., Funae Y.: High performance liquid chromatography technique for resolving multiple forms of hepatic membrane-bound cytochrome P-450. *Proc. Nat. Acad. Sci.* 1980, **77**: 6473–6475.

38 Kremers P., Goujon F., De Graeve J., Van Cantfort J., Gielen J. E.: Multiplicity of cytochrome P-450 in primary fetal hepatocytes in culture. *Eur. J. Biochem.* 1981, **116**: 67–72.

39 Kremers P., Letawe-Goujon F., De Graeve J., Duvivier J., Gielen J. E.: The expression of different mono-oxygenases supported by cytochrome P-450 in neonatal rat and in primary fetal hepatocytes in culture. *Eur. J. Biochem.* 1983, **137**: 603–608.

40 Kremers P., Beaune P., Gielen J. E.: Induction of different cytochrome P450 isozymes in cultured fetal rat hepatocytes. (Submitted.)

41 Laemmli U. K.: Cleavage of structural proteins during the assembly of the head of bacteriophage T_4. *Nature* 1970, **227**: 680–683.

42 Lambiotte M., Sjovall J.: Hydroxylation and sulfatation of bile acids in rat hepatoma cultures under influence of glucocorticoids. *Biochem. Biophys Res. Common.* 1979, **86**: 1089–1095.

43 Lambiotte M., Thierry N.: Induction par les glucocorticoïdes dans les cultures de foie foetal et d'hepatome de la morphogenèse des canalicules, de l'hydroxylation des acides biliaires et de l'activation de l'alfatoxine B. *In: Les Colloques de l'INSERM: Pharmacologie due Développement*: INSERM, Paris, 1979, vol. 89, 113–124.

44 Meyer U. A.: Regulation of drug metabolism. Biochemical aspects. *In: Les Colloques de l'INSERM: Pharmacologie due Développement*: INSERM, Paris 1979, vol. 89, 127–138.

45 Moldeus P., Grundin R., Von Bahr C., Orrenius S.: Studies on drug-cytochrome P-450 interaction in isolated rat liver cells. *Biochem. Biophys. Res. Commun.* 1973, **55**: 937–944.

46 Nakamura T., Yoshimoto K., Nakayama Y., Tomita Y., Ichihara A.: Reciprocal modulation of growth and differentiated functions of mature rat hepatocytes in primary culture by cell-cell contact and cell membranes. *Proc. Nat. Acad. Sci.* 1983, **80**: 7229–7233.

47 Nebert D. W., Gelboin H. V.: Substrate-inducible microsomal aryl hydroxylase in mammalian cell culture. Assay and properties of induced enzyme. *J. Biol. Chem.* 1968, **243**: 6242–6249.

48 Nebert D. W., Gielen J. E.: Aryl hydrocarbon hydroxylase induction in mammalian liver cell culture. II. Effects of actinomycin D and cycloheximide on induction processes by phenobarbital or polycyclic hydrocarbons. *J. Biol. Chem.* 1971, **246**: 5199–5206.

49 Omura R. A., Sato R.: The carbon monoxide-binding pigment of liver microsomes. Evidence for its hemoprotein nature. *J. Biol. Chem.* 1964, **239**: 2370–2385.

50 Owens I. S., Nebert D. W.: Aryl hydrocarbon hydroxylase induction in mammalian liver-derived

cell cultures. Stimulation of 'cytochrome P-450 associated' enzyme activity by many inducing compounds. *Molec. Pharmacol.* 1974, **11**: 94–104.

51 Paine A. J., Villa P.: Ligands maintain cytochrome P-450 in liver cell culture by affecting its synthesis and degradation. *Biochem. Biophys. Res. Commun.* 1980, **97**: 744–750.

52 Paine A. J., Villa P., Hockin L. J.: Evidence that ligand formation is a mechanism underlying the maintenance of cytochrome P-450 in rat liver cell culture potent maintenance by metyrapone. *Biochem. J.* 1980, **188**: 937–939.

53 Paine A. J., Hockin L. J., Allen C. M.: Long-term maintenance and induction of cytochrome P-450 in rat liver cell culture (technical note). *Biochem. Pharmacol.* 1982, **31**: 1175–1178.

54 Paye M., Beaune P., Kremers P., Guengerich F. P., Letawe-Goujon F., Gielen J. E.: Quantification of two cytochrome P-450 isozymes by an enzyme-linked immunoabsorbent assay (Elisa). *Biochem. Biophys. Res. Commun.* 1984, **122**: 137–142.

55 Pelkonen O., Korkonen P., Jouppila P., Karki N.: Induction of aryl hydrocarbon hydroxylase in human fetal liver cell and fibroblast cultures by polycyclic hydrocarbons. *Life Sci.* 1975, **16**: 1403–1410.

56 Pelkonen O.: Metabolism of benzo (a) pyrene in human adult and fetal tissues. *Carcinogenesis* 1976, **1**: 9–20.

57 Pelkonen O., Korkonen P.: The metabolism of benzo (a) pyrene in cell cultures and homogenates from different human fetal tissues. *In: Microsomes and Drug Oxidations*, V. Ullrich (Ed.): Pergamon Press, Oxford, 1977, pp 411–417.

58 Phillipson C. E., Godden P. M. M., Lum P. Y., Ioannides C., Parke D. V.: Determination of cytochrome P-448 activity in biological tissues. *Biochem. J.* 1984, **221**: 81–88.

59 Rauvala H.: Cell surface carbohydrates and cell adhesion. *Trends Biol. Sci.* 1983, **96**: 323–325.

60 Sato R., Omura T.: *Cytochrome P-450*: Kondansh LID, Academic Press, New York, 1978.

61 Schmassman H. V., Glatt H. R., Oesch F.: A rapid assay for epoxide hydratase activity with benzo (a) pyrene-4, 5-(K-region) oxide as substrate. *Anal. Biochem.* 1976, **74**: 94–103.

62 Schneider J., Sassa S., Kappas A.: Metabolism of estradiol in liver cell culture. Differential responses of C-2 and C-16 oxidations to drugs and other chemicals that induce selective species of cytochrome P-450. *J. Clin. Invest.* 1983, **72**: 1420–1426.

63 Shawver L. K., Seidel S. L., Krieter P. A., Shires T. K.: An enzyme-linked immunoabsorbent assay for measuring cytochrome b_5 and NADPH-cytochrome P-450 reductase in rat liver microsomal fractions. *Biochem. J.* 1984, **217**: 623–632.

64 Shiverick K., Neims A. H.: Multiplicity of testosterone hydroxylase in a reconstituted hepatic cytochrome P-450 system from uninduced male rat. *Drug Metab. Disp.* 1979, **7**: 290–295.

65 Sies H.: The use of perfusion of liver and other organs for the study of microsomal electron transport and cytochrome P-450 systems. *In: Methods in Enzymology*, S. P. Colowick, N. O. Kaplan (Eds): Academic Press, New York, 1978, pp 48–59.

66 Sinclair J. F., Sinclair P. R., Smith E. L., Bement W. J., Pomeroy J., Bonkowsky H.: Ethanol mediated increase in cytochrome P-450 in cultured hepatocytes. *Biochem. Pharmacol.* 1981, **30**: 2805–2809.

67 Song B. J., Fujino T., Park S. S., Friedman F. P., Gelboin H. V.: Monoclonal antibody-directed radioimmunoassay of specific cytochrome P-450. *J. Biol. Chem.* 1984, **259**: 1394–1397.

68 Stammati A. P., Silano V., Zucco F.: Toxicology investigation with cell culture systems. *Toxicology* 1981, **20**: 91–153.

69 Suolinna E. M.: Isolation and culture of liver cells and their use in the biochemical research of xenobiotics. *Med. Biol.* 1982, **60**: 237–254.

70 Thomas P. E., Reik L. M., Ryan D. E., Levin W.: Characterization of nine monoclonal antibodies against rat hepatic cytochrome P-450. *J. Biol. Chem.* 1984, **259**: 3890–3899.

71 Thurman R. G., Kauffman F. C.: Factors regulating drug metabolism in intact hepatocytes. *Pharmacol. Rev.* 1980, **31**: 229–251.

72 Ullrich V., Weber P.: The O-dealkylation of 7-ethoxycoumarin by liver microsomes. *Hoppe Seyler's Z. Physiol. Chem.* 1972, **353**: 1171–1177.

73 Ullrich V., Kremers P.: Multiple forms of cytochrome P-450 in the microsomal mono-oxygenase system. *Arch. Toxicol.* 1977, **39**: 41–50.

74 Van Cantfort J., De Graeve J., Gielen J. E.: Radioactive assay for aryl hydrocarbon hydroxylase. Improved method and biological importance. *Biochem. Biophys. Res. Commun.* 1977, **79**, 505–512.

75 Van Cantfort J., Goujon F., Gielen J. E.: Benzo (α) pyrene metabolism in rat fetal hepatocytes in culture. Improved methodology and effect of substrate concentration. *Chem.-Biol. Interactions* 1979, **28**: 147–160.

76 Van Cantfort J., Leonard-Poma M., Sele-Doyen J., Gielen J. E.: Differences in the biochemical properties of aldrin epoxidase, a cytochrome P-450 dependent mono-oxygenase in various tissues. *Biochem. Pharmacol.* 1983, **32**: 2697–2702.

77 Wolff T., Deml E., Wanders H.: Aldrin epoxidation, a highly sensitive indicator specific for cytochrome P-450 dependent mono-oxygenase activities. *Drug Metab. Disp.* 1979, **7**: 301–305.

Research in *Isolated and cultured hepatocytes* A. Guillouzo & C. Guguen-Guillouzo eds., pp. 313–332.
© 1986 John Libbey Eurotext Ltd./INSERM

14

Use of isolated and cultured hepatocytes for xenobiotic metabolism and cytotoxicity studies

André GUILLOUZO

Unité de Recherches Hépatologiques U49, INSERM, Hôpital Pontchaillou, 35033 Rennes Cédex, FRANCE

SUMMARY

Isolated and cultured adult hepatocytes have been increasingly used over the past ten years for pharmacotoxicological studies. Isolated hepatocytes express most of the functional activities of the intact liver, and are therefore suitable for investigating xenobiotic metabolism, cytotoxicity and the effects of drugs on cellular metabolism. Cultured hepatocytes allow longer studies but the rapid loss of cytochrome P-450 and drug metabolizing enzymes represent evident shortcomings. Despite a number of attempts to modify medium composition, conditions of culture allowing long-term maintenance of all cytochrome P-450 isoenzymes in rodent hepatocytes have not yet been defined. However, drug induction of *de novo* synthesis of cytochrome P-450 isozymes has been demonstrated during culture. Adult human hepatocytes are much more stable in culture than rodent hepatocytes. In standard culture, human cells showed only a slow decrease in cytochrome P-450 levels, while in co-culture with rat liver epithelial cells they maintain a relatively stable concentration of total cytochrome P-450 and of two major isoenzymes for at least 10 days. Furthermore, these cells are able to metabolize drugs according to Phase I and Phase II drug metabolizing enzyme pathways. Cultured human hepatocytes, particularly when placed in co-culture, should become a suitable model for predicting hepatic metabolic pathways and hepatotoxicity of new drugs in man.

Introduction

The liver is the primary organ involved in metabolism of xenobiotics. Many compounds are taken up by hepatocytes and converted to pharmacologically inactive, active or toxic metabolites. Xenobiotic metabolism occurs according to various pathways which are classified into two groups. Phase I reactions which include oxidations, reductions and hydrolyses; and Phase II conjugation reactions. One major Phase I pathway is represented by the cytochrome P-450 dependent mono-oxygenases located in membranes of the endoplasmic reticulum. The mono-oxygenase system has three main components: a group of hemoproteins collectively called cytochrome P-450, a NADPH requiring flavoprotein (NADPH cytochrome P-450 reductase) and a lipid moiety which is a constitutive part of the membrane. The multiple forms of cytochrome P-450 account for the wide substrate specificity of the mixed-function oxidase system. Conjugating enzymes (Phase II) are located either in membranes, (UDP-glucuronyltransferase) or in the cytosol (sulfotransferase).

Complex regulatory processes, involving both endogenous and exogenous factors are exerted on hepatic metabolism *in vivo* and so, a number of investigators have turned to simpler *in vitro* experimental models for studying drug metabolism and toxicity. In particular, isolated and cultured hepatocytes have been increasingly used over the past ten years. Most of the studies have been carried out with rodent cells and the results of these have been extrapolated to humans. However, in view of the qualitative and quantitative interspecies differences which commonly exist in hepatic metabolism of xenobiotics, the validity of such extrapolation is open to question.

This paper summarizes recent developments in the use of isolated and cultured adult hepatocytes from various species, including man, in pharmacotoxicological research. The results with fetal cells as well as the use of cultured hepatocytes for carcinogenesis and mutagenesis studies are reviewed in other chapters.

Drug metabolism in isolated hepatocytes

Various methods have been devised to isolate hepatocytes from different species with considerable variations in cell yields and in maintenance of functional activities. Viable hepatocytes are now easily obtained in high yields by enzymatic treatment of the liver. The advantages of the use of freshly isolated hepatocytes are the homogeneity of the suspension, functional similarities with the *in vivo* state and the ability to analyse multiple parameters from the same parent suspension.

Several aspects of drug metabolism have been investigated using freshly isolated rat hepatocytes. The cytochrome P-450 concentration, measured by a spectral assay, was found to be close to that of the parent tissue in an oxidized non-substrate-bound state (62). The addition of hexobarbital, lidocaine or nortriptyline resulted in rapid binding to cytochrome P-450 as revealed by the formation of a Type I spectral change (62). A number of drug metabolizing enzymes were also present at levels observed in the liver. These included aminopyrine-N-demethylase, p-nitrosoanisole-O-demethylase, aniline hydroxylase (40) and NADPH cytochrome c reductase (22). Suspensions of adult hepatocytes remain active for a few hours in performing metabolism of variety of xenobiotic substrates, whether Phase I or Phase II drug metabolizing enzymes are involved. Metabolites generated by the cytochrome P-450 mono-oxygenase system have been shown to be subsequently conjugated with glucuronic acid (11, 17, 44, 97), sulfate (11) or glutathione (11, 44). Inhibitors of drug metabolism such as SKF 525 A and metyrapone, also produced similar inhibitory patterns in isolated hepatocytes and in liver microsomes (7, 61).

As expected, spectral changes in cytochrome P-450 and changes in various enzyme activities were enhanced in hepatocytes prepared after treating animals with inducers. The profile of stimulated xenobiotic-metabolizing activities in hepatocytes was in general closely related to that shown by subcellular liver fractions from the same animals (7, 61, 62). This was recently well illustrated for the glucuronidation pathway. Glucuronidation is catalysed by multiple forms of UDP-glucuronyltransferase that are differently inducible by xenobiotics. Ullrich & Bock (89) have studied glucuronidation of various substrates in isolated hepatocytes from untreated rats and from rats treated with methylcholanthrene or phenobarbital. Glucuronidation of 1-naphthol and 3-hydroxybenzo(a)pyrene was enhanced in methylcholanthrene-treated hepatocytes while that of chloramphenicol and bilirubin was increased in phenobarbital-treated cells. Glucuronidation of other compounds including paracetamol and oxazepam was not markedly altered by either inducer. These observations are in agreement with differential induction of UDP-glucuronyltransferase activities measured in liver microsomes from normal and treated animals.

The metabolic rates of substrates are often similar or slightly lower in isolated hepatocytes than in corresponding 9000×g supernatant or microsomes. Thus, drugs such as α1-acetyl-methadol (7) and alprenolol (61) were metabolized at a similar rate, while others including ethinimate (7) and ethylmorphine (7, 20) were more slowly metabolized in isolated hepatocytes. In the latter experiments, either V_{max} (7) or Km (7, 20) values were decreased. These slower rates of drug metabolism in intact hepatocytes did not appear to be due to an insufficiency of cellular NADPH (45, 95). Such an early decline could be related to differential alterations of drug metabolizing enzymes (or isozymic forms). Thus, glucuronidation of morphine declined at a more rapid rate than that of naphtnol in suspended rat hepatocytes, suggesting a differential lability of the glucuronyltransferase isozymic forms (78).

In fact, in intact cells drug metabolism is intimately related to other cellular events. Thurman & Kauffman (85) have distinguished at least four types of regulation that can be imposed upon mixed function oxidation: induction, substrate and co-factor supply, activation and inhibition by effectors and competing reactions. These authors reported a number of examples of the regulation of drug metabolism in isolated hepatocytes. Thus, compounds which affect intermediary metabolism may have profound effects on rates and patterns of drug biotransformation. They may act by a variety of mechanisms which include direct inhibition of specific enzyme activities, competition for co-factors and uncoupling of oxidative phosphorylation (85). These mechanisms will not be illustrated in the present review. However, it is important to emphasize the influence of the nutritional status of the liver *in vivo* before hepatocyte isolation, and also of the *in vitro* environment when using freshly isolated hepatocyte suspensions. Profound alterations in the nutritional status could considerably affect metabolic rates of substrates. This point is particularly important to consider with adult human hepatocytes obtained from kidney donors (35). It has been shown that the absence of perfusion with glucose between trauma and kidney removal may result in striking alterations of various energy parameters (43). The incubation conditions of hepatocyte suspensions may also be critical. Aldrin epoxidation to dieldrin was maintained stable for 6 h when rat hepatocytes were incubated at 20°C with continuous bubbling of 95%0_2–5%CO_2, but was considerably decreased when the cells were placed at 37°C or incubated at 27°C with gentle introduction of the gas mixture on the surface of the suspension (49). Physiological concentrations of Ca^{++} increased the glucuronidation of harmol while higher concentrations caused a decrease. The sulphation pathway was not affected (4). Since *in vitro* the environment incubation is subject to dramatic changes over a few hours, some attempts have been made to use a perifusion system. No obvious difference was reported in either oxidative or conjugative metabolism when this perifusion incubation system was compared with isolated cells incubated in conventional conditions (65).

The conjugation of metabolites generated by the mixed oxidation system can be step-limiting in the overall metabolism of drugs, particularly when compounds that decrease ATP production (menadione, 2,4-dinitrophenol) or increase NADH content (ethanol) are involved. These compounds are powerful inhibitors of glucuronidation and/or sulphation in isolated hepatocytes from rats (60, 97). Depletion of cellular ATP could lead to a reduction of the cellular levels of uridine diphosphate glucuronic acid (UDPGA) and 3'-phosphoadenosine 5'-phosphosulfate (97). On the other hand, an increased cellular NADH concentration might inhibit the (NAD+) requiring enzyme UDP-glucose dehydrogenase, thereby preventing synthesis of UDPGA (60).

However, the capacity of isolated hepatocytes to regenerate UDPGA appears to remain quite high. Administration of phenobarbital to suspensions of rat hepatocytes stimulated the UDPGA pathway, within 90 min probably as a result of the inhibition of glycogen synthesis (64). The most sensitive conjugation pathway to environment appears to be the glutathione transferase, which has raised increasing interest since glutathione protects the liver against necrosis due to acetaminophen. Reduced glutathione content of rat hepatocytes decreased to one half of that in the intact liver during the isolation process but addition of ethylene guanosine tetraacetic acid to the perfusion medium prevented its loss (94). Intracellular glutathione levels were also increased by methionine or homocysteine in the incubation medium (3).

Drug metabolism in hepatocyte suspensions may be influenced by other compounds. A number of studies have dealt with the effects of ethanol on the mixed function oxidation. In general high concentrations of ethanol inhibit drug oxidation, while low concentrations may have a stimulating effect (29). Thus, alprenol oxidation in rat hepatocytes was increased in the presence of low concentration of ethanol, and inhibited by 10 mM (28).

Drug metabolizing enzyme activities may vary with sex and age. Several studies are consistent with an age decline in the mixed oxidation system in rats. The rate of aflatoxin B_1 metabolism by isolated rat hepatocytes was found to decline to about 50% between the 6th and the 30th month (74). No qualitative changes in the pattern of digitoxin metabolites was observed in hepatocytes isolated from 3- and 30-month-old male rats but the V_{max} decreased by about 30% in cells from older rats (90, 91). Both reactions are mediated by cytochrome P-450-dependent mono-oxygenases.

It is accepted that several drug metabolizing enzymes are heterogeneously distributed within the lobule. This heterogeneity appears to be retained after hepatocyte isolation. Gumucio *et al.* (37) measured cytochrome P-450 in two hepatocyte subpopulations separated in a continuous density gradient after 3 days of phenobarbital administration. They found a 5-fold induction of cytochrome P-450 in the population of light density cells, corresponding to centrilobular hepatocytes while the heavy density population, corresponding to periportal hepatocytes, did not show any increase of their cytochrome P-450 level, compared with the same hepatocyte subpopulation from untreated animals. Tonda & Hirata (87) separated adult rat hepatocytes from untreated, phenobarbital- or 3-methylcholanthrene-treated rats into four subpopulations according to cell density by using a discontinuous Percoll gradient and found differences in glucuronidation and sulphation of p-nitrophenol between the subpopulations.

In summary, isolated hepatocytes exhibit Phase I and Phase II drug enzyme activities that reflect the *in vivo* state and are, therefore, a valuable system for assessing hepatic drug metabolism. A major advantage is that multiple parameters may be analysed in cells from the same organ, ie dose-response, effects of inhibitors. However, isolated hepatocytes show severe degenerative changes within a few hours, which limit their use and favour the choice of hepatocyte culture systems (79). Indeed, long-term *in vitro* maintenance of hepatocytes requires cell attachment to a support.

Drug metabolism in cultured hepatocytes

Rodent hepatocytes

Most of the studies have been performed on rat hepatocytes. In conventional culture conditions these cells usually survive for 1–3 weeks (for reviews see references 9, 33 and 79) but a number of studies have shown that their total cytochrome P-450 rapidly declines. The level is significantly altered within a few hours and is not more than 10 to 40% of the initial value after 24 or 48 hours of culture (21, 22, 40, 50). The loss of cytochrome P-450 can be temporarily prevented by supplementing the culture medium with a variety of compounds, such as hormones, ligands and heme precursors. A mixture of hormones and nutrients including hydrocortisone, estradiol, testosterone, insulin, thyroxine and fatty acids delays cytochrome P-450 loss for 24 or 48 hours (13, 14). Paine *et al.* demonstrated that nicotinamide (71), isonicotinamide (68), metyrapone (50) or methionine in a cyst(e)ine-free medium (3, 66) promoted cytochome P-450 maintenance. Dexamethasone (55), adrenal corticosteroids (57), ascorbic acid (8), 5-aminolaevulinic acid (13, 39), and glycerol or fructose (41) are also capable of slowing down the decline in the level of cytochrome P-450. Maintenance is not improved by the presence of serum or insulin (22, 58). Other authors cultured rat hepatocytes on organic substrates or in association with other cell types. Michalopoulos *et al.* (56) measured the level of cytochrome P-450 comparatively in rat hepatocytes cultured on collagen-coated plates, floating collagen gels and on human fibroblasts. They found that cytochrome P-450 was better maintained in cells cultured on human fibroblasts and on collagen gels than in cells cultured on collagen-coated plates. Recently, Bégué *et al.* (5) showed that the cytochrome P-450 level remained relatively stable for at least 10 days in adult rat hepatocytes co-cultured with another liver cell type (Fig. 1).

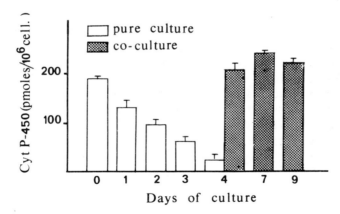

Fig. 1: **Cytochrome P-450 content of adult rat hepatocytes cultured alone or with rat liver epithelial cells for various times.** The results are expressed as pmoles per 10^6 hepatocytes. Data from reference 5.

Changes in cytochrome P-450 concentration can result from alterations in degradation and/or synthesis rate of heme and/or apoprotein. The loss in cytochrome P-450 is associated with a parallel rise in the activity of microsomal heme oxygenase, the enzyme which converts heme to bile pigment, indicating an excess of free heme. However, the two events are not related. Paine *et al.* (69) found that high levels of cytochrome P-450 can be maintained in the presence of high levels of heme oxygenase activity. 5-Aminolaevulenic acid synthetase (ALAS) activity, the rate-limiting enzyme in the biosynthetic pathway of heme, rapidly increases in culture: after 19–24 h it reached about 8-times the initial activity and remained 3- to 4-fold elevated after 4 days (21). Such an induction can be interpreted as a lack of heme or a disturbance along the biosynthetic pathway. This conclusion is suggested not only by the enhanced maintenance of 5-aminolaevulinic acid (13, 39) but also by the inhibition of ALAS activity in a dose-dependent fashion by exogenous heme (21). Degradation of cytochrome P-450 is inhibited by cycloheximide suggesting that this process required protein synthesis (38). Paine & Villa (70) have shown that maintenance of cytochrome P-450 resulted from a balance between the rates of synthesis and degradation of the hemoproteins.

During the first 24–48 h of culture microsomal mono-oxygenase activities also decline but to different extents in hepatocytes whether isolated from normal rat liver (22) or from rat liver 4 to 6 days after partial hepatectomy (40). A decline parallel with that of cytochrome P-450 was observed for aminopyrine-N-demethylase and aniline hydroxylase while NADPH-cytochrome c reductase and aryl hydrocarbon hydroxylase are moderately reduced and p-nitroanisole-O-demethylase remains unchanged (40). Culture conditions which favour cytochrome P-450 maintenance delay the decrease in associated mono-oxygenase activities (5, 14, 56); but all mono-oxygenase activities are not equally maintained (51). These observations are consistent with a differential *in vitro* stability of cytochrome P-450 subspecies. This interpretation is sustained by recent finding from Guengerich and coworkers (31). These authors used an immunochemical method to quantify eight cytochrome P-450 isoenzymes in freshly isolated and 66 h cultured rat hepatocytes, and showed that the different cytochrome P-450 isoenzymes had varying stabilities depending on culture conditions. Williams' E medium with or without metyrapone and a cysteine-free medium were tested. The effects of metyrapone could not be correlated with the ability of the compound to bind as a ligand to isolated P-450 isoenzymes.

Various inducers may increase the level of cytochrome P-450 and/or several mono-oxygenase enzyme activities in cultured adult rat hepatocytes. Maximum induction is usually observed following addition of the inducer to 2-or 3-day cultures, the cells being relatively unresponsive during the first 24 h after attachment (18, 63). Some drugs induced a spectrum of cytochrome P-450 forms different from that induced *in vivo* (22, 51). Fetal forms are preferentially induced *in vitro*. This is the case with phenobarbital (22, 51), although as observed *in vivo* this compound stimulates proliferation of the smooth endoplasmic reticulum in culture (57). In contrast, other drugs appear to retain the capacity to induce specific forms of cytochrome P-450. Thus, after 2 days exposure of rat hepatocytes to clofibrate, lauric acid hydroxylation was markedly stimulated, while there was little effect on three other cytochrome P-450 dependent oxidases, namely ethylmorphine N-demethylase, 7-ethoxycoumarin O-deethylase and 7-ethoxyresorufin-O-deethylase (52). This drug is known to induce a form of cytochrome P-450 relatively specific for hydroxylation of lauric acid in the rat. Villa *et al.* (92) provided evidence that co-cultured rat hepatocytes treated once daily for 3 days with erythromycin estolate exhibited increased cytochrome P-450 and stable complexed cytochrome P-450 as reported *in vivo*. As observed with cytochrome P-450 levels, mono-oxygenases activities may also exhibit differences in their response to inducers in cultured hepatocytes by comparison with the *in vivo* situation (18).

In a number of studies cytochrome P-450 was measured by non-specific assay methods which reflect net changes only of the heme moiety without regard to metabolism of the apoprotein portion. Guzelian's group was the first to demonstrate *de novo* synthesis of specific forms of cytochrome P-450 after addition of pregnenolone 16-α carbonitrile (PCN) and phenobarbital (PB) to non-proliferating rat hepatocytes cultured in a serum-free medium. However, the cells contained a lower concentration of total cytochrome P-450 than do freshly isolated counterparts (19, 63). Using specific quantitative immunoassays, these authors found that the rate of synthesis was 9-fold higher for cytochrome P-450-PCN, and as much as 20-fold higher for cytochrome P-450-PB in rat hepatocytes exposed for 72 h to pregnenolone 16-α carbonitrile and phenobarbital respectively. The magnitude of this increase was less that observed *in vivo* (63). However, addition of selenium to phenobarbital-treated cultures resulted in a 2-fold increase in the rate of synthesis of the cytochrome P-450-PB form (63). This indicates that various factors could be important for maximum induction of cytochrome P-450 forms *in vitro*. Associated mono-oxygenase activities were concomitantly increased (19, 63). Recently, the same group reported that *de novo* synthesis of the cytochrome P-450-PCN form was also stimulated by dexamethasone and other glucocorticoids (77).

Another way to evaluate drug metabolizing capacity of cultured hepatocytes is to perform qualitative and quantitative determination of metabolites of drugs formed at various times of culture. Adult rat hepatocytes have been shown to metabolize a number of xenobiotics including p-chloromethylaniline (16), aflatoxin B$_1$ (13), ketotifen (53), benzo(a)pyrene (76). Ketotifen is biotransformed according to the same pathways as found *in vivo*, namely reduction and demethylation (53). However, as expected, metabolite production rapidly decreases during time in culture in parallel with the loss of cytochrome P-450 and various drug enzyme metabolizing activities. Further evidence of the occurrence of altered drug metabolizing capacity of hepatocytes during culture is provided by differences in the response to inducers. A 2.6-fold induction of benzo(a)pyrene metabolism occurred in hepatocytes treated with 2,3,7,8-tetrachloro-dibenzo-p-dioxin from 49 to 55 h compared to a 1.2-fold induction from 31 to 37 h after cell seeding (82).

A similar decline in cytochrome P-450 concentration and drug enzyme activities during time in culture was found in postnatal rat hepatocyte cultures (1) and in cultured adult hepatocytes from the rodent species. However, it may be noted that in newborn rat hepatocyte cultures, phenobarbital induced proliferation of smooth endoplasmic reticulum and increased cell survival (36). Renton *et al.* (73) reported a 90 and 97% loss respectively in aryl hydrocarbon hydroxylase and aminopyrine N-demethylase activity in mouse hepatocytes during the first 24 h of culture. Maslansky & Williams (54) measured cytochrome P-450 levels at various times between 0 and 24 h in hepatocytes from rat, mouse, hamster and rabbit cultured in Williams' E medium. The most rapid decline was found in mouse hepatocytes; the decline being slightly greater than in rat cells. About 50% and 80% of the initial value of cytochrome P-450 was still retained in hamster and rabbit hepatocytes respectively after 24 h. This shows that species-differences exists in the *in vitro* stability of cytochrome P-450. However, the stability of cytochrome P-450 in rabbit hepatocytes is only temporary and a marked decline is also observed between 24 and 72 h after cell plating (53).

Much less attention has been paid to the ability of hepatocyte cultures to conjugate the primary metabolites generated by the mono-oxygenases with glucuronic acid, sulfate and glutathione. As observed with the cytochrome P-450 dependent mono-oxygenases, the activities of conjugating enzymes rapidly decline in cultured rat hepatocytes. However, these cells are capable of forming oxidative and conjugative metabolites of benzo(a)pyrene over the first 24 h after plating (76). Rabbit hepatocytes formed sulfoconjugates from ketotifen for at least 7 days in culture (53; Bégué *et al.*, unpublished results). Gluthatione concentration falls by 70% within 24 h in rat hepatocytes cultured in a cysteine-free medium (3). However, it is maintained at the normal level by the addition of methionine. Interestingly, Rojkind *et al.* (75) were able to demonstrate detectable activity of glutathione S-transferase in rat hepatocytes after 6–8 weeks when these cells were cultured on a connective tissue biomatrix extracted from rat liver.

Thus, despite a number of attempts, satisfactory maintenance of cytochrome P-450 levels for several days without changes in the isoenzymic pattern and with preservation of the differential response to inducers of these enzymes has not yet been achieved in rodent hepatocyte cultures. Indeed, hepatocytes tend towards a more fetal-like state and even when normal values of cytochrome P-450 could be maintained for some days, alterations in drug metabolizing enzyme activities were observed suggesting that key regulatory factors remain to be elucidated.

Human hepatocytes

Procedures for isolation of adult human hepatocytes have been devised only recently (see Chapter 1) and studies on drug metabolism are still very limited. We have measured total cytochrome P-450 in adult human hepatocytes cultured alone or in association with rat liver epithelial cells for 10 days. In conventional culture, cytochrome P-450 is much more stable than in rodent hepatocytes. After 6–8 days, it still represented around 50% of the initial value (34). In contrast, as observed in co-cultured rat hepatocytes, the cytochrome P-450 content was maintained close to the initial value in co-cultured human hepatocytes for at least 10 days (Fig. 2). Addition

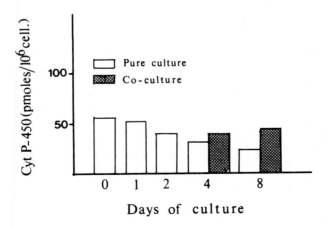

Fig. 2. Cytochrome P-450 content of adult human hepatocytes cultured alone or with rat liver epithelial cells for various times. The results are expressed as pmoles per 10^6 hepatocytes. Data from reference 34.

of phenobarbital resulted in a net increase of cytochrome P- 450, particularly in co-culture (1.7- to 2.1-fold). Moreover, two major cytochrome P-450 isoenzymes were demonstrated by immunostaining after polyacrylamide gel electrophoresis of microsomal proteins and transfer to nitrocellulose. These isoenzymes were quantified by densitometry over the first 10 days and were found to remain relatively stable in both pure and mixed cultures (34). More recently, we have confirmed the maintenance of these two isoenzymes using the immunoperoxidase technique and shown that cultured human hepatocytes retain the heterogeneity of cytochrome P-450 isoenzymic distribution which was observed in the lobules of the liver *in vivo* (72).

That cultured human hepatocytes remain able to metabolize drugs *in vitro* for several days was further demonstrated by the findings obtained with ketotifen. This drug is mainly metabolized in man by two pathways, namely reduction and glucuronidation. Metabolites were analysed by high pressure liquid chromatography in pure and mixed cultures after a 24 h incubation with ^{14}C-ketotifen at various times of culture and their structure was confirmed by mass spectrometry. The glucuronidation which was still active after 3 weeks in co-culture was no longer demonstrated after 4 days in pure culture (6). Recently, two other compounds, namely pindolol and fluperlapine, were also found to be metabolized in human hepatocyte cultures according to the same major pathways as *in vivo* (unpublished observations).

Isolated hepatocytes in toxicity assessment

A number of xenobiotics, either directly or after conversion to more toxic compounds, may impair hepatocellular and other functions. Cell injury may be initiated by the formation of a stable (non-covalent) complex with a protein or another intracellular compound, or via the formation of highly reactive chemical species or by inducing physicochemical changes within the cell or its environment (10). Cell damage is limited or prevented by a variety of defence systems which include drug metabolizing enzymes, binding proteins, antioxidants and active oxygen metabolizing enzymes.

Isolated hepatocytes have been widely used as an experimental model for toxicity assessment (25, 27, 47). They may serve as a screening test for toxic agents. Cytotoxicity is usually evaluated by the measurement of cytosolic enzyme leakage, morphologic changes visualized at the light microscopic level and/or determination of cell viability by the trypan blue exclusion test. Lactate dehydrogenase has been considered the most representative of the cytosolic enzymes liberated into the medium during membrane damage. Some authors have emphasized the importance of cellular metabolic competence as an indicator of cytotoxicity. Glycogen and protein synthesis levels (26, 41, 48), urea content (81) and lactate to pyruvate ratio (81) have been proposed as good markers of cellular metabolic competence. In our laboratory we are routinely using determination of the rate of albumin secretion as a criterion of metabolic activity of isolated and cultured hepatocytes.

Cell injury can be greatly influenced by the environment and the ability of the cells to take up the compound. Environmental parameters, particularly oxygen tension and composition of the incubation medium must be carefully defined. Thus, the concentation of Ca^{++} has a critical role in the magnitude of toxicity induced by various compounds in hepatocyte suspensions. Toxicity is potentiated in the absence of extracellular Ca^{++} (23, 80); this is possibly linked to an increase in lipid peroxidation and in glutathione depletion (23). The uptake process of a compound can be altered by interaction with or biotransformation of another chemical, or by pretreatment of the liver. Corona *et al.* (12) have reported that pre-exposure of rabbits to amitryptiline resulted in a decreased uptake of the drug by hepatocytes after isolation, suggesting that the chronic *in vivo* treatment had induced changes in the plasma membrane.

Hepatocyte suspensions have been used to study morphological and biochemical alterations induced by a variety of compounds. This model is suitable for analysing molecular events related to the toxicity of hepatotoxins. Compounds which require metabolic activation to exert their toxic effects often induce similar toxicity as observed in the intact animal. Examples include toxicity induced by bromobenzene (83, 84), paracetamol (42) and thioacetamide (30). Tyson *et al.* (88) tested a number of compounds and found that all but two correlated to *in vivo* results. Cellular damage provoked by bromobenzene and paracetamol required previous depletion of glutathione content (42, 84). Species differences are visualized *in vitro* to a similar extent as observed *in vivo*; isolated mouse hepatocytes are more susceptible to paracetamol than rat hepatocytes (59).

Most of the toxic agents induce liver damage *in vivo* in a predictable manner and can be considered as true (predictable) hepatotoxins. However, a few compounds produce hepatic injury only in unusually susceptible humans and have been named idiosyncracy-dependent (unpredictable) toxins (98). Among the drugs which may cause liver damage in conditions suggesting a drug allergy response, are sulfonamides, halothane, erythromycin estolate and chlorpromazine. For some drugs, toxic effects have been attributed to hypersensitivity coupled to a certain degree of intrinsic hepatotoxicity (98). Use of isolated rat hepatocytes has demonstrated a positive correlation between the adverse effects of the drugs on liver cells and their ability to cause injury in man. For example, chlorpromazine, which is far more likely to cause jaundice than promazine, is approximately 10-fold more toxic to isolated hepatocytes than is promazine (99).

Cultured hepatocytes in toxicity assessment

Hepatocytes in suspension have a short life, thus preventing their use for studies on chronic effects of hepatotoxins. Such chronic investigations can be carried out with hepatocyte primary cultures. However, it must be kept in mind that the drug metabolizing enzyme activities undergo alterations during culture. In addition, compounds which are toxic *in vivo* may exert their toxic effects either in the cell where they are formed or after transport to other cells or organs.

After one or two days in culture there is a rapid decline in the level of cytochrome P-450 and a number of enzyme activities, so that after this time the cells do not reflect the *in vivo* situation (33) (see the section on drug metabolism in cultured hepatocytes). This explains why toxicological studies are usually performed on rodent hepatocyte cultures during the first two days following cell plating. As for isolated hepatocytes, the environment plays a critical role in the cytotoxic potential of hepatotoxins to hepatocyte cultures. Under anoxic conditions the covalent binding of carbon tetrachloride and halothane, which undergo reductive biotransformation *in vivo*, to cultured hepatocytes is enhanced, whereas that of chloroform and 1,1,2-trichoroethane, which undergo oxidative biotransformation, is decreased (15). The toxicity of erythromycin estolate is increased in rat hepatocyte cultures maintained in a medium deprived of proteins (93).

Problems caused by the lack of extrahepatic release of toxic compounds and accumulation of compounds in the culture medium have been emphasized by Paine & Hockin (67). These authors have studied the effects of three groups of toxins on cultured rat hepatocytes maintained under conditions that resulted in either a low or a high concentration of cytochrome P-450. As predicted, toxins (ethionine, galactosamine) which are not metabolized by cytochrome P-450 were equally toxic regardless of the cytochrome P-450 concentration. In contrast, the behaviour of the two other groups of compounds was not predictable. Indeed, compounds that are activated by cytochrome P-450 (carbon tetrachloride, bromobenzene, cyclo-phosphamide, paracetamol) and those which are detoxified by cytochrome P-450 (strychnine, pentobarbital) were also equally toxic regardless of the cytochrome P-450 content of the cells after a 24 h incubation. Only when the treatment was limited to 1-4 h, and followed by a 20 h incubation in a toxin-free medium, was carbon tetrachloride more toxic to cultured hepatocytes containing high levels of cyto-chrome P-450. These results indicate that accumulation of toxic compounds in the medium can be a limitation to the use of cultured hepatocytes in toxicity tests.   ·

Some authors proposed that this problem of the lack of extrahepatic release and accumulation of toxic compounds, may be overcome by co-culturing rat hepatocytes with fibroblasts (2, 24, 25). An example is provided by the toxicity of cyclo-phosphamide which is converted by the mono-oxygenase system into cytotoxic metabolites that non-specifically alkylate DNA and cellular proteins. By day 3 after a 24 h exposure to 1×10^{-4}M to 1×10^{-3}M cyclophosphamide, a 40% decrease in cell number and total proteins was found in postnatal rat hepatocyte cultures. Moreover, dramatic morphological changes were observed in hepatocytes because of fibroblast destruction (2). Cytotoxicity was prevented by SKF 525A, an inhibitor of the mono-oxygenase system. Similar observations were made by using adult rat hepatocyte cultures for cyclophosphamide (24) and various other chemicals (25, 96). We have preliminary evidence that the co-culture system which associates hepa-tocytes with rat liver epithelial cells (32) also represents a suitable model for this purpose.

Rat hepatocyte cultures have also been used for studying the effects of several compounds which have been reported to be unusually hepatotoxic in man. Thus, sodium salicylate was hepatotoxic and the degree of cellular damage was dose-dependent and influenced by the medium concentration of albumin (86). Two of its metabolites were also found hepatotoxic in a dose-related fashion (46). Villa *et al.* (92, 93) compared the effects of erythromycin estolate and erythromycin base in rat hepatocyte cultures, in addition to cultures of other hepatic cell types. As observed *in vivo*, erythromycin estolate was found to be more toxic than erythromycin base and the degree of cytotoxicity decreased with the culture time in conventional hepatocyte cultures. This was not related to the loss of cytochrome P-450. These antibiotics were equally toxic to liver fibroblastic and epithelial cells which did not contain detectable amounts of cytochrome P-450, as well as to co-cultured rat hepatocytes which retained a normal level of cytochrome P-450 that responded to phenobarbital addition (Fig. 3). Erythromycin estolate was also more toxic than erythromycin base to cultured adult human hepatocytes (35).

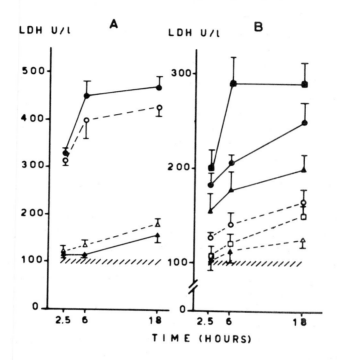

Fig. 3. **Time- and dose-dependent effects of erythromycins on lactic dehydrogenase leakage from co-cultured rat hepatocytes (A) and other hepatic and non-hepatic cell cultures (B).** (A) 8×10^{-4}M erythromycin base (EB) (▲—▲,△ - - - △) and 4×10^{-4}M erythromycin estolate (EE) (●—●,○ - - - ○) were added to co-cultures at 4 (———) and 8 (- - - -) days after plating and lactic dehydrogenase (LDH) leakage was measured at 2.5, 6 and 18 h after antibiotic addition. (B) 8×10^{-4}M EB (○ - - - ○,□ - - - □,△ - - - △) and 4×10^{-4}M EE (●—●,■—■,▲—▲) were added to rat liver epithelial cells (○ - - - ○,●—●) and human skin fibroblasts (□ - - - □,■—■) and LDH leakage was measured at 2.5, 6 and 18 h after antibiotic addition. Cells lines were used 3 or 4 days after seeding. LDH leakage from control cultures with 0.5% DMSO (/////). Mean values ± S.E. of 3 cultures. Data from reference 92.

Conclusions

Several aspects of xenobiotic metabolism have been studied using freshly isolated or short-term cultured hepatocytes from untreated and treated rodents. These models appear suitable for studying hepatic metabolism pathways and acute toxicity of chemicals. However, longer term investigations are not possible because of the rapid alteration of the cytochrome P-450 level and drug metabolizing enzymes. Addition of various factors, eg hormones, to media enhances the maintenance of cytochrome P-450 but long term expression of a stable enzymatic pattern in rodent hepatocytes has not yet been achieved. However, species differences have been observed in the *in vitro* behaviour of adult hepatocytes. Human adult hepatocytes are much less sensitive to the *in vitro* environment than rodent hepatocytes. Especially when co-cultured with rat liver epithelial cells, they retain high levels of total cytochrome P-450, two major cytochrome P-450 isozymes and the capability to metabolize drugs according to Phase I and Phase II drug metabolizing enzyme pathways for several days. It may be assumed that maintenance of drug metabolizing enzymes will be further improved in co-culture when the composition of media is better defined.

The first results with cultured adult human hepatocytes suggest that this system will become a suitable model for predicting hepatic metabolic pathways and hepatotoxicity of new drugs in man. It could partly replace and reduce the use of experimental animals for pharmacotoxicological studies. Of course, this model needs to be further characterized. For example, it is important to determine whether the entire drug enzymatic equipment is present at normal hepatic levels and remains inducible. Moreover, it is necessary to determine whether individual differences in metabolism, particularly those between 'high' and 'low' metabolizers, are retained in culture. A rate-limiting step is the availability of human hepatocytes. This difficulty could, at least partly, be overcome by the cryopreservation of the cells. Several laboratories, including ours, have already succeeded in freezing adult hepatocytes within recent months and it will undoubtedly soon be possible to routinely freeze adult hepatocytes which, after thawing, will remain viable and be able to attach and survive in culture.

ACKNOWLEDGMENTS

The author thanks Professor M. Bourel and Drs P. Beaune, J. M. Bégué, D. Ratanasavanh and P. Villa for the critical reading of the manuscript and is indebted to Mrs A. Vannier for typing. Personal research described in this review was supported by INSERM, MRT, FRM and the Foundation Langlois.

REFERENCES

1 Acosta D., Anuforo D. C., McMillin R., Soine N. H., Smith R. G.: Comparison of cytochrome P-450 levels in adult rat liver, postnatal rat liver and primary cultures of postnatal rat hepatocytes. *Life Sci.* 1979, **25**: 1413–1418.
2 Acosta D., Mitchell D. B.: Metabolic activation and cytotoxicity of cyclophosphamide in primary cultures of postnatal rat hepatocytes. *Biochem. Pharmacol.* 1981, **30**: 3225–3230.
3 Allen C. M., Hockin L. J., Paine A. J.: The control of glutathione and cytochrome P-450 in hepatic parenchymal cell culture and the stimulation of haem oxygenase activity. *Biochem. Pharmacol.* 1981, **30**: 2739–2742.
4 Andersson B., Jones D. P., Orrenius S.: Effect of calcium ions on ethanol oxidation and drug glucuronidation in isolated hepatocytes. *Biochem. J.* 1979, **184**: 709–711.
5 Bégué J. M., Guguen-Guillouzo C., Pasdeloup N., Guillouzo A.: Prolonged maintenance of active cytochrome P-450 in adult rat hepatocytes co-cultured with another liver cell type. *Hepatology* 1984, **4**: 839–842.

6 Bégué J. M., Le Bigot J. F., Guguen-Guillouzo C., Kiechel J. R., Guillouzo A.: Cultured human adult hepatocytes: a new model for drug metabolism studies. *Biochem. Pharmacol.* 1983, 32: 1643–1646.

7 Billings R. E., McMahon R. E., Ashmore J., Wagle S. R.: The metabolism of drugs in isolated rat hepatocytes: A comparison with *in vitro* drug metabolism and drug metabolism in subcellular liver fractions. *Drug Metab. Dispos.* 1977, 5: 518–526.

8 Bissell D. M., Guzelian P. S.: Ascorbic acid deficiency and cytochrome P-450 in adult rat hepatocytes in primary monolayer culture. *Arch. Biochem. Biophys.* 1979, 192: 569–576.

9 Bissell D. M. Guzelian P. S.: Phenotypic stability of adult rat hepatocytes in primary monolayer culture. *Ann. N.Y. Acad. Sci.* 1980, 349: 85–98.

10 Bridges J. W., Benfort D. U., Hubbard S. A.: Mechanisms of toxic injury. *Ann. N.Y. Acad. Sci.* 1983, 407: 42–63.

11 Burke M. D., Vadi H., Jernstrom B., Orrenius S.: Metabolism of benzo(a)pyrene with isolated hepatocytes and the formation and degradation of DNA-binding derivatives. *J. Biol. Chem.* 1977, 252: 6424–6431.

12 Corona G. L., Santagostino G., Facino R. M., Pirillo D.: Cell membrane modifications in rabbit isolated hepatocytes following a chronic amitryptiline treatment. *Biochem. Pharmacol.* 1973, 22: 849–856.

13 Decad G. M., Hsieh D. P. H., Byard J. L.: Maintenance of cytochrome P-450 and metabolism of aflatoxin B_1 in primary hepatocyte cultures. *Biochem. Biophys. Res. Commun.* 1977, 78: 279–287.

14 Dickens M., Peterson R. E.: Effects of a hormone-supplemented medium on cytochrome P-450 content and mono-oxygenase activities of rat hepatocytes in primary culture. *Biochem. Pharmacol.* 1980, 29: 1231–1238.

15 Direnzo A. B., Gandolfi A. J., Sipes I. G., Brendel K., Byard J. L.: Effects of O_2 tension on the bioactivation and metabolism of aliphatic halides by primary rat-hepatocyte cultures. *Xenobiotica* 1984, 14: 521–525.

16 Dougherty K. K., Spilman S. D., Green C. E., Steward A. R., Byard J. L.: Primary cultures of adult mouse and rat hepatocytes for studying the metabolism of foreign chemicals. *Biochem. Pharmacol.* 1980, 29: 2117–2124.

17 Dybing E., Soderlund E., Haug L. T., Thorgeirsson S. S.: Metabolism and activation of 2-acetylaminofluorene in isolated rat hepatocytes. *Cancer Res.* 1979, 39: 3268–3275.

18 Edwards A. M., Glistak M. L., Lucas C. M., Wilson P. A.: 7-Ethoxycoumarin deethylase activity as a convenient measure of liver drug metabolizing enzymes: regulation in cultured rat hepatocytes. *Biochem. Pharmacol.* 1984, 33: 1537–1546.

19 Elshourbagy N. A., Barwick J. L., Guzelian P. S.: Induction of cytochrome P-450 by pregnenolone-16-α-carbonitrile in primary monolayer cultures of adult rat hepatocytes and in cell-free translation system. *J. Biol. Chem.* 1981, 256: 6060–6068.

20 Erickson R. R., Holtzman J. L.: Kinetic studies on the metabolism of ethylmorphine by isolated hepatocytes from adult rats. *Biochem. Pharmacol.* 1976, 25: 1501–1506.

21 Evarts R. P., Marsden E., Thorgeirsson S. S.: Regulation of heme metabolism and cytochrome P-450 levels in primary culture of rat hepatocytes in a defined medium. *Biochem. Pharmacol.* 1984, 33: 565–569.

22 Fahl, W. E., Michalopoulos G., Sattler G. L., Jefcoate C. R., Pitot H. C.: Characteristics of microsomal enzyme controls in primary cultures of rat hepatocytes. *Arch. Biochem. Biophys.* 1979, 192: 61–72.

23 Fariss M. W., Olafsdottir K., Reed D. J.: Extracellular calcium protects isolated rat hepatocytes from injury. *Biochem. Biophys. Res. Commun.* 1984, 121: 102–110.

24 Fry J. R., Bridges J. W.: A novel mixed hepatocyte-fibroblast culture system and its use as a test for metabolism-mediated cytotoxicity. *Biochem. Pharmacol.* 1977, 26: 969–973.

25 Fry J. R., Bridges J. W.: Use of primary hepatocyte cultures in biochemical toxicology. *Rev. Biochem. Toxicol.* 1979, 1: 201–247.

26 Goethals F., Krack G., Deboyser D., Vossen P., Roberfroid M.: Critical biochemical functions of isolated hepatocytes as sensitive indicators of chemical toxicity. *Fund. Appl. Toxicol.* 1984, 4: 441-450.

27 Grisham J. W.: Use of hepatic cell cultures to detect and evaluate the mechanisms of action of toxic

chemicals. Int. Rev. Exp. Pathol. 1979, **20**: 123–210.

28 Grundin R.: Metabolic interaction of ethanol and alprenolol in isolated liver cells. *Acta Pharmacol. Toxicol.* 1975, **37**: 185–200.

29 Grundin R., Moldeus P., Vadi H., Orrenius S., Von Barh C., Backstrom D., Ehrenberg A: Drug metabolism in isolated rat liver cells. *Adv. Exp. Med. Biol.* 1975, **58**: 251–269.

30 Gudzinowicz M., Neal R. A.: Biochemical effects and metabolism of thiocetamide (TAA) and thioacetamide-S-oxide (TAAO) by isolated rat liver cells. *Pharmacologist* 1979, **21**: 186.

31 Guengerich F. P.: Factors involved in the regulation of the levels and activities of rat liver cytochromes P-450. *Biochem. Soc. Trans.* 1984, **12**: 68–70.

32 Guguen-Guillouzo C., Clement B., Baffet G., Beaumont C., Morel-Chany E., Glaise D., Guillouzo A.: Maintenance and reversibility of active albumin secretion by adult rat hepatocytes co-cultured with another liver epithelial cell type. *Exp. Cell Res.* 1983, **143**: 47–54.

33 Guguen-Guillouzo C., Guillouzo A.: Modulation of functional activities in cultured rat hepatocytes. *Molec. Cell. Biochem.* 1983, **53/54**: 35–56.

34 Guillouzo A., Beaune P., Gascoin M. N., Bégué J. M., Campion J. P., Guengerich F. P., Guguen-Guillouzo C.: Maintenance of cytochrome P-450 in cultured adult human hepatocytes. *Biochem. Pharmacol.* 1985, **34**: 2991–2995.

35 Guillouzo A., Bégué J. M., Campion J. P., Gascoin M. N., Guguen-Guillouzo C.: Human hepatocyte cultures: a model for pharmaco-toxicological studies. *Xenobiotica* 1985, **15**: 635–647.

36 Guillouzo A., Guguen-Guillouzo C., Boisnard M., Bourel M., Benhamou J. P.: Smooth endoplasmic reticulum proliferation and increased cell multiplication in cultured hepatocytes of the newborn rat in the presence of phenobarbital. *Exp. Molec. Path.* 1978, **28**: 1–9.

37 Gumucio J., De Mason L. J., Miller D. L., Krezoski S. O., Keener M.: Induction of cytochrome P-450 in a selective subpopulation of hepatocytes. *Am. J. Physiol.* 1978, **234**: C102–C109.

38 Guzelian P. S., Barwick J. L.: Inhibition by cycloheximide of degradation of cytochrome P-450 in primary cultures of adult rat liver parenchymal cells and *in vivo. Biochem. J.* 1979, **180**: 621–630.

39 Guzelian P. S., Bissell D. M.: Effect of cobalt on synthesis of heme and cytochrome P-450 in the liver. Studies of adult rat hepatocytes in primary monolayer culture and *in vivo. J. Biol. Chem.* 1976, **251**: 4421–4427.

40 Guzelian P. S., Bissell D. M., Meyer U. A.: Drug metabolism in adult rat hepatocytes in primary monolayer culture. *Gastroenterology* 1977, **72**: 1232–1239.

41 Gwynn J., Fry J. R., Bridges J. W.: The effect of paracetamol and other foreign compounds on protein synthesis in isolated adult rat hepatocytes. *Biochem. Soc. Trans.* 1979, **7**: 117–119.

42 Hogberg J., Kristogenson A.: A correlation between glutathione levels and cellular damage in isolated hepatocytes. *Eur. J. Biochem.* 1977, **74**: 77–82.

43 Houssin D., Capron M., Celier C., Cresteil T., Demaugre F., Beaune P.: Evaluation of isolated human hepatocytes. *Life Sci.* 1983, **33**: 1805–1809.

44 Jones C. A., Moore B. P., Cohen G. M., Fry J. R., Bridges J. W.: Studies on the metabolism and excretion of benzo(a)pyrene in isolated adult rat hepatocytes. *Biochem. Pharmacol.* 1978, **27**: 693–702.

45 Junge O., Brand K.: Mixed function oxidation of hexobarbital and generation of NADPH by the hexose monophosphate shunt in isolated rat liver cells. *Arch. Biochem. Biophys.* 1975, **171**: 398–406.

46 Kingsley E. D., Gray P., Tolman K. G., Tweedale R.: The toxicity of metabolites of sodium valproate in cultured hepatocytes. *J. Clin. Pharmacol.* 1983, **23**: 178–185.

47 Klaassen C. D., Stacey N. H.: Use of isolated hepatocytes in toxicity assessment. In: *Toxicology of the Liver*, G. Plaa, W. R. Hewitt (Eds): Raven Press, New York, 1982, pp 147–179.

48 Krack G., Goethals F., Deboyser D., Roberfroid M.: Metabolic competence of isolated hepatocytes in suspension: a new tool for *in vitro* toxicological evaluation. In: *Isolation, Characterization and Use of Hepatocytes*, R. A. Harris, N. W. Cornell (Eds): Elsevier Biomedical, New York, 1983, pp 391–398.

49 Kurihara N., Hori N., Ichinose R.: Cytochrome P-450 content and aldrin epoxidation to dieldrin in isolated rat hepatocytes. *Pest. Biochem. Physiol.* 1984, **21**: 63–74.

50 Lake B. G., Paine A. J.: The effect of hepatocyte culture conditions on cytochrome P-450 linked drug metabolizing enzymes. *Biochem. Pharmacol.* 1982, **31**: 2141–2144.

51 Lake B. G., Paine A. J.: Induction of hepatic cytochrome P-450 and drug metabolism by metyrapone in the rat: relevance to its effects in rat-liver cell culture. *Xenobiotica* 1983, **13**: 725–730.

52 Lake B. G., Tim J. B., Stubberfield C. R., Beamand J. A., Gangolli S. D.: Induction of lauric acid hydroxylation and maintenance of cytochrome P-450 content by clofibrate in primary cultures of rat hepatocytes. *Life Sci.* 1983, **33**: 249–254.

53 Le Bigot J. F., Bégué J. M., Kiechel J. R., Guillouzo A.: Species differences in metabolism of ketotifen in rat, rabbit and man: demonstration of similar pathways *in vivo* and in cultured hepatocytes. (Submitted.)

54 Maslansky C. J., Williams G. M.: Primary cultures and the levels of cytochrome P-450 in hepatocytes from mouse, rat, hamster and rabbit liver. *In Vitro.* 1982, **18**: 683–693.

55 Michalopoulos G., Pitot H. C.: Primary culture of parenchymal cells on collagen membranes: morphological and biochemical observations. *Exp. Cell Res.* 1975, **94**: 70–78.

56 Michalopoulos G., Russel F., Biles C.: Primary cultures of hepatocytes on human fibroblasts. *In Vitro* 1979, **15**: 796–806.

57 Michalopoulos G., Sattler C. A., Sattler G. L., Pitot H. C.: Cytochrome P-450 induction by phenobarbital and 3-methylcholanthrene in primary cultures of hepatocytes. *Science* 1976, **193**: 907–909.

58 Michalopoulos G., Sattler G. L., Pitot H. C.: Maintenance of microsomal cytochrome b5 and P-450 in primary culture of parenchymal liver cells on collagen membranes. *Life Sci.* 1976, **18**: 1139–1144.

59 Moldeus P.: Paracetamol metabolism and toxicity in isolated hepatocytes from rat and mouse. *Biochem. Pharmacol.* 1978, **27**: 2859–2863.

60 Moldeus P., Andersson B., Norling A.: Interaction of ethanol oxidation with glucuronidation in isolated hepatocytes. *Biochem. Pharmacol.* 1978, **27**: 2583–2588.

61 Moldeus P., Grundin R., Vadi H., Orrenius S.: A study of drug metabolism linked to cytochrome P-450 in isolated rat liver cells. *Eur. J. Biochem.* 1974, **46**: 351–360.

62 Moldeus P., Grundin R., Von Barh C., Orrenius S.: Spectral studies on drug cytochrome P-450 interaction in isolated rat liver cells. *Biochem. Biophys. Res. Commun.* 1973, **55**: 937–944.

63 Newman S., Guzelian P. S.: Stimulation of *de novo* synthesis of cytochrome P-450 by phenobarbital in primary non proliferating cultures of adult rat hepatocytes. *Proc. Natl. Acad. Sci.* 1982, **79**: 2922–2926.

64 Notten W. R. F., Henderson P. T., Kuyper C. M. A.: Stimulation of the glucuronic acid pathway in isolated rat liver cells by phenobarbital. *Int. J. Biochem.* 1975, **6**: 713–718.

65 Orton T. C., Sorman A. E., Crisp D. N., Sturdee A. P.: Dynamics of xenobiotic metabolism by isolated rat hepatocytes using a multichannel perifusion system. *Xenobiotica* 1983, **13**: 743–753.

66 Paine A. J., Hockin L. J.: Nutrient imbalance causes the loss of cytochrome P-450 in liver cell culture: formulation of culture media which maintain cytochrome P-450 at *in vivo* concentrations. *Biochem. Pharmacol.* 1980, **29**: 3215–3218.

67 Paine A. J., Hockin L. J.: The maintenance of cytochrome P-450 in liver cell culture: recent studies on P-450 mediated mechanisms of toxicity. *Toxicology* 1982, **25**: 41–45.

68 Paine A. J., Hockin L. J., Legg R. F.: Relationship between the ability of nicotinamide to maintain nicotinamide adenine dinucleotide in rat liver cell culture and its effect on cytochrome P-450. *Biochem. J.* 1979, **184**: 461–463.

69 Paine A. J., Legg R. F.: Apparent lack of correlation between the loss of cytochrome P-450 in hepatic parenchymal cell culture and the stimulation of haem oxygenase activity. *Biochem. Biophys. Res. Commun.* 1978, **81**: 672–679.

70 Paine A. J., Villa P.: Ligands maintain cytochrome P-450 in liver cell culture by affecting its synthesis and degradation. *Biochem. Biophys. Res. Commun.* 1980, **97**: 744–750.

71 Paine A. J., Williams L. J., Legg R. F.: Apparent maintenance of cytochrome P-450 by nicotinamide in primary cultures of rat hepatocytes. *Life Sci.* 1979, **24**: 2185–2192.

72 Ratanasavanh D., Beaune P., Baffet G., Rissel M., Kremers P., Guengerich F. P., Guillouzo A.: Immunocytochemical evidence of the maintenance of cytochrome P-450 isozymes, NADPH cytochrome *c* reductase and epoxide hydrolase in pure and mixed primary cultures of adult human hepatocytes. *J. Histochem Cytochem.* 1986, **34**: (in press).

73 Renton K. W., Deloria L. B. Mannering G. J.: Effects of polyriboinosinic acid-polyribocytidylic

acid and a mouse interferon preparation on cytochrome P-450 dependent mono-oxygenase systems in cultures of primary mouse hepatocytes. *Molec. Pharmacol.* 1978, **14**: 672–681.

74 Richardson A., Sutter M. A., Jayaraj A., Webb J. M.: Age-related changes in the ability of hepatocytes to metabolize aflatoxin B_1. *In: Liver and Aging — Liver and Drugs*, K. Kitani (Ed.): Elsevier Biomedical Press, Amsterdam, 1982, pp 119–132.

75 Rojkind M., Gatmaitan Z., Mackensen S., Giambrone M., Ponce P., Reid L. M.: Connective tissue biomatrix: Its isolation and utilization for long-term cultures of normal rat hepatocytes. *J. Cell Biol.* 1980, **87**, 255–263.

76 Schmeltz W. I., Tosk J., Williams G. M.: Comparison of the metabolic profiles of benzo(a)pyrene obtained from primary cell cultures and subcellular fractions derived from normal and methyl-cholanthrene-induced rat liver. *Cancer Lett.* 1978, **5**: 81–89.

77 Schuetz E. G., Wrighton S. A., Barwick J. L., Guzelian P. S.: Induction of cytochrome P-450 by glucocorticoids in rat liver. *J. Biol. Chem.* 1984, **259**: 1999–2006.

78 Schwarz L. R., Gotz R., Wolff T., Wiebel F. J.: Mono-oxygenase and glucuronyltransferase activities in short-term cultures of isolated rat hepatocytes. *FEBS Lett*, 1979, **98**: 203–206.

79 Sirica A. E., Pitot H. C.: Drug metabolism and effects of carcinogens in cultured hepatic cells. *Pharmacol. Rev.* 1980, **31**: 205–228.

80 Smith M. T., Thor H., Orrenius S.: Toxic injury to isolated hepatocytes is not dependent on extracellular calcium. *Science* 1981, **213**: 1257–1259.

81 Sorensen E. M., Acosta D.: Protective effects of calcium on cadmium-induced cytotoxicity in cultured rat hepatocytes. *In Vitro* 1982, **18**: 288.

82 Steward A. R., Byard J. L.: Induction of benzo(a)pyrene metabolism by 2,3,7,8-tetrachloro-dibenzo-p-dioxin in primary cultures of adult rat hepatocytes. *Tox. Appl. Pharmacol.* 1981, **59**: 603–616.

83 Thor H., Moldeus P., Kristofenson A., Hogberg J., Reed D. J., Orrenius S: Metabolic activation and hepatotoxicity: metabolism of boromobenzene in isolated hepatocytes. *Arch. Biochem. Biophys.* 1978, **188**: 114–121.

84 Thor H., Orrenius S.: The mechanism of bromobenzene-induced cytotoxicity studied with isolated hepatocytes. *Arch. Toxicol.* 1980, **44**: 31–43.

85 Thurman R.G, Kauffman F. C.: Factors regulating drug metabolism in intact hepatocytes. *Pharmacol. Rev.* 1980, **31**: 229–251.

86 Tolman K. G., Peterson P., Gray B. S. Hammar S. P.: Hepatotoxicity of salicylates in monolayer cell cultures. *Gastroenterology* 1978, **74**: 205–208.

87 Tonda K., Hirata M.: Glucuronidation and sulfation of p-nitrophenol in isolated rat hepatocyte subpopulations. Effects of phenobarbital and 3-methylcholanthrene pretreatment. *Chem. Biol. Inter.* 1983, **47**: 277–287.

88 Tyson C. A., Mitoma C., Kalivoda J.: Evaluation of hepatocytes isolated by a nonperfusion technique in a prescreen for cytotoxicity. *J. Toxicol. Environ. Health.* 1980, **6**: 197–205.

89 Ullrich D., Bock K. W.: Glucuronide formation of various drugs in liver microsomes and in isolated hepatocytes from phenobarbital and 3-methylcholanthrene-treated rats. *Biochem. Pharmacol.* 1984, **33**: 97–101.

90 Van Bezooijen C. F. A., Soekawa Y., Ohta M., Nokubo M., Kitani K.: Metabolism of digitoxin by isolated rat hepatocytes. *Biochem. Pharmacol.* 1980, **29**: 3023–3025.

91 Van Bezooijen C. F. A., Sakkee A. N., Boonstra-Nieveld I. H. S., Bégué J. M., Guillouzo A., Knook D. L.: The effect of age on digitoxin biotransformation in isolated hepatocytes. *In: Liver and Aging – Liver and drugs*, K. Kitani (Ed.): Elsevier Biomedical Press, Amsterdam, 1982, pp 162–176.

92 Villa P., Bégué J. M., Guillouzo A.: Effects of erythromycin derivatives on cultured rat hepatocytes. *Biochem. Pharmacol.* 1984 **33**: 4098–4101.

93 Villa P., Bégué J. M., Guillouzo A.: Erythromycin toxicity in primary cultures of rat hepatocytes. *Xenobiotica.* 1985, **15**: 767–773.

94 Vina J., Hems R., Krebs H. A.: Maintenance of glutathione content in isolated hepatocytes. *Biochem. J.* 1978, 627–630.

95 Weigl K., Sies H.: Drug oxidations dependent on cytochrome P-450 in isolated hepatocytes: The role of the tricarboxylates and the aminotransferases in NADPH supply. *Eur. J. Biochem.* 1977, **77**: 401–408.

96 Wiebkin P., Fry J. R., Bridges J. W.: Metabolism mediated cytotoxicity of chemical carcinogenesis and non carcinogenesis. *Biochem. Pharmacol.* 1978, **27**: 1849–1851.

97 Wiebkin P., Parker, G. L., Fry J. R., Bridges J. W.: Effects of various metabolic inhibitors on biphenyl metabolism in isolated rat hepatocytes. *Biochem. Pharmacol.* 1979, **28**: 3315–3321.

98 Zimmerman H. J.: Chemical hepatic injury and its detection. *In: Toxicology of the Liver*, G. Plaa, W. R. Hewitt (Eds), Raven Press, New York, 1982, pp 1–45.

99 Zimmerman H. J., Abernathy C. O.: Structural determinants of toxic effects of phenothiazines and other tricyclics on hepatocytes *in vitro. Hepatology* 1983, **3**: 1088.

Research in *Isolated and cultured hepatocytes* A. Guillouzo & C. Guguen-Guillouzo eds., pp. 333–352.
© 1986 John Libbey Eurotext Ltd./INSERM

15

Use of hepatocytes for studies of mutagenesis and carcinogenesis

George K. MICHALOPOULOS, Steven C. STROM and
Randy L. JIRTLE

*Departments of Pathology (GKM) and Radiology (SCS, RLJ), Duke
University Medical School, Durham, North Carolina, 27710, USA*

SUMMARY

This article reviews the applications of primary cultures of hepatocytes for studies of carcinogenesis. Specifically, hepatocytes have been used as endpoints in genotoxicity bioassays or as tools for the study of the mechanisms of carcinogenesis *per se*. Despite the decline of microsomal functions in hepatocytes in culture, more activity and a wider spectrum of mixed function oxidase activities are preserved in hepatocytes than in any other type of cell in culture. Unscheduled DNA synthesis, measurement of DNA damage and hepatocyte mediated mutagenesis are the most commonly used genotoxicity bioassays with hepatocytes. These techniques have been also applied to cultures of human hepatocytes isolated by collagenase perfusion. Replicating hepatocytes in primary culture are sensitive to the presence of chemical carcinogens. Inhibition of the DNA synthesis is seen with very low concentrations of xenobiotics known to generate large DNA adducts. DNA synthesis in initiated hepatocytes is inhibited much less than that of the normal cells. Replicating hepatocytes have also been used as bioassays for the growth factors that control liver regeneration and neoplasia.

Introduction

Several unique features of hepatic biology make liver a suitable tissue to be used as a model for carcinogenesis studies. These are the following:

1) Liver is one of the sites of formation of solid tumours in most instances when carcinogens are administered through the food or the drinking water to rodents.
2) Hepatocyte microsomes contain mixed function oxidases that are capable of catalysing enzymatic reactions resulting in the 'bioactivation' of most pro-carcinogens to their active carcinogenic form.
3) Liver is endowed with a high capacity for regenerative growth. This can be induced following simple stimuli such as partial hepatectomy or administration of necrogenic toxins.
4) Last, but not least, there is a large data bank of the biochemistry of the hepatic tissue, due to the facility with which liver can be subjected to cellular fractionation procedures. This data bank on normal liver provides a background on which aspects of biochemistry of neoplasia can be studied.

The wide use of liver for carcinogenesis studies prompted the application of hepatocyte cultures for studies in this area. These studies have mainly focused on the measurement of the expression of the enzymes involved with carcinogen metabolism and the measurement of specific endpoints of genotoxicity in response to the addition of chemical carcinogens to hepatocyte cultures. The most commonly used geno-toxicity endpoints have been unscheduled DNA synthesis (UDS), and hepatocyte mediated mutagenesis. These approaches have been now applied to both rodent and human hepatocytes. A major missing link interfering with the direct study of liver carcinogenesis *in vitro* has been the lack of systems in which clonal growth of hepatocytes (analogous to the clonal growth seen with cells such as fibroblasts, endothelial cells etc) can be maintained. This makes it currently impossible to conduct direct mutagenesis assays on the hepatocytes themselves. It also makes it impossible to design systems for the *in vitro* study of the steps involved in the neoplastic transformation of these cells. Recent progress in the induction of hepatocyte growth *in vitro* provides hope that systems that allow clonal growth of hepatocytes may be developed in the near future. The present review will discuss a summary of the findings that resulted from the use of hepatocyte cultures for studies relating to carcinogenesis and consider the new approaches that now appear to emerge and could be explored further in future studies.

DNA damage and unscheduled DNA synthesis induced by chemical carcinogens in cultures of hepatocytes

The studies reviewed in this chapter have used genotoxic agents, usually chemical carcinogens, to quantitate DNA damage induced by these agents in cultures of hepatocytes. Repair DNA synthesis is monitored as unscheduled DNA synthesis (UDS). Many such similar studies have been conducted using other cell systems. In most cell systems however, the lack of sufficient capabilities to carry out the 'bioactivation' of procarcinogens (the majority of chemical carcinogens) has allowed only the study of genotoxicity induced by direct acting carcinogens or activated derivatives of procarcinogens. Hepatocytes have become of interest because they have the capability to 'activate' procarcinogens through the microsomal and cytosolic enzymes associated with drug metabolism. There is a large data bank on the effect of most of these procarcinogens as inducers of hepatic tumourigenesis. The studies reviewed in this section have attempted to provide *in vitro* models which would allow quantitation of several parameters of hepatocarcinogenesis that are difficult or impossible to quantitate *in vivo*.

Several techniques have been used to demonstrate DNA damage in cultures of hepatocytes. These include mainly velocity sedimentation of DNA in alkaline sucrose gradients, and elution of isolated DNA from filters in an alkaline environment. Using these techniques several investigators (5, 14, 16, 50, 75) have shown that administration of carcinogens in hepatocyte cultures is associated with the development of alkali-labile sites which result in fragmented DNA and affect the sedimentation properties in gradients or the rate of elution from filters. The appearance of low molecular weight DNA forms in combination with UDS can be even further enhanced by addition of the chain terminator dideoxythymidine (77). In most instances the DNA used was prelabelled by subjecting the donor animals to partial hepatectomy followed by injections of tritiated thymidine. The donor animals were kept at least for two weeks after hepatectomy before being used as donors for hepatocyte isolation. At that point after hepatectomy it is assumed that the hepatocytes have reverted to the pre-hepatectomy state. An additional problem with the development and use of this technique is the finding that the DNA of hepatocytes in culture is more fragmented than in the liver *in vivo* (61). It is not well understood whether this condition is a result of the environment of the culture and the presence of genotoxic compounds such as free radicals etc or whether the DNA fragmentation is analogous to the development of single strand breaks seen in other cell types during changes in their differentiation (23, 34). The spontaneous fragmentation of the DNA in hepatocytes in culture may interfere with the sensitivity of these techniques in situations where it would be used as a genotoxicity bioassay.

A more direct approach to measure DNA damage and repair has been the measurement of the rate of formation and removal of DNA adducts. There is more literature available in this area with whole liver *in vivo*. The formation and removal of

DNA adducts in different hepatic populations has been measured *in vivo* by Lewis & Swenberg (45). Pegg and coworkers measured the formation and removal of O-6-guanine in isolated hepatocytes and found that the rates were comparable to *in vivo* values (91). Strom *et al.* demonstrated that the carcinogens benzo(a)pyrene (BP) and N-2-acetylaminofluorene (AAF) bind to hepatocyte DNA (85, 86, 87), though higher concentrations were found to be bound to the DNA of human fibroblasts co-cultured with the hepatocytes. In more detail studies the formation removal of RNA and DNA adducts after exposure to N-OH AAF was monitored by Howard *et al.* (29). It was found that the dG-C-AF adduct was the principal adduct formed (60% of total) as opposed to only 20% of adducts accounted by this form in the liver *in vivo*. Using specific anti-DNA-AAF adduct antibodies, Poirier *et al.* demonstrated that whereas in most other cell types the C8-AAF adducts exist in the deacetylated form, in hepatocytes 80% of the adducts was in the acetylated form (68). Detailed analysis of the types of adducts generated by BP was also performed by Ashurst *et al.* (11). Stairs *et al.* showed that much of the BP adducts could be accounted by binding to the mitochondrial DNA (78). The binding to the latter (on a per unit length basis) was 4–15 times more than that of the nuclear DNA. The overall importance of the DNA adducts formed on mitochondrial DNA has not as yet been fully evaluated *in vitro* or *in vivo*. Recent studies by Loretz & Pariza (47) have focused on the role of glutathione and sulfate levels as determinants of the binding of AAF metabolites on macromolecules of hepatocytes in primary culture. Considering the voluminous literature on the formation and removal of DNA adducts in the liver *in vivo* much more remains to be done to characterize the differences between the hepatocytes *in vivo* and *in vitro* in this area. Reflecting the overall decrease in microsomal mixed function oxidase levels seen in *in vitro* hepatocytes, the recent finding by Novicki *et al.* (64) that the formation of AAF adducts decreases with hepatocytes in culture is not surprising. It should be of interest however, to compare the decline in the rate of formation of specific DNA adducts with the decline of specific cytochrome P-450 forms.

Measurement of UDS in hepatocytes in culture was attempted much earlier, before studies on the quantitation of adduct formation and removal had been attempted. It was first reported by Williams (95, 96) that UDS in response to carcinogens could be measured in hepatocytes in culture using autoradiographic techniques. Similar results were also reported by Michalopoulos *et al.* (54) and Yager *et al.* (97) by measuring UDS with liquid scintillation. The principle in either approach is that 'activation' of a procarcinogen to the directly carcinogenic form is followed by formation of adducts with DNA. These adducts are perceived by the proper cellular enzymatic systems as DNA damage and excised, along with a variable length patch of the adjacent DNA. The excised patch of DNA is resynthesized and thymidine incorporation can be used to follow this process. For reviews on the mechanisms underlying this phenomenon please see references 80 and 81. In a typical UDS measurement, hepatocyte cultures are incubated with a chemical carcinogen and tritiated thymidine (together or in succession). The incorporation of thymidine induced by the chemical is monitored and compared to control cultures. When the incorporation of thymidine is monitored by autoradiography, the results are usually expressed as grains per nucleus, after subtraction of the grains of an area equivalent to the size of the nucleus, in the same culture, and after subtraction of the grains of nuclei from other cultures used as control. Frequently, especially in cultures of hepatocytes, numerous grains are seen over the cytoplasm. Convincing evidence has been presented by Lonati-Calligani *et al.* that these counts are due to mitochondrial DNA repair and they should be recorded for their own merit (46). Combinations of microscopes and computerized video imaging have been introduced to improve the accuracy of the grain counting and the correction for control counts (56). Cells that are in scheduled DNA synthesis (S-phase) appear with black nuclei and are ignored. The grains due to the induction of UDS are more sparse, uniformly distributed throughout the culture and are counted individually in order to measure the UDS. Since it is relatively easy to distinguish between cells in S-phase and cells in UDS, there is no need to use agents that suppress the regular (scheduled) DNA synthesis. When UDS is assayed by liquid scintillation spectrometry, agents such as hydroxyurea are frequently used to suppress the regular (semiconservative) DNA synthesis (98). Concerns have been expressed, however, that hydroxyurea itself can be a cause of artifacts (9, 31).

The autoradiographic technique introduced by Williams has been extensively used as a bioassay for genotoxicity of xenobiotics. A comprehensive validation of this technique was undertaken by Probst *et al.* (69). In that study, 218 compounds were compared using the Ames system of bacterial mutagenesis (8) and the UDS in hepatocyte cultures measured by autoradiography. There was excellent correlation between UDS in hepatocytes and bacterial mutagenesis for polycyclic aromatic hydrocarbons, aromatic amines, biphenyls, nitrosamines, azo compounds, acridines, halogenated compounds, nitrosoureas, quinolines, pyridines, purines, pyrimidines and carbamates. Nitrocompounds that were active in the bacterial mutagenesis, probably due to bacterial nitroreductase, were weak inducers of UDS. The authors concluded that: 'The results . . . indicate the usefulness of hepatocyte UDS system as a component in a battery of short-term predictive tests for mutagens/carcinogens'. The reliability of this method was also evaluated by Williams *et al.* (93). In another separate study of the literature on UDS in hepatocytes conducted under the US Environmental Protection Agency Gene-Tox Program, it was concluded that testing through UDS was appropriate as a component in mutagenicity/carcinogenicity testing programmes (60). It was pointed out, however, that more work needed to be performed to understand the nature of the differences between hepatocyte preparations. Recently, several technical improvements have been published on the measurement of hepatocyte UDS by liquid scintillation. Althaus *et al.* have introduced methodology that allows rapid quantitation of the induced UDS in a matter of hours after the addition of carcinogens (6). Use of filters for the trapping of the DNA also allows rapid quantitation, as shown by Hsia *et al.* (87). The sensitivity of the technique can also be enhanced by isolation of nuclei prior to the measurement of the thymidine incorporation, as demonstrated by Olson *et al.* (65). Use of special supplements in the culture medium may allow study of the compounds that require activation by the colonic flora. This was shown in a study by Williams *et al.* (94) in which addition of cycasin elicited no UDS response unless β-glucosidase was also added to the cultures. The amount of induced UDS was dependent on the amount of β-glucosidase added. This is in accordance with the findings on the metabolism of this carcinogen which clearly indicate that this compound is activated by the colonic flora through a hydrolytic step that requires the action of *β*-glucosidase.

Other studies have focused not so much on the value of UDS in hepatocytes as a predictor of carcinogenicity but rather on the mechanisms of the phenomenon. Studies by Michalopoulos *et al.* have shown that the UDS induced by procarcinogens declines as a function of the time in culture and is at all points less for the cells in primary cultures compared to suspensions of freshly isolated cells (54). This is probably due to decrease in the capability of the cells in culture to activate chemical carcinogens, because of the decline of the levels of microsomal enzymes. Bermudez (15) demonstrated that the repair of hepatocyte DNA is inhibited after addition of aphidicolin. This clearly demonstrates the participation of the DNA polymerase alpha, for which aphidicolin is a specific inhibitor. This is of interest, in view of the fact that in most other mammalian cells it is the beta polymerase that has been implicated with DNA repair synthesis. Studies by Althaus *et al.* (4, 7) have emphasized the role of ADP-ribosyl transferase on the late aspects of the repair process in hepatocytes. Similar results had been previously shown for other cell types (83). ADP-ribosyl transferase increases rapidly soon after the hepatocytes are placed in primary culture. Inhibition of this enzyme with 3-aminobenzamide or other inhibitors resulted in enhanced removal of single strand breaks and UDS after exposure to methyl methanesulfonate or ultraviolet light. Inhibition of ADP-ribosyl transferase or addition of nicotinamide also suppressed the expression of fetal phenotype. The role of the ADP-ribosyl transferase appears important in several processes occurring in cultured hepatocytes and UDS may be just one of these processes (3). Studies by Sirica *et al.* (76) have shown that in late cultures, addition of hydrocortisone and glucagon enhances the UDS response. This is of interest in view of the fact that there has not been any other study of the possible hormonal regulation of this phenomenon and use of hepatocyte cultures may provide unique information in this area. Zurlo & Yager have demonstrated that under proper conditions not only excision repair but also SOS-type repair can be induced in hepatocyte cultures (99). In this type of repair, first documented for bacteria and later for eucaryotic cells, DNA synthesis is allowed to proceed even on a damaged template. The result is enhanced cell survival at the risk of higher mutagenesis due to fixation of the lesion of the damaged template. The phenomenon can be demonstrated as increased survival of UV-irradiated viruses in carcinogen treated cells. This phenomenon was demonstrated in hepatocyte cultures in the above study using Herpes simplex virus (type 1). The demonstration of SOS-type repair in hepatocytes is of considerable importance in view of several previous reports that hepatocarcinogenesis is enhanced after induction of hepatic regeneration following carcinogen treatment. The study by Zurlo & Yager provides a molecular explanation for the nature of the 'fixation' of the mutagenic process during regeneration and it demonstrates the value of using hepatocyte cultures to perform studies on the molecular processes involved in hepatocarcinogenesis that would be impossible to carry *in vivo*.

Previous reports have demonstrated a decreased carcinogen metabolism and UDS response in hepatocyte cultures compared to the liver *in vivo*. In view of these findings, a recent (59) modification of the UDS genotoxicity bioassay by Mirsalis & Butterworth is of considerable interest. In this assay, carcinogens or substances intended for testing are given at sufficient dose to rats *in vivo*. At specified times after the administration of the chemical the liver is perfused with collagenase and the hepatocyte cultures are assayed for UDS. In this manner the activation of the chemical and the presumed genotoxic damage are allowed to occur *in vivo* when the normal complement of enzymes involved in carcinogen metabolism and 'activation' are still present. This technique has been validated with several genotoxic compounds. Of interest is the case of 2,6 dinitrotoluene, a powerful liver carcinogen which was not found to be genotoxic by any other assay, including the induction of UDS in hepatocyte cultures. This compound was found to be a potent inducer of UDS following the *in vivo – in vitro* approach (57). Further studies published by the same team showed that the compound is 'activated' by metabolism by the gut flora and becomes thus carcinogenic for the liver (58). This technique has so far been validated with a variety of carcinogens and it is a very promising test for genotoxicity. It also allows for testing of compounds with pre-treated rats using microsomal enzyme inducers such as phenobarbital and 3-methylcholanthrene. This approach has also been recently extended to pancreatic cells (79).

Hepatocyte mediated genotoxicity assays

As mentioned above, there are currently no systems available that allow clonal growth of hepatocytes in culture. As a result, it is impossible to conduct *in vitro* mutagenesis and neoplastic transformation studies directly on hepatocytes. To overcome this obstacle, several attempts have been made to use co-cultivation systems in which hepatocytes are maintained together with cells that can be used in *in vitro* clonal assays. Such cells have been frequently used as indicators in mutagenesis or cell transformation bioassays. The combined cultures are exposed to indirect acting genotoxic agents. The hepatocytes provide the 'metabolic activation' and supply the direct acting mutagenic/carcinogenic metabolites. These metabolites are transported to the adjacent cells and induce measurable genotoxicity. Most of the cell systems used directly for genotoxicity bioassays (V79 cells, C3H10T1/2 cells, CHO cells, human fibroblasts) have very limited capability to metabolize mutagenic/ carcinogenic chemicals. In a standard assay format, control cultures that are composed of the indicator cells alone, without hepatocytes, are used. The genotoxicity induced by a specific carcinogen in the cultures without hepatocytes is subtracted from the genotoxicity induced in the mixed cultures. The difference between these two values is the genotoxicity mediated by the hepatocytes. The use of intact hepatocytes was prompted by the realization that the profiles of metabolites of chemical carcinogens generated by intact cells are in most instances different than those generated by hepatocyte homogenates. The problems associated with the use of homogenates as activators in mutagenesis bioassays have been presented in several publications (10, 12, 62, 74). Lack of small molecular weight co-factors, altered ratios of enzymes involved in competing metabolic pathways and other artifacts introduced by the cell rupture and the use of buffers prompted the thought that intact hepatocytes should have several advantages over homogenates as activators in mutagenesis bioassays. Use of intact hepatocytes also allows studies of the intercellular transfer of xenobiotic metabolites, a phenomenon which appears to play a significant role in carcinogenesis in the whole animal.

Fry & Bridges (24) first employed hepatocytes for this type of study prepared by enzymatic digestion of fragments of hepatic tissue. The results presented showed that the cultures used were contaminated with non-parenchymal elements. Nevertheless, in the presence of hepatocytes, cyclophosphamide was toxic to rat fibroblasts maintained in co-cultivation. Parenchymal hepatocytes prepared by collagenase perfusion of the rat liver were first employed in studies of cell mediated mutagenesis by Langenbach and his co-workers (40). Hepatocytes were maintained in mixed cultures with V79 cells. The latter is a hamster cell line often used in mutagenesis bioassays. In the presence of hepatocytes the carcinogens diethyl-and dimethyl-nitrosamine as well as aflatoxin B1 induced point mutations in the Na^+, K^+, ATPase identified as ouabain resistant mutants. Non-carcinogenic analogues of these compounds failed to induce mutagenesis. The induced mutagenic frequency was dependent on the number of hepatocytes. In further studies (39) by the same team it was shown that hepatocytes were more efficient in inducing V79 mutants with aflatoxin than with benzo(a)pyrene. To the contrary, fibroblasts were more efficient in inducing V79 mutants after activation with benzo(a)pyrene as opposed to aflatoxin. These results indicated that cell mediated bioassays can be used to demonstrate and study the mechanisms of cell specificity in carcinogen metabolism and its effects on adjacent cells. Comparisons with lung cells (44) also demonstrated the induction of V79 mutants by compounds that were recognized as specific carcinogens for the tissue from which the activator cells were derived. Thus, aflatoxin B1 was weakly mutagenic when lung cells were used as mediators but was strongly mutagenic when hepatocytes were used as mediators. The opposite was seen with polycyclic aromatic hydrocarbons. Similar results were found in comparisons of hepatocytes with urinary bladder epithelial cells (42). Similar studies were conducted with hamster hepatocytes by Katch *et al.* (37). Bermudez *et al.* (13) used the same approach with Chinese hamster ovary (CHO) cells studying mutations of the locus of hypoxanthine-guanine-phosphoribosyl-transferase (HPRT). HPRT was also the target for hepatocyte mediated mutagenesis in co-cultures of rat hepatocytes and human fibroblasts, studied by Michalopoulos *et al.* (55). Human fibroblasts have been used in mutagenesis studies with the rationale that they furnish information relevant to the human genome. Human fibroblasts by themselves however can only be used in to study the effect of direct acting carcinogens (1). The co-culture of these cells with rat hepatocytes allows the extension of previous studies and the study of mutagenesis induced on human fibroblasts by procarcinogens. In the presence of rat hepatocytes, diethylnitrosamine induced mutations in the human fibroblasts. A similar approach has also been followed by Tong *et al.* for polycyclic aromatic hydrocarbons (89). In subsequent studies by Strom *et al.* these results were also applied to benzo(a)pyrene and AAF (85, 86, 87). This system has been recently extended by Strom *et al.* to co-cultivation of human hepatocytes and human fibroblasts (88). This approach allows the design of a mutagenesis screen composed entirely of human cells and will be presented in more detail in the section on human hepatocytes of this chapter.

In addition to the above cells used for co-cultures, hepatocytes have also been combined with bacterial strains used in the mutagenesis assay designed by Ames *et al.* Pariza and coworkers demonstrated the feasibility of this approach (26). In the presence of hepatocytes, aflatoxin B1 was mutagenic to *Salmonella* strains. In addition to mutagenesis, the same study demonstrated the presence of aflatoxin adducts to hepatocyte macromolecules. These studies were also applied to the carcinogens 2-amido–3-methylimidazo {4, 5-f} quinoline and 2-aminofluorene (25).

Mixed hepatocyte cultures have also been applied to study other indicators of genotoxicity, including neoplastic transformation. Poiley *et al.* utilized hamster hepatocytes in conjunction with hamster embryo cells (67). The latter cells have been frequently used in transformation bioassays. In the presence of the hepatocytes the carcinogens diethylnitrosamine, 2-nitrofluorene and 4-aminoazobenzene were capable of inducing neoplastic transformation *in vitro* in the populations of the embryo cells. To our knowledge, this is the only application of mixed hepatocyte cultures for the study of neoplastic transformation. Sister chromatid exchange as an endpoint was studied in mixed hepatocyte cultures with human fibroblasts (38), V79 cells (41) and CHO cells (17). Another interesting approach with applications to the study of chemotherapeutic agents was also taken by Alley *et al.* (2). In their study, hepatocytes were combined with the soft agar assay for clonal growth of tumour stem cells. Hepatocytes improved the cytotoxic efficacy of cyclophosphamide, indicine-N-oxide and procarbazine but reduced the effect of several chemo-therapeutic agents that appeared to be active without metabolic activation. The decreased efficacy of these compounds was presumably due to the binding of these agents to the hepatocytes, resulting in decreased availability of the drug to the tumour cells. Other agents were unaffected. This model should be of use for the study of the mode of action of agents used in tumour chemotherapy.

The studies reviewed above document that the mixed cultures of non-proliferating hepatocytes with other proliferating cell types can be used in a variety of applications. The multiplicity of the models employed has made it difficult to conduct comparative analysis of the performance of the hepatocytes in the combined cultures. Often the emphasis is in the achievement of the end result (mutagenesis, cytotoxicity etc) without complete analysis of the conditions that would optimize the performance of the hepatocytes in the several assays. In most instances, the levels of the microsomal enzymes and other such indices in these co-cultures were never analysed. Although hepatocytes seem able to mediate a genotoxic response under a variety of circumstances and with several endpoints, we do not know whether the effects were mediated under optimal hepatocyte performance. Several studies have been conducted however with some of these systems to study the biology of the hepatocyte in the mixed culture environment. In studies mentioned above by Michalopoulos *et al.* (53) it was shown that hepatocytes maintained on top of a monolayer of human fibroblasts maintained decreased but measurable and inducible levels of cytochrome P450, in a manner comparable to hepatocytes maintained on collagen gels. Cytochrome P450 was induced by phenobarbital and 3-methyl-cholanthrene and cytochromes P450 and P448 were seen with each of the inducers. Previous studies had also shown that the attachment of hepatocytes on top of other monolayers is selective. Hepatocytes readily align themselves on top of fibroblasts whereas they do not attach on top of the so called 'clear epithelial cells' (Michalopoulos, unpublished observations). In similar studies, Langenbach *et al.* (43) demonstrated that hepatocytes maintained on a monolayer of irradiated C3H/10T1/2 cells were capable of metabolizing the carcinogen AAF at 70% of the day 1 level even at 14 days in culture. In addition, tyrosine aminotransferase could be induced until day 10 in culture. Hepatocytes maintained on plastic dishes lost both of these functions after day 5 in culture. These studies and subsequent studies by Reid and co-workers (22) using hepatic biomatrix emphasize the determinant role of the substratum of attachment on the differentiation of hepatocytes in culture.

The effect of hepatocyte numbers per dish on the final genotoxic/cytotoxic effect of the carcinogen tested seems to vary with the carcinogen type and the cell line used in the co-cultivation. The frequency of the ouabain resistant mutants induced by dimethylnitrosamine in the system described by Langenbach *et al.* increased proportionate to the hepatocyte number (40). In co-cultures with *Salmonella* strains in the system described by Pariza and co-workers (26) increasing density of hepatocytes decreased the mutagenic frequency induced in the bacteria. This was found when intact hepatocytes were used. When permeabilized hepatocytes were used, the opposite results were found. Increased frequency of mutants was seen with increased numbers of hepatocytes. The above results prompt the consideration of the complicated and mutually competing interactions between the activated carcinogenic metabolites and the cell populations present in the culture. More hepatocytes would presumably create a larger initial concentration of active mutagenic species. The increased numbers of hepatocytes could, however, also result in deactivation of the active species through conjugation reactions. Alternatively, the larger numbers of hepatocytes could reduce the numbers of active mutagenic molecules available to the cell line because the active mutagenic molecules may interact with the hepatocyte macromolecules and thus not be available to interact with the cell line and cause mutations. Analogous considerations also apply to the effect of the promutagen concentration. Large concentrations may result in hepatocyte death and thus decrease the final concentration of active mutagenic species because there are not enough hepatocytes available to carry out the activation. This was demonstrated in the study by Michalopoulos *et al.* (55). These findings demonstrate that the viability of the hepatocytes is an important consideration in these systems and should be considered in the design of the bioassays. The finding (26) that permeabilized hepatocytes are more efficient in co-culture mutagenesis bioassays is of interest and may relate to the results of the studies by Jones *et al.* (35, 36). In these studies it was shown that hepatocytes prepared from enzymatic digestion of hepatic slices were more efficient in mediating mutagenesis than hepatocytes prepared by the collagenase perfusion technique. The results obtained with this system show excellent correlation between mutagenic and carcinogenic potency for 26 nitrosamines tested. Activation of other carcinogens, such as aflatoxin B1, has also been shown. The most interesting feature of this system is its enhanced sensitivity compared to other hepatocyte mediated bioassays. There is at least a 10–fold increase in minimal effective mutagenic nitrosamine concentration with hepatocytes prepared by digestion of hepatic slices as compared to those prepared by collagenase perfusion. The authors have not demonstrated increased maintenance of microsomal enzymes or other enzymes involved in xenobiotic metabolism in these cells. The findings by Pariza *et al.* using permeabilized hepatocytes (26) and the previous studies demonstrating the increased viability of hepatocytes prepared by collagenase perfusion as compared to those prepared from digestion of slices (73) raises the question whether the improved sensitivity and excellent performance of the system described by Jones *et al.* may be due to increased permeability of the hepatocytes used in the bioassay.

The factors that regulate the distribution of xenobiotic metabolites between the hepatocytes and the co-cultured cell line need to be further investigated. The role of serum in the medium is difficult to predict. Serum may enhance the viability of the hepatocytes and thus result in enhanced activation capability. It also may facilitate the maintenance of the xenobiotic in solution, thus making it more available to the hepatocytes. On the other hand, the serum proteins may act as binding sites for the activated xenobiotic species and reduce the number of active molecules available to induce mutations in the cell line. There are no comprehensive *in vitro* studies on the mode utilized for the export of the active mutagenic xenobiotic species from the hepatocytes. Hepatocyte cultures have been shown to produce numerous products that they secrete in the medium, among them albumin and lipoproteins (92). Several studies have demonstrated the fact that non-polar carcinogens such as polycyclic aromatic hydrocarbons or some aromatic amines are transported in the serum of animals bound to lipoproteins (18, 19). It is quite likely that the same molecules produced by hepatocytes in culture can be utilized for the transport of activated xenobiotic mutagens. These bound forms can be carried to the cell lines used as the endpoint for the mutagenesis assay. Strom *et al.* have studied the distribution of the genotoxic damage in the two cell populations of the mixed cultures, namely rat hepatocytes and human fibroblasts (86). Carcinogens that are known to induce primarily liver tumours (AAF and diethylnitrosamine) induced more UDS on the hepatocytes as compared to the fibroblasts. The carcinogen benzo(a)pyrene that is metabolized by the liver but does not induce liver tumours in long term feeding regimens induced more UDS on the fibroblasts than the hepatocytes. These studies show the value of UDS as a predictor of tissue specific carcinogenesis (also previously shown by Stich *et al.* (80)). In the same (86) and in a subsequent (87) study it was also shown that the carcinogen benzo(a)pyrene induced more DNA adducts on the fibroblasts than the hepatocytes. Similar findings were shown in a later study for the carcinogen AAF (85). Analogous findings were also reported by Umbenhauer *et al.* (90) in a study in which naked DNA was added to the hepatocyte cultures. Addition of dimethylnitrosamine resulted in more overall methylation and formation of O-6-guanine was seen in the extracellular DNA compared to the intranuclear hepatocyte DNA. These studies demonstrate the existence of protective mechanisms for the hepatocyte that result in export of the most of the carcinogenic metabolites to the external environment and offer relative protection to the intranuclear hepatocyte DNA. The nature of these protective mechanisms has not been studied in detail but it is undoubtful, in view of the *in vivo* evidence (18, 19) that the albumin and the lipoproteins secreted by the hepatocytes to the external environment must play a role in this process. The role of lipoproteins as transport carriers in the induction of UDS on lymphocytes was recently shown by Busbee (33). In the absence of lipoproteins, the administered active benzo(a)pyrene metabolites could not enter the cell to induce UDS. It is well known that most cells possess lipoprotein receptors. Since lipoproteins can act as stabilizers and carriers for carcinogens activated by the hepatocytes (18, 19), the mode of export of the ultimate carcinogenic species from their site of activation in the hepatocytes to the rest of the body via lipoproteins should be an important phenomenon to study. The mixed hepatocyte cultures can be used to great advantage to study these and other intercellular aspects of carcinogenesis focusing on specific cell targets and specific carcinogens. An example of this approach is the recent study by Ottenwalder *et al.* (66). Isolated hepatocytes and hepatic endothelial cells were co-incubated with vinyl chloride. More vinyl chloride adduct formation was observed in the endothelial cells than in the hepatocytes. Since glutathione has been speculated as having an important role in vinyl chloride carcinogenesis it was interesting to show, as the authors did, that the addition of glutathione reduced the formation of vinyl chloride adducts in both the hepatocytes and the endothelial cells.

Human hepatocytes in carcinogenesis studies

Primary cultures of human hepatocytes have been described several times in the last decade. In most instances these attempts utilized hepatocytes derived from protease digestion of very small hepatic biopsies, usually needle biopsies. The numbers of hepatocytes obtained were very low and there was no methodology available which would utilize the principles of the collagenase perfusion technique that has so successfully been applied to the rat liver. The first adaptations of the collagenase perfusion technique for large human hepatic fragments were described by Byard *et al.* (70) and Strom *et al.* (84). These techniques allowed for the first time production of large numbers of human hepatocytes that could be maintained in many replicate cultures and used for experimentation analogous to the rodent hepatocyte systems. Though these techniques differ in detail, the basic principle was the same. Catheters are inserted into the vascular orifices exposed at the cut surface of the liver. Fragments are selected that are surrounded by capsule on most of their available surface with a limited cut surface, so that the perfusate is forced to recirculate through the specimen and perfuse a substantial portion of the hepatic fragment. The two-step collagenase perfusion technique as described by Seglen is employed in principle. The first perfusate is Ca^{++}-free so that it depletes the liver of calcium ions. In the second step, calcium ions are reintroduced along with the collagenase. The report by Strom *et al.* emphasized the need for accurate monitoring of the temperature delivered to the hepatic parenchyma. In general the temperature should be kept higher than 32°C. Similar techniques were subsequently also described by Guguen-Guillouzo *et al.* (27). In this section we will describe only the applications of cultures of human hepatocytes for carcinogenesis studies. For more details on the techniques of isolation and culture, see references 27, 70, 84.

In comparison to the rather precipitous drop of cytochrome P450 in rat hepatocytes, the human hepatocytes appear to maintain at least 50% of their cytochrome P450 in primary culture. In the authors' experience human hepatocytes in general survive more than the rat hepatocytes in primary culture, especially if they are kept as a dense monolayer culture in serum free media. Such a culture of human hepatocytes has been shown in Fig. 1.

Unscheduled DNA synthesis can be induced in human hepatocytes with a list of chemical carcinogens (84). These now include nitrosamines, AAF, benzo(a)pyrene, aflatoxin, nitropyrenes etc. Of interest was the fact that in a study by Butterworth and co-workers (20), aflatoxin B1 was the strongest inducer of UDS on human hepatocytes. Despite substantial epidemiological evidence for the implication of aflatoxin B1 in human liver cancer, this finding is the first direct demonstration of the

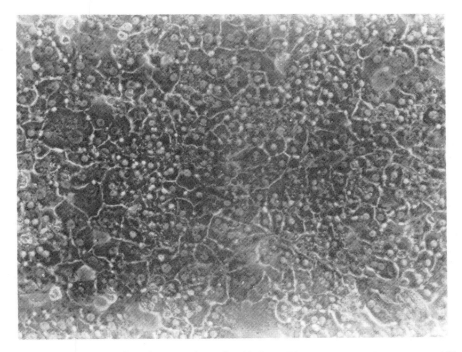

Fig. 1. Human hepatocytes in primary culture for 28 days. Phase contrast microscopy, ×200

genotoxic capabilities of aflatoxin for the human genome. This simple test, directly applied from similar techniques for the rat hepatocytes, should be as valid for the human as much as it has been validated for the rodent systems. Refinements of the technique such as the use of video imaging for automatic subtraction of the background, they have been recently applied (56), should enhance the accuracy of the technique.

Measurement of UDS furnishes data on the extent of repair of the induced DNA damage. It is essential to also obtain a measure of the amount of DNA damage that has escaped the repair process. Such evidence is furnished by mutagenesis bioassays. The fixed genetic damage, measured as induced mutation frequency on a specific gene locus, is directly assayed. It is impossible at this point to make clonal assays of hepatocytes in culture. The only clonal assays available for hepatocytes, either rat or human, utilize transplantation techniques, as described by Jirtle *et al.* (32). Thus, direct assays of mutagenesis induced on hepatocytes cannot be performed at this point. To obviate this difficulty, we have introduced the system of combined cultures of human hepatocytes and human fibrobasts (88), in direct analogy to the system of rat hepatocytes and human fibroblasts also described from our laboratories and mentioned above (55). Due to the fact that this system is composed entirely of human cells one of which can be cloned and the other (hepatocyte) can activate chemical pro-carcinogens, results obtained by pro-carcinogens in this system have direct applicability to the human situation. Using this technique we have shown dose-dependent induced mutagenesis for diethylnitrosamine (88), and benzo(a)pyrene (Michalopoulos, unpublished observations).

Cultures of replicating hepatocytes in studies of carcinogenesis

Despite the lack of systems in which clonal growth of hepatocytes can be sustained in a manner analogous to cells such as fibroblasts, endothelial cells etc, there have been several systems described recently that allow DNA synthesis and mitosis for a limited number of cycles in hepatocytes in culture. For a complete review of these systems please see the chapter on *Hepatocyte proliferation in culture* by McGowan in this volume. The system defined in our laboratories has been used for *in vitro* studies of the factors that control liver regeneration and also for carcinogenesis studies. We and others have found so far that in normal rat and human serum, the factors that stimulate hepatocyte proliferation in otherwise non-proliferating hepatocytes are:
1) Epidermal growth factor (EGF) (28, 49).
2) Hepatopoietin A (HPTA), a large molecular weight protein that is activated by serine proteases. It interacts in an additive manner with EGF (52).
3) Hepatopoietin B (HPTB), a small serum polypeptide that interacts in a synergistic manner with either HPTA or EGF (52).
4) Norepinephrine. This catecholamine acts through the alpha-1 receptor and requires the presence of both insulin and EGF (21).
5) Vasopressin (72) as well as a factor derived from platelets (82) that stimulates hepatocyte proliferation have been studied by Bucher, McGowan and co-workers.

We have also recently described the synergistic interaction between proline or other non-essential amino acids and EGF (28). The effect of EGF is strongly dependent on the presence of proline and, secondarily, tyrosine and phenylalanine.

Of interest for carcinogenesis studies is recent findings by Luetteke in our laboratory that dialysed conditioned media from hepatoma cell lines also stimulate hepatocyte proliferation (Michalopoulos, unpublished observations). The factor(s) responsible are between 20 000 and 60 000 in molecular weight and they compete with EGF for binding to the EGF receptor on both A431 cells and rat hepatocytes. Thus, it appears rat hepatic carcinogenesis is associated with the acquisition of the capability to produce growth factors that stimulate normal hepatocytes to proliferation. This whole study has been conducted using sparse cultures of rat hepatocytes as the bioassay and it highlights one of several potential applications that cultures of replicating hepatocytes can have for the investigation of the mechanisms that lead to hepatic neoplasia.

Another use of replicating hepatocytes for carcinogenesis studies has been the measurement of the inhibition of DNA synthesis induced by the addition of chemical carcinogens on replicating hepatocyte cultures by Novicki *et al.* (64). In this system, cultures of replicating hepatocytes were used as described by Michalopoulos *et al.* (51). Chemical procarcinogens were added to hepatocytes that were stimulated to proliferate with rat serum. Different degrees of inhibition of DNA synthesis were observed, dependent on the type of the carcinogen and dose used. At high doses, cytotoxicity was seen. This was assayed by the use of hepatocytes whose DNA had been prelabelled by performing partial hepatectomy followed by injection of tritiated thymidine on the donor animals as previously described (71). Loss of prelabelled

DNA was used as the measurement of cytotoxicity induced by the chemical. Inhibition of DNA synthesis was estimated when no demonstrable cell death could be measured by the prelabelled hepatocyte assay. The carcinogens AAF and aflatoxin B1 were the strongest inhibitors of DNA synthesis. The 50% inhibitory dose was at 10^{-9} M for aflatoxin B1 and 10^{-7} M for AAF. Higher doses associated with cytotoxicity were required for the nitrosamines. Benzo(a)pyrene induced 50% inhibition at 10^{-5} M. The results with AAF and aflatoxin B1 are of interest because at the concentrations mentioned above there is no evidence of genotoxicity with any other assay utilizing hepatocyte cultures. The increased sensitivity of this assay may be due to the fact that large sections of DNA are rendered inaccessible to the DNA polymerase during DNA synthesis when bulky DNA adducts are present. Thus, a decrease in thymidine uptake can be easily monitored. In the same study it was also shown that the replicating hepatocytes in sparse cultures are as capable as the non-replicating hepatocytes in monolayers in terms of activation of carcinogens. When radiolabelled AAF was used, equal amounts per mg DNA were bound to the DNA of the non-replicating *vs* the replicating hepatocytes. Another aspect of the same study that directly relates to studies of hepatic carcinogenesis was the use of cultures from rat livers carrying clones of initiated hepatocytes. These clones were developed by injection of diethylnitrosamine after partial hepatectomy, as in standard protocols (63). The initiated hepatocytes can be recognized by histochemical stains for the enzyme gamma-glutamyl transpeptidase (63) and they can be distinguished easily on autoradiographic studies of DNA synthesis on that basis. In this way, direct comparisons of the replication of the normal and initiated hepatocytes can be made within the same culture dish. The findings of this study showed that the initiated hepatocytes were uniformly more resistant to the inhibitory effects of all carcinogens tested. Inhibition of DNA synthesis of initiated hepatocytes was seen however with most of the carcinogens, even though it was less than that seen on the normal hepatocytes.

Conclusions

Primary cultures of hepatocytes have been used extensively to study aspects of mutagenesis and carcinogenesis. Historically, the first applications of these systems have been in design of bioassays for genotoxicity of procarcinogens, such as measurement of UDS and hepatocyte mediated mutagenesis. The application of these techniques on human hepatocytes should furnish unique information, previously not available directly for the human liver. The establishment now of systems that allow hepatocyte replication expands the horizon for the use of these cells in carcinogenesis studies. The effects of carcinogens or the study of the replication of the initiated hepatocytes can be directly studied. The use of these cultures as bioassays for the study of growth factors associated with liver regeneration and carcinogenesis should also provide useful new information. It is hoped that with the proper combination of growth factors, media supplements and substrate modifications, the proper conditions will be arrived at in the future that would allow hepatocytes to be grown in a clonal manner. At that point, direct assays on hepatocytes, rather than the hepatocyte mediated assays available today, should be possible, and direct studies on mutagenesis and neoplastic transformation of hepatocytes should become feasible.

ACKNOWLEDGEMENTS

Part of the work presented in this review was supported by NIH Grants CA30241, CA35373, CA25951 and EPA CRA R811687010.

REFERENCES

1 Albertini R. J., Demars R.: Diploid azaguanine-resistant mutants of cultured human fibroblasts. *Science* 1970, **169**: 482–485.
2 Alley M. C., Powis G., Appel P. L., Kooistra K. L., Lieber M. M.: Activation and inactivation of cancer chemotherapeutic agents by rat hepatocytes cocultured with human tumor cell lines. *Cancer Res.* 1984, **44**: 549–556.
3 Althaus F. R., Lawrence S. D., He Y. Z., Sattler G. L., Tsukada Y., Pitot H. C.: Effects of altered [ADP-ribose]n metabolism on expression of fetal functions by adult hepatocytes. *Nature* 1982, **300**: 366–368.
4 Althaus F. R., Lawrence S. D., Sattler G. L., Pitot H. C.: ADP-ribosyltransferase activity in cultured hepatocytes. Intractions with DNA repair. *J. Biol. Chem.* 1982, **257**: 5528–5535.
5 Althaus F. R., Lawrence S. D., Sattler G. L., Pitot H. C.: DNA damage produced by the antihistaminic drug methapyrilene hydrochloride. *Mutat. Res.* 1982, **103**: 213–218.
6 Althaus F.R., Lawrence S. D., Sattler G. L., Longfellow D. G., Pitot H. C.: Chemical quantification of unscheduled DNA synthesis in cultured hepatocytes as an assay for the rapid processing of potential chemical carcinogens. *Cancer Res.* 1982, **42**: 3010–3015.
7 Althaus F. R., Pitot H. C.: Consequences of altered poly(ADP-ribose) metabolism on hepatocyte functions *in vitro*. *Int. Symp. Princess Takamatsu Cancer Res. Fund*, 1983, **13**: 321–331.
8 Ames B. N., McCann J., Yamasaki E.: Methods for detecting carcinogens and mutagens with the Salmonella/mammalian-microsome mutagenicity test. *Mutat. Res.* 1975, **31**: 347–364.
9 Andreae U., Greim H.: Induction of DNA repair replication by hydroxyurea in human lymphoblastoid cells mediated by liver microsomes and NADPH. *Biochem. Biophys. Res. Commun.* 1979, **87**: 50–58.
10 Ashby, J., Styles J. A.: Does carcinogenic potency correlate with mutagenic potency in the Ames assay? *Nature* 1978, **271**: 452–455.
11 Ashurst S. W., Cohen G. M.: A benzo(a)pyrene-7,8-dihydrodiol-9,10-epoxide is the major metabolite involved in the binding of benzo(a)pyrene to DNA in isolated viable rat hepatocytes. *Chem. Biol. Interact.* 1980, **29**: 117–127.
12 Baird W. M., Dipple A., Grover P., Sims P., Brookes P.: Studies on the formation of hydrocarbon-deoxyribonucleoside products by the binding of derivatives of 7-methylbenz-(a)anthracene to DNA in aqueous solution and in mouse embryo cells in culture. *Cancer Res.* 1973, **33**: 2386–2392.
13 Bermudez E., Couch D. B., Tillery T.: The use of primary rat hepatocytes to achieve metabolic activation of promutagens in the Chinese hamster ovary/hypoxanthine-guanine phosphoribosyl transferase mutational assay. *Environ. Mutagen.* 1982, **4**: 55–64.
14 Bermudez E., Mirsalis J. C., Eales H. C.: Detection of DNA damage in primary cultures of rat hepatocytes following *in vivo* and *in vitro* exposure to genotoxic agents. *Environ. Mutagen.* 1982, **4**: 667–669.
15 Bermudez E.: The inhibition of DNA repair in primary rat hepatocyte cultures by aphidicolin: Evidence for the involvement of the alpha polymerase in the repair process. *Biochem. Biophys. Res. Commun.* 1982, **109**: 275–281.
16 Bradley M. O., Dysart G., Fitzsimmons K., Harbach P., Lewin J., Wolf G.: Measurements by filter elution of DNA single- and double-strand breaks in rat hepatocytes: effects of nitrosamines and gamma-irradiation. *Cancer Res.* 1982, **42**: 2592–2597.

17 Brat V., Williams G. M.: Hepatocyte-mediated production of sister chromatid exchange in co-cultured cells by acrylonitrile: Evidence of extracellular transport of a table reactive intermediate. *Cancer Lett.* 1982, **17**: 213–216.

18 Busbee D., Joe C. O., Rankin P. W., Ziprin R. L., Wilson R. D.: Benzo(a)pyrene uptake by lymph: a possible transport mode for immunosuppressive chemicals. *J. Toxicol. Environ. Hlth* 1984, **13**: 43–51.

19 Busbee D. L., Rankin P. W., Payne D. M., Jasheway D. W.: Binding of benzo(a)pyrene and intracellular transport of a bound electrophilic benzo(a)pyrene metabolite by lipoproteins. *Carcinogenesis* 1982, **3**: 1107–1112.

20 Butterworth B. E., Doolittle D. J., Working P. K., Strom S. C., Jirtle R. L., Michalopoulos G.: *Chemically induced DNA repair in rodent and human cells*, Banbury Report 13: Indicators of genotoxic exposure: Cold Spring Harbor Laboratory, 1982, 1–14.

21 Cruise J. L., Houck K. A., Luetteke N. C., Thaler F. J., Kilts K., Jirtle R. L., Michalopoulos G.: Stimulation of hepatocyte proliferation by norepinephrine and serum factors. *Fed. Proc.* 1984, **43**: 373.

22 Enat R., Jefferson D. M., Ruiz-Opazo N., Gatmaitan Z., Leinwand L. A., Reid L. M.: Hepatocyte proliferation *in vitro*: Its dependence on the use of serum-free hormonally defined medium and substrata of extracellular matrix. *Proc. Natl. Acad. Sci.* 1984, **81**: 1411–1415.

23 Farzaneh F., Zalin R., Brill D., Shall S.: DNA strand breaks and ADP-ribosyl transferase activation during cell differentiation. *Nature* 1982, **300**: 362–366.

24 Fry J. R., Bridges J. W.: A novel mixed hepatocyte-fibroblast culture system and its use as a test for metabolism-mediated genotoxicity. *Biochem. Pharmacol.* 1977, **26**: 969–973.

25 Gayda D. P., Pariza M. W.: Activation of 2-amino–3-methylimidazo[4,5-f]quinoline and 2-aminofluorene for bacterial mutagenesis by primary monolayer cultures of adult rat hepatocytes. *Mutat. Res.* 1983, **118**: 7–14.

26 Gayda D. P., Pariza M. W.: Activation of aflatoxin B1 by primary cultures of adult rat hepatocytes: effects of hepatocyte density. *Chem. Biol. Interact.* 1981, **35**: 255–265.

27 Guguen-Guillouzo C., Campion J. P., Brissot P., Glaise D., Launois B., Bourel M., Guillouzo A.: High yield preparation of isolated human adult hepatocytes by enzymatic perfusion of the liver. *Cell Biol. Intern. Rep.* 1982, **6**: 625–628.

28 Houck K. A., Michalopoulos G.: Proline is required for the stimulation of DNA synthesis in hepatocyte cultures by EGF. *Rapid Commun. Cell Biol.* (In Press.)

29 Howard P. C., Casciano D. A., Beland F. A., Shaddock J. G.: The binding of N-hydroxy-2-acetylaminofluorene to DNA and repair of the adducts in primary hepatocyte cultures. *Carcinogenesis* 1981, **2**: 97–102.

30 Hsia M. T. S., Kreamer B. L., Dolara P.: A rapid and simple method to quantitate chemically induced unscheduled DNA synthesis in freshly isolated rat hepatocytes facilitated by DNA retention of membrane filters. *Mutat. Res.* 1983, **122**: 177–185.

31 Irwin J., Strauss B.: Use of hydroxyurea in the measurement of DNA repair by the BND cellulose method. Environ. *Mutagen.* 1980, **2**: 381–388.

32 Jirtle R. L., Michalopoulos G., McLain J. R., Crowley J.: Transplantation system for determining clonogenic survival of parenchymal hepatocytes exposed to ionizing radiation. *Cancer Res.* 1981, **41**: 3512–3518.

33 Joe C. O., Rankin P. W., Busbee D. L.: Human lymphocytes treated with r-7, t-8-dihydroxy-t-9, 10-epoxy-7,8,9,10-tetrahydrobenzo(a)pyrene require low density lipoproteins for DNA excision repair. *Mutat. Res.* 1984, **131**: 37–43.

34 Johnstone A. P., Williams F. T.: Role of DNA breaks and ADP-ribosyl transferase activity in eukaryotic differentiation in human lymphocytes. *Nature* 1982, **300**: 368–370.

35 Jones C. A., Huberman E.: A sensitive hepatocyte mediated assay for the metabolism of nitrosamines to mutagens for mammalian cells. *Cancer Res.* 1980, **40**: 406–411.

36 Jones C. A., Marlino P. J., Lijinsky W., Huberman E.: The relationship between the carcinogenicity and the mutagenicity of nitrosamines in a hepatocyte-mediated mutagenicity assay. *Carcinogenesis* 1981, **2**: 1075–1077.

37 Katoh Y., Tanaka M. , Takayama S.: Higher efficiency of hamster hepatocytes than rat hepatocytes for detecting dimethylnitrosamine and diethylnitrosamine in hepatocyte-mediated Chinese hamster V79 cell mutagenesis bioassays. *Mutat. Res.* 1982, **105**: 265–269.

38 Kligerman A. D., Michalopoulos G.: Sister chromatid exchange studies in human fibroblast-rat hepatocyte co-cultures. *Environ. Mutagen.* 1980, 2: 157–166.

39 Langenbach R., Freed H. J., Huberman E.: Cell specificity in metabolic activation of aflatoxin B1 and benzo(a)pyrene to mutagens for mammalian cells. *Nature* 1978, **276**: 277–280.

40 Langenbach R., Freed H. J., Huberman E.: Liver cell mediated mutagenesis of mammalian cells by liver carcinogens. *Proc. Natl. Acad. Sci.* 1978, **75**: 2864–2867.

41 Langenbach R., Hix C., Oglesby L., Allen L.: Cell mediated mutagenesis of Chinese hamster V79 cells and *Salmonella typhimurium*. *Ann. N.Y. Acad. Sci.* 1983, **407**: 258–266.

42 Langenbach R., Malick L., Nesnow S.: Rat bladder cell-mediated mutagenesis of Chinese hamster V79 cells and metabolism of benzo(a)pyrene. *J. Natl. Cancer Inst.* 1981, **66**: 913–917.

43 Langenbach R., Malick L., Tompa A., Kuszynski C., Freed H., Huberman E.: Maintenance of adult rat hepatocytes on C3H10T1/2 cells. *Cancer Res.* 1979, **39**: 3509–3514.

44 Langenbach R., Nesnow S., Tompa A., Gingell R., Kuszynski C.: Lung and liver cell mediated mutagenesis systems: specificities in the activation of chemical carcinogens. *Carcinogenesis* 1981, 2: 851–858.

45 Lewis J. G., Swenberg J. A.: Differential repair of 0(6)-methylguanine in DNA of rat hepatocytes and nonparenchymal cells. *Nature* 1980, **288**: 185–187.

46 Lonati-Calligani M., Lohman P. H. M., Berends F.: The validity of the autoradiographic method for detecting DNA repair synthesis in rat hepatocytes in primary cultures. *Mutat. Res.* 1983, **113**: 145–160.

47 Loretz L. J., Pariza M. W.: Effect of glutathione levels, sulfate levels, and metabolic inhibitors on covalent binding of 2-amino-3-methylimidazo[4,5-f]quinoline and 2-acetylaminofluorene to cell macromolecules in primary cultures of adult rat hepatocytes. *Carcinogenesis* 1984, 5: 895–899.

48 Martelli A., Cavanna M., Gambino V., Robbiano L., Brambilla G.: Genotoxicity of cimetidine in primary cultures of rat hepatocytes. *Mutat. Res.* 1983, **120**: 133–137.

49 McGowan J. A., Strain A. N., Bucher N. R. L.: DNA synthesis in primary cultures of adult rat hepatocytes in a defined medium: effects of epidermal growth factor, insulin, glucagon and cyclic AMP. *J. Cell Phys.* 1981, **108**: 353–363.

50 Mendoza-Figueroa T., Lopez-Revilla R., Villa-Trevino S.: Dose dependent DNA ruptures induced by the procarcinogen dimethylnitrosamine on primary liver cultures. *Cancer Res.* 1979, **39**: 3254–3257.

51 Michalopoulos G., Cianciulli H. D., Novotny A. R., Kligerman A. D., Strom S. C., Jirtle R. L.: Liver regeneration studies with rat hepatocytes in primary culture. *Cancer Res.* 1982, **42**: 4673–4682.

52 Michalopoulos G., Houck K. A., Dolan M. L., Luetteke N. C.: Control of hepatocyte proliferation by two serum factors. *Cancer Res.* 1984, **44**: 4414–4419.

53 Michalopoulos G., Russell F., Biles C.: Primary cultures of hepatocytes on human fibroblasts. *In Vitro* 1979, **15**: 796–805.

54 Michalopoulos G., Sattler G. L., O'Connor L., Pitot H. C.: Unscheduled DNA synthesis induced by procarcinogens in suspensions and primary cultures of hepatocytes on collagen membranes. *Cancer Res.* 1978, **38**: 1866–1871.

55 Michalopoulos G. K., Strom S. C., Kligerman A. D., Irons G. P., Novicki D. L.: Mutagenesis induced by procarcinogens at the hypoxanthine-guanine phosphoribosyl transferase locus on human fibroblasts cocultured with rat hepatocytes. *Cancer Res.* 1981, **41**: 1873–1878.

56 Mirsalis J. C., Tyson C. K., Butterworth B. E.: Detection of genotoxic carcinogens in the *in vivo-in vitro* hepatocyte DNA repair assay. *Environ. Mutagen.* 1982, 4: 553–562.

57 Mirsallis J. C., Butterworth B. E.: Induction of unscheduled DNA synthesis in rat hepatocytes following *in vivo* treatment with dinitrotoluene. *Carcinogenesis* 1982, 3: 241–245.

58 Mirsallis J. C., Hamm T. E., Sherrill J. M., Butterworth B. E.: Role of the gut flora in the genotoxicity of dinitrotoluene. *Nature* 1982, **295**: 322–323.

59 Mirsallis J. C., Tyson C. K., Butterworth B. E.: Detection of genotoxic carcinogens in the *in vivo-in vitro* hepatocyte DNA repair assay. *Environ. Mutagen.* 1982, 4: 667–669.

60 Mitchell A. D., Casciano D. A., Meltz M. L., Robinson D. E., San R. H. C., Williams G. M., Von Halle E. S.: Unscheduled DNA synthesis test: A report of the U.S. Environmental Protection Agency Gene-Tox program. *Mutat. Res.* 1983, **123**: 363–410.

61 Moir R. D., Smith G. J., Stewart B. W.: Structural defects in DNA from primary hepatocyte

cultures. *Cell Biol. Intern. Rep.* 1983, **7**: 227–235.

62 Newbold R. F., Wigley C. B., Thompson M. H., Brookes P.: Cell mediated mutagenesis in cultured Chinese hamster cells by carcinogenic polycyclic hydrocarbons. Nature and extent of the associated DNA reaction. *Mutat. Res.* 1977, **43**: 101–106.

63 Novicki D. L., Jirtle R. P., Michalopoulos G.: Establishment of two rat hepatoma cell strains produced by a carcinogen initation, phenobarbital promotion protocol. *In Vitro* **19**: 191–201.

64 Novicki D. L., Rosenberg M. R., Michalopoulos G.: Inhibition of DNA synthesis by chemical carcinogens in cultures of initiated and normal proliferating hepatocytes. *Cancer Res.* (In press.)

65 Olson J. M., Casciano D. A., Pounds J. G.: A method for rapid, sensitive quantitation of short-patch repair in cultured rat hepatocytes. *Mutat. Res.* 1983, **119**: 381–386.

66 Ottenwalder H., Kappus H., Bolt H. M. : Covalent protein binding of vinyl chloride metabolites during co-incubation of freshly isolated hepatocytes and hepatic sinusoidal cells of rats. *Arch. Toxicol.* [Suppl] 1983, **6**: 266–270.

67 Poiley J., Raineri R., Pienta R. J.: Use of hamster hepatocytes to metabolize carcinogens in an *in vitro* bioassay. *J. Natl. Cancer Inst.* 1979, **63**: 514–523.

68 Poirier M. C., Yuspa S. H.: Detection and quantitation of acetylated and deacetylated N-2-fluorenylacetamide-DNA adducts by radioimmunoassay. *Natl. Cancer Inst. Monogr.* 1981, **58**: 211–216.

69 Probst G. S., McMahon R. E., Hill L.El, Thompson C. Z., Epp J. K., Neal S. B.: Chemically induced unscheduled DNA synthesis in primary rat hepatocyte culture: A comparison with bacterial mutagenicity using 218 compounds. *Environ. Mutagen.* 1981, **3**: 11–32.

70 Reese J. A., Byard J. L.: Isolation and culture of adult hepatocytes from liver biopsies. *In Vitro* 1981, **17**: 935–940.

71 Rosenberg M. R., Strom S. C., Michalopoulos G.: Effect of hydrocortisone and nicotinamide on gamma-glutamyl transferase in primary cultures of hepatocytes. *In Vitro* 1982, **18**: 775–781.

72 Russel W. E., Bucher N. R. L.: Vasopressin augments growth factor stimulated DNA synthesis in primary cultures of adult hepatocytes. *Endocrinology* 1982, **110**: 162.

73 Seglen P. O.: Preparation of isolated rat liver cells. *Methods Cell Biol.* 1976, **18**: 29–83.

74 Selkirk J. K.: Divergence of metabolic activation systems for short term mutagenesis bioassays. *Nature* 1977, **270**: 604–607.

75 Sina J. F., Bean C. L., Dysart G. R., Taylor V. I., Bradley M. O.: Evaluation of the alkaline elution/rat hepatocyte assay as a predictor of carcinogenic/mutagenic potential. *Mutat. Res.* 1983, **113**: 357–391.

76 Sirica A. E., Hwang C. G., Sattler G. L., Pitot H. C.: Use of primary cultures of adult rat hepatocytes on collagen gel-nylon mesh to evaluate carcinogen-induced unscheduled DNA synthesis. *Cancer Res.* 1980, **40**: 3259–3267.

77 Smith G. J., Charlton R. K., Grisham J. W., Kaufman D. G.: Increased sensitivity for detection of carcinogen-induced DNA repair with the chain terminator dideoxythymidine. *Biochem. Biophys. Res. Commun.* 1978, **83**: 1538–1544.

78 Stairs P. W., Guzelian P. S., Van Tuyle G. C.: Benzo(a)pyrene differentially alters mitochondrial and nuclear DNA synthesis in primary hepatocyte cultures. *Res. Commun. Chem. Pathol. Pharmacol.* 1983, **42**: 95–106.

79 Steinmetz K. L., Mirsallis J. C.: Induction of unscheduled DNA synthesis in primary cultures of rat pancreatic cells following *in vivo* and *in vitro* treatment with genotoxic agents. *Environ. Mutagen.* 1984, **6**: 321–330.

80 Stich H. F., Kieser D.: Use of DNA repair systems in detecting organotropic actions of chemical carcinogens. *Proc. Soc. Exptl. Biol. Med.* 1974, **145**: 1339–1342.

81 Stich H. F., Laishes B. A.: DNA repair and chemical carcinogens. *Pathobiol. Ann.* 1973, 341–376.

82 Strain A. J., McGowan J. A., Bucher N. R. L.: Stimulation of DNA synthesis in primary cultures of adult rat hepatocytes by rat platelet associated substances. *In Vitro* 1982, **18**: 108–116.

83 Strauss B. S.: The interaction of u.v.- and methyl methanesulfonate-induced DNA repair synthesis: a role for poly(ADP-ribose)? *Carcinogenesis* 1984, **5**: 577–582.

84 Strom S. C., Jirtle R. L. , Jones R. S., Novicki D. L., Rosenberg M. R., Novotny A., Irons G., McLainn J. R., Michalopoulos G.: Isolation, culture and transplantation of human hepatocytes. *J. Natl. Cancer Inst.* 1982, **68**: 771–777.

85 Strom S. C., Jirtle R. L., Michalopoulos G.: Genotoxic effects of 2-acetylaminofluorene on rat and

human hepatocytes. *Environ. Hlth Persp.* 1983, **49**: 165–170.

86 Strom S. C., Kligerman A. D., Michalopoulos G.: Comparisons of the effects of chemical carcinogens in mixed cultures of rat hepatocytes and human fibroblasts. *Car-cin* **2**: 709–715.

87 Strom S. C., Michalopoulos G.: Mutagenesis and DNA binding of benzo(a)pyrene in cocultures of rat hepatocytes and human fibroblasts. *Cancer Res.* 1982, **42**: 4519–4524.

88 Strom S. C., Novicki D. L., Novotny A., Jirtle R., Michalopoulos G.: Human hepatocyte mediated mutagenesis and DNA repair activity. *Carcinogenesis* 1983, **4**: 683–686.

89 Tong C., Fazio M., Williams G. M.: Rat hepatocyte mediated mutagenesis of human cells by carcinogenic polycyclic aromatic hydrocarbons but not organochlorine pesticides. *Proc. Soc. Exp. Biol. Med.* 1981, **167**: 572–575.

90 Umbenhauer D. R., Pegg A. E.: Alkylation of intracellular and extracellular DNA by dimethylnitrosamine following activation by isolated rat hepatocytes. *Cancer Res.* 1981, **41**: 3471–3474.

91 Umbenhauer D. R., Pegg A. E.: Metabolism of dimethylnitrosamine and subsequent removal of 06–methylguanine from DNA by isolated rat hepatocytes. *Chem. Biol. Interact.* 1981, **33**: 229–238.

92 Vance D. E., Weinstein D. B., Steinberg B.: Isolation and analysis of lipoproteins secreted by rat liver hepatocytes. *Biochim. Biophys. Acta* 1984, **792**: 39–47.

93 Williams G. M., Laspia M. F., Dunkel V. C.: Reliability of the hepatocyte culture/DNA repair test in testing coded carcinogens and noncarcinogens. *Mutat. Res.* 1982, **97**: 359–370.

94 Williams G. M., Laspia M. F., Mori H., Hirono I.: Genotoxicity of cycasin in the hepatocyte culture/DNA repair test supplemented with beta-glucosidase. *Cancer Lett.* 1981, **12**: 329–333.

95 Williams G. M.: Carcinogen-induced DNA repair in primary rat liver cell cultures; a possible screen for chemical carcinogens. *Cancer Lett.* 1976, **1**: 231–236.

96 Williams G. M.: Detection of chemical carcinogens by unscheduled DNA synthesis in rat liver primary cultures. *Cancer Res.* 1977, **37**: 1845–1851.

97 Yager J. D., Miller J. A.: DNA repair in primary cultures of rat hepatocytes. *Cancer Res.* 1978, **38**: 4385–4394.

98 Young C. W., Schochetman G., Hodas S., Balis E.: Inhibition of DNA synthesis by hydroxyurea: structure-activity relationships. *Cancer Res.* 1967, **27**: 535–540.

99 Zurlo J., Yager J. D.: U.V.-enhanced reactivation of U.V.-irradiated herpes virus by primary cultures of rat hepatocytes. *Carcinogenesis* 1984, **5**: 495–500.

Research in *Isolated and cultured hepatocytes* A. Guillouzo & C. Guguen-Guillouzo eds., pp. 353–376.
© 1986 John Libbey Eurotext Ltd./INSERM

16

Use of isolated and cultured hepatocytes in studies on bile formation

Rolf GEBHARDT

*Physiologisch-chemisches Institut der Universität Tübingen, Hoppe-Seyler-Strasse 1,
D-7400 Tübingen, FEDERAL REPUBLIC OF GERMANY*

SUMMARY

Isolated and cultured hepatocytes have proved useful tools for investigating a wide variety of hepatocellular functions related to bile formation as well as phenomena related to intrahepatic cholestasis. Freshly isolated cells have mainly been used in studies on biosynthetic and uptake processes especially facilitating the kinetic analysis of the latter, while their advantage for investigations on excretory mechanisms appears limited because of an at least partially disturbed membrane heterogeneity. These particular limitations may be overcome by cultured hepatocytes which either retain (undissociated cell groups) or regain (initially separated cells) a structurally and functionally intact biliary polarity. The culture approach renders it possible to detect and examine phenomena intimately associated with the apical pole such as canalicular motility and allows it for the first time to directly measure the transport of solutes into single bile canaliculi.

Introduction

Bile formation is one of the major hepatic functions and plays a central role not only in digestion but also in the elimination of numerous endogenous and exogenous compounds. This exocrine secretory function is coupled to a unique hepatocellular polarity. The anatomical limitations of this architecture precluding the application of classic transport techniques are at least partly responsible for the poor understanding of the mechanisms involved in bile secretion (20, 78). The complexity of the enterohepatic circulation as well as of the endocrine system, on the other hand, has impeded attempts to directly determine bile acid synthesis and examine its regulation *in vivo*. For these and other reasons there is a demand for isolated cell preparations which circumvent the problems of blood flow, hemodynamics, different distributional compartmentation, cellular diversity etc but retain sufficient integrity to perform the cellular functions involved in bile formation. However, during the isolation of cellular entities not only the normal orientation of the hepatocytes in the liver acinus is lost but also the complex tissue architecture which forms the basis of a separate biliary compartment. Obviously, the possible structural and functional alterations manifesting on the level of single hepatocytes are of considerable importance for any evaluation of isolated cell preparations as model systems for biliary transport processes. Only a thorough consideration of structural changes resulting from both tissue dispersion (60) and cultivation (16) in connection with careful comparative functional studies (24, 91) will provide a basis for the correct interpretation of metabolic and transport data obtained *in vitro*.

The present review discusses the advantages and the drawbacks of currently available systems, namely isolated liver parenchymal cells in suspension and in primary culture, traces possible future developments and describes the extent to which our knowledge of hepatic bile formation has been advanced by studies using these systems.

Biosynthetic functions

The liver is concerned with the synthesis of a variety of bile constituents, particularly of bile acids, phospholipids, cholesterol and bile pigments. In this section only the synthesis of bile acids will be reviewed, whereas that of phospholipids and cholesterol, the possible biliary secretion of which is unknown so far *in vitro*, will not be discussed. There is also little information about the synthesis of bile pigments such as bilirubin (18) despite the fact that heme catabolism is increased in cultured hepatocytes due to an enhanced level of heme oxygenase (19). Biotransformation which is often closely related to the biliary secretion of xenobiotics will also not be considered except for some selected aspects of conjugation.

Bile acid synthesis

The rates of synthesis reported for different bile acids (conjugates) in both isolated and cultured hepatocytes are listed in Table 1 and compared with some determinations *in vivo*. Leaving aside some early studies (4, 50) which have been corrected by more advanced techniques (12, 168), the production rates found in isolated cells are fairly comparable to *in vivo* estimates (Table 1). In contrast, rates of synthesis in primary cultured hepatocytes are lower (one-half to one-fifth) than those in isolated hepatocytes (34) probably due to limited cholesterol availability. Nevertheless, bile acid synthesis appears as one of the most stable functions in cultured hepatocytes (34). Bile acid synthesis in isolated cells could be stimulated by 7α-hydroxycholesterol (25). It was also greatly enhanced when donor animals were pretreated with cholestyramine (25, 76, 168) or subjected to biliary drainage (28, 33).

Table 1. **Rates of bile acid synthesis determined in isolated and cultured hepatocytes by different techniques.**

	Rate of synthesis $nmol \times mg^{-1} \times h^{-4}$	Assay technique[a]	Incubation medium[b]	References
Isolated hepatocytes:				
Cholic acid	13.9[c]	EA	SS	(4)
	0.25	GC	SS	(168)
	0.1–0.2	RIA	SS	(25)
	0.12[c]	EA	SS	(76)
Total bile acids	0.19–0.23[c]	GC	CM	(171)
	12–30	EA	SS	(50)
	0.09[c]	RIA	SS	(27)
Cultured hepatocytes:				
Cholic acid	0.012[c]	GC	CM	(34)
Total bile acids	0.021[c]	GC	CM	(34)

[a] EA: enzymatic assay; GC; gas chromatography; RIA: radioimmunoassay.
[b] SS: salt solution; CM: complex medium.
[c] Values normalized from results reported in respective sources.

Some conflicting results exist concerning the spectrum of bile acid production *in vitro*. Undoubtedly, cholic acid is one of the major forms synthesized by isolated and cultured hepatocytes (Table 1). However, substantial amounts of chenodeoxycholic acid (CDCA) have been identified only in some studies using isolated hepatocytes (4, 27, 171) but not in others (76, 77) as well as in cultured hepatocytes (34, Kempen & Gebhardt, unpublished observations). Instead, these workers reported the production of β-muricholic acid (27, 34, 76) in line with the high capacity of both isolated and cultured hepatocytes to convert CDCA to β-muricholic acid, presumbaly via an efficient 6-β hydroxylation (26, 34).

With respect to the quantitative spectrum, it thus appears that bile acid synthesis *in vitro* is well comparable to that *in vivo* (32, 59), particularly if it is taken into account that a biliary compartment draining the newly formed CDCA is missing. On the other hand, 6-β hydroxylation may be somewhat enhanced in preparations *in vitro* as reported for perfused rat liver (98, 126) and may depend on the pretreatment of donor rats (eg with cholestyramine or cholesterol diet) (26, 76).

The question on how hepatic bile acid synthesis may be regulated has not yet been satisfactorily answered *in vivo*. The long-standing hypothesis that bile acids exert feedback control on their own synthesis could be rejected by results from both isolated (29) and cultured hepatocytes (33). On the other hand, evidence for a control of cholesterol synthesis by bile salts has been presented (10). The availability of cholesterol has been found to be a major determinant of bile acid synthesis (33, 34, 77). A direct relation between lipoprotein uptake and bile acid production has been demonstrated (34). Furthermore, different cholesterol pools seem to be used for the synthesis of different bile acids (77). Dibutyryl-cAMP has been shown to increase the synthesis of cholic acid (27) – apparently by stimulating the conversion of cholesterol (155) – and to reduce the extent of β-muricholate production (27).

Conjugation of cholephilic compounds

Conjugation is a major event preceding the biliary excretion of many endogenous and exogenous compounds. Several aspects of conjugation in isolated hepatocytes have been reviewed (158). In the following discussion additional information is considered concerning the conjugation of bile acids and some other compounds.

Newly synthesized bile acids appear in the incubation medium mainly in conjugated form (25, 100), the taurine conjugate being more abundant than that of glycine (76, 171). Supplemented bile acids are conjugated as well (80). The spectrum of conjugation seems to depend strongly upon the nature of bile acid and on substrate availability (76). In cultured hepatocytes bile acid conjugation with taurine is maintained by both exogenous and biosynthesized taurine, whereas that of glycine is affected by biosynthesized glycine only (100). Conjugation is poorly developed in cultured fetal hepatocytes but can be stimulated by treatment with dexamethasone (80).

Organic anions are predominantly secreted as conjugates with glutathione or glucuronic acid. Conjugation of bromosulphophthalein (BSP) with glutathione has been reported to proceed more slowly than the uptake but faster than the release from the cells (137). Intracellularly about 40% of BSP are bound to ligandin (160).

Glucuronidation has been studied in the case of bilirubin where the formation of bilirubin-diglucuronide (BDG) is still a matter for debate. Using cultured hepatocytes Bissell & Billing (17) found evidence for a sequential formation of BDG from bilirubin-monoglucuronide (BMG). In addition, they detected a separate apparently stable pool of BMG (17). Formation of BMG and BDG has also been described in isolated cells together with its stimulation by pretreatment of donor rats with spironolactone (97).

Information on glucuronidation and sulphation is also available for several other compounds (39, 96, 127). In general, these processes are controlled by the concentration of UDP-glucuronic acid or inorganic sulphate (127, 146). During short-term cultivation a decay in glucuronyltransferase activity has been noted (132), which might be due to the absence of stabilizing hormones.

Transcellular biliary transport

The fate of the biliary polarity

In their pioneer study on the isolation of liver parenchymal cells Berry & Friend (15) recognized that the splitting of desmosomes induced by removal of calcium is one of the key events of the separation procedure. In contrast, gap and tight junctions seem to resist to the removal of calcium (152), but for other reasons they also disappear during tissue dispersion. As a result of its different stability, the tight junctional complex may sometimes be retained by one cell (eg after mechanical separation of cells). It seems to be this particular situation which may occasionally lead to the preservation of intact bile canaliculi associated with single cells as observed by Phillips *et al.* (111) and Wisher & Evans (169).

In general, however, hepatocytes isolated by collagenase dispersion appear as spheres uniformly decorated with numerous microvilli when examined by scanning or transmission electron microscopy (60, 106, 145, 166). On these spheres neither a contiguous nor a bile canalicular domain of the plasma membrane is discernible by morphological criteria only (40, 106, 165).

Randomization of the hepatocyte plasma membrane may be brought about mainly by lateral movement of components within the plane of the membrane. Sometimes proteolytic degradation of selected membrane constituents might be involved (19). This has been claimed for leucine aminopeptidase (LAP) on the basis of cyto-chemical results (162). Biochemical measurements indicating no loss of LAP activity (Gebhardt, unpublished observations), however, support the view that only spreading over the cell membrane has occurred as found for other marker enzymes of the bile canalicular membrane (60) which retain their activities as well (75). Redistribution has also been described for LAP after treatment of cultured hepatocytes with vinblastine (52) and, indeed, a rearrangement of cytoskeleton elements might play a role in the dislocation of domain-specific components and in the disappearance of tight junctions (*cf* 120).

Contrasting with the view of a totally randomized cell surface there is some biochemical and functional evidence suggesting the preservation of at least remnants of the canalicular membrane domain. Wisher & Evans (169) claim the isolation of sinusoidal and bile canalicular membrane fractions, but unfortunately there is no clear-cut separation of respective marker enzymes. Functional evidence is derived mainly from differential effects of experimental conditions on uptake and release of bile acids or organic anions by the hepatocytes (see below). However, these differences can also be explained by the existence of different carrier systems, even if these do not reside within their natural specialized membrane environment.

In addition to membrane randomization, the disappearance of the intracellular biliary polarity characterized by the distribution of Golgi complexes and lysosomes has been claimed (15, 40, 165, 166). In contrast, the preservation of this polarity in isolated cells has been documented in a careful study by Groothuis *et al.* (60), explaining also the apparent persistence of bond-like patterns of ectoenzymes reported previously (162). In conclusion, isolated hepatocytes apparently do not maintain their original membrane heterogeneity, but a general evaluation as to what extent remnants of the bile canalicular domain are preserved seems impossible particularly since even minor differences between cell isolation procedures may be of great influence.

In primary cultures of rat hepatocytes the presence of bile canaliculi has been noted in numerous reports (see references 55, 166). Although some of these canaliculi may originate from undissociated pairs of cells, clear-cut evidence that bile canaliculi can be formed *de novo* in culture has been presented (165, 166). This unique property has rendered the culture approach a valuable system for the investigation of the events and mechanisms involved in the recovery of hepatocyte membrane heterogeneity and cell-cell interactions (16).

Although the exact sequence of events underlying the reassociation of cultured hepatocytes has not yet been determined, it is believed that pre-existent remnants of contact points such as hemi-desmosomes trigger this process (40). Once a smooth contiguous membrane has reformed between adjacent hepatocytes, heavy inter-digitating subdomains characterized by the accumulation of huge amounts of cholesterol seems to initiate the formation of bile canaliculi (55). It has been suggested that the cholesterol is inserted by fusion of Golgi vesicles with the lateral membrane (120). The designated 'luminal' part is subsequently encirculated by tight junctions. The formation *in vitro* of tight junctions has been described in detail (45, 121, 166). In some studies they were observed apically and near the upper surface (45, 123) whereas in others an exclusively apical localization was found (55, 121). Interestingly, 'surface' tight junctions were found to develop in response to vinblastine (120).

Maturation of bile canaliculi proceeds via intermediate vesicular forms to the full developed canaliculi within a period of 12 to 24 h. Finally, they are studded with microvilli (55, 166; Fig. 1) and sealed by tight junctions excluding ruthenium red (166). Furthermore, at this stage the cells unequivocally show an intracellular biliary polarity which seems not to be acquired in the presence of antimicrotubular agents (35). Subsequently, the mature bile canaliculi may convert to larger smooth-surfaced biliary spaces (Fig. 1) which probably can also originate from the intermediate stages (55, 71). Although these enlarged spaces are morphologically similar to bile canaliculi of cholestatic rats they are still capable of secreting fluorescein (54).

The initiation of bile canalicular differentiation is most frequent during the first and second day of cultivation but does not completely cease during later periods, whereas the large dilated forms accumulate continuously (55, 71). Dexamethasone does not stimulate the development of bile canaliculi in cultures from adult hepatocytes as it does in those from fetal hepatocytes (81) but this hormone seems to affect various secretory events. After 1 or 2 weeks in culture most canaliculi suddenly disappear. However, in co-cultures prepared according to the method of Guguen-Guillouzo *et al.* (61) an intact biliary polarity persists at least for 2 months (Gekeler & Gebhardt, unpublished observation).

The differentiation of bile canaliculi is associated with changing activities of marker enzymes (phosphatases) at the canalicular membrane (71) in agreement with observations *in vivo* (37). On the other hand, the same enzyme activities reside for a

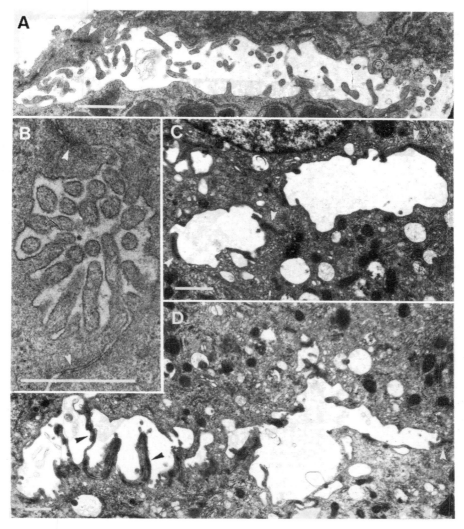

Fig. 1. Types of bile canaliculi most frequently observed in cultures of adult rat hepatocytes maintained for 2 to 3 days. A, B: bile canaliculi of group V (71) containing many microvilli. C: dilated bile canaliculi (group IV) lacking microvilli. D: series of segmented bile canaliculi of an intermediate type (group III). Arrow heads point to tight junctions. Bars: 1 μM. (B, C taken from reference 70).

long time and to a variable extent on the sinusoidal and the lateral membranes of individual cells (71) – most probably a consequence of the randomization process taking place during cell isolation. Furthermore, biochemical measurements indicate alterations in the activities of these marker enzymes as well as of γ-GT (71, 75) which all vary in response to hormones and other effectors (31, 71, 75, 122). It is still unknown whether the induction of γ-GT observed in late cultures (85, 122, 147) is related to changes of the biliary polarity (as in cholestasis), to phenotypic alterations ('fetalization') of the cultured cells, or to both. Cultivation seems also to be associated with alterations of other membrane components and membrane functions (46, 157). Thus, despite the reformation of a biliary polarity, the cultured hepatocytes restore their original membrane topography and composition only to a certain extent which has to be further characterized in future studies.

Undissociated cells and aspects of canalicular motility

The cultivation of undissociated pairs or groups of hepatocytes carrying almost intact bile canaliculi between them may provide a new approach for studies on biliary secretion. In particular, the determination of parameters related to the secretory process (eg transmembrane potentials) is facilitated in this system (58g). The potency of this approach in closing the gap between structure and function is illustrated by the recent discovery of active contractions of such preformed canaliculi at early stages of monolayer formation by use of time-lapse cinephotomicrography (104). From histograms of contraction intervals it could be determined that there is a peak of contractile activity every 5.5 min (112). Interestingly, the transmembrane potential of cultured liver cells was found to oscillate within a similar range of 4–6 min (170). The coincidence of these time periods might suggest that both phenomena are associated, but so far they have not been recorded at comparable cultivation periods.

Canalicular contractions were found to be increased in number by taurocholate (95). They were greatly inhibited by administration of cytochalasin (114) or pretreatment of donor rats with phalloidin (167) suggesting the participation of actin microfilaments (113).

Until now, canalicular contractions have not been described in bile canaliculi of certainly new origin in culture. At least for the large dilated canaliculi a contractile activity can be definitively excluded. In this respect it is interesting to note that the initial reorganization of actin microfilaments takes abut 24 h (93) and that abnormal accumulations of actin filaments may occur under certain conditions (89, 123). It thus remains to be determined whether a normal organisation of actin microfilaments is reestablished in cultured hepatocytes.

Uptake of bile salts

The uptake of bile salts has been the subject of numerous studies using isolated and cultured hepatocytes. In principle, three different components have been shown to participate in the uptake of bile salts and their conjugates: 1) a non-saturable, 2) a saturable Na^+-independent, and 3) a saturable Na^+-dependent component which seems to be the most important one (2, 124, 130). In addition, a non-specific and specific adsorption to the plasma membrane has been reported (8, 66, 130), but the relationship between binding and uptake is unclear.

The unsaturable portion of the uptake is quite small at physiological bile salt concentrations (2, 124) and seems to represent diffusion through the plasma membrane. Uptake via this component at higher concentrations correlates well with lipophilicity of the free and conjugated compounds (14, 66, 138) which may also determine non-specific binding to plasma membrane lipids (8, 66).

The saturable Na^+-independent component has been identified only in a few

Table 2. Kinetic constants of saturable bile salt uptake determined in different experimental systems.

Bile salt	K_m μM	V_{max} $nmol \times mg^{-1} \times min^{-1}$	Sodium dependence	References
Isolated hepatocytes:				
Cholate	58–74	0.57–1.17	+	(5, 6)
	13	0.83	+	(66)
	39	0.6	–	(2)
	67	1.43	–	(101)
Glycocholate	3.7	1.21	+	(66)
Taurocholate	19	1.7	+	(130)
	15–26	1.34–1.53	+	(2, 5)
	39	1.04	+	(94)
	40	n.r.[a]	+	(102)
	11	26.1[b]	+	(116)
	21–42	1.3	+	(21, 22)
	3.7	1.21	+	(66)
	57	0.74	–	(2)
Chenodeoxycholate	32.8	4.35	+	(66)
	33	4.8	+	(14)
Cultured hepatocytes:				
Taurocholate	16–28	1.93[b]	+	(129, 133)
	36	0.42	+	(124)
	$nmol \times g^{-1}$	$nmol \times g^{-1} \times min^{-1}$		
Perfused liver:				
Cholate	526	1494[b]	+	(118)
	436	327	+	(38)
Taurocholate	90–258	1200–1950[b]	+	(117, 118)
	61	299	+	(38)
Chenodexoycholate	236	684[b]	+	(118)

[a] nr: not reported
[b] Values normalized from results reported in the respective sources.

studies (2, 3, 83). This route may be shared by bile salts and other organic anions (see below).

Corresponding to its importance for the uptake of bile salts and their conjugates a saturable Na^+-dependent component has been identified in almost all studies. A comparison of kinetic constants determined for several bile salts and their conjugates is given in Table 2. Obviously, there is a striking difference between the values determined in isolated and cultured cells and those found in the isolated perfused rat liver illustrating the difference between parameters meaningful either with respect to kinetics or to physiology. Direct comparison of the apparent K_m values of several bile salts and their conjugates revealed that the taurine conjugates have a higher affinity (14, 66). Based on saturation kinetics and Na^+-dependence this transport component is considered to be carrier-mediated and driven by a Na^+-gradient established by Na^+, K^+-ATPase. Support for this assumption is found in the activation energy determined to 13 kcal/mol (124) or 26 kcal/mol (101) for cholate and 29 kcal/mol for taurocholate (130), the inhibitory effect of ouabain (2, 124, 129, 130) and the influence of various respiratory chain inhibitors and uncouplers (2, 6,

99, 101, 129, 130). In addition, dissipation of the Na^+-gradient by substrates that undergo Na^+-dependent transport via different transport systems reduces bile salt uptake (22) as do the loop diuretics bumetanide and furosemide whose influence has been ascribed to an inhibition of Na^+-coupled transport in isolated hepatocytes despite their lack of effect on the uptake of α-methylamino-isobutyric acid (21).

The question of existence of different carrier-systems for bile acids is controversial (5, 101, 133). It appears likely that the answer to this question cannot be provided on the basis of kinetic approaches and equilibrium studies only, but must await the identification of carrier molecules, such as the bile salt binding polypeptides recently detected by photo-affinity labelling in isolated plasma membranes and intact hepatocytes (79, 161) or by other affinity labels (172). It seems established, however, that the Na^+-dependent carrier system is not shared by other organic anions (94, 140).

There are many indications from studies *in vivo* that structural elements other than membrane carriers (eg microfilaments, microtubules, Golgi apparatus) participate in the transport of bile acids (for reviews see references 20 and 78). In isolated hepatocytes, taurocholate uptake was competitively inhibited by cytochalasin B (116) and, less effectively, non-competitively, by colchicine (116) or vinblastine (102). The mechanistic implications of these findings still await further investigation. Studies comparing isolated and cultured hepatocytes could provide new insights, since in the latter an as yet unexplained deterioration of the uptake of desmethylphalloidin (which presumably shares a common carrier with bile acids (47)) has been observed (44, 90).

The hormonal regulation of bile acid uptake is not well understood at present. Both secretin and cholecystokinin octapeptide were found to decrease taurocholate uptake by a common mechanism mediated by cAMP (102). In cultured hepatocytes dexamethasone and tocopherol were found to prevent the loss in transport capacity for cholate as well as for BSP during cultivation (49). The progressive increase in taurocholate uptake with age (157) might also be controlled by glucocorticoids.

Uptake of organic anions

Bromosulphophthalein (BSP) has been shown to be selectively taken up and conjugated by isolated parenchymal cells but not by isolated Küpffer cells (151). At low substrate concentrations, a saturable uptake process seems to be involved (83, 84, 140, 160) which, in hepatocytes from fed animals, apparently follows simple Michaelis-Menten kinetics (84, 140). However, on the basis of inhibition of BSP uptake by taurocholate (83, 84, 162, 163; but not in 140) a separate transport component with a higher affinity has been detected (83, 84). In hepatocytes from fasted rats, these two components are directly revealed by kinetic analysis and show an increased K_m (50%) of the low affinity component (84). At higher concentrations, BSP uptake was found to deviate from linearity (140). BSP is transported much faster than its GSH-conjugate which may compete with BSP for the same carrier (131) but conjugation itself does not influence the uptake rate (128).

The nature of the uptake process is far from clear. Contrasting results concerning the influence of inhibitors of energy metabolism (no effect (140) versus inhibition

(160)) and concerning the dependence on temperature (140, 160) have been reported. Depending on either result, an active carrier-mediated mechanism has been postulated (160) or partially questioned (140). The latter authors suggested a combined binding and diffusion process as an alternative (140). There is no doubt, however, that BSP uptake is Na^+-independent (140). Whatever the mechanism of uptake may be, binding to distinct translocation sites seems to be essential (140), as stressed also by the negative influence of poor viability on BSP uptake (139, 160) associated with a decrease in binding sites and association constants (139).

DBSP which, in contrast to BSP, is not metabolized in rat liver is also taken up by a saturable process with an activation energy of 26 kcal/mole at 1 μM suggesting the involvement of a membrane carrier (23). Uptake was partially dependent on metabolic energy but not on a Na^+-gradient.

A marked dependence upon metabolic energy was also found for iodipamide which is supposed to share a transport system with cholate (110). The route of uptake of iopanoic acid studied in cultured hepatocytes is unknown (9). It is unique in so far as a saturable uptake component could be demonstrated only in the presence of albumin suggesting that a carrier-mediated mechanism depended on an albumin-iopanoic acid-hepatocyte interaction. In the absence of albumin, only a non-saturable uptake was found. Extracellular sodium was not required for uptake (9).

In contrast to the above mentioned organic anions, unconjugated bilirubin has been found to gain access to the cytoplasm by diffusion only, and accumulation has been explained by a high intracellular binding (67). While the latter seems compatible with the results of Bissell *et al.* (18), a diffusion mediated uptake is not in line with many studies *in vivo* (see reference (78)) and with the identification of a possible carrier protein for bilirubin (88).

Uptake of other solutes and xenobiotics

Chloride transport has been studied in cultured hepatocytes (125) because of its potential contribution to bile acid independent bile flow. Although the possible existence of a Na^+-coupled chloride transport could not be excluded, evidence against a specific chloride requirement for bile formation has been presented (125).

Ouabain, a cardiac glycoside, has been used to probe into the mechanisms of the biliary transport of neutral compounds. The uptake process seemed to be saturable, concentrative and energy-dependent (41, 144) and was proposed to be mediated either by the Na^+-independent bile acid carrier or by the uptake system for steroids (144). The participation of the taurocholate-carrier is unlikely because of the differential effect of maturation (149) or of microsomal enzyme inducers (43) on both transport systems which seem to differ also in their lobular distribution (150). In contrast to taurocholate, ouabain seems to be released from hepatocytes simply by a passive mechanism (144).

A saturable, energy-dependent uptake process has been found also for the organic cation procaine amide ethobromide (42). Interestingly, the quaternary nitrogen seems not to be the main determinant for the specificity of this uptake (42).

In addition, studies on the uptake and metabolism of various other natural or synthetic compounds have been performed including estrogens (115, 141), morphine and nalorphine (68) and rifampicine (82), which all meet the requirements of carrier-mediated transport, and of naphthol (142) or lidocaine (30), which seem to be taken up by diffusion.

Aspects of the secretion of bile salts and organic anions

As pointed out in a previous section studies on biliary secretion, using isolated hepatocytes may suffer from the absence of the original membrane heterogeneity. However, if this fact is taken into account studies using isolated hepatocytes may lead to interesting implications for the efflux mechanism. According to Schwarz *et al.* (135) the efflux of taurocholate is a saturable process with an activation energy of about 12 kcal/mol. It is dependent on metabolic energy as judged from inhibition by antimycin A and CCCP but seems not to be affected by ouabain (135). The release of taurocholate is stimulated by catecholamines via an α-adrenergic mechanism (58) and by vasopressin whose influence is potentiated by ocytocin (58).

Excretion of the GSH-conjugate of BSP has also been found to be saturable and energy-dependent (137). It proceeds more slowly (6%) than the uptake and it has been suggested that this is mediated by a carrier different from that involved in the uptake (137). The same may be true for DBSP (23).

These examples demonstrate that separate secretory mechanisms still operate in isolated hepatocytes but quantitative conclusions can hardly be drawn from those studies until the equivalence to the *in vivo* situation has been demonstrated (24).

In cultured hepatocytes which newly form a biliary polarity a situation closer to the *in vivo* state seems to be established. However, in this case it is also conceivable that transport systems involved in secretion do not gather exclusively at the apical pole but still remain active to some extent in the basolateral part of the plasma membrane (Ugele & Gebhardt, unpublished observations).

The functional integrity of the newly established biliary polarity in cultured rat hepatocytes has been demonstrated for the secretion of organic anions but so far not for that of bile acids. Using fluorescein, Lambiotte (80) originally described the accumulation of fluorescence over structures supposed to represent bile canaliculi under the phase contrast microscope. This initial approach has been corroborated and extended in two recent communications (13, 54) demonstrating a striking similarity between sequential staining of cytoplasm and bile canaliculi recorded *in vitro* and the events observed by intra-vital microscopy (64). Furthermore, independent evidence for a true transcellular secretory process has been provided including the discharge of stained canaliculi by a short exposure to 1M sucrose (54) and the apparent inhibition of secretion but not of uptake by taurolithocholate (13, 54).

The functional integrity of bile canaliculi seems unique to primary cultures of hepatocytes since a number of hepatoma cells failed to secrete intracellularly formed fluorescein (11), despite their morphologically well developed bile canaliculi.

Recently, we have introduced a family of derivatives of N-fluoresceinyl-thiourea superior to fluorescein as model substrates for organic anion transport in cultured hepatocytes (70, 72). The N-fluoresceinyl, N-glycyl-thiourea (FGTU), a highly anionic compound, is rapidly transferred to the biliary compartment without significantly staining the cytoplasm of the hepatocytes at concentrations below 60 μM (Fig. 2 *a*, *b*). FGTU is taken up by a saturable, Na^+-independent system.

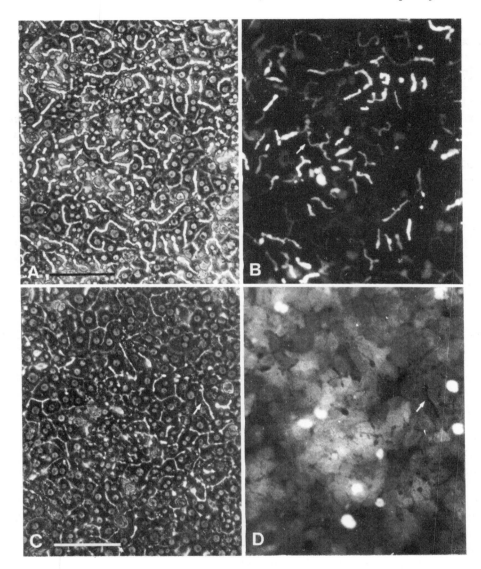

Fig. 2. **Biliary secretion of the organic anion FGTU in primary cultures of hepatocytes.** A, B: Phase contrast and fluorescence micrographs of a culture incubated with 60 μM FTGU for 20 min. Fluorescence is detectable only in bile canaliculi (arrow). C, D: Culture incubated with FGTU in the presence of 120 μM fluoresceinamine for 60 min. Fluorescence due to FGTU is seen in the cytoplasm but not in bile canaliculi (arrow) indicating a complete inhibition of the secretory event. Bars: 100 μM. (Taken from reference 70.)

A non-saturable process becomes dominating at concentrations above 300 μM (159). The biliary secretion of FGTU is completely blocked by fluorescein amine, a non-fluorescent structural analogue, whereas the uptake is inhibited to a lesser extent (72, 159). As a consequence, fluorescence appears in the cytoplasm, indicating a higher intracellular concentration, whereas the bile canaliculi are not stained at all (Fig. 2 *c, d*).

These results suggest the existence of different carrier systems for uptake and secretion of these organic anions (72, 159). The carrier mediating the export into the biliary compartment presumably prefers more anionic molecules explaining the different behaviour of FGTU and fluorescein which is supposed to be glucuronidated before being secreted (Ugele & Gebhardt, unpublished observations).

The advantages of these N-fluoresceinyl-thiourea-derivatives and the easy accessibility of the bile canalicular compartment in the monolayer approach has rendered it possible for the first time to measure the secretion of cholephilic compounds into single bile canaliculi by using fluorescence microphotolysis (Gebhardt & Peters, to be published). As shown in Fig. 3, the transport of FGTU into a pre-equilibrated bile

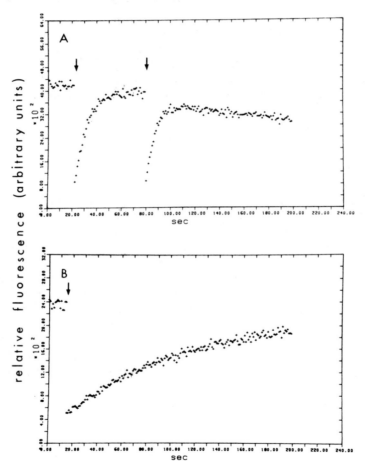

Fig. 3. Cytoplasmic-bile canalicular flux of the organic anion FGTU determined by fluorescence microphotolysis. Cultures were preincubated with 80 μM FGTU for 90 min. The three steps of the measurement are easily distinguished: measurement of fluorescence in a pre-equilibrated bile canaliculus before bleaching, reduction of fluorescence by bleaching, and flux of the dye into the canaliculus after bleaching. Panels A and B demonstrate the heterogeneity of the secretory events in two different bile canaliculi of the same culture. (For details of fluorescence microphotolysis see Peters (107).)

canaliculus whose fluorescent content has been partially bleached out can easily be measured allowing the determination of the rate constants of the secretory process. Different bile canaliculi in culture may show a large variation in their ability to perform secretion (Fig. 3), demonstrating their heterogeneous nature from a functional point of view.

Transport of proteins

The majority of serum proteins taken up by hepatocytes via endocytosis are transferred to the lysosomal compartment for degradation and appear in bile only in low amounts. Asialoglycoproteins, for instance, follow this pathway and their binding, endocytosis and intracellular fate has been studied in great detail particularly in isolated hepatocytes (*cf* 153). These interesting studies cannot be reviewed herein, but it should be mentioned that in the case of gold-labelled galactosylated bovine serum albumin the delivery of a small fraction of the ligand to the bile canaliculi has been demonstrated in hepatocyte cultures (36).

On the other hand, some endocytosed serum proteins such as immunoglobulin A (IgA) escape the lysosomal degradation and are excreted in a selective and concentrated manner into bile. Isolated and cultured hepatocytes have served as potent tools in elucidating some mechanistic details involved in uptake, intracellular processing and canalicular secretion of IgA. Several reports have shown that secretory component (SC), the receptor for IgA, is synthesized by these cells (87, 148), exposed on the cell surface (51, 69, 87, 103, 148) and to some extent released into the culture medium (87). Strong evidence has accumulated that IgA binds specifically to SC (86, 103) and that this binding is an ultimate requirement for uptake (51, 69, 86, 87) which proceeds via endocytosis into vesicles (69, 86). Once internalized, IgA may be digested to some extent (86), while a major part is found as secretory IgA in the culture medium (86) and accumulates in the newly formed bile canaliculi, as demonstrated immunocytochemically (51), as well as at the ultra-structural level using gold-conjugated IgA (57). However, these cytochemical studies (57) as well as the biochemical results of Limet *et al.* (86) have revealed some transfer of IgA to the lysosomal compartment which may exceed the extent observed *in vivo*. Using the same techniques, evidence for the participation of both microtubules and microfilaments in the transcellular transport of IgA has been provided (53, 56, 57). These results not only demonstrate the existence of a functional transcellular and biliary transport of IgA in cultured hepatocytes, but also promise further insight into this process for future studies.

Functional and structural studies related to cholestasis

Despite a growing understanding of the normal physiology of bile formation, little is known about the pathophysiology of intrahepatic cholestasis (78, 119). There are now several lines of evidence demonstrating that isolated and cultured hepatocytes provide valuable new experimental approaches for the investigation of the pathogenesis of drug-induced cholestasis.

A first aspect concerns the interaction of cholestatic agents with the transport of cholephilic compounds. Cholestatic compounds have been applied either *in vivo* (giving rise to 'cholestatic' hepatocytes (156, 164)) or directly *in vitro*. The cholestatic bile salt taurolithocholate (TLC) was found to inhibit taurocholate uptake directly in isolated hepatocytes in a non-competitive manner (133, 143). This type of inhibition together with the well-known detergent activity of TLC suggest non-specific membrane perturbations. Some steroids (eg norethandrolone, 17β-estradiol) which cause various types of jaundice, also inhibited taurocholate uptake pre-sumably by a similar mechanism (134, 136). However, these membrane interactions seemed to be specific in so far only that the uptake, but not the secretion, of taurocholate was inhibited by these compounds (133, 134, 136, 143). In cultured hepatocytes, on the other hand, TLC apparently inhibited the secretion of fluorescein into bile canaliculi without impairing uptake (13, 54) and morphological alterations at the canalicular membrane were prominent (73). These results suggest strikingly different interactions of TLC at the basolateral and the apical membrane, but direct comparative studies are required to verify these findings in one and the same experimental system.

Non-competitive inhibition of the uptake of cholate and taurocholate in isolated hepatocytes has also been found for the antibiotics rifamycin SV and rifampicin (7). In contrast, fusidates which show some structural similarity to bile acids, inhibited the uptake of the same two bile salts in a competitive way suggesting a more direct interference with the bile acid carrier (1).

Studies in isolated hepatocytes have contributed to the understanding of the hepatotoxicity of phalloidin. Interchangeable inhibition of uptake between bile salts and phalloidin or its derivatives has been demonstrated suggesting that phalloidin is taken up by the hepatic bile salt carrier (48, 108, 109, 172). This may explain the organospecificity of this toxin (47). Another cyclopeptide, antamanide, also seems to share this route (110).

A second aspect, as yet rarely illustrated, concerns the consequences of the cholestatic state for the biosynthetic activity. The demonstration that enhanced levels of taurocholate may be responsible for the rise of alkaline phosphatase in cholestasis (65) is one of the most straightforward examples in this direction.

Finally, a third aspect covers the structural alterations of cell organelles and membranes induced by cholestatic compounds. Taurolithocholate has been shown to cause characteristic deformations of the canalicular membrane as it does *in vivo*, and the role of cholesterol in this process could be specified (73). Characteristic structural changes induced by chlorpromazine have also been described *in vitro* (74). In this study, evidence has been presented for a primary action of this drug restricted to the sinusoidal surface of the plasma membrane (74). Several studies have focused on the influence of antimicrotubular drugs indicating structural dissolution of the bile canaliculi (52, 120) similar to *in vivo*, or the inability of the cultured cells to re-establish their biliary polarity (35, 52). Antimicrofilamentous drugs, on the other hand, have been found to disturb the canalicular motility (114, 167).

Conclusions

It is obvious from this review that studies using currently available isolated and cultured hepatocyte preparations have provided valuable information with respect to many aspects of biliary secretion and cholestasis. The usefulness of these systems will become even greater if the structural and functional alterations associated with the isolated and cultured state are defined more precisely. Moreover, it will be the challenge of future studies to minimize such alterations by establishing more adequate culture conditions (eg those provided by co-cultivation (62)). This is particularly important for the culture approach which may open a new round of research on biliary excretion because of the preservation of an intact cellular polarity and the easy accessibility of the bile canalicular compartment. It must be kept in mind, however, that these biliary spaces are tightly sealed thus representing blind pouches after some time in culture. Therefore, the possibility that 'cholestasis' may be an inherent feature of the culture system which is responsible for some of the phenotypic alterations should carefully be investigated (16, 71).

ACKNOWLEDGEMENTS

I wish to express my thanks to Dr H. J. M. Kempen (Gaubius Instituut, Leiden), Dr H. Robenek (Universität Münster) and Dr R. Peters (Max-Planck-Institut für Biophysik, Frankfurt) for the stimulating and fruitful collaboration in different fields of bile acid production and biliary secretion in cultured hepatocytes. I am indebted to Professor Dr D. Mecke for his continuous interest and encouragement. Many thanks are due to Dr G. Michalopoulos for critical reading of the manuscript. This work was supported by the Deutsche Forschungsgemeinschaft.

REFERENCES

1 Anwer M. S., Hegner D.: Interaction of fusidates with bile acid uptake by isolated rat hepatocytes. *Naunyn-Schmiedberg's Arch. Pharmacol.* 1978, **302**: 329–332.

2 Anwer M. S., Hegner D.: Effect of Na^+ on bile acid uptake by isolated rat hepatocytes. *Hoppe Seyler's Z. Physiol. Chem.* 1978, **359**: 181–192.

3 Anwer M. S., Hegner D.: Effect of organic anions on bile acid uptake by isolated rat hepatocytes. *Hoppe Seyler's Z. Physiol. Chem.* 1978, **359**: 1027–1030.

4 Anwer M. S., Kroker R., Hegner D.: Bile acid secretion and synthesis by isolated rat hepatocytes. *Biochem. Biophys. Res. Commun.* 1975, **64**: 603–609.

5 Anwer M. S., Kroker R., Hegner D.: Effect of albumin on bile acid uptake by isolated rat hepatocytes. Is there a common bile acid carrier? *Biochem. Biophys. Res. Commun.* 1976, **73**: 63–71.

6 Answer M. S., Kroker R., Hegner D.: Cholic acid uptake into isolated rat hepatocytes. *Hoppe Seyler's Z. Physiol. Chem.* 1976, **357**: 1477–1486.

7 Anwer M. S., Kroker R., Hegner D.: Inhibition of hepatic uptake of bile acids by rifamycins. *Naunyn-Schmiedeberg's Arch. Pharmacol.* 1978, **302**: 19–24.

8 Anwer M. S., Kroker R., Hegner D., Petter A.: Cholic acid binding in isolated rat liver plasma membranes. *Hoppe Seyler's Z. Physiol. Chem.* 1977, **358**: 543–553.

9 Barnhart J. L., Witt B. L., Hardison W. G., Berk R. N.: Uptake of iopanoic acid by isolated rat hepatocytes in primary culture. *Am. J. Physiol.* 1983, **244**: G630–G636.

10 Barth C. A., Hillmar I.: Taurocholate inhibits the glucocorticoid-induced rise of 3-hydroxy-3-methylglutaryl-CoA reductase in primary culture of hepatocytes. *Eur. J. Biochem.* 1980, **110**: 237–240.

11 Barth C. A., Wiebel F., Schwarz L. R.: Transcellular transport of biliary compounds in primary cultures of adult rat hepatocytes, but not in hepatoma lines. *In: Isolation, Characterization and Use of Hepatocytes*, R. A. Harris, N. W. Cornell (Eds): Elsevier Science Publishing, New York, 1983, pp 267–270.

12 Barth C. A., Wirthensohn K.: Enzymatic determination of bile acids from liver cells with 3β-

hydroxysteroid dehydrogenase – a warning. *J. Lipid Res.* 1981, **22**: 1025–1027.

13 Barth C. A., Schwarz L. R.: Transcellular transport of fluorescein in hepatocyte monolayers: evidence for functional polarity of cells in culture. *Proc. Natl. Acad. Sci.* 1982, **79**: 4985–4987.

14 Bartholomew T. C., Billing B. H.: The effect of 3-sulphation and taurine conjugation on the uptake of chenodeoxycholic acid by rat hepatocytes. *Biochem. Biophys. Acta* 1983, **754**: 101–109.

15 Berry M. N., Friend D. S.: High-yield preparation of isolated rat liver parenchymal cells. A biochemical and fine structural study. *J. Cell Biol.* 1969, **43**: 506–520.

16 Bissell D. M.: Hepatocellular function in culture: the role of cell-cell interaction. *In: Isolation, Characterization and Use of Hepatocytes*, R. A. Harris, N. W. Cornell (Eds): Elsevier Science Publishing, New York, 1983, pp 51–58.

17 Bissell D. M., Billing B. H.: Bilirubin metabolism in primary hepatocyte culture. *In: The Liver: Quantitative Aspects of Structure and Function*, R. Preisig, J. Bircher (Eds): Editio Cantor, Aulendorf, 1979, pp 110–117.

18 Bissell D. M., Deal D. R., Hammaker L. E.: Determinants of bilirubin transport into bile. *Gastroenterology* 1975, **69**: A-9/809.

19 Bissell D. M., Guzelian P. S.: Phenotypic stability of adult rat hepatocytes in primary monolayer culture. *Ann. N.Y. Acad. Sci.* 1980, **349**: 85–98.

20 Blitzer B. L., Boyer J. L.: Cellular mechanisms of bile formation. *Gastroenterology* 1982, **82**: 346–357.

21 Blitzer B. L., Ratoosh S. L., Donovan C. B., Boyer J. L.: Effects of inhibitors of Na^+-coupled ion transport on bile acid uptake by isolated rat hepatocytes. *Am. J. Physiol.* 1982, **243**: G4–G53.

22 Blitzer B. L., Ratoosh S. L., Donovan C. B.: Amino acid inhibition of bile acid uptake by isolated rat hepatocytes: relationship to dissipation of transmembrane Na^+-gradient. *Am. J. Physiol.* 1983, **245**: G399–G403.

23 Blom A., Keulemans K., Meijer D. K. F.: Transport of dibromosulphophthalein by isolated rat hepatocytes. *Biochem. Pharmacol.* 1981, **30**: 1809–1816.

24 Blom A., Scaf A. H., Meijer D. K. F.: Hepatic drug transport in the rat. A comparison between isolated hepatocytes, the isolated perfused liver and the liver *in vivo. Biochem. Pharmacol.* 1982, **31**: 1553–1565.

25 Botham K. M., Beckett G. J., Percy-Robb I. W., Boyd G. S.: Bile acid synthesis in isolated rat liver cells. The effect of 7α-hydroxycholesterol. *Eur. J. Biochem.* 1980, **103**: 299–305.

26 Botham K. M., Boyd G. S.: The metabolism of chenodeoxycholic acid to β-muricholic acid in rat liver. *Eur. J. Biochem.* 1983, **134**: 191–196.

27 Botham K. M., Boyd G. S.: The effect of dibutyryladenosine 3',5'-monophosphate on the synthesis of bile salts in isolated hepatocytes from rat. *Eur. J. Biochem.* 1983, **134**: 313–319.

28 Botham K. M., Lawson M. E., Beckett G. J., Percy-Robb I. W., Boyd G. S.: Portal blood concentrations of conjugated cholic and chenodeoxycholic acids. Relationship to bile salt synthesis in liver cells. *Biochem. Biophys. Acta* 1981, **665**: 81–87.

29 Botham K. M., Lawson M. E., Beckett G. J., Percy-Robb I. W., Boyd G. S.: The effect of portal blood bile salt concentrations on bile salt synthesis in rat liver. Studies with isolated hepatocytes. *Biochem. Biophys. Acta* 1981, **666**: 238–245.

30 Chen C.-P., Vu V. T., Cohen S. D.: Lidocaine uptake in isolated rat hepatocytes and effects of dl-propranolol. *Toxicol. Appl. Pharmacol.* 1980, **55**: 162–168.

31 Coloma J., Gómez-Lechón M. J., García M. D., Felíu J. E., Báguena J.: Effect of glucocorticoids on the appearance of gamma-glutamyl transpeptidase activity in primary cultures of adult rat hepatocytes. *Experientia*, 1981, **37**: 941–943.

32 Cronholm T., Sjövall J.: Bile acids in portal blood of rats fed different diets and cholestyramine. *Eur. J. Biochem.* 1967, **2**: 375–383.

33 Davis R. A., Highsmith W. E., Malone-McNeal M., Archambault-Schexnayder J., Kuan C. W.: Bile acid synthesis by cultured hepatocytes. *J. Biol. Chem.* 1983, **258**: 4079–4082.

34 Davis R. A., Hyde P. M., Kuan J.-C. W., Malone-McNeal M., Archambault-Schexnayder J.: Bile acid secretion by cultured rat hepatocytes. Regulation by cholesterol availability. *J. Biol. Chem.* 1983, **258**: 3661–3667.

35 De Brabander M., Wanson J.-C., Mosselmans R., Geuens G., Drochmans P.: Effects of antimicrotubular compounds on monolayer cultures of adult rat hepatocytes. *Biol. Cellulaire* 1978, **31**: 127–140.

36 Deschuyteneer M., Prieels J.-P., Mosselmans R.: Galactose-specific adsorptive endocytosis: an ultrastructural qualitative and quantitative study in cultured rat hepatocytes. *Biol. Cell* 1984, **50**: 17–30.

37 De Wolf-Peeters C., De Vos R., Desmet V., Bianchi L., Rohr H. P.: Electron microscopy and morphometry of canalicular differentiation in fetal and neonatal rat liver *Exp. Mol. Path.* 1974, **21**: 339–350.

38 Dietmaier A., Gasser R., Graf J., Peterlik M.: Investigations on the sodium dependence of bile acid fluxes in the isolated perfused rat liver. *Biochim. Biophys. Acta* 1976, **443**: 81–91.

39 Driscoll J. L., Hayner N. T., Williams-Holland R., Spies-Karotkin G., Galletti P. M., Jauregui H. O.: Phenolsulfonphthalein (phenol red) metabolism in primary monolayer cultures of adult rat hepatocytes. *In Vitro* 1982, **18**: 835–842.

40 Drochmans P., Wanson J. C., May C., Bernaert D.: Ultrastructural and metabolic studies of isolated and cultured hepatocytes. *In: Hepatotrophic Factors*, Ciba Foundation Symposium 55, Elsevier/Excerpta Medica/North Holland, 1978, pp 7–29.

41 Eaton D. L., Klaassen C. D.: Carrier-mediated transport of ouabain in isolated hepatocytes. *J. Pharmacol. Exp. Therap.* 1978, **205**: 480–488.

42 Eaton D. L., Klaassen C. D.: Carrier-mediated transport of the organic cation procain amide ethobromide by isolated rat liver parenchymal cells. *J. Pharmacol. Exp. Therap.* 1978, **206**: 595–606.

43 Eaton D. L., Klaassen C. D.: Effect of microsomal enzyme inducers on carrier-mediated transport systems in isolated rat hepatocytes. *J. Pharmacol. Exp. Therap.* 1979, **208**: 381–385.

44 Faulstich H., Trischmann H., Mayer D.: Preparation of tetra-methylrhodaminyl-phalloidin and uptake of the toxin into short-term cultured hepatocytes by endocytosis. *Exp. Cell Res.* 1983, **144**: 73–82.

45 Feltkamp C. A., Van Der Waerden A. W. M.: Junction formation between cultured normal rat hepatocytes. An ultrastructural study on the presence of cholesterol and the structure of developing tight-junction strands. *J. Cell Sci.* 1983, **63**: 271–286.

46 Ferayorni L. S., McMillan P. N., Raines L., Gerhardt C. O., Jauregi H. O.: Lectin binding to adult rat liver *in situ*, isolated hepatocytes, and hepatocyte cultures. *In: Isolation, Characterization and Use of Hepatocytes*, R. A. Harris, N. W. Cornell (Eds): Elsevier Science Publishing, New York, 1983, pp 271–276.

47 Frimmer M.: Organotropism by carrier-mediated transport. *Trends Pharmacol. Sci.* 1982, 395–397.

48 Frimmer M., Petzinger E., Rufeger U., Veil L. B.: The role of bile acids in phalloidin poisoning. *Naunyn-Schmiedeberg's Arch. Pharmacol.* 1977, **301**: 145–147.

49 Galivan J.: Stabilization of cholic acid uptake in primary cultures of hepatocytes by dexamethasone and tocopherol. *Arch. Biochem. Biophys.* 1982, **214**: 850–852.

50 Gardner B., Chenouda M. S.: Studies of bile acid secretion by isolated rat hepatocytes. *J. Lipid Res.* 1978, **19**: 985–991.

51 Gebhardt R.: Primary cultures of rat hepatocytes as a model system of canalicular development, biliary secretion, and intrahepatic cholestasis. III. Properties of the biliary transport of immunoglobulin A revealed by immunofluoescence. *Gastroenterology* 1983, **84**: 1462–1470.

52 Gebhardt R.: Disappearance of visible bile canaliculi caused by vinblastine in primary cultures of rat hepatocytes. *Exp. Cell Res.* 1983, **144**: 218–223.

53 Gebhardt R.: Participation of microtubules and microfilaments in the transcellular biliary secretion of immunoglobulin A in primary cultures of rat hepatocytes. *Experientia*, 1984, **40**: 269–271.

54 Gebhardt R., Jung W.: Biliary secretion of sodium fluorescein in primary monolayer cultures of adult rat hepatocytes and its stimulation by nicotinamide. *J. Cell Sci.* 1982, **56**: 233–244.

55 Gebhardt R., Jung W., Robenek H.: Primary cultures of rat hepatocytes as a model system of canalicular development, biliary secretion, and intrahepatic cholestasis. I. Distribution of filipin-cholesterol complexes during *de novo* formation of bile canaliculi. *Eur. J. Cell Biol.* 1982, **29**: 68–76.

56 Gebhardt R., Robenek H.: Ligand-induced patch formation of IgA-secretory component-complexes induced by cytochalasin B on the surface of cultured rat hepatocytes. (Submitted.)

57 Gebhardt R., Robenek H.: Primary cultures of rat hepatocytes as a model system of biliary

secretion. VI. Surface binding, endocytosis and biliary secretion of IgA-gold conjugates in normal and vinblastine-treated cultures. (Submitted.)

58 Gewirtz D. A., Randolph J. K., Goldman I. D.: Induction of taurocholate release from isolated rat hepatocytes in suspension by α-adrenergic agents and vasopressin: Implications for control of bile salt secretion. *Hepatology* 1984, **4**: 205–212.

58a Graf J., Gautam A., Boyer J. L.: Isolated rat hepatocyte couplets: A primary secretory unit for electrophysiologic studies of bile secretory function. *Proc. Natl. Acad. Sci.* 1984, **81**: 6516–6520.

59 Greim H., Trülzsch D., Roboz J., Dressler K., Czygan P., Hutterer F., Schaffner F., Popper H.: Mechanism of cholestasis. 5. Bile acids in normal rat livers and in those after bile duct ligation. *Gastroenterology* 1972, **63**: 837–845.

60 Groothuis G. M. M., Hulstaert C. E., Kalicharan D., Hardonk M. J.: Plasma membrane specialization and intracellular polarity of freshly isolated rat hepatocytes. *Eur. J. Biochem.* 1981, **26**: 43–51.

61 Guguen-Guillouzo C., Clement B., Baffet G., Beaumont C., Morel-Chany E., Glaise D., Guillouzo A.: Maintenance and reversibility of active albumin secretion by adult rat hepatocytes co-cultured with another liver epithelial cell type. *Exp. Cell Res.* 1983, **143**: 47–54.

62 Guguen-Guillouzo C., Guillouzo A.: Modulation of functional activities in cultured rat hepatocytes. *Molec. Cell. Biochem.* 1983, **53/54**: 35–56.

63 Guzelian P. S., Bissell D. M., Meyer U. A.: Drug metabolism in adult rat hepatocytes in primary monolayer culture. *Gastroenterology* 1977, **72**: 1232–1239.

64 Hanzon V.: Liver cell secretion under normal and pathologic conditions studied by fluorescence microscopy on living rats *Acta Physiol. Scand.* 1952, **28** (Suppl 101): 1–268.

65 Hatoff D. E., Hardison W. G. M.: Induced synthesis of alkaline phosphatase by bile acids in rat liver cell culture. *Gastroenterology* 1979, **77**: 1062–1067.

66 Iga T., Klaassen C. D.: Uptake of bile acids by isolated rat hepatocytes. *Biochem. Pharmacol.* 1982, **31**: 211–216.

67 Iga T., Eaton D. L., Klaassen C. D.: Uptake of unconjugated bilirubin by isolated rat hepatocytes. *Am. J. Physiol.* 1979, **236**: C9–C14.

68 Iwamoto K., Eaton D. L., Klaassen C. D.: Uptake of morphine and nalorphine by isolated rat hepatocytes. *J. Pharmacol. Exp. Therap.* 1978, **206**: 181–189.

69 Jones A. L., Huling S., Hradek G. T., Gaines H. S., Christansen W. D., Underdown B. J.: Uptake and intracellular disposition of IgA by rat hepatocytes in monolayer culture. *Hepatology* 1982, **2**: 769–776.

70 Jung W.: Primärkulturen von Rattenhepatocyten als Modellsystem zur Untersuchung der biliären Sekretion und der intrahepatischen Cholestase. Thesis, Tübingen, 1983.

71 Jung W., Gebhardt R., Mecke D.: Alterations in activity and ultrastructural localization of several phosphatases on the surface of adult rat hepatocytes in primary monolayer culture. *Eur. J. Cell Biol.* 1982, **27**: 230–241.

72 Jung W., Gebhardt R., Mecke D.: Transport von organischen Anionen in Primärkulturen von Rattenhepatocyten. *Hoppe-Seyler's Z. Physiol. Chem.* 1983, **364**: 343.

73 Jung W., Gebhardt R., Robenek H.: Primary cultures of rat hepatocytes as a model system of canalicular development, biliary secretion, and intrahepatic cholestasis. II. Taurolithocholate-induced alterations of canalicular morphology and of the distribution of filipin-cholesterol complexes. *Eur. J. Cell Biol.* 1982, **29**: 77–82.

74 Jung W., Gebhardt R., Robenek H.: Primary cultures of rat hepatocytes as a model system of canicular development, biliary secretion, and intrahepatic cholestasis. V. Disturbance of the cellular membrane and bile canalicular ultrastructure induced by chlorpromazine. *Virchows Arch. [Cell Pathol.]* 1985, in press.

75 Kato S., Aoyama K., Nakamura T., Ichihara A.: Biochemical studies on liver functions in primary cultured hepatocytes of adult rats. III. Changes of enzyme activities on cell membranes during culture. *J. Biochem.* 1979, **86**: 1419–1425.

76 Kempen. H. J. M., Vos-Van Holstein M. P. M., De Lange J.: Bile acids and lipids in isolated rat hepatocytes: content synthesis, and release, as affected by cholestyramine treatment of the donor rats. *J. Lipid Res.* 1982, **23**: 823–830.

77 Kempen H. J., Vos-Van Holstein M., De Lange J.: Bile acids and lipids in isolated rat hepatocytes. II. Source of cholesterol used for bile acid formation, estimated incorporation of

tritium from tritiated water, and by effect of ML-236B. *J. Lipid Res.* 1983, **24**: 316–323.

78 Klaassen C. D., Watkins III J. B.: Mechanisms of bile formation, hepatic uptake, and biliary excretion. *Pharmacol Rev.* 1984, **36**: 1–67.

79 Kramer W., Bickel U., Buscher H.-P., Gerok W., Kurz G.: Bile salt-binding polypeptides in plasma membranes of hepatocytes revealed by photoaffinity labelling. *Eur. J. Biochem.* 1982, **129**: 13–24.

80 Lambiotte M.: Glucocorticoid influence on morphological differentiation and bile acid metabolism in rat liver cell culture. *In: Bile Acid Metabolism in Health and Disease*, G. Paumgartner, A. Stiehl (Eds): University Park Press, Baltimore, 1977, pp 33–47.

81 Lambiotte M., Vorbrodt A., Benedetti E. L.: Expression of differentiation of rat foetal hepatocytes in cellular culture under the action of glucocorticoids: appearance of bile canaliculi. *Cell Diff.* 1973, **2**: 43–53.

82 Laperche Y., Graillot C., Arondel J., Berthelot P.: Uptake of rifampicin by isolated rat liver cells. Interaction with sulphobromophthalein uptake and evidence for separate carriers. *Biochem. Pharmacol.* 1979, **28**: 2065–2069.

83 Laperche Y., Preaux A. M., Berthelot P.: Two systems are involved in the sulfobromophthalein uptake by rat liver cells: one is shared with bile salts. *Biochem. Pharmacol.* 1981, **30**: 1333–1336.

84 Laperche Y., Preaux A.-M., Feldmann G., Mahu J., Berthelot P.: Effect of fasting on organic anion uptake by isolated rat liver cells. *Hepatology* 1981, **1**: 617–621.

85 Leffert J., Moran T., Sell S., Skelly H., Ibsen K., Mueller M., Arias I.: Growth state-dependent phenotypes of adult hepatocytes in primary monolayer culture. *Proc. Soc. Natl. Acad. Sci.* 1978, **75**: 1834–1838.

86 Limet J. N., Schneider Y.-J., Vaerman J.-P., Trouet A.: Binding, uptake and intracellular processing of polymeric rat immunoglobulin A by cultured rat hepatocytes. *Eur. J. Biochem.* 1982, **125**: 437–443.

87 Limet J. N., Schneider Y.-J., Trouet A., Vaerman J.-P.: Binding, uptake and processing of polymeric IgA by cultured rat hepatocytes. *In: Current Topics in Veterinary Medicine and Animal Science*, J. Bourne (Ed.): Martinus Nijhoff, London, 1981, Vol 12, pp 43–86.

88 Lunazzi G. C., Tiribelli C., Gazzin B., Sottocasa G. L.: Further studies on bilitranslocase, a plasma membrane protein involved in hepatic organic anion uptake. *Biochim. Biophys. Acta* 1982, **685**: 117–122.

89 Mak W. W.-N., Sattler C. A., Pitot H. C.: Accumulation of actin microfilaments in adult rat hepatocytes cultured on collagen gel/nylon mesh. *Cancer Res.* 1980, **40**: 4552–4564.

90 Mayer D., Faulstich H.: Two sites of intracellular localization of rhodaminyl-phalloidin in hepatocytes. *Biol. Cell* 1983, **48**: 143–150.

91 Meijer D. K. F., Blom A.: Hepatic transport of organic anions and organic cations in the rat *in vivo*, isolated perfused rat livers and isolated rat hepatocytes. *In: The Liver: Quantitative Aspects of Structure and Function*, R. Preisig, J., Bircher (Eds): Editio Cantor, Aulendorf, 1979, pp 77–86.

92 Meijer D. K. F., Blom A., Weitering J. G.: The influence of phenobarbital pretreatment on the subcellular distribution in liver and transport rate in isolated hepatocytes of dibromosulphophthalein. *Biochem. Pharmacol.* 1982, **31**: 2539–2542.

93 Miettinen A., Virtanen I., Linder E.: Cellular actin and junction formation during reaggregation of adult rat hepatocytes into epithelial cell sheets. *J. Cell Sci.* 1978, **31**: 341–353.

94 Minder E., Paumgartner G.: Disparate Na$^+$-requirement of taurocholate and indocyanine green uptake by isolated hepatocytes. *Experientia* 1979, **35**: 888–890.

95 Miyairi M., Oshio C., Watanabe S., Smith C. S., Yousef I. M., Phillips M. J.: Taurocholate accelerates bile canalicular contractions in isolated rat hepatocytes. *Gastroenterology* 1984, **87**: 788–792.

96 Moldéus P., Dock L., Cha Y.-N., Berggren M., Jernstöm B.: Elevation of conjugation capacity in isolated hepatocytes from BHA-treated mice. *Biochem Pharmacol.* 1982, **31**: 1907–1910.

97 Mottino A. D., Guibert E. E., Carnovale C., Morisoli L. S.,Rodriguez Garay E. A.: Formation of bilirubin monoglucuronide and diglucuronide in isolated rat hepatocytes. Effect of spironolactone. *Biochem. Pharmacol.* 1983, **32**: 3157–3161.

98 Ogura M., Goto M., Ayaki Y.: Formation of bile acids in hemoglobin-free perfused rat livers. *J. Biochem.* 1978, **83**: 527–535.

99 Ohkuma S.: Biochemical and pharmacological analyses on mechanism of conjugated bile acids

formation in hepatocytes. I. Characteristics of uptake of taurine, glycine and cholic acid by freshly isolated hepatocytes and hepatocytes in primary culture. *Kyoto-furitsu Ika Daigaku Zasshi* 1982, **91**: 1243–1269.

100 Ohkuma S.: Biochemical and pharmacological analyses on mechanism of conjugated bile acid formation in hepatocytes. II. Mechanisms of formation of conjugated bile acids in freshly isolated hepatocytes and hepatocytes in primary culture. *Kyoto-furitsu Ika Daigaku Zasshi* 1982, **91**: 1271–1282.

101 Ohkuma S., Kuriyama K.: Uptake of cholic acid by freshly isolated rat hepatocytes: presence of a common carrier for bile acid transports. *Steroids* 1982, **39**: 7–19.

102 Olinger E. J., Hercker E. S., Ostrow J. D.: Cellular regulation of taurocholate uptake by isolated rat hepatocytes. *In: The Liver: Quantitative Aspects of Structure and Function*, R. Preisig, J. Bircher (Eds): Editio Cantor, Aulendorf, 1979, pp 97–98.

103 Orlans E., Peppard J., Fry J. F., Hinton R. H., Mullock B. M.: Secretory component as the receptor for polymeric IgA on rat hepatocytes. *J. Exp. Med.* 1979, **150**: 1577–1581.

104 Oshio C., Phillips M. J.: Contractility of bile canaliculi: implications for liver function. *Science* 1981, **212**: 1041–1042.

105 Paumgartner G., Reichen J.: Different pathways for hepatic uptake of taurocholate and indocyanine green. *Experientia* 1975, **31**: 306–308.

106 Penasse W., Bernaert D., Mosselmans R., Wanson J. C., Drochmans P.: Scanning electron microscopy of adult rat hepatocytes *in situ*, after isolation of pure fractions by elutriation and fate in culture. *Biol. Cell.* 1979, **34**: 175–186.

107 Peters R.: Nucleo-cytoplasmic flux and intracellular mobility in single hepatocytes measured by fluorescence microphotolysis. *EMBO J.* 1984, **3**: 1831–1836.

108 Petzinger E.: Competitive inhibition of the uptake of demethylphalloidin by cholic acid in isolated hepatocytes. *Naunyn-Schmiedeberg's Arch. Pharmacol.* 1981, **316**: 345–349.

109 Petzinger E., Frimmer M.: Comparative studies on the uptake of ^{14}C-bile acids and ^{3}H-demethylphalloin in isolated rat liver cells. *Arch. Toxicol.* 1980, **44**: 127–135.

110 Petzinger E., Joppen C., Frimmer M.: Common properties of hepatocellular uptake of cholate, iodipamide and antamanide, as distinct from the uptake of bromosulphophthalein. *Naunyn-Schmiedeberg's Arch. Pharmacol.* 1983, **322**: 174–179.

111 Phillips M. J., Oda M., Edwards V. D., Greenberg G. R., Jeejeebhoy K. N.: Ultrastructural and functional studies of cultured hepatocytes. *Lab. Invest.* 1974, **31**: 533–542.

112 Phillips M. J., Oshio C., Miyairi M., Katz H., Smith C. R.: A Study of bile canalicular contractions in isolated hepatocytes. *Hepatology* 1982, **2**: 763–768.

113 Phillips M. J., Oshio C., Miyairi M., Watanabe S., Smith C. R.: What is actin doing in the liver cell? *Hepatology* 1983, **3**: 433–436.

114 Phillips M. J., Oshio C., Miyairi M., Smith C. R.: Intrahepatic cholestasis caused by cytochalasin may be a canalicular motility disorder. *Lab Invest.* 1983, **48**: 205–211.

115 Rao M. L., Rao S., Breuer H.: Uptake of estrone, estradiol-17β and testosterone by isolated rat liver cells. *Biochem. Biophys. Res. Commun.* 1977, **77**: 566–573.

116 Reichen J., Berman M. D., Berk P. D.: The role of microfilaments and of microtubules in taurocholate uptake by isolated rat liver cells. *Biochim. Biophys. Acta* 1981, **643**: 126–133.

117 Reichen J., Paumgartner G.: Kinetics of taurocholate uptake by the perfused rat liver. *Gastroenterology*, 1975, **68**: 132–136.

118 Reichen J., Paumgartner G.: Uptake of bile acids by perfused rat liver. *Am. J. Physiol.* 1976, **231**: 734–742.

119 Reichen J., Simon F. R.: Cholestasis. *In: The Liver: Biology and Pathobiology*, I. Arias, H. Popper, D. Schachter, D. A. Shafritz (Eds): Raven Press, New York, 1982, pp 785–800.

120 Robenek H., Gebhardt R.: Primary cultures of rat hepatocytes as a model system of canalicular development, biliary secretion, and intrahepatic cholestasis. IV. Disintegration of bile canaliculi and disturbance of tight junction formation caused by vinblastine. *Eur. J. Cell Biol.* 1983, **31**: 283–289.

121 Robenek H., Jung W., Gebhardt R.: The topography of filipin-cholesterol complexes in the plasma membrane of cultured hepatocytes and their relation to tight junction formation. *J. Ultrastruct. Res.* 1982, **78**: 95–106.

122 Rosenberg M. R., Strom S. C., Michalopoulos G.: Effect of hydrocortisone and nicotinamide on

gamma glutamyltransferase in primary cultures of rat hepatocytes. *In Vitro* 1982, **18**: 775–782.
123 Sattler C. A., Michalopoulos G., Sattler G. L., Pitot H. C.: Ultrastructure of adult rat hepatocytes cultured on floating collagen membranes. *Cancer Res.* 1978, **38**: 1539–1549.
124 Scharschmidt B. F., Stephens J. E.: Transport of sodium, chloride, and taurocholate by cultured rat hepatocytes. *Proc. Natl. Acad. Sci.* 1981, **78**: 986–990.
125 Scharschmidt B. F., Van Dyke R. W., Stephens J. E.: Chloride transport by intact rat liver and cultured rat hepatocytes. *Am. J. Physiol.* 1982, **242**: G628–G633.
126 Schoelmerich J., Kitamura S., Miyai K.: Changes of the pattern of biliary bile acids during isolated rat liver perfusion. *Biochem. Biophys. Res. Commun.* 1983, **115**: 518–524.
127 Schwarz L. R.: Modulation of sulfation and glucuronidation of 1-naphthol in isolated rat liver cells. *Arch. Toxicol.* 1980, **44**: 137–145.
128 Schwarz L. R.: Conjugation does not influence initial rates of uptake of sulphobromophthalein into isolated hepatocytes. *Hoppe Seyler's Z. Physiol. Chem.* 1982, **363**: 1225–1230.
129 Schwarz L. R., Barth C. A.: Taurocholate uptake by adult rat hepatocytes in primary culture. *Hoppe Seyler's Z. Physiol. Chem.* 1979, **360**: 1117–1120.
130 Schwarz L. R., Burr R., Schwenk M., Pfaff E., Greim H.: Uptake of taurocholic acid into isolated rat-liver cells. *Eur. J. Biochem.* 1975, **55**: 617–623.
131 Schwarz L. R., Götz R., Klaassen C. D.: Uptake of bromosulphophthalein-glutathione conjugate by isolated hepatocytes. *Am. J. Physiol.* 1980, **239**: C118–C123.
132 Schwarz L. R., Götz R., Wolff T., Wiebel F. J.: Mono-oxygenase and glucuronyltransferase activities in short-term cultures of isolated rat hepatocytes. *FEBS Lett.* 1979, **98**: 203–206.
133 Schwarz L. R., Schwenk M., Barth C., Greim H.: Studies with isolated liver cells: effect of taurolithocholate on the transport of taurocholate and bromosulphophthalein. *In: Biological Effects of Bile Acids*, G. Paumgartner, A. Stiehl, W. Gerok (Eds): University Park Press, Baltimore, 1979, pp 127–133.
134 Schwarz L. R., Schwenk M., Greim H.: Effects of cholestatic steroids on uptake and release of taurocholate in isolated hepatocytes. *In: Bile Acid Metabolism in Health and Disease*, G. Paumgartner, A. Stiehl (Eds): University Park Press, Baltimore, 1976, pp 145–150.
135 Schwarz L. R., Schwenk M., Pfaff E., Greim H.: Excretion of taurocholate from isolated hepatocytes. *Eur. J. Biochem.* 1976, **71**: 369–373.
136 Schwarz L. R., Schwenk M., Pfaff E., Greim H.: Cholestatic steroid hormones inhibit taurocholate uptake into isolated rat hepatocytes. *Biochem. Pharmacol.* 1977, **26**: 2433–2437.
137 Schwarz L. R., Summer K.-H., Schwenk M.: Transport and metabolism of bromosulphophthalein by isolated rat liver cells. *Eur. J. Biochem.* 1979, **94**: 617–622.
138 Schwenk M.: Transport systems of isolated hepatocytes. Studies on the transport of biliary compounds. *Arch. Toxicol.* 1980, **44**: 113–126.
139 Schwenk M., Burr R., Pfaff E.: Influence of viability on bromosulphophthalein uptake by isolated hepatocytes. *Naunyn-Schmiedeberg's Arch. Pharmacol.* 1976, **295**: 99–102.
140 Schwenk M., Burr R., Schwarz L. R., Pfaff E.: Uptake of bromosulphophthalein by isolated liver cells. *Eur. J. Biochem.* 1976, **64**: 189–197.
141 Schwenk M., López Del Pino V., Bolt H. M.: The kinetics of hepatocellular transport and metabolism of estrogens (comparison between estrone sulfate, estrone and ethinylestradiol). *J. Steroid Biochem.* 1979, **10**: 37–41.
142 Schwenk M., López Del Pino V., Remmer H.: An experimental model for the study of hepatic transport and metabolism of toxic compounds. *Arch. Toxicol.* Suppl 2, 1979, 339–343.
143 Schwenk M., Schwarz L. R., Greim H.: Taurolithocholate inhibits taurocholate uptake by isolated hepatocytes at low concentrations. *Naunyn-Schmiedeberg's Arch. Pharmacol.* 1977, **298**: 175–179.
144 Schwenk M., Wiedmann T., Remmer H.: Uptake, accumulation and release of ouabain by isolated rat hepatocytes. *Naunyn-Schmiedeberg's Arch. Pharmacol.* 1981, **316**: 340–344.
145 Seglen P. O.: Preparation of isolated rat liver cells. *Methods Cell. Biol.* 1976, **13**: 29–83.
146 Singh J., Schwarz L. R.: Dependence of glucuronidation rate on UDP-glucuronic acid levels in isolated hepatocytes. *Biochem. Pharmacol.* 1981, **30**: 3252–3254.
147 Sircia A. E., Richards W., Tsukada Y., Sattler C. A., Pitot H. C.: Fetal phenotypic expression by adult rat hepatocytes on collagen gel/nylon meshes. *Proc. Natl. Acad. Sci.* 1979, **76**: 283–287.
148 Socken D. J., Jeejeebhoy K. N., Bazin H., Underdown B. J.: Identification of secretory

component as an IgA receptor on rat hepatocytes. *J. Exp. Med.* 1979, **50**: 1538–1548.

149 Stacey N. H., Klaassen C. D.: Uptake of ouabain by isolated hepatocytes from livers of developing rats. *J. Pharmacol. Exp. Therap.* 1979, **211**: 360–363.

150 Stacey N. H., Klaassen C. D.: Uptake of galactose, ouabain and taurocholate into centrilobular and periportal enriched hepatocyte subpopulations. *J. Pharmacol. Exp. Therap.* 1981, **216**: 634– 639.

151 Stege T. E., Loose L. D., Di Luzio N. R.: Comparative uptake of bromosulphophthalein by isolated Küpffer and parenchymal cells. *Proc. Soc. Exp. Biol. Med.* 1975, **149**: 455–461.

152 Stevenson B. R., Goodenough D. A.: Zonulae occludentes in junctional complex-enriched fractions from mouse liver; preliminary morphological and biochemical characterization. *J. Cell Biol.* 1984, **98**: 1209–1221.

153 Stockert R. J., Morell A. G.: Endocytosis of glycoproteins. *In: The Liver: Biology and Pathobiology*, I. Arias, H. Popper, D. Schachter, D. A. Shafritz (Eds): Raven Press, New York, 1982, pp 205–217.

154 Suchy F. J., Balisteri W. F.: Uptake of taurocholate by hepatocytes isolated from developing rats. *Pediatr. Res.* 1982, **16**: 282–285.

155 Sundaram G. S., Rothman V., Margolis S.: Stimulation of bile acid synthesis by dibutyryl cyclic AMP in isolated rat hepatocytes. *Lipids* 1983, **18**: 443–447.

156 Tarao K., Olinger E. J., Ostrow J. D., Balisteri W. F.: Impaired bile acid efflux from hepatocytes isolated from the liver of rats with cholestasis. *Am. J. Physiol.* 1982, **243**: G253–G258.

157 Tarentino A. L., Galivan J.: Membrane characteristics of adult rat liver parenchymal cells in primary monolayer culture. *In Vitro* 1980, **16**; 833–846.

158 Thurman R. G., Kauffman F. C.: Factors regulating drug metabolism in intact hepatocytes. *Pharmacol. Rev.* 1980, **31**: 229–251.

159 Ugele B., Jung W., Gebhardt R.: Fluorescein analogs as probes for biliary transport of organic anions in primary cultures of rat hepatocytes. *Hepatology* 1984, **4**: 776.

160 Van Bezooijen C. F. A., Grell T., Knook D. L.: Bromosulphophthalein uptake by isolated liver parenchymal cells. *Biochem. Biophys. Res. Commun.* 1976, **69**: 354–361.

161 Von Dippe P., Levy D.: Characterization of the bile acid transport system in normal and transformed hepatocytes. *J. Biol. Chem.* 1983, **258**: 8896–8901.

162 Vonk R. J., Jekel P. A., Meijer D. K. F., Hardonk M. J.: Transport of drugs in isolated hepatocytes. The influence of bile salts. *Biochem. Pharmacol.* 1978, **27**: 397–405.

163 Vonk R. J., Von Doorn A. B. D., Meijer D. K. F.: The influence of bile salts on hepatocellular transport. *In: Biological Effects of Bile Acids*, G. Paumgartner, A. Stiehl, W. Gerok (Eds): University Park Press, Baltimore, 1979, pp 121–126.

164 Walli K., Wieland E., Wieland Th.: Phalloidin uptake by the liver of cholestatic rats *in vivo*, isolated perfused liver and isolated hepatocytes. *Naunyn-Schmiedeberg's Arch. Pharmacol.* 1981, **316**: 257–261.

165 Wanson J. C., Bernaert D., May C.: Morphology and functional properties of isolated and cultured hepatocytes. *In: Progress in Liver Diseases*, H. Popper, F. Schaffner (Eds): Vol. VI, Grune & Stratton, New York, 1979, pp 1–22.

166 Wanson J.-C., Drochmans P., Mosselmans R., Ronveaux M.-F.: Adult rat hepatocytes in primary monolayer culture. Ultra-structural characteristics of intercellular contacts and cell membrane differentiations. *J. Cell Biol.* 1977, **74**: 858–877.

167 Watanabe S., Miyari M., Oshio C., Smith C. R., Phillips M. J.: Phalloidin alters bile canalicular contractility in primary monolayer cultures of rat liver. *Gastroenterology* 1983, **85**: 245–253.

168 Whiting M. J., Edwards A. M.: Measurement of cholic acid synthesis and secretion by isolated rat hepatocytes. *J. Lipid Res.* 1979, **20**: 914–918.

169 Wisher M. H., Evans W. H.: Preparation of plasma-membrane subfractions from isolated rat hepatocytes. *Biochem J.* 1977, **164**: 415–422.

170 Wondergem R.: Transmembrane potential of rat hepatocytes in primary monolayer culture. *Am. J. Physiol.* 1981, **241**: C209–C214.

171 Yousef I. M., Ho J., Jeejeebhoy K. N.: Bile acid synthesis in isolated rat hepatocytes. *Can. J. Biochem.* 1978, **56**:780–783.

172 Ziegler K., Frimmer M., Möller W., Fasold H.: Chemical modification of membrane proteins by brominated taurodehydrocholate in isolated hepatocytes; relationship to the uptake of cholate and of phalloidin and to the sensitivity of hepatocytes to phalloidin. *Naunyn-Schmiedeberg's Arch. Pharamcol.* 1982, **319**: 254–261.

Research in *Isolated and cultured hepatocytes* A. Guillouzo & C. Guguen-Guillouzo eds, pp. 377–398.
© 1986 John Libbey Eurotext Ltd./INSERM

17

Use of cultured hepatocytes in parasitology

Dominique MAZIER

Département de Santé Publique, Parasitologie et Médecine Tropicale, Hôpital de la Salpêtrière, 47 bd de l'hôpital, 75013 Paris, FRANCE

SUMMARY

Among the numerous parasites which transit through or remain in the liver, only the *Haemosporididea* divide in the hepatocyte. Among this group, only the genus *Plasmodium* has been studied using cultures of functional hepatocytes. The hepatic stages of the mammalian *Plasmodia* cycle are by far those for which our knowledge is the most fragmentary, particularly in human malaria. For over 40 years, the difficulties in studying the liver phase of these parasites *in vivo* have stimulated attempts to recreate *in vitro* the conditions which allow parasite development. Hepatic schizogony was obtained both in a few cell lines and in primary cultures of hepatocytes, first for rodent parasites, and recently for two human *Plasmodia*. Nevertheless, up to now, only human hepatocytes are able to support the growth of the malignant human parasite *Plasmodium falciparum*. Liver cells cultures have also additionally provided insight into the life cycle of *Isospora*.

Various technical aspects are discussed in this chapter: hepatocyte dependent factors (species, age, sex of the donor) and culture medium (sera, cortisteroids etc.). The advantages of culturing hepatic stages in liver parenchymal cells or in cells lines are compared. It is obvious that this model is very promising for biological, biochemical and ultrastructural studies, for host-parasite relationships, species susceptibility, and so forth. Culture of mammalian hepatocytes has already proved of value in investigations of tissue schizontocidal drugs and the functional properties of antibodies which interact with sporozoite penetration and development in the hepatocyte.

Introduction

Many parasites, from protozoans to helminths, have a liver phase in their life cycle. Some simply transit through the liver on their journey to other more permanent sites. However, many may remain there for varying periods of time where they undergo partial or complete maturation. In a few instances, the liver is the site of parasite multiplication, but only rarely do parasites invade the parenchymal cell to undergo division. This phenomenon is restricted to a small group of sporozoans belonging to the *Haemosporididea* (see Table 1).

Because malaria is one of the greatest killers of the human race, most of the studies concern the genus *Plasmodium* and, with the exception of some experiments with *Isospora* (58), culture of functional hepatocytes was only used for mammalian genera of *Plasmodiidae*.

Table 1. Parasites for which division in hepatocytes is obligatory or facultative

Division is obligatory	Division is facultative
Mammalian genera of Plasmodiidae	*Leucocytozoidae*
— Genus *Plasmodium* (Rodent-primate-human)	— *Leucocytozoon simondi* (duck)
Mammalian genera of Haemoproteidae	multiplication also occurs in macrophages of
— *Hepatocystis*	spleen, liver and bone marrow
(Monkey-bat-squirrel-hyppopotamus-mouse deer)	
— *Nycteria* (Bat)	
— *Biguetiella* (Bat)	

Malaria

Hepatic stages of mammalian malaria follow the bite of an infected *Anopheles* mosquito (represented schematically in Table 2). Injected sporozoites are rapidly cleared from the blood and invade liver parenchymal cells where they undergo a cycle of asexual division (hepatic schizogony). When mature, these exoerythrocytic schizonts (EES) release merozoites which, in turn, may invade red blood cells and initiate repeated cycles of asexual development. Some erythrocytic parasites differentiate into gametocytes, the sexual forms. When a mosquito sucks gametocyte-containing blood, the ingested gametocytes reproduce in the gut where they develop into sporozoites.

The cycle is basically the same for the different plasmodia. However, two human malaria parasites, (*P. vivax* and *P. ovale*), and some malaria parasites of apes and monkeys cause true relapses for several years. In preference to the continuous cycle theory of Shortt & Garnham (73), there is experimental evidence for the existence in *P. cynomolgi* (44) and *P. vivax* (43) of a dormant uninucleated liver form, called hypnozoite.

The hepatic stages, a silent phase of the plasmodia life cycle, were discovered simultaneously by Shortt & Garnham (72) and Hawking *et al.* (28) in 1948, almost 50 years after erythrocytic stages and sporozoites were discovered by Laveran and Ross, respectively.

Because of its clinical relevance and its ready availability, the blood schizogonic

Table 2. Plasmodium sp *cycle (from Gentilini).*

EES: exoerythroctic schizont; S: sporozoite; H: hepatocyte; zm; merozoite; Hy: hypnozoite; T: trophozoite; ES: erythrocytic schizont; Gy: gametocyte; Ok: ookinete; Oc: oocyst; Gt: gamete; SG: salivary glands.

cycle has thus far been the most exhaustively studied phase. Furthermore, *in vitro* cultivation of these stages (29, 80) has led, since 1976, to major improvements in the possibilities of studying these stages.

Despite studies on EES in primate hosts (10) and discovery in 1964 of the conditions required for cyclical transmission of the rodent parasite in the laboratory (84), intrahepatic schizogony is by far the stage for which our knowledge is the most fragmentary, particularly in human malaria. This is not surprising in view of the difficulty in investigating humans with a parasite located in the liver.

Recourse to animals models has been tempered by a lack of host species susceptible to human malaria parasites. Although it now appears that some species of monkeys, other than those able to sustain blood infections, may be susceptible to the liver stages (18), this approach has been limited in large part by difficulties in producing sporozoites. Large numbers of sporozoites are necessary for experimental work on this part of the plasmodia life cycle.

Because of these difficulties, an alternate approach, *in vitro* exoerythrocytic schizogony, became increasingly attractive. Avian malaria parasites will not be discussed here since exoerythrocytic division occurs in endothelial cells. Nevertheless, it should be noted that *in vitro* cultivation of the EES of avian plasmodia has led to major advances in the knowledge of their morphology, drug sensitivity and immunology.

Historical aspects

Culture of the hepatic stages of rodent malaria. In contrast to the avian model in use since 1955 (15), it was only in 1978 that rodent pre-erythrocyte forms could be cultivated (22).

As pointed out by Huff in 1963 (37), progress was impeded by the assumptions that EES are rigidly host cell specific and that hepatic parenchymal cells do not grow well in culture. About 10 years later both these notions were revised, leading to breakthrough in the cultivation of rodent EES.

The concept of parasite-host cell specificity was greatly undermined in 1974 (7) by successful cultivation of an avian parasite in mammalian cells. This finding illustrated that the presumed host specificity did not necessarily hold true, at least for *in vitro* systems. It led, in 1979, to the first successful cultivation of EES of a rodent plasmodium, *P. berghei*, in fibroblasts derived from embryonic rat brain and liver, or from embryonic turkey brain (78). Other results subsequently confirmed the ability of cell lines to support the growth of rodent EES (74), in particular the obtention in 1981 by Hollingdale *et al.* of the complete cycle of *P. berghei* in human embryonic lung cells (34) and later in a hepatoma cell line (36).

The second assumption, the impossibility of cultivating hepatic parenchymal cells, was refuted by improvements in enzymatic isolation and culture of functional hepatocytes (8, 70). These improvements opened the way to cultivating the EES in their natural host cell, the hepatocyte.

The first step was the maintenance *in vitro* of liver cells previously infected *in vivo*. By modifying the enzymatic liver dissociation technique of Bonney *et al.* (8), Foley *et al.* obtained suspensions of parasitized hepatocytes with viable and infective EES of *P. berghei* (22); these suspensions were utilized to initiate primary cell cultures.

Though no morphological entities clearly identifiable as EES were ever observed in the cell cultures, these cultures remained infectious for recipient rodents for up to 44 hours *in vitro*. This time span corresponds to the incubation period of this parasite in the rat host.

The next step was the initiation *in vitro* of the sporozoite infection achieved in 1981 by Lambiotte *et al.* (45). Salivary glands of *Anopheles stephensi* containing *P. yoelii yoelii* sporozoites were disrupted and added to primary cultures originating from the liver of an adult rat perfused with a collagenase solution. Forty-seven hours after *in vitro* inoculation, numerous well-developed and normal looking schizonts were found in the hepatocyte monolayer. In 1982, the complete *in vitro* cycle was demonstrated by Mazier *et al.* (53) using hepatocytes of *Thamnomys gazellae*, an African rodent which, *in vivo*, is an excellent experimental host for the EES of *P. yoelii yoelii*. Viable merozoites were released by the schizonts as demonstrated by the parasitaemia observed in mice infected with culture supernatants. Similar results were obtained by Pirson (63) using rat hepatocytes and *P. berghei* sporozoites isolated by the Hypaque-discontinuous gradient centrifugation technique, and by Meiss *et al.* who in 1984 described for the first time the ultrastructure of maturing EES of *P. berghei* in primary cultures of Brown Norway rat hepatocytes (57).

Culture of the hepatic stages of human malaria. Culture of human EES was achieved only recently for three reasons. The first was the difficulty in obtaining infectious sporozoites of human malaria. Until the recent breakthrough in the culture of infectious gametocytes of *P. falciparum* (12, 38, 64), it was necessary to feed mosquitoes with gametocytes containing blood collected from patients. The scarcity of such patients in temperate climates made it difficult to duplicate experiments. The second was the problem of the host cell: failure to obtain the complete development in cell lines comforted us in the idea that the hepatocyte was indeed the cell of choice. Rodent hepatocytes were rapidly found inappropriate and it became obvious that one had to use human hepatocytes, the isolation and culture of which had been developed only in 1982 (27). The third reason was the fact that, unlike rodent plasmodia, the human hepatic cycle is long, lasting more than one week, which multiplies the risks of contamination from the mosquitoes, and the maintainance of functional hepatocytes.

In 1976, Doby & Barker (16) demonstrated that at least the first developmental stages of *P. vivax* could occur after inoculation of sporozoites into human liver cell cultures. In 1983, using primary cultures of human hepatocytes dissociated by canulation and perfusion of a small vessel of a biopsy specimen, Mazier *et al.* obtained the complete cycle of *P. vivax*, up to the release of merozoites able to invade red blood cells (52). The problem caused by the length of hepatic cycle of this human plasmodium was resolved by cocultivating hepatocytes with a rat liver epithelial cell line, a procedure known to improve their viability for several weeks (26). In 1984, two groups of investigators simultaneously reported the *in vitro* growth of *P. falciparum*. In primary cultures of human hepatocytes, Smith *et al.* (76) followed the development of EES up to 72 hours. Using the same type of cells, we obtained complete *in vitro* development of this plasmodium (50, 51) as demonstrated by the presence of intraerythrocytic forms in red blood cells added at the 7th day post infection to the hepatocyte culture dishes.

In the case of *P. falciparum*, unlike *P. vivax*, the existence of cultures which assure the development of the sexual erythrocytic stages, the gametocytes, has permitted an orderly production of infectious sporozoites as noted above. Thus, it is now possible to initiate, on a regular basis, the hepatic cycle of *P. falciparum* and perform experiments aimed at studying schizontocidal drugs and immunologic processes.

Involvement of Küpffer cells

Shin *et al.* (71), having observed sporozoites of *P. berghei* within hepatocytes 2 minutes after *in vivo* inoculation, considered this brief lag-time as a proof of direct hepatocyte invasion by the sporozoites. Verhave & Meis (81), however, present both direct and indirect evidence for a prior passage through the Küpffer cells: the existence of an anatomical barrier between the sinusoidal capillary and the hepatocyte (87, 88); the demonstration that blockade of the RES or destruction of the Küpffer cells result in decreased blood clearance of sporozoites accompanied by a reduction in the number of EES in parenchymal cells (75, 83). Lastly, ultrastructural studies showed that sporozoites, taken up by Küpffer cells, can escape into Disse's space and penetrate into the hepatocyte (55).

Under EES culture conditions, sporozoites do not transit through the Küpffer cells which could contaminate hepatocyte cultures. However, the percentage of sporozoites found intracellularly is low (0.1 to 0.5% in our experiments with *P. falciparum*); it is currently impossible to state whether only few of the sporozoites are truly infectious, whether only certain hepatocytes are susceptible to penetration, and whether a transit through a Küpffer cell would increase the infectiousness of the parasite.

Comments

A review of reports dealing with *in vitro* culture of EES of mammalian plasmodia shows that development of several rodent parasite is possible in functional hepatocytes: *P. yoelii* (45, 53), *P. berghei* (57, 63), *P. chabaudi* (49), *P. vinckei petteri* (47), as well as two human parasites, *P. vivax* (52) and the malignant *P. falciparum* (51, 76). The complete cycle can be obtained up to release of merozoites capable of infective recipient rodents (53, 57, 63) or human red blood cells (51, 52). Light microscopy (Figs 1 & 2) and ultrastructural studies (Figs 3 & 4) demonstrate that the parasite growing *in vitro* has the same basic morphological organization as *in vivo*, and that the organelles are not significantly different from those of EES developing *in vivo*, although peculiar vesicles, not previously described in *in vivo* infection, are identified (Fig. 4.5). Quantitative differences, however, do exist. The parasites grow at a slower rate *in vitro* than *in vivo*. This was first observed for the rodent parasite *P. yoelii* (53), since full maturation was delayed (60 to 66 hours) as compared to *in vivo*. Similar observations were made with *P. berghei* (57) as with human parasites *P. vivax* (52) and *P. falciparum* (51). Moreover, some schizonts while reaching total maturity *in vitro* remain smaller than *in vivo*. This smaller size may be due to the shape of the cells in culture. Not all schizonts reach maturity, but similar results were obtained *in vivo* with a *Saimiri sciureus* monkey infected with sporozoites of *P. falciparum*. Aside some altered mitochondria (Fig. 4.6), which are sometimes more electrodense and more slender than those of non-infected hepatocytes, no signs of cell degeneration are recorded.

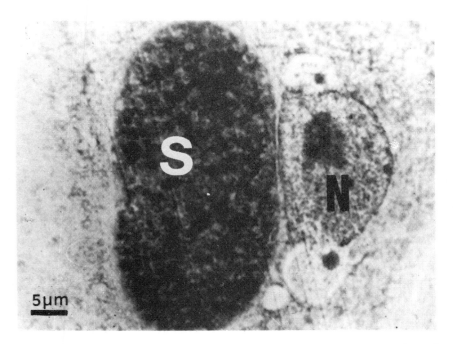

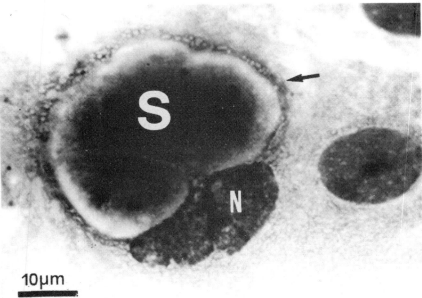

Fig. 1. Exoerythrocytic parasites in cultural hepatocytes. Schizonts are generally located close to the nucleus of the host cell which appears unaltered by the presence of the parasite except for a condensed area surrounding a clear space around the schizont (arrow).

Top: a 48-h schizont of *P. yoelii yoelii* in a *Thamnomys gazellae* hepatocyte (reprinted with permission from reference 53).

Bottom: schizont of *P. vivax* in a human hepatocyte containing about 300 nuclei. Schizonts are regularly found in binuclear hepatocytes. It is not known whether sporozoites develop better after invading tetraploid hepatocytes. Culture fixed 7 days after sporozoite inoculation (Reprinted with permission from reference 52).

N, hepatocyte nucleus; S, schizont.

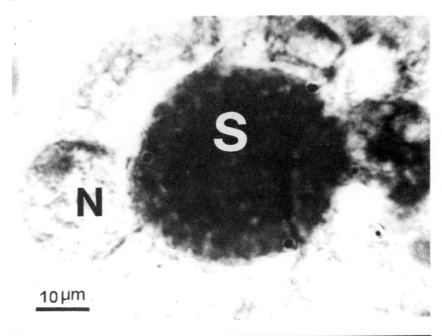

10 μm

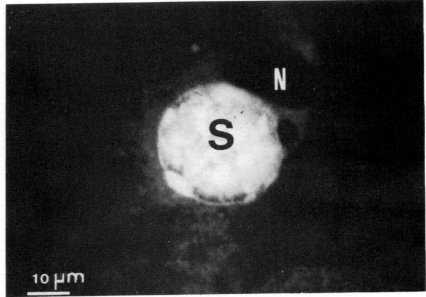

10 μm

Fig. 2. Seven-day schozonts of *P. falciparum* in human hepatocytes

Top: giemsa staining. This late schizont contains several hundred merozoites. There is no clear area surrounding the parasite as was found in *P. vivax* culture (Reprinted with permission from reference 54).

Bottom: indirect fluorescent antibody test (IFAT). Culture is incubated with a diluted hyperimmune serum from an African adult, then with a fluorescein-conjugated antiserum to human immunoglobulins G, M and A.

N, hepatocyte nucleus; S, schizont.

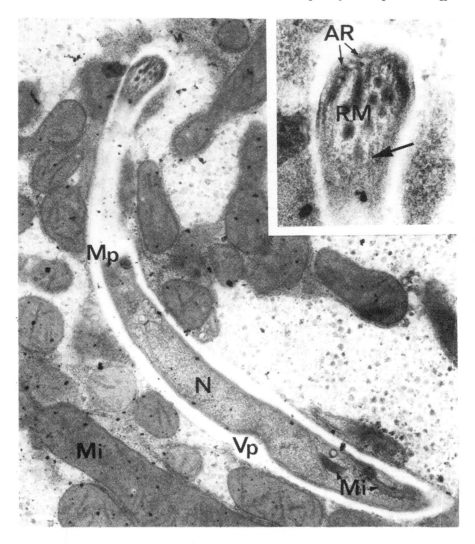

Fig. 3. Sporozoite of *P. falciparum* inside a human hepatocyte *in vitro*, **one hour after depositing the salivary glands on the liver culture.** It is located in a parasitophorous vacuole (Vp). A long nucleus (N) mitochondrion (Mi) and a micropore (Mp) are visible ($\times$ 20 000). Insert : a higher magnification of the apex showing 2 apical rings (AR), part of the rhoptry-microneme complex (RM) and sub-pellicular microtubule (arrow) ($\times$ 60 000) (plate Y. Boulard et al.).

Hepatocyte-dependent factors. 1) *Species. In vivo*, various species and strains of rodents vary widely in their susceptibility to rodent malaria as demonstrated by the number and size of EES.

In vitro, this difference also exists, often correlated with the *in vivo* observations. Nonetheless, some hypotheses proposed for the *in vivo* susceptibility are becoming irrelevant *in vitro*. For example, the ability of sporozoites to reach hepatocytes seems to depend on the rat strain particularly the ease with which the oxidative burst by

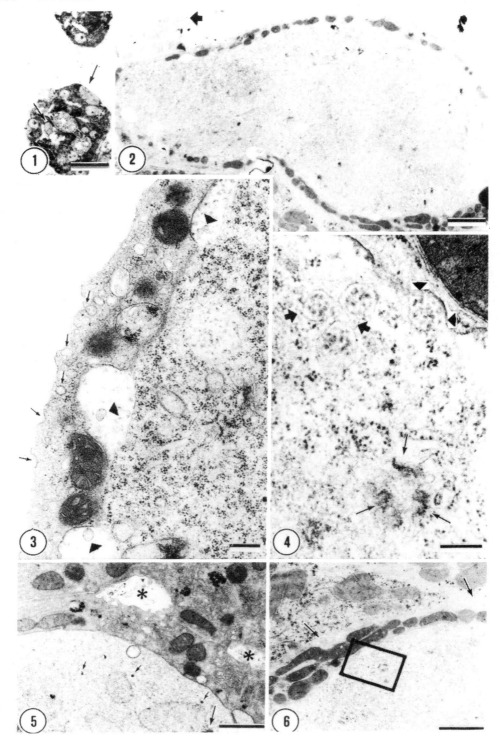

Küpffer cells can be triggered (81).

In vivo, as *in vitro*, the hepatocytes of *Thamnomys gazellae*, an African rodent close to the natural host, seems to be the most appropriate cell for *P. yoelii*. Hamster and Wistar rat hepatocytes are less susceptible (48, 49). The low recovery of mouse hepatocytes is most probably due to the fragility of this cell in culture. Brown Norway rats have a high susceptibility for *P. berghei* sporozoite infection, *in vitro*, as *in vivo* (57).

Up to now, human hepatocytes appear to be the most appropriate host cell for *P. vivax* and *P. falciparum*. Rat hepatocytes, however, permitted penetration of *P. falciparum* sporozoites: after 24 hours in culture, the fluorescence pattern and size are the same as in human hepatocytes, but the parasites do not develop further, the size at 48 hours being similar to that seen at 24 hours (unpublished results).

The culture system should therefore be of help in unravelling the problem of host specificity, at least at the hepatocyte level.

2) *Age*. Two problems have to be considered: age of the donor from which hepatocytes are isolated and age of the hepatocyte cultures at time of infestation. The age of the host is important *in vivo*, since adult rats and mice are more resistant to sporozoite infection than four-week-old animals (85). However, in the same studies it was noted that embryonic parenchymal liver cells were refractory. The age of the donor is not as critical *in vitro*; one of the best *P. falciparum* cultures we obtained was in hepatocytes from a 83-year-old donor!

In vivo refractoriness may be explained by the fact that embryonic cells contain more glycogen than adult parenchymal cells. Indeed, it has been shown that EES are distributed in the afferant zones of the lobules where the glycogen content is minimal. In rodents, Verhave *et al.* found that EES number can be increased more than 2-fold after 48 hours of starvation (81). Similar results have been obtained with *P. cynomolgi* in starved monkeys (11) and after treatment with phlorhizin which

---

Fig. 4.   Semithin section showing rat hepatocyte clusters.*1*. Developing *P. berghei* parasites appeared as lighter stained intracellular bodies (arrows). Scale bar 30 μm.
2. Thin section of a parasite growing in rat hepatocyte *in vitro*. The EES is structurally similar to parasites grown *in vivo*. Note mosquito muscle (arrow). Scale bar 3 μm.
3. Detail of the host/parasite interface and extracellular compartment of the culture medium. Many small coated vesicles are present in the hepatocyte (thin arrows) indicating an exchange of products between medium and host cell. In addition to the well known floccular substance, vesicular structures are visible in the parasitophorous vacuole (arrow heads). Scale bar 0.5 μm.
4. Host/parasite interface showing small peripheral vesicles (thick arrows) with floccular content which is deposited in the parasitophorous vacuole between the parasite plasmalemma and the hepatocyte membrane (arrow heads). A Golgi-complex with budding vesicles is distinctly visible (thin arrows). This figure is a higher magnification of the rectangle indicated in 6. Scale bar 0.5 μm.
5. Part of a parasite grown *in vivo*. Note that there is no morphological difference between the mitochondria of the parasitized hepatocyte and those of the neighbouring cells. Asterisks show bile canaliculi. Small electron-dense granules are visible (thin arrow) which are not particularly associated with Golgi complexes (arrows). Scale bar 2 μm.
6. Host/parasite interface *in vitro*. Note the difference in size and electron-density between the mitochondria of the infected and those of the uninfected hepatocyte. Bile canaliculus-like regions can be recognized between the two hepatocytes (arrows). Scale bar 2 μm.
(Reproduced from Meis et al., Cell Biol. Int. Rep., 1984, by permission of the author and publisher).

depletes the liver of glycogen (81). However, very preliminary results with hepatocyte cultures maintained without insulin (insulin acts by transforming glucose to glycogen in the cell), indicate that *P. yoelii* schizonts did not survive.

Concerning the age of the hepatocyte culture, Meis *et al.* infect rat cells 3 hours after seeding of the hepatocytes. This is surely too short an interval for human hepatocytes because of their fragility during the first 24 hours of culture. Twenty-four to 48 hours seems to be optimal, but cultures of human hepatocytes initiated 5 days earlier can support the growth of *P. falciparum* until maturity without any problem.

3) *Sex of the donor. In vivo*, female rats, particularly when pregnant, are less susceptible to sporozoite infection. This can be correlated with the decrease in the number of EES when the level of an oestrogenic hormone (diethyl stilboestrol) increases (82). To establish *in vitro* correlations between the sex of the donor and susceptibility to the EES is difficult when working with human *Plasmodia* in human hepatocytes, since all parameters vary from one experiment to another. An anecdotal point: the 83-year-old-donor was a female! It can be argued that at this age oestrogen levels are relatively low. It should also be considered that a hormonal effect may disappear under culture conditions.

Culture medium. Different media can be used: Ham F12-NCTC 109 (45) MEM (53), modified Eagle's (H 16) (63), William's medium E (57). All these media supplemented with bovine insulin (53, 57) and with bovine serum albumin (53), support development of the EES. Hollingdale *et al.* (35), with different cell lines, used various culture media: MLM, NCTC 135, MEM, RPMI 1640, all of which with the exception of RPMI supported the complete EE cycle, indicating that the role of the medium is essentially to maintain the host cell in a functional state. The reasons for the poor results obtained with RPMI 1640 are unclear. We confirmed this observation with *P. yoelii* in rodent hepatocytes (unpublished).

One real difficulty encountered in the development of EES derives from the fact that salivary glands of mosquitoes often contain bacteria and yeasts which contaminate the cultures. Streptomycin is known to inhibit the erythrocytic stages of *P. falciparum* cultures. However, high dose of this antibiotic (200 μg/ml) in association with penicillin (200 IU/ml) does not damage EES development and usually prevents bacterial growth.

More difficult is the problem of yeasts. In our hands, however, 5-fluoro-cytosine (Ancotil®)(5 μg/ml) can be used without deleterious effects on schizont development and will prevent a great deal of contamination. Higher doses are toxic and do not seem to be more efficient (unpublished).

The use and choice of sera is of fundamental importance, especially with regard to infestation. In mammalian cells, specific biological recognition sites have been detected on the glycoprotein and glycolipid components of the plasma membrane, particularly the carbohydrate moieties of these macromolecules (86). Hepatocytes have receptor sites for glycoproteins which are rapidly taken up by the liver (3). With the aid of lectins, Schulman *et al.* (77) reported that sporozoites, when incubated in serum, especially serum from hosts susceptible to sporozoite infection, combine with a glycoprotein or a glycolipid component of this serum. These authors speculate that the bound serum components may play a role in liver invasion by functioning as recognition sites for receptors present on the surface membrane of the host liver cells being invaded.

Several teams, therefore, are dissecting salivary glands in undiluted homologous sera (34, 57). Hollingdale observed that *P. falciparum* and *P. vivax* sporozoites invaded WI 38 cells only in the presence of 1% human serum. The hepatoma cell line Hep G_2 A16, however, did not require this additive (6, 32). In our experience, homologous serum is not required for penetration of rodent or human malaria sporozoites into homologous hepatocytes or into other cells.

Another important point pertains to the addition of corticosteroids, hydrocortisone (45, 53) or dexamethasone (57) to the media. *In vivo* experiments have shown that in rats pretreated with dexamethasone, parasite densities were 4-times higher than in control rats (81). It has been proposed that dexamethasone, which has a membrane stabilizing effect on the phagocytic cells and inhibits the fusion of lysosomes and phagocytic vacuoles, delays intracellular killing (81). *In vitro* the influence of dexamethasone on parasite growth may be related to the deservation of Princen *et al.* (65) that this hormone enhances specific protein synthesis and prevents the decomposition of mRNA in cultured rat hepatocytes. α-Interferon was also found to be able to act at the pre-erythrocytic phase of the disease and could protect mice infected with sporozoites of *P. berghei* (39, 40, 41). Corticosteroids may thus facilitate the *in vitro* growth of the parasite by preventing synthesis of interferon by Küpffer cells present in hepatocyte cultures.

Advantages of cultivating EES in hepatocytes or in cell lines. The problems are quite different depending on whether rodent or human EES are considered.
Rodent EES. Complete *P. berghei* cycle can be obtained in human embryonic lung cells (34) and in the hepatoma cell line Hep G_2 A16 (36). Moreover, ultrastructural studies demonstrated that in this cell line, the sporozoites transform in a manner morphologically identical to that seen *in vivo* (2). The advantages of a cell line allowing EES growth are obvious: easier manipulation, better reproducibility since individual particularities exist in individual donors, even in standardized experiments. However, it may be found that a homologous, functional hepatocyte is the cell of choice for certain applications, such as chemotherapeutic studies which would be best performed using the cell type involved in the metabolism of the drugs under study.
Human EES. One problem with human parasites is the length of the hepatic cycle, more than one week. Thus, difficulties may be encountered with cells maintaining rapid growth, even at confluence. This can be controlled, as shown recently, by using irradiated hepatoma cells to cultivate *P. vivax* (33). Regarding *P. falciparum*, two points must be considered: penetration of the sporozoite, and its development. Sporozoites of this species are known to penetrate in human embryonic lung, Hep G_2 A16, VERO, MRC 9 and rhesus monkey cells (32). Smith *et al.* found these sporozoites capable of entering several cell types (76) and we noticed invasion of rat hepatocytes and a melanoma cell line (unpublished). But, until now, full development was not achieved except in human hepatocytes (51). These results suggest that *P. falciparum* culture might depend on the specific metabolic profile of the human hepatocyte rather than of the presence of specific host cell receptors.

Expected developments

Useful in basic studies of rodent parasite species, EES culture are especially suited for human plasmodia. Biology, metabolism, biochemistry, host-parasite relationships, species susceptibility and ultrastructure of the parasite can be studied *in vitro*. A few points will be considered further.

Research in the field of tissue schizontocidal drugs. Apart from a few experiments in the avian culture system (1, 5, 79), the EES drugs could only be tested in *in vivo* models.

Attention must be drawn to two factors. First, it is difficult to study drug effects at the hepatic level (9, 62), therefore new drugs are identified by their ability to prevent the development of the erythrocytic stage. Secondly, two kinds of activity have to be detected since the schizont, which manifests an intense anabolic activity, is extremely sensitive to metabolic inhibitors in contrast to the hypnozoite, the dormant form, in which little biosynthetic activity occurs.

Rodent models have proved of value for the detection of hepatic schizontocidal activity (61) but, until now, they have not been used to identify drugs that might be effective against *P. vivax* infections, although hepatic schizonts found several months after infestation indicate that hypnozoite may exist in *Thamnomys rutilans* (46). Chemosensitivity of human plasmodia has been studied in *Aotus* (68) and *Saimiri* monkeys (68, 69) but *P. cynomolgi* in the *Rhesus monkey* remains the principal model for the evaluation of potential hypnozoitocides. The cost and availability of monkeys are serious hindrance to *in vivo* evaluation of new drugs prior to clinical assays. However, the developing resistance of human malaria strains to blood schizontocidal drugs, and the toxicity of primaquine, the only compound reliably active against EES stresses the necessity for new compounds. As *in vitro* cultivation of the erythrocytic stages of *P. falciparum* (29, 80) has opened the way for screening the blood schizontocidal action of molecules, the alternative approach of testing tissue schizontocidal drugs in hepatocytes is an attractive one. Preliminary experiments demonstrate that *in vitro* results using hepatocytes infested with *P. yoelii* are in concordance with those obtained *in vivo* (59). The human culture system, particularly the co-culture system, should be appropriate for testing anti-relapse compounds on *in vitro* grown hypnozoites.

Research in the field of immunology. We would like to outline some future possibilities offered by EES culture in hepatocytes.
Antigenic studies of the hepatic stages. The complex developmental cycle of malaria parasites involves morphologically as well as antigenically different forms. These modifications raise questions about the control mechanisms as well as the stage-specificity of immunity to this disease. Stage specific antigens, located on the surfaces of the *Plasmodium*, have been identified in sporozoites (60), erythrocytic merozoites (21) and gametes (66). These antigens are considered to be the best candidates for vaccine production.

Recently, Druilhe *et al.* (19) demonstrated that in addition to antigens of broad specificity shared with blood stages and other malaria species, the EES of *P. falciparum* exhibit stage and species specific antigens which are located at the periphery of the schizont. As EES of avian parasites have been shown to induce strong protective immunity (23, 30, 31), it is of great interest to test mammalian EES for their ability to induce immunological protection. Culture systems might provide a means for isolating these stages more easily than from livers infected *in vivo*, particularly the merozoites released from the hepatic schizont. In the same way, production of monoclonal antibodies against EES is now possible. These antibodies would act as probes to detect, in genomic DNA of *Plasmodium*, the gene coding for EES antigens.

Assessment of defence mechanisms against sporozoites. Vaccination experiments against human malaria using whole irradiated sporozoites were promising (13, 67), but further insight into immunization with purified molecules has been hampered by the unavailability of the appropriate immunogens.

Recently, two groups (14, 20) succeeded in cloning and sequencing a surface protein of the sporozoite, the circumsporozoite (CS) protein, leading to the production in usable amounts of both recombinant and synthetic peptides. As a preliminary step before carrying out immunization experiments in human volunteers antibodies raised in mice against several recombinant and synthetic peptides were evaluated for protective activity in Hep G_2 A16 cells (4, 89) and human hepatocyte culture (54). With both, the ability of antibodies to block the penetration of sporozoites could be measured, but the human hepatocyte culture system had the advantage of showing that antibodies continue to exert an effect on schizont development, after sporozoite penetration. This inhibition may result from an alteration by antibodies of some sporozoites in a way that does not prevent penetration. Alternatively antibodies may exert an effect on trophozoites at the intracellular level. Whether or not antibodies directed against the parasite can enter hepatocytes directly is not known. Thus the *in vitro* culture of the liver stages of *P. falciparum* provides a new and useful tool to evaluate the level of protection, naturally acquired or induced by immunization in animals and in man. Such studies will be particularly beneficial before challenge with live organisms, and will make possible functional studies of anti-malaria antibodies, with special emphasis on their interaction with sporozoite penetration and development in the hepatocyte.

Other parasites

In vivo studies on the life cycle of *Isospora sp.* (24) were supplemented by *in vitro* assays. To study the sequence of asexual schizogony in the sparrow (*Passer domesticus*), Millet *et al.* (58) infected primary cultures of the canary (*Serinus canarius*) hepatocytes with sporozoites of *Isospora* sp. (Fig. 5).

Several schizogonic cycles occur during the extra-intestinal phase of *Isospora*. Some of the released merozoites are able to transform into 'dormant' trophozoites. Thus, the intestinal phase could be initiated from those forms stocked during the prepatent phase in the reticulo-endothelial system. This mechanism appears, therefore, to be very similar to those of some *Haemosporididea* such as *Plasmodium vivax* or *P. cynomolgi* (43, 44); this hypothesis is strongly supported by the finding that primaquine selectively eliminates the 'dormant' stage of both *P. cynomolgi* (42) and *Isospora* sp (25).

We have already mentioned the difficulty of testing drugs with potential effects on

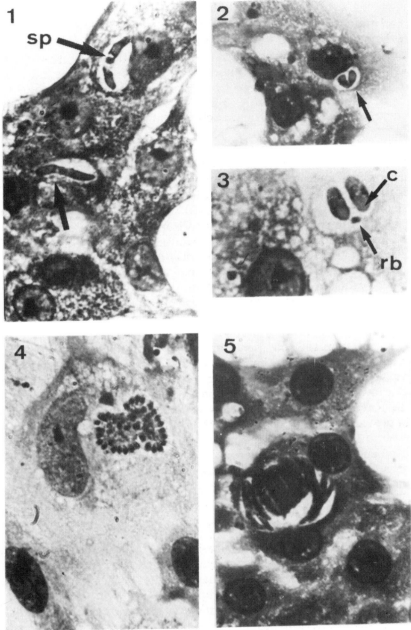

Fig. 5. **Culture of *Isospora* sp in primary cultures of canary hepatocytes.** *1–4: extra-intestine phase*
1. sporozoites (sp) in hepatocytes.
2. sporozoite undergoes a primary division (arrow)
3. sporozoite division results into two similar semi-sporozoites and a small residual body (rb)
c: cristalloide
4. mature schizont with short merozoites.
5. *Plain intestinal cycle* The sporozoites transform directly in schizonty with long merozoites
(plate Landau I. and Millet P.).

relapses of *P. vivax* (ie active against the hypnozoite) in small laboratory animals. For those laboratories having difficulties in obtaining human hepatocytes and *P. vivax* sporozoites, the *Isospora* model is perhaps another way to study the latent stages of protozoans.

Conclusions

Functional hepatocytes have proven to be a valuable support for the exo-erythrocytic development of *Plasmodia in vitro*. Infection with *P. vivax* and *P. falciparum* as well as with animal parasites has been successful; it is, therefore, not presumptuous to envisage that *P. malariae* and *P. ovale*, the other two human parasites, will also undergo complete schizogony *in vitro* when their corresponding sporozoites are available. Although the hepatocyte is the cell of choice for the development of exo-erythrocytic stages, particularly in the case of human malaria, the validity of the model remains to be confirmed. A simple example is instructive: *in vitro* we found that the circumsporozoite (CS) protein, the predominant surface protein of the sporozoite of *P. falciparum*, persists throughout schizogony (unpublished results); *in vivo*, in the *Saimiri* monkey, the CS protein is undetectable, at least by the 3rd day post-infection (17). Is this phenomenon connected to the simian hepatocyte itself, the monkey being an artificial host for *P. falciparum*? Or, is the CS protein lost *in vivo* at time of Küpffer cell invasion as suggested by Meis (56)? This question is of central importance since the strategy of antisporozoite vaccines is based on the production of protective anti-CS protein antibodies.

However, although caution should be exercised when extrapolating from cell culture to *in vivo* situations, the good correlations between *in vivo* and *in vitro* chemotherapeutic studies demonstrate the usefulness of this approach.

ACKNOWLEDGEMENTS

This work was supported by Institut National de la Santé et de la Recherche Médicale grant 841018, United Nations Development Programme/World Bank/World Health Organization Special Program on training and Research in Tropical Diseases grant 840105, the French Minister of Research and Industry (82-L-0760 and 82-L-0787), Conseil Scientifique Pitié-Salpêtrière and Naval Medical Research and Development Command work unit 3M 162770A870 AF312. We thank D. Frommel for reviewing the manuscript and S. Mellouk, B. Texier, B. Burel and G. Lecso for their co-operation.

REFERENCES

1 Aikawa M., Beaudoin R. L.: Morphological effects of 8-aminoquionolines on the exoerythrocytic stages of *Plasmodium fallax. Military Med.* 1969, **134**: 985–999.
2 Aikawa M., Schwartz A., Uni S., Nussenzweig R., Hollingdale M.: Ultrastructure of *in vitro* cultured exoerythrocytic stage of *Plasmodium berghei* in a Hepatoma cell line. *Am. J. Trop. Med. Hyg.* 1984, **33**: 792–799.
3 Ashwell G., Morell A.: The role of surface carbohydrates in the hepatic recognition and transport of circulating glycoproteins. *Adv. Enzymol.* 1974, **41**: 99–128.
4 Ballou W. R., Rothbard J., Wirtz R. A., Gordon D. M., Williams J. S., Gore R. W., Schneider I., Hollingdale M. R., Beaudoin R. L., Maloy W. L., Miller L. H., Hockmeyer W. T.:

immunogenicity of synthetic peptides from circumsporozoite protein of *Plasmodium falciparum*. *Science* 1985, **228**: 996–999.

5   Beaudoin R. L., Aikawa M.: Primaquine-induced changes in morphology of exoerythrocytic stages of malaria. *Science* 1968, **160**: 1233–1234.

6   Beaudoin R. L., Mazier D., Hollingdale M. R.: *In vitro* cultivation of the exoerythrocytic stages of malaria parasites. *In: Textbook of Malaria*, W. Wernsdorfer, I. McGregor (Eds): Churchill Livingstone, Edinburgh. (In press.)

7   Beaudoin R. L., Strome C. P. A., Clutter W. G.: Cultivation of exoerythrocytic stages of malaria in mammalian liver cells. *Exp. Parasitol.* 1974, **36**: 355–359.

8   Bonney R. J., Becker J. E., Walker P. R., Potter V. R.: Primary monolayer cultures of adult rat liver parenchymal cells suitable for study of the regulation of enzyme synthesis. *In Vitro* 1974, **9**: 399–413.

9   Boulard Y., Landau I., Miltgen F., Ellis D. S., Peters W.: The chemotherapy of rodent malaria XXXIV causal prophylaxis. Par III: Ultrastructural changes induced in exoerythrocytic schizonts of *Plasmodium yoelii yoelii* by primaquine. *Ann. Trop. Med. Parasitol* 1983, **77**: 555–568.

10 Bray R. S.: *Studies on the Exoerythrocytic Cycle in the Genus* Plasmodium: London School of Hygiene & Tropical Medicine, Memoir No 12, Lewis & Co, London,1957, 84–149.

11 Bray R. S.: *Studies on the Exoerythrocytic Cycle in the Genus* Plasmodium: London School of Hygiene & Tropical Medicine, Memoir No 12, Lewis & Co, London, 1–92.

12 Campbell C. C., Chin W., Collins W. E., Moss D. M.: Infection of *Anopheles freeborni* by gametocytes of cultured *Plasmodium falciparum*. *Trans. Roy. Soc. Trop. Med. Hyg.* 1980, **74**: 668–669.

13 Clyde D. F., McCarthy V. C., Miller R. M., Woodward W. E.: Immunisation of man against *falciparum* and *vivax* malaria by use of attenuated sporozoïtes. *Am. J. Trop. Med. Hyg.* 1975, **24**: 397–401.

14 Dame J. B., Williams J. L., McCutchan T. F., Weber J. L., Wirtz R. A., Hockmeyer W. T., Maloy W. L., Haynes J. D., Schneider I., Roberts D., Sanders G. S., Reddy E. P., Diggs C. L., Miller L. H.: Structure of the gene encoding the immunodominant surface antigen on the sporozoite of the human malaria parasite *Plasmodium falciparum*. *Science* 1984, **225**: 593–599.

15 De Oliveira M. X., Meyer H.: *Plasmodium gallinaceum* in tissue culture. Observations after one year of cultivation. *Parasitology* 1955, **45**: 1–4.

16 Doby J. M., Barker R.: Essais d'obtention *in vitro* des formes préérythrocytaires de *Plasmodium vivax* en cultures de cellules hépatiques humaines inoculées par sporozoïtes. *C.R. Séances Soc. Biol.* (Rennes) 1976, **170**: 661-665.

17 Druilhe P.: Intérêt des nouveaux tests immunologiques appliqués à l'étude de l'épidémiologie du Paludisme humain. International Colloquium Malaria in Africa. Changes in continuity. Antwerp, 1984.

18 Druilhe P., Miligen F., Landau I., Rinjard J., Gentilini M.: Schizogonie hépatique de *Plasmodium falciparum* chez le singe *Cebus apella*. *C.R. Acad. Sc. Paris* 1982, **294**, Série III: 511–513.

19 Druilhe P., Puebla R. M., Miltgen F., Perrin L., Gentilini M.: Species and stage-specific antigens in exoerythrocytic stages of *Plasmodium falciparum*. *Am. J. Trop. Med. Hyg.* 1984, **33**: 336–341.

20 Enea V., Ellis J., Zavala F., Arnot D. E., Asavanich A., Masuda A., Quakyi I., Nussenzweig R. S.: DNA cloning of *Plasmodium falciparum* circumsporozoite gene: amino acid sequence of repetitive epitope. *Science* 1984, **225**: 628–629.

21 Epstein N., Miller L. H., Kaushel D. C., Udeinya I. J., Renner J., Howard R. J., Asorsky R., Aikawa M., Hess R. L.: Monoclonal antibodies against a specific surface determinant on malaria (*Plasmodium knowlesi*) merozoites block erythrocyte invasion. *J. Immunol.* 1981, **127**: 212–220.

22 Foley D. A., Kennard J., Vanderberg J. P.: *P. berghei*: infective exoerythrocytic schizonts in primary monolayer cultures of rat liver cells. *Exp. Parasitol.* 1978, **46**: 166–178.

23 Graham H. A., Palczuk N. C., Stauber L. A.: Immunity to exoerythrocytic forms of malaria. II. Passive transfer of immunity to exoerythrocytic forms. *Exp. Parasitol.* 1973, **34**: 372–381.

24 Grulet O., Landau I., Millet P., Baccam D.: Les *Isospora* de Moineau. II. Etudes sur la biologie. *Ann. Parasitol. Hum. Comp.* 1985. (In press.)

25 Grulet O., Landau I., Millet P., Baccam D.: Les *Isospora* de Moineau. III. Action sélective de la primaquine sur les formes d'attente. *Ann. Parasitol. Hum. Comp.* 1985. (In press.)

26 Guguen-Guillouzo C., Baffet G., Clement B., Bégue J. M., Glaise D., Guillouzo A.: Human adult

hepatocytes: isolation and maintenance at high levels of specific functions in a co-culture system. *In*: *Isolation, Characterization and Use of Hepatocytes*, R. A. Harris, N. W. Cornell (Eds): Elsevier, Amsterdam, 1983, pp 105–110.

27 Guguen-Guillouzo C., Campion J. P., Brissot P., Glaise D., Launois B., Bourel M., Guillouzo A.: High yield preparation of isolated human adult hepatocytes by enzymatic perfusion of the liver. *Cell. Biol. Int. Rep.* 1982, **6**: 625–628.

28 Hawking F., Perry W. L. M., Thurston J. P.: Tissue forms of a malaria parasite, *Plasmodium cynomolgi*. *Lancet* 1948, **i**: 783.

29 Haynes J. D., Diggs C. L., Hines F. A., Desjardins R. E.: Culture of human malaria parasites, *Plasmodium falciparum*. *Nature* 1976, **263**: 767–769.

30 Holbrook T. W., Palczuk N. C., Stauber L. A.: Immunity to exoerythrocytic forms of malaria. III. Stage-specific immunization of turkeys against exoerythrocytic forms of *Plasmodium fallax*. *J. Parasitol.* 1974, **60**: 248–354.

31 Holbrook T. W., Spitalny G. L., Palczuk N. C.: Stimulation of resistance in mice to sporozoite-induced *Plasmodium berghei* malaria by injections of avian exo-erythrocytic forms. *J. Parasitol.* 1976, **62**: 670–675.

32 Hollingdale M. R.: *In vitro* invasion of cultured cells by sporozoites of primate and human species. Abstracts of 2nd Conference on Malaria and Babesiosis, 19–22 September 1983, Annecy, France.

33 Hollingdale M. R., Collins W. E., Campbell C. C., Schwartz A. L.: *In vitro* culture of two populations (dividing and non-dividing) exoerythrocytic parasites of *Plasmodium vivax*. *Am. J. Trop. Med. Hyg.* 1985, **34**: 216–222.

34 Hollingdale M. R., Leef J. L., McCullough M., Beaudoin R. L.: *In vitro* cultivation of the exoerythrocytic stage of *Plasmodium berghei* from sporozoïtes. *Science* 1981, **213**: 1021–1022.

35 Hollingdale M. R., Leland P., Leef J. L., Beaudoin R. L.: The influence of cell type and culture medium on the *in vitro* cultivation of exoerythrocytic stages of *Plasmodium berghei*. *J. Parasit* 1983, **69**: 346–352.

36 Hollingdale M. R., Leland P., Schwartz A. L.: *In vitro* cultivation of the exoerythrocytic stage of *Plasmodium berghei* in a hepatoma cell line. *Am. J. Trop. Med. Hyg.* 1983, **32**: 682–684.

37 Huff C. G.: Experimental research on avian malaria. *In*: *Advances in Parasitology*, B. Dawes, London, Academic Press, 1963, Vol. 1, 1–65.

38 Ifediba T., Vanderberg J. P.: Complete *in vitro* maturation of *Plasmodium falciparum* gametocytes. *Nature* 1981, **294**: 364–366.

39 Jahiel R. I., Nussenzweig R. S., Vanderberg J., Vilcek J.: Anti-malarial effect of interferon inducers at different stages of development of *Plasmodium berghei* in the mouse. *Nature* 1968, **220**: 710–711.

40 Jahiel R. I., Vilcek J., Nussenzweig R. S.: Exogenous interferon protects mice against *Plasmodium berghei* malaria. *Nature* 1970, **227**, 1350–1351.

41 Jahiel R. I., Vilcek J., Nussenzweig R., Vanderberg J.: Interferon inducers protect mice against *Plasmodium berghei* malaria. *Science* 1968, **61**: 802–803.

42 Krotoski W. A., Bray R. S., Garnham P. C. C., Gwadz R. W., Killick-Kendrick R., Draper C. C., Targett G. A. T., Krotoski D. M., Guy M. W., Koontz L. C., Cogswell F. B.: Observations on early and late post-sporozoite tissue stages in primate malaria. II. The hypnozoite of *Plasmodium cynomolgi bastianellii*. *Am. J. Trop. Med. Hyg.* 1982, **31**: 211–225.

43 Krotoski W. A., Collins W. E., Bray R. S., Garnham P. C. C., Cogswell F. B., Gwadz R. W., Killick-Kendrick R., Wolf R., Sinden R., Koontz L. C., Stanfill P. S.: Demonstration of hypnozoites in sporozoite-transmitted *Plasmodium vivax* infection. *Am. J. Trop. Med. Hyg.* 1982, **31**: 1291–1293.

44 Krotoski W. A., Krotoski D. M., Garnham P. C. C., Bray R. S., Killick-Kendrick R., Draper C. C., Targett G. A. T., Guy M. W.: Relapses in primate malaria: discovery of two populations of exoerythrocytic stages. Preliminary note. *Br. Med. J.* 1980, **280**: 153–154.

45 Lambiotte M., Landau I., Thierry N., Miltgen F.: Développement de schizontes dans des hépatocytes de rat adulte en culture après infestation *in vitro* par des sporozoïtes de *Plasmodium yoelii*. *C.R. Acad. Sc. Paris* 1981, **293**: 431–433.

46 Landau I.: Exoerythrocytic schizonts of a rodent *plasmodium* in the liver of a wild *Thamnomys rutilans*. *Trans. Roy. Soc. Trop. Med. Hyg.* 1966, **60**, 5.

47 Landau I.: Personal communication.

48 Landau I., Mazier D., Baxter J., Millet P., Miltgen F., Druilhe P.: Sur la culture des schizontes de *Plasmodium* dans les hépatocytes. World Health Organization. 1985. (In press.)

49 Landau I., Mazier D., Baxter J., Millet P., Miltgen F., Druilhe P., Gentilini M.: Sur la culture des schizontes de *Plasmodium* dans les hépatocytes. XI International Congress for Tropical Medicine and Malaria. Calgary, Canada, 1984, Sept. 16–22.

50 Mazier D., Beaudoin R. L., Mellouk S., Druilhe P., Texier B., Trosper J., Miltgen F., Landau I., Paul C., Brandicourt O., Guguen-Guillouzo C., Langlois P., Gentilini M.: Obtention *in vitro* des stades hépatiques de *Plasmodium falciparum*. *Ann. Parasitol. Hum. Comp.* 1984, **59**: 525–526.

51 Mazier D., Beaudoin R. L., Mellouk S., Druilhe P., Texier B., Trosper J., Miltgen F., Landau I., Paul C., Brandicourt O., Guguen-Guillouzo C., Langlois P., Gentilini M.: Complete development of hepatic stages of *Plasmodium falciparum in vitro*. *Science* 1985, **227**: 440–442.

52 Mazier D., Landau I., Druilhe P., Miltgen F., Guguen-Guillouzo C., Baccam D., Baxter J., Chigot J. P., Gentilini M.: Cultivation of the liver forms of *Plasmodium vivax* in human hepatocytes. *Nature* 1984, **307**: 367–369.

53 Mazier D., Landau I., Miltgen F., Druilhe P., Lambiotte M., Baccam D., Gentilini M.: Infestation *in vitro* d'hépatocytes de *Thamnomys* adulte par des sporozoïtes de *Plasmodium yoelii*: schizogonie et libération de mérozoïtes infestants. *C.R. Acad. Sc. Paris* 1982, **294**: 963–965.

54 Mazier D., Mellouk S., Beaudoin R. L., Texier B., Druilhe, P., Hockmeyer W. T., Trosper J., Paul C., Young J. F., Miltgen F., Galley B., Brandicourt O., Chedid L., Charoenvit Y., Chigot J. P., Gentilini M.: Effect of antibodies to recombinant and synthetic peptides on development of *P. falciparum* sporozoïtes *in vitro*. *Science* 1985 (in press).

55 Meis J. F. G. M., Verhave J. P., Jap P. H. K., Meuwissen J. H. E. T.: An ultrastructural study on the role of Kupffer cells in the process of infection by *Plasmodium berghei* sporozoites in rats. *Parasitology* 1983, **86**, 231–242.

56 Meis J.: Exoerythrocytic development of a rodent malaria parasite. Thesis, Nijmegen, 1984, p. 9.

57 Meis J. F. G. M., Verhave J. P., Meuwissen J. H. E. T., Jap P. H. K., Princen H. M. G., Yap S. K.: Fine structure of *Plasmodium berghei* exoerythrocytic forms in cultured primary rat hepatocytes. *Cell Biol. Int. Rep.* 1984, **8**: 755–765.

58 Millet P., Baxter J., Landau I.: Division initiale de sporozoïtes d'une *Isospora* de Moineau en culture cellulaire. *Ann. Parasitol. Hum. Comp.* 1984, **59**: 321–322.

59 Millet P., Landau I., Baccam D., Miltgen F., Mazier D., Peters W.: Mise au point d'un modèle expérimental 'rongeur' pour l'étude *in vitro* des schizonticides exoérythrocytaires. *Ann. Parasitol. Hum. Comp.* 1985. **60**: 211–212.

60 Nardin E. H., Nussenzweig V., Nussenzweig R. S., Collins W. E., Harinasuta K. T., Tapchaisri P., Chomcharn Y.: Circumsporozoïte proteins of human malaria parasites *Plasmodium falciparum* and *Plasmodium vivax*. *J. Exp. Med.* 1982, **156**: 20–30.

61 Peters W., Davies E. E., Robinson B. L.: The chemotherapy of rodent malaria XXIII. Causal prophylaxis part 2. Practical experience with *Plasmodium yoelii nigeriensis* in drug screening. *Ann. Trop. Med. Parasit.* 1975, **65**: 311–328.

62 Peters W., Ellis D., Boulard Y., Landau I.: The chemotherapy of rodent malaria XXXVI. Causal prophylaxis. Part IV. The activity of a new 8-aminoquinoline WR 225, 448 against exoerythrocytic schizonts of *Plasmodium yoelii yoelii*. *Ann. Trop. Med. Parasitol.* 1984, **78**: 467–478.

63 Pirson P.: Culture of the exoerythrocytic liver stages of *Plasmodium berghei* sporozoites in rat hepatocytes. *Trans. Roy. Soc. Trop. Med. Hyg.* 1982, **76**: 422.

64 Ponnudurai T., Meuwissen J. H. E. Th, Leeuwenberg A. D. E. M., Verhave J. P., Lensen A. H. W.: The production of mature gametocytes of *Plasmodium falciparum* in continuous cultures of different isolates infective to mosquitoes. *Trans. Roy. Soc. Trop. Med. Hyg.* 1982, **76**: 242–250.

65 Princen H. M. G., Moshage H. J., Dehaard H. J. W., Vangemert P. J. C., Yap S. H.: The influence of glucocorticoid on the fibrinogen messenger RNA content of rat liver *in vivo* and in hepatocyte suspension culture. *Biochem. J.* 1984, **220**: 631–637.

66 Rener J., Carter R., Rosenberg Y., Miller L. H.: Antigamete monoclonal antibodies synergistically block transmission of malaria by preventing fertilization in the mosquito. *Proc. Natl. Acad. Sci.* 1980, **77**: 6797–6799.

67 Rieckmann K. H., Beaudoin R. L., Cassells J. S., Sell K. W.: Use of attenuated sporozoites in the immunization of human volunteers against *falciparum* malaria. *Bull. WHO* 1979, **57**: 261–265.

68 Rossan R. N., Young M. D., Baerg D. C.: Chemotherapy of *Plasmodium vivax* in *Saimiri* and *Aotus*

models. *Am. J. Trop. Med. Hyg.* 1975, **24**: 168–173.

69 Schmidt L. H.: Infections with *Plasmodium falciparum* and *Plasmodium vivax* in the owl monkey-model systems for basic biological and chemotherapeutic studies. *Trans. R. Soc. Trop. Med. Hyg.* 1973, **67**: 446–474.

70 Seglen P. O.: Preparation of rat liver cells. III Enzymatic requirements for tissue dispersion. *Exp. Cell. Res.* 1973, **82**: 391–398.

71 Shin S. C. J., Vanderberg J. P., Terzakis J. A.: Direct infection of hepatocytes by sporozoites of *Plasmodium berghei. J. Protozool.* 1982, **29**: 448–454.

72 Shortt H. E., Garnham P. C. C.: The pre-erythrocytic development of *P. cynomolgi* and *P. vivax. Trans. Roy. Soc. Med. Hyg.* 1948, **41**: 785–795.

73 Shortt H. E., Garnham P. C. C.: Demonstration of a persisting exoerythrocytic cycle in *Plasmodium cynomolgi* and its bearing on the production of relapses. *Br. Med. J.* 1948, **1**: 1225–1232.

74 Sinden R. E., Smith J. E.: Culture of the liver stages (exoerythrocytic schizonts) of rodent malaria parasites from sporozoites *in vitro. Trans. Roy. Soc. Trop. Med. Hyg.* 1980, **74**: 134–136.

75 Sinden R. E., Smith J. E.: The role of the Küpffer cell in the infection of rodents by sporozoites of *Plasmodium*: uptake of sporozoites by perfused liver and the establishment of infection *in vivo. Acta Trop.* 1982, **39**: 11–27.

76 Smith J. E., Meis J. F. G. M., Ponnudurai T., Verhave J. P., Moshage H. J.: *In-vitro* culture of exoerythrocytic form of *Plasmodium falciparum* in adult human hepatocytes. *Lancet* 1984, **ii**: 757–758.

77 Shulman S., Oppenheim J. D., Vanderberg J. P.: *Plasmodium berghei* and *Plasmodium knowlesi*: serum binding to sporozoites. *Exp. Parasitol.* 1980, **49**: 420–429.

78 Strome C. P. A., De Santis P. L., Beaudoin R. L.: The cultivation of the exoerythrocytic stages of *Plasmodium berghei* from sporozoites. *In Vitro*, 1979, **15**: 531–536.

79 Tonkin I.: The testing of drugs against exoerythrocytic forms of *P. gallinaceum* in tissue culture. *Br. J. Pharmacol.* 1946, **1**: 163.

80 Trager W., Jensen J. B.: Human malaria parasites in continuous culture. *Science* 1976, **193**: 673–675.

81 Verhave J. P., Meis J. F. G. M.: The biology of tissue forms and other asexual stages in mammalian plasmodia. *Experientia* 1984, **40**: 1317–1329.

82 Verhave J. P., Meis J. F. G. M.: The delivery of exoerythrocytic malaria parasites. International Colloquium Malaria in Africa. Changes in Continuity. Antwerp, 1984.

83 Verhave J. P., Meuwissen J. H. E. Th., Golenser J.: The dual role of macrophages in the sporozoite-induced malaria infection. A hypothesis. *Int. J. Nuclear Med. Biol.* 1980, **7**: 149–156.

84 Yoeli M., Most H., Bone G.: *Plasmodium berghei*: cyclical transmission by experimentally infected *Anopheles quadrimaculatus. Science* 1964, **144**: 1580.

85 Wery M.: Studies on the sporogony of rodent malaria parasites. *Ann. Soc. Belge Med. Trop.* 1968, **48**: 1–137.

86 Winzler R. J.: Carbohydrates in cell surfaces. *Int. Rev. Cytol.* 1970, **29**: 77–125.

87 Wisse E., De Zanger R., Jacobs R.: Lobular gradients in endothelial fenestrae and sinusoïdal diameter favour centralobular exchange processes in scanning EM study. *In: Sinusoidal Liver Cells*, D. L. Knook, E. Wisse (Eds): Elsevier Biomedical Press, Amsterdam, 1982, pp 61–67.

88 Wisse E., De Zanger R., Jacobs R., McCuskey R. S.: Scanning electron microscope observations on the structure of portal veins, sinusoids and central veins in rat liver. *Scanning Electron Microscopy* III, 1983: 1441–1452.

89 Young J. F., Hockmeyer W. T., Gross M., Ballou W. R., Wirtz R. A., Trosper J. H., Beaudoin R. L., Hollingdale M. R., Miller L. H., Diggs C. L., Rosenberg M.: Expression of *P. falciparum* circumsporozoïte protein in *E. coli* for a human malaria vaccine. *Science* 1985, **228**: 958–962.

Index

α₂u-Globulin 162, 163, 167, 269
Glucagon 25, 26, 27, 29, 44, 52, 68, 70, **71**,
73, 74, 90, 91, 93, 94, 95, 99, 101, **128**, 160,
180, 182, 189, 190, 191, 192, 196, 199, **200**,
235, 338
  receptor 196
Glucocorticoids 29, 44, 49, 51, 68, 73, 93,
162, 189, 190, 191, 192, 202, 211, 216, 217,
242, 269, 272, 277, 299, 302, 305, 320, 362
Glucokinase 269
Gluconeogenesis **64-78**, 94, 103, 191
Glucose 17, **64-78**, 100, 101, 180, 388
  in the culture medium 9, 16, 288
  dehydrogenase 316
  6-phosphatase 16, 17, 19, 23, 99, 183
  6-phosphate 64
  6-phosphate dehydrogenase 192, 202,
  266, 269
Glucosidase 337
Glucuronic acid 245, 286, 315, 320, 356
Glucuronidation 286, 297, 315, 316, 322,
356
Glucuronyltransferase 314, 315, 316, 357
Glutamate 69, 71
Glutamine 37, 71, 78, 159
Glutathione 286, 315, 316, 317, 321, 323,
344, 362, 364
  transferase 316, 321, 356
Glyceraldehyde-3-phosphate dehydroge-
nase 75
Glycerol 94, 118, 318
  in gluconeogenesis **64-78**
  3-phosphate 70, 94
  phosphate acyltransferase 94
Glycine 356
Glycogen 180, 316, 322, 387
  phosphorylase 99
  synthetase 99
Glycogenolysis 181, 196, 197, 198, 199
Glycolatte 162
Glycolipid 265, 338
Glycolysis 64, 94, 101
Glycoprotein 115, 122, 166, 265, 271, 338
Glycosamine 166
Glycosaminoglycan 218, 236, **245**, 265
Glycosidase 265
Glycosylation 117, 121, 122, 166, 202, 211,
241, 248
Glycosyltransferase 265
Golgi apparatus **116**, 117, 118, 120, 121,
124, 156, 157, 161, 166, 242, 248, 357, 358,
362
Growth factor **14-32**, 229, 231, 235, 270
  hormone 160, 163, 192, 235, 270
GTP 197
O-6-Guanine 336, 343
Guinea-pig 3, 67, 75, 76, 77, 78

Halothane 323, 324
Hamster 3, 320, 340, 341, 387
Haptoglobin 160, 161, 164, 166
Harmol 316
HDL 115-130, 136-150
  receptor 146
Heart 136, 137, 143
Hela cell 41, 139
Heme 292, 300, 318, 319
  oxydase 355
Hemidesmosome 56, 358
Hemoglobin 202
Hemopexin 159, 160, 161, 164, 179
Heparan sulfate 219, **246-249**
Heparin 27, 29, **246**, 248
Hepatectomy 3, 17, 23, 25, 26, 29, 138, 143,
319, 335, 347
Hepatic stimulator substance 32
Hepatitis 241
Hepatoma cell 32, 56, 73, 141, 145, 146,
164, 166, 189, 191, 194, 195, 204, 242, 246,
249, 343, 344, 346, 364, 380, 389
Hepatonectin 239
Hepatopoietin 346
Hepatotrophic factor **14-38**
HEPES **2-9**
Hexanoate 75
Hexobarbital 315
Hexosamine 245
Hexose-6-phosphate 72
Histidine 159
Histone 191
Homocysteine 317
Hormonally defined medium **226-249**, 276
Hormone
  in cell differentiation **226-249**, 270, 318
  in cell proliferation **14-32**
Human 90, 121, 144, 147, 156, 164, 182,
219, 241, 299, 316, 318, **321**, 323, 324, 336,
340, 341, 343, **344**, **378-393**
  adult, cell isolation 3
  fetal, cell isolation 8
Hyaluronic acid 219, **246**
Hyaluronidase 2, 8, 172
Hybridization (in situ) 157, 215, 242
Hydrocarbon 286, 287, 289, 294, 304, 337,
340, 343
Hydrocortisone 29, 160, 162, 163, 164, 165,
179, 216, 318, 338, 389
Hydrolase 140, 141
3-Hydroxybenzo(a)pyrene 315
3-Hydroxybutyrate 88
Hydroxycitrate 102
7α-Hydroxycholesterol 355
Hydroxylase 303
Hydroxylation 211, 214, 241, 290, 294, 295,
299, 303, 355, 356

α-Methylamino-isobutyric acid 362
2-(3-Methylcinnamyl hydrazono)-
   propionate 78
1-Methyl-isobutylxanthine 199
3-Methyl-isobutyryl-xanthine 28
Methyl-methane-sulfonate 338
Methylprednisolone 216
Metrizamide **6**
Metyrapone 292, 295, 302, 305, 306, 315,
   318, 319
Microfilament **41**, **45**, 47, 48, 50, 360, 362
Microsomes 90, 94, 115, 246, 290, 291, 299,
   301, 302, 315
Microtrabecular lattice 41
Microtubule **41**, 56, **118**, 140, 166, 211, 218,
   362
   associated proteins 41
Mitochondrion 45, 67, 69, 75, 76, 77, 78, 88,
   90, 94, 96, 102, 104, 129, 269, 336, 337,
   382
   β oxydation **103**
Mitosis **14-32**, 44
Monensin 166, 248
Monkey 382, 387
Monocyte 164
Mono-oxygenase 286, 288, 290, 299, **300**,
   301, 314, 315, 317, 319, 320, 324
Morphine 316, 363
Mouse 25, 74, 76, 78, 162, 163, 164, 178,
   246, 262, 308, 323, 381, 382, 387
   cell isolation 3
   embryo cell (3H/10T1/2) 161
β-Muricholic acid 355, 356
Muscle 136, 139, 246, 248
Myocyte 264
Myristate 124

Na$^+$ 31, 363
NADH 65, 75, 96, 316
NADPH 192, 193, 314, 315
   cytochrome c reductase 315, 319
Nalorphine 363
Naphthol 315, 364
Naphtoflavone 295, 300, 301, 302, 305, 306
Neonatal liver 16, 19, 192, 196
Neuraminidase 2
Neuron 216, 278
Nicotinamide 292, **300**, 318, 338
2-Nitrofluorene 341
p-Nitrophenol 317
Nitropyrene 344
Nitroreductase 37
p-Nitrosoanisole-O-demethylase 315, 319
Nitrosourea 337
Noradrenaline (see norepinephrine)

Norepinephrine 27, 28, 93, 346
Norethandrolone 368
Nortriptyline 315
5'-Nucleotidase 145
Nucleus 41, 51, 68, 270, 275, 336

Obesity 101, 129
Octanoate 75, 78, 96, 100, 104
Octanoylcarnitine 96, 98, 100
Octaploid hepatocyte 22
Octylglucoside 194, 203
Ocytocin 364
Oleate 90, 91, 93, 96, 98, 100, 101, 104, 124,
   125
Oleic acid 128
Oligosaccharide 166, 249
Oncogene 32, 57
Ornithine 16, 178
   carbamoyl transferase 16
   decarboxylase 183
Orotic acid 117
Osmolarity 6, 31, 160
Ouabain 342, 361, 363, 364
Oval cell 53, 54
Ovariectomy 162
Oxaloacetate 67, 71, 103, 104
Oxazepam 315
Oxytetracycline 288

Palmitate 91, 93, 96, 100
Palmitic acid 138
Palmitoleate 124
Palmitoyl-carnitine 78, 99, 100
   -CoA 78, 100
Pancreatic cell 116, 278, 39
Papain 2
Paracetamol 315, 317, 323, 324
D-Penicillamine 211, 218
Pentenoic acid 75
Pentobarbital 324
Pepsin 2, 239, 244
Pepstatin **201**
Peptidase 211
Periportal hepatocyte 6, 7, 156, 317
Peroxidation 323
Pertussis toxin 196
Phalloidin 360, 368
Phenobarbital 6, 286, 287, 288, 290, 294,
   295, 297, 299, 300, 302, 304, 305, 306, 315,
   316, 317, 320, 322, 325, 339
Phenol 297, 299
Phenozybenzamine 189
Phenylalanine 159
2-(Phenylalkyl)-oxirane-2-carboxylate 78

Urea 16, 75, 269, 299, 322
Uridine diphosphate glucuronic acid 316
Uvomorulin 263

Vasopressin **28**, 29, 69, 70, 71, 80, 93, 346
Velocity sedimentation 7
Vimentin 41, 43, 56
Vinblastine 140, 211, 357, 358, 362
Vinculin 41, 45
Vinyl chloride 344
Vitamin 270
Vitellin 163
VLDL **14-130**, **136-150**

Xylitol 77
β-Xyloside 248

Yohimbine 189